Medical-Surgical Nursing

made Incredibly Easy!

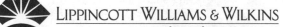

LIPPINCOTT WILLIAMS & WILKINS

A **Wolters Kluwer** Company

Philadelphia • Baltimore • New York • London
Buenos Aires • Hong Kong • Sydney • Tokyo

Staff

Publisher
Judith A. Schilling McCann, RN, MSN

Editorial Director
David Moreau

Clinical Director
Joan M. Robinson, RN, MSN

Senior Art Director
Arlene Putterman

Art Director
Mary Ludwicki

Clinical Editors
Jana L. Sciarra, RN, MSN, CRNP (clinical project manager); Marguerite S. Ambrose, DNSC, APRN, BC; Wanda H. Jones, RN, BSN, MJ; Anita Lockhart, RN, C, MSN; Kate McGovern, RN, MSN, CCRN

Editors
Tracy S. Diehl (senior associate editor), Marylou Ambrose, Kathy Goldberg, Judd Howard, Brenna Mayer

Copy Editors
Kimberly Bilotta (supervisor), Scotti Cohn, Tom DeZego, Heather Ditch, Amy Furman, Shana Harrington, Pamela Wingrod

Designers
Lynn Foulk, Jacalyn B. Facciolo

Illustrator
Bot Roda

Digital Composition Services
Diane Paluba (manager), Joyce Rossi Biletz, Richard Eng

Manufacturing
Patricia K. Dorshaw (senior manager), Beth Janae Orr

Editorial Assistants
Megan Aldinger, Tara Carter-Bell, Linda Ruhf

Indexer
Karen C. Comerford

MSNIE—D N O S A
05 04 03   10 9 8 7 6 5 4 3 2 1

Library of Congress Cataloging-in-Publication Data
Medical-surgical nursing made incredibly easy.
   p.; cm.
   Includes bibliographical references and index.
   1. Surgical nursing — Handbooks, manuals, etc. 2.
   Nursing — Handbooks, manuals, etc. [DNLM: 1. Nursing
   Care — methods — Handbooks. 2. Perioperative
   Nursing — methods — Handbooks. WY 49
   M4896 2004] I. Lippincott Williams & Wilkins.

RT51.M436 2004
610.73—dc21
ISBN 1-58255-269-X (pbk.: alk. paper)   2003011172

Contents

Contributors and consultants

Jane E. Ashley, RN, PhD
Associate Professor
Boston College
Chestnut Hill, Mass.

Margaret E. Barnes, RN, MSN
Staff RN – Emergency Room
Samaritan Hospital
Ashland, Ohio

Roseanne Baughman, RN, MSN, CRNP
Nurse Practitioner
Central Bucks Internal Medicine
Doylestown, Pa.

Cheryl L. Brady, RN, MSN
Adjunct Faculty
Youngstown (Ohio) State University

Anne Walendy Davis, RN, PhD, BC
Professor of Nursing
Department of Nursing, East Central University
Ada, Okla.

Linda Fuhrman, MSN, ANCC
Nurse Practitioner
San Francisco VA Medical Center

Arlinda Garner, RN, MS
Professor of Nursing
College of the Mainland
Texas City, Tex.

René A. Jackson, RN, BSN
RN, Special Procedures
Charlotte Regional Medical Center
Punta Gorda, Fla.

Eleftheria T. Karapas, RN, MS
Clinical Consultant
Lemont, Ill.

Lakshmi McRae, RN,C, BA (H)
Staff Nurse
Doctor's Outpatient Surgical Center
Pasadena, Tex.

Jennifer McWha, RN, MSN
Nursing Instructor
Del Mar College
Corpus Christi, Tex.

Brenda H. Owens, APRN, PhD, BC, FNP
Coordinator, Nurse Practitioner Programs
Loyola University New Orleans

Catherine Shields, RN, BSN
Instructor of Practican Nursing
Ocean County Vocational School
Lakehurst, N.J.

Russlyn A. St. John, RN, MSN
Associate Professor
St. Charles Community College
St. Peters, Mo.

Carol A. Stephenson, RN,C, EdD, CHPN
Emeritus Associate Professor
Texas Christian University
Ft. Worth
Case Manager
St. Paul Hospice
Dallas

Patricia D. Weiskittel, RN, MSN, CNN, CS
Renal Transplant Clinical Nurse Specialist
University Hospital
Cincinnati

Foreword

While we all start out as students in the medical-surgical arena, many of us find ourselves at home in this hectic, chaotic world and build a career in medical-surgical nursing. Some of us may leave the field, only to return to the exciting profession years later.

In fact, the majority of nurses will find themselves at the bedside in hospital nursing at some point in their lives. Hospitals continue to be the main employer of all registered nurses; approximately 59% of all registered nurses work in the hospital setting.

Medical-surgical nursing is a vast and complex area of nursing that encompasses many subspecialties. For this reason, medical-surgical nurses — whether they are students, practicing nurses, or those returning to the field — need education materials that offer current, relevant clinical information in an easy-to-understand format. *Medical-Surgical Nursing Made Incredibly Easy* covers the fundamental kernels of such varied nursing subjects as fluid and electrolyte balance, nursing process, and health history and physical assessment of patients — all essential to the medical-surgical nurse.

Everyday problems associated with various body systems are presented in a clear, common-sense manner. Quite frankly, *Medical-Surgical Nursing Made Incredibly Easy* is just that — an easy read!

Some highlights of the book include:
• quick-scan tables, illustrations, and flowcharts that focus on crucial information
• lighthearted humor and whimsical cartoon characters that enhance presentation of content
• logos that attract attention and point you to essential information
• quick quizzes with rationales that help you see what you've learned and help explain difficult concepts.

Medical-Surgical Nursing Made Incredibly Easy begins with the essentials necessary to understand and provide medical-surgical nursing care. It then covers nearly 300 disorders across 13 body system–oriented chapters, with additional overview chapters on the nursing process and perioperative care. Other topics include pain management, gerontologic care, and cancer care.

Key features of the book help to make referencing and learning information simple and user-friendly. Some of these features include:

 Education edge — patient-teaching tips and checklists to promote wellness and prevent complications

 A closer look — overviews of complex disease pathways

What do I do?—identification of potential crises and emergency actions the nurse must take.

For the novice nursing student, this book can enhance her classroom and clinical instruction as well as help her study for NCLEX exams. Seasoned nurses can use it to orient new nurses as well as to refresh their own knowledge.

The art of teaching is the ability to be clear and straightforward with material that's often complex. This book offers content in understandable terms and facilitates learning with illustrations and humor.

Medical-Surgical Nursing Made Incredibly Easy has succeeded admirably in finding commonalties for all medical-surgical units and in providing a step-by-step approach to learning.

Linda Honan Pellico, PhD(c), APRN
Medical-Surgical Nursing Coordinator
Graduate Entry Prespecialty in Nursing
Yale University
New Haven, Conn.

Medical-surgical nursing practice

Just the facts

In this chapter, you'll learn:

♦ which roles and functions the medical-surgical nurse performs

♦ how to define health and illness

♦ the importance of health promotion in patient care.

A look at medical-surgical nursing

Medical-surgical nursing focuses on adult patients with acute or chronic illness and their responses to actual or potential alterations in health. Medical-surgical nursing is one of many specialties in nursing, yet its scope is much broader than such specialties as cardiovascular or orthopedic nursing.

Thanks to the Academy

The Academy of Medical-Surgical Nurses was created in 1991 and now has more than 20 chapters across the United States. Medical-surgical nurses assume diverse roles and responsibilities. They may work in any health care setting, but most are employed by acute care facilities.

What you need to know

Because they care for a wide range of patients in terms of age and illness, medical-surgical nurses need a broad knowledge of the biological, psychological, and social sciences. In addition, because the typical medical-surgical patient is older than age 65, a strong background in gerontology is required.

The typical med-surg patient is over age 65, so I need a strong background in gerontology.

Roles and functions

Recent changes in health care reflect changes in the populations requiring nursing care and a philosophical shift toward health promotion rather than treatment of illness. The role of the medical-surgical nurse has broadened in response to these changes. Medical-surgical nurses are caregivers, as always, but now they're also educators, advocates, leaders and managers, change agents, and researchers.

Caregiver

Nurses have always been caregivers, but the activities this role encompasses changed dramatically in the 20th century. Increased education of nurses, expanded nursing research, and the consequent recognition that nurses are autonomous and informed professionals have caused a shift from a dependent role to one of independence and collaboration. (See *Critical thinking: An essential skill.*)

A model of independence

Unlike earlier models, medical-surgical nurses now conduct independent assessments and implement patient care based on their knowledge and skills. They

Med-surg nurses implement patient care based on their own knowledge and skills.

Critical thinking: An essential skill

In the complex, rapidly changing health care environment, critical thinking is a skill necessary for providing safe, effective nursing care. Critical thinking takes basic problem solving one step further by considering all related factors, including the patient's unique needs as well as any of the nurse's thoughts and beliefs that may influence her decision-making ability. Critical-thinking skills enable the nurse to take a step outside of the situation and look at the whole picture more objectively.

Truth seekers
Critical thinkers have the desire to seek truth and actively pursue answers to questions to

obtain this complete picture. They're also open-minded and creative, and can draw from past clinical experience to come up with all possible alternatives and then zero in on the best solution for the patient.

Practice for your practice
Books, articles, and online courses are available to hone nurses' critical-thinking skills. Check out *www.nclex.com/ctabout.asp* for more information. When nurses engage in critical thinking, their patients have the best chances for success!

also collaborate with other members of the health care team to implement and evaluate that care.

Educator

With greater emphasis on health promotion and illness prevention, the nurse's role as educator has become increasingly important. The nurse assesses learning needs, plans and implements teaching strategies to meet those needs, and evaluates the effectiveness of the teaching. To be an effective educator, the nurse must have effective interpersonal skills and be familiar with principles of adult learning.

Before you go

Patient teaching is also a major part of discharge planning. Along with teaching come responsibilities for making referrals, identifying community and personal resources, and arranging for necessary equipment and supplies for home care.

Advocate

As an advocate, the nurse helps the patient and his family members interpret information from other health care providers and make decisions about his health-related needs. The nurse must accept and respect a patient's decision, even if it differs from the decision the nurse would make.

Coordinator

All nurses practice leadership and manage time, people, resources, and the environment in which they provide care. They carry out these tasks by directing, delegating, and coordinating activities. (See *How to delegate safely*, page 4.)

Call a huddle

All health care team members, including the nurse, provide patient care. Although the doctor is usually considered the head of the team, the nurse plays an important role in coordinating the efforts of all team members to meet the patient's goals and may conduct team conferences to facilitate communication among team members.

The nurse plays an important role in coordinating efforts of all health care team members.

How to delegate safely

Nurses must have a clear understanding of their responsibilities to ensure that delegating is done safely and successfully. Nurses must remember that although responsibility for a task has been delegated, accountability hasn't. Nurses should receive regular updates from the person assigned the task, ask specific questions, and evaluate the outcome.

Five "rights"

The National Council of State Boards of Nursing identifies five "rights" of delegation that must be satisfied by the delegating nurse:

Right task—The task being assigned or transferred must be within the scope of abilities and practice of the individual receiving the responsibility.

Right circumstance—The individual variables involved (patient condition, environment, caregiver training) must be appropriate for delegation.

Right person—The individual receiving the responsibility must have the legal authority to perform the task. Institutional policies regarding delegation must be consistent with the law.

Right direction and communication—Instructions and expectations must be clear and understood.

Right supervision and follow-up—The delegating nurse must supervise, guide, and evaluate the performance of individuals to whom she delegates. In addition to ensuring that a particular task has been successfully carried out, the delegating nurse must also provide additional training and feedback to coworkers who function under her direction.

Change agent

As a change agent, the nurse works with the patient to address his health concerns, and with staff members to address organizational and community concerns. This role demands a knowledge of change theory, which provides a framework for understanding the dynamics of change, human responses to change, and strategies for effecting change.

Doing what's right

In the community, nurses serve as role models and assist consumers in bringing about changes to improve the environment, work conditions, or other factors that affect health. Nurses also work together to bring about change through legislation by helping to shape and support the laws that mandate the use of car safety seats and motorcycle helmets.

Discharge planner

As a discharge planner, the nurse assesses the patient's needs at discharge, including the patient's support systems and living situation. The nurse also links the patient with available community resources.

Researcher

The primary tasks of nursing research are to promote growth in the science of nursing and to develop a scientific basis for nursing practice. Every nurse should be involved in nursing research and apply research findings to her nursing practice.

Identify and incorporate

Although not all nurses are trained in research methods, each nurse can participate by remaining alert for nursing problems and asking questions about care practices. Many nurses who give direct care identify such problems, which then serve as a basis for research investigation. Nurses can improve nursing care by incorporating research findings into their practice and by communicating the research to others.

We can improve nursing care by incorporating research findings in our practice and telling others.

The health-illness continuum

How people view themselves—as individuals and as part of the environment—affects the way health is defined. Many people view health as a continuum, with wellness—the highest level of function—at one end and illness and death at the other. All people are somewhere on this continuum and, as their health status changes, their location on the continuum also changes.

Health defined

Throughout history, the definition of health has changed depending on the knowledge and beliefs of the time and culture. Some people have regarded health and disease as reward or punishment for their actions. Others have viewed health as soundness or wholeness of the body.

What is it?

Although health is a commonly used term, definitions abound. No single definition is universally accepted. A common one describes health as a disease-free state, but this presents an either-or situation: A person is either healthy or ill.

We may talk about health all the time, but defining the word isn't easy!

WHO says...

The World Health Organization (WHO) calls health "a state of complete physical, mental, and social well-being and not merely the absence of disease or infirmity." This definition doesn't allow for degrees of health or illness. It also fails to reflect the concept of health as dynamic and constantly changing.

It's about culture

Sociologists view health as a condition that allows for the pursuit and enjoyment of desired cultural values. These include the ability to carry out activities of daily living, such as working and performing household chores.

It's about levels

Many people view health as a level of wellness. According to this definition, a person is striving to attain his full potential. This allows for a more holistic and subjective view of health.

Factors affecting health

One of the nurse's primary functions is to assist patients in reaching an optimal level of wellness. When assessing patients, the nurse must be aware of factors that affect their health status and plan to tailor interventions accordingly. Such factors include:
• genetics (biological and genetic makeup that causes illness and chronic conditions)
• cognitive abilities (which affect a person's view of health and ability to seek out resources)
• demographic factors, such as age and sex (certain diseases are more prevalent in a certain age-group or sex)
• geographic locale (which predisposes a person to certain conditions)
• culture (which determines a person's perception of health, the motivation to seek care, and the types of health practices performed)
• lifestyle and environment (such as diet, level of activity, and exposure to toxins)
• health beliefs and practices (which can affect health positively or negatively)
• previous health experiences (which influence reactions to illness and the decision to seek care)
• spirituality (which affects a person's view of illness and health care)
• support systems (which affect the degree to which a person adapts and copes with a situation).

Illness defined

Nurses must understand the concept of illness, particularly how illness may affect the patient. Illness may be defined as a sickness or deviation from a healthy state. It's considered a broader concept than disease. Disease commonly refers to a specific biological or psychological problem that's supported by clinical manifestations and results in a body system or organ malfunction. (See *Disease development*.) Illness, on the other hand, occurs when a person is no longer in a state of perceived "normal" health. A person may have a disease, but not be ill all the time because his body has adapted to the disease.

What does it mean to you?

Illness also encompasses how the patient interprets the disease's source and importance, how the disease affects his behavior and relationships with others, and how he tries to remedy the problem. Another significant component is the meaning that a person attaches to the experience of being ill.

Unlike *illness*, the word *disease* refers to a specific problem that results in body system or organ malfunction. Ouch!

Disease development

A disease is usually detected when it causes a change in metabolism or cell division that causes signs and symptoms. How the cells respond to disease depends on the causative agent and the affected cells, tissues, and organs. In the absence of intervention, resolution of the disease depends on many factors functioning over a period of time, such as extent of disease and the presence of other diseases. Manifestations of disease may include hypofunction, hyperfunction, or increased or decreased mechanical function.

Disease stages

Typically, diseases progress through the following stages:

- exposure or injury—target tissue exposed to a causative agent or injury

- latency or incubation period—no evident signs or symptoms

- prodromal period—generally mild nonspecific signs and symptoms

- acute phase—disease at its full intensity, possibly with complications; called the subclinical acute phase if the patient still functions as though the disease weren't present

- remission—second latency phase that occurs in some diseases and is commonly followed by another acute phase

- convalescence—progression toward recovery

- recovery—return of health or normal functioning; no remaining signs or symptoms of disease.

Types of illness

Illness may be acute or chronic. Acute illness usually refers to a disease or condition that has a relatively abrupt onset, high intensity, and short duration. If no complications occur, most acute illnesses end in a full recovery, and the person returns to the previous or a similar level of functioning.

Regain and maintain

Chronic illness refers to a condition that typically has a slower onset, less intensity, and a longer duration than acute illness. The goal is to help the patient regain and maintain the highest possible level of health, although some patients fail to return to their previous level of functioning.

Effects of illness

When a person experiences an illness, one or more changes occur that signal its presence. These may include:
- changes in body appearance or function
- unusual body emissions
- sensory changes
- uncomfortable physical manifestations
- changes in emotional status
- changes in relationships.

Most people experience a mild form of some of these changes in their daily lives. However, when the changes are severe enough to interfere with usual daily activities, the person is usually considered ill.

Perception and reaction

People's reactions to feeling ill vary. Some people seek action immediately and others take no action. Some may exaggerate their symptoms and others may deny that their symptoms exist. A patient's perception and reaction to illness is unique and is usually based on his culture, knowledge, view of health, and previous experiences with illness and the health care system.

Effects of illness on family

The presence of illness in a family can have a dramatic effect on the functioning of the family as a unit. The type of effect depends on the following factors:
- which member is ill
- the seriousness and duration of the illness

When changes in health interfere with daily activities, a person is considered ill.

I figured the "no skin or organs" thing would be a problem.

• the family's social and cultural customs (each member's role in the family and the tasks specific to that role).

Which member?

The types of role change that occur also vary, depending on the family member affected. For example, if the affected member is the primary breadwinner, other members may need to seek employment to supplement the family income. As the primary breadwinner assumes a dependent role, the rest of the family must adjust to new roles. If the affected family member is a working single parent, serious economic and child care problems may result. That person must depend on support systems for help or face additional stress.

Health promotion

Research shows that poor health practices contribute to a wide range of illnesses, a shortened life span, and increased health care costs. Good health practices have the opposite effect: fewer illnesses, a longer life span, and lower health care costs.

Better late than never

Good health practices can benefit most people no matter when they're started. Of course, the earlier in life good practices are started, the fewer poor habits have to be overcome. Even so, later is better than never. For example, stopping cigarette smoking has immediate and long-term benefits. Immediately, the patient will experience improved circulation, pulse rate, and blood pressure. After 10 years without smoking, he'll cut his risk of dying from lung cancer in half.

Better late than never. Stopping smoking now could save us in the long run!

What is health promotion?

Quite simply, health promotion is teaching good health practices and finding ways to help people correct their poor health practices.

But what specifically should you teach? The project Healthy People 2010 sets forth comprehensive health goals for the nation with the aim of reducing mortality and morbidity in all ages. These objectives make a useful teaching plan. (See Healthy People 2010: *Selected objectives*, page 10.)

Healthy People 2010: Selected objectives

Launched in January 2000 by the U.S. Department of Health and Human Services, *Healthy People 2010* sets forth two major goals for U.S. citizens: to increase the quality and years of life and to eliminate health disparities among segments of the population (for example, those that occur by gender, race, education, disability, geographic location, or sexual orientation).

The following are important target objectives that will help to measure the nation's progress toward achieving these goals.

Increase
• To at least 30% the proportion of people age 18 and older who engage in physical activity that promotes the development and maintenance of cardiopulmonary fitness 3 or more days per week for 20 minutes or more per occasion

• To at least 96% the proportion of people of all ages who have access to a specific source of primary care
• To at least 50% the proportion of adults age 18 and older with recognized depression who receive treatment

Decrease
• To no more than 15% the incidence of obese adults age 20 and older
• To no more than 12% the incidence of cigarette smoking among adults age 18 and older
• To no more than 9.2 per 100,000 people deaths caused by motor vehicle accidents
• To no more than 6% the incidence of adults age 18 or older who report binge drinking in the past 30 days

---

Adult health care

Adults between ages 25 and 64 may fall victim to several health problems, including heart disease and cancer. Although some of these problems stem from genetic predisposition, many are linked to unhealthy habits, such as overeating, smoking, lack of exercise, and alcohol and drug abuse. Your teaching can help an adult recognize and correct these habits to ensure a longer, healthier life.

Geriatric health care

Today, people live longer than ever before. In the past century, life expectancy in the United States has increased from 47 years to about 76 years. Fortunately, most elderly people maintain their independence, with few needing to be institutionalized.

Cope and avoid

Even so, most elderly people suffer from at least one chronic health problem. With the nurse's help, they can cope with existing health problems and learn to avoid new ones. Doing so will improve their quality of life and allow them to continue contributing to society.

State of mind

Aging is a state of mind and body.

Emphasize that aging is a state of mind as well as of body. Urge the elderly patient to continue as many activities as possible, depending on his mobility. Also, help him explore new interests or hobbies. Recommend that he attend a hospital- or community-sponsored seminar on retirement. Such seminars usually cover topics like budgeting and health and fitness.

Quick quiz

1. Which of the following isn't a characteristic of a critical thinker?
   A.   Practical, situation-oriented decision making
   B.   Creativity
   C.   Open-mindedness
   D.   Desire for truth

Answer: A. Critical thinkers actively pursue answers to questions and consider all alternatives in making a decision. This requires creativity, a desire for truth, and being open-minded.

2. A nurse who is preparing to delegate:
   A.   can delegate a task to whomever she chooses.
   B.   can delegate whichever task she chooses.
   C.   has no responsibility for follow-up.
   D.   makes sure the person she delegates to has the legal authority to perform the task.

Answer: D. To delegate safely, nurses must observe several "rights": the right task, right circumstance, right person, right direction and communication, and right supervision and follow-up.

3. Which of the following is an example of health promotion?
   A.   Administering antibiotics to a patient
   B.   Splinting a patient's fractured bone
   C.   Assisting a patient in stopping smoking
   D.   Inserting an I.V. catheter

Answer: C. Health promotion involves teaching good health practices as well as helping people correct their poor health practices. Helping a patient to stop smoking helps him to correct a poor health practice.

4. The effect of illness on a family unit depends on several factors, including:

    A.   when the illness occurs.

    B.   which family member is affected.

    C.   whether the illness is due to poor health habits.

    D.   at what point the patient sought care.

Answer: B. The effect of illness on a family unit depends on which family member is affected, the seriousness and duration of the illness, and the family's social and cultural customs.

Scoring

☆☆☆ If you answered all four items correctly, super! You surge ahead of the pack in med-surg!

☆☆ If you answered three items correctly, great! You sure have been practicing your nursing practice!

☆ If you answered fewer than three items correctly, don't despair! Reviewing the chapter will promote your healthy understanding!

Nursing process

Just the facts

In this chapter, you'll learn:

♦ the five key steps of the nursing process

♦ how to effectively communicate with your patient while taking a health history

♦ what components the health history contains

♦ how to perform inspection, palpation, percussion, and auscultation.

A look at the nursing process

One of the most significant advances in nursing has been the development and acceptance of the nursing process. This problem-solving approach to nursing care offers a structure for applying your knowledge and skills in an organized, goal-oriented manner. It serves as the cornerstone of clinical nursing by providing a systematic method for determining the patient's health problems, devising a care plan to address those problems, implementing the plan, and evaluating the plan's effectiveness.

Process pluses

When used effectively, the nursing process offers several important advantages:
• The patient's specific health problems, not the disease, become the focus of health care. This emphasis promotes the patient's participation and encourages his independence and compliance—factors important to a positive outcome.
• Identifying a patient's health problems improves communication by providing

Staying goal-oriented is the cornerstone of clinical nursing!

EVALUATION
IMPLEMENTATION
PLANNING
NURSING DIAGNOSIS
ASSESSMENT

nurses who care for the patient with a common list of recognized problems.

• The nursing process provides a consistent and orderly professional structure. It promotes accountability for nursing activities based on evaluation and, in so doing, leads to quality assurance.

Common phases

The five phases of the nursing process are dynamic and flexible. Because they're interrelated, they often overlap. Together, they resemble the steps that many other professions rely on to identify and correct problems. They include:

 assessment

 nursing diagnosis

 planning

 implementation

 evaluation.

Dynamic and flexible, that's me — and the nursing process!

Assessment

Assessment involves data collection used to identify a patient's actual and potential health needs. According to American Nurses Association guidelines, data should accurately reflect the patient's life experiences and his patterns of living. To accomplish this, you must assume an objective and nonjudgmental approach when gathering data. You can obtain data through a health history, a physical examination, and a review of pertinent laboratory and medical information.

The accuracy and completeness of your patient's answers largely depend on your interview skills.

Health history

A health history is used to gather subjective data about the patient and explore past and present problems. First, ask the patient about his general physical and emotional health; then ask him about specific body systems and structures. Information may come from the patient himself, from the patient's significant other, or from other health care professionals.

The accuracy and completeness of your patient's answers largely depend on your skill as an interviewer. Before you start asking questions, review the communication guidelines in the following sections.

Interview techniques to avoid

Some interview techniques create communication problems between nurse and patient. Techniques to avoid include:
• asking "why" or "how" questions
• asking probing or persistent questions
• using inappropriate language
• giving advice
• giving false reassurance
• changing the subject or interrupting.
   Also avoid using clichés or stereotypical responses, giving excessive approval or agreement, jumping to conclusions, or using defensive responses.

Effective techniques

To obtain the most benefit from a health history interview, try to ensure that the patient feels comfortable and respected and believes he can trust you. Use effective interview techniques to help the patient identify resources and improve problem-solving abilities. Remember, however, that successful techniques in one situation may not be effective in another. Your attitude and the patient's interpretation of your questions can vary. In general, you should:
• allow the patient time to think and reflect
• encourage the patient to talk
• encourage the patient to describe a particular experience
• indicate that you have listened to the patient such as through paraphrasing the patient's response.

Know right from wrong

Although there are many right ways to communicate with a patient, there are also some wrong ways that can hamper your interview. (See *Interview techniques to avoid*.)

Conducting the interview

Physical surroundings, psychological atmosphere, interview structure, and questioning style can all affect the interview flow and outcome; so can your ability to adopt a communication style to fit each patient's needs and situation. Close the door to help prevent interruptions, and try to arrange yourself so you're facing the patient, slightly offset from him, to create a friendly feeling.

Start at the very beginning

Begin by introducing yourself. Establish an interview time frame, and ask if the patient has questions about the interview procedure. Spend a few minutes chatting informally before beginning the interview.

A note on notes

Lengthy note taking may distract the patient, who may wonder if you're listening. If you must take notes, tell the patient before the interview starts. Finish the interview by summarizing salient interview points, telling the patient the interview results, explaining how the physical assessment will be conducted, and discussing follow-up plans.

My name is Joy. I'll be asking you questions about your health for the next 10 minutes or so. Do you have any questions before we start?

Short and sweet

A patient who is ill, experiencing pain, or sedated may have difficulty completing the health history. In such instances, obtain only the information pertaining to the immediate problem. To avoid tiring a seriously ill patient, obtain the history in several sessions or ask a close relative or friend to supply essential information.

Two types

Typically, the health history includes two types of questions: open-ended, which permit more subtle and flexible responses, and closed-ended, which require only a yes-or-no response. Open-ended questions usually result in the most useful information and give patients the feeling that they're actively participating in and have some control over the interview. Closed-ended questions help eliminate rambling conversations. They're also useful when the interview requires brevity — for example, when a patient reports extreme pain or digresses frequently.

Open-ended questions usually result in the most useful information.

Logical and patient

Whatever question type you use, move logically from one history section to the next. Allow the patient to concentrate and give complete information on a subject before moving on.

Obtaining health history data

The health history has five major sections: biographic data, health and illness patterns, health promotion and protection patterns, role and relationship patterns, and a summary of health history data.

Biographic data

Begin obtaining the patient's health history by collecting personal information. This data section identifies the patient and provides important demographic information. By filling out a form, you usually gather facts, such as the patient's address, telephone number, age, sex, birth date, Social Security number, place of birth, race, nationality, marital status, occupation, education, religion, cultural background, and emergency contact person.

Health and illness patterns

This information includes the patient's chief complaint; current, past, and family health history; status of physiologic systems; and developmental considerations.

Mind his P's and Q's

Determine why the patient is seeking health care by asking, "What brings you here today?" If the patient has specific symptoms, record that information in the patient's own words. Ask the patient with a specific symptom or health concern to describe the problem in detail, including the suspected cause. To ensure that you don't omit pertinent data, use the PQRST mnemonic device, which provides a systematic approach to obtaining information. (See *PQRST: What's the story?* page 18.)

For a patient who seeks a health maintenance assessment, health counseling, or health education, expect to take few notes. Ask the patient about recent minor illnesses or health concerns.

Ask the patient with a specific concern to describe the problem in detail.

Think back

Next, record childhood and other illnesses, injuries, previous hospitalizations, surgical procedures, immunizations, allergies, and medications taken regularly.

Tell me about your mother

Information about the patient's relatives can also unmask potential health problems. Some diseases, such as cardiovascular disease, alcoholism, depression, and cancer, may be genetically linked. Others, such as hemophilia, cystic fibrosis, sickle cell anemia, and Tay-Sachs disease, are genetically transmitted.

Genogram and grampa, too

Determine the general health status of the patient's immediate family members, including maternal and paternal grandparents,

PQRST: What's the story?

Use the PQRST mnemonic device to fully explore your patient's chief complaint. When you ask the questions below, you'll encourage him to describe his symptom in greater detail.

Provocative or palliative

Ask the patient:
- What provokes or relieves the symptom?
- Do stress, anger, certain physical positions, or other things trigger the symptom?
- What makes the symptom worsen or subside?

Quality or quantity

Ask the patient:
- What does the symptom feel like, look like, or sound like?
- Are you having the symptom right now? If so, is it more or less severe than usual?
- To what degree does the symptom affect your normal activities?

Region or radiation

Ask the patient:
- Where in the body does the symptom occur?
- Does the symptom appear in other regions? If so, where?

Severity

Ask the patient:
- How severe is the symptom? How would you rate it on a scale of 1 to 10, with 10 being the most severe?
- Does the symptom seem to be diminishing, intensifying, or staying about the same?

Timing

Ask the patient:
- When did the symptom begin?
- Was the onset sudden or gradual?
- How often does the symptom occur?
- How long does the symptom last?

---

parents, siblings, aunts, uncles, and children. If any are deceased, record the year and cause of death. Use a genogram to organize family history data. Information about the patient's past and current physiologic status (also called review of systems) is another health history component. A careful assessment helps identify potential or undetected physiologic disorders.

Health promotion and protection patterns

What a patient does or doesn't do to stay healthy is affected by such factors as health beliefs, personal habits, sleep and waking patterns, exercise and activity, recreation, nutrition, stress and coping, socioeconomic status, environmental health patterns, and occupational health patterns. To help assess health promotion and protection patterns, ask the patient to describe a typical day and inquire about which behaviors the patient believes are healthful.

Role and relationship patterns

A patient's role and relationship patterns reflect his psychosocial (psychological, emotional, social, spiritual, and sexual) health. To assess role and relationship patterns, investigate the patient's self-concept, cultural influences, religious influences, family role and relationship patterns, sexuality and reproductive patterns, social support patterns, and other psychosocial considerations. Each of these patterns can influence the patient's health.

Summary of health history data

Conclude the health history by summarizing all findings. For the well patient, list the patient's health promotion strengths and re-sources along with defined health education needs. If the inter-view points out a significant health problem, tell the patient what it is and begin to address the problem. This may involve referral to a doctor, education, or plans for further investigation.

Physical assessment

During the physical assessment, use drapes so only the area being examined is exposed. Develop a pattern for your assessments, starting with the same body system and proceeding in the same sequence. Organize your steps to minimize the number of times the patient needs to change position. By using a systematic approach, you'll be less likely to forget an area.

Count 'em — four

No matter where you start your physical assessment, you'll use four techniques:

 inspection

 palpation

 percussion

 auscultation.

Use these techniques in sequence except when you perform an abdominal assessment. Because palpation and percussion can alter bowel sounds, the sequence for assessing the abdomen is inspection, auscultation, per-cussion, and palpation. Let's look at each step in the se-quence.

Palpation and percussion can alter bowel sounds, so they come after inspection and auscultation when assessing the abdomen.

Percussion types

You can perform percussion using the direct or indirect method. Direct percussion reveals tenderness. Indirect percussion elicits sounds that give clues to the makeup of the underlying tissue.

Direct percussion

Using one or two fingers, tap directly on the body part. Ask the patient to tell you which areas are painful and watch his face for signs of discomfort. This technique is commonly used to assess an adult patient's sinuses for tenderness.

Indirect percussion

Press the distal part of the middle finger of your nondominant hand firmly on the body part. Keep the rest of your hand off the body surface. Flex the wrist of your dominant hand. Using the middle finger of your dominant hand, tap quickly and directly over the point where your other middle finger touches the patient's skin. Listen to the sounds produced.

Inspection

Inspect the patient using vision, smell, and hearing to observe normal conditions and deviations. Performed correctly, inspection can reveal more than other techniques.

Inspection begins when you first meet the patient and continues throughout the health history and physical examination. As you assess each body system, observe for color, size, location, movement, texture, symmetry, odor, and sounds.

Palpation

Palpation requires you to touch the patient with different parts of your hands, using varying degrees of pressure. To do this, you need short fingernails and warm hands. Always palpate tender areas last. Tell your patient the purpose of your touch and what you're feeling with your hands.

Sounds and their sources

As you practice percussion, you'll recognize different sounds. Each sound is related to the structure underneath. This chart offers a quick guide to percussion sounds and their sources.

Sound	Quality of sound	Where it's heard	Source
Tympany	Drumlike	Over enclosed air	Air in bowel
Resonance	Hollow	Over areas of part air and part solid	Normal lung
Hyperresonance	Booming	Over air	Lung with emphysema
Dullness	Thudlike	Over solid tissue	Liver, spleen, heart
Flatness	Flat	Over dense tissue	Muscle, bone

Palpate to evaluate

As you palpate each body system, evaluate the following features:
- texture — rough or smooth?
- temperature — warm, hot, or cold?
- moisture — dry, wet, or moist?
- motion — still or vibrating?
- consistency of structures — solid or fluid-filled?

Percussion

Percussion involves tapping your fingers or hands quickly and sharply against parts of the patient's body, usually the chest or abdomen. The technique helps you locate organ borders, identify organ shape and position, and determine if an organ is solid or filled with fluid or gas. (See *Percussion types*.)

Do you hear what I hear?

Percussion requires a skilled touch and an ear trained to detect slight variations in sound. Organs and tissues, depending on their density, produce sounds of varying loudness, pitch, and duration. For instance, air-filled cavities such as the lungs produce markedly different sounds than do the liver and other dense tissues. (See *Sounds and their sources*.)

As you percuss, move gradually from areas of resonance to those of dullness and then compare sounds. Also, compare sounds on one side of the body with those on the other side.

Little things make a big difference! Always be sure to warm your hands and instruments before assessing a patient.

Auscultation

Auscultation, usually the last assessment step, involves listening for various breath, heart, and bowel sounds with a stethoscope. To prevent the spread of infection among patients, clean the heads and end pieces of the stethoscope with alcohol or a disinfectant after every use.

Diagnostic test findings

Diagnostic test findings complete the objective database. Together with the nursing history and physical examination, they form a significant profile of the patient's condition.

Analyzing the data

The final aspect of assessment involves data you've compiled. In your analysis, include the following steps:
• Group significant data into logical clusters. You'll base your nursing diagnosis not on a single sign or symptom but on a cluster of assessment findings. By analyzing the clustered data and identifying patterns of illness-related behavior, you can begin to perceive the patient's problem or risk of developing other problems.
• Identify data gaps. Signs, symptoms, and isolated incidents that don't fit into consistent patterns can provide the missing facts you need to determine the overall pattern of your patient's problem.
• Identify conflicting or inconsistent data. Clarify information that conflicts with other assessment findings, and determine what's causing the inconsistency. For example, a diabetic patient who says that she complies with her prescribed diet and insulin administration schedule, but whose serum glucose is greatly elevated, may need to have her treatment regimen reviewed or revised.
• Determine the patient's perception of normal health. A patient may find it harder to comply with the treatment regimen when his idea of normality doesn't agree with yours.
• Determine how the patient handles his health problem. For instance, is the patient coping with his health problem successfully, or does he need help? Does he deny that he has a problem, or does he admit it but lack solutions to the problem?
• Form an opinion about the patient's health status. Base your opinion on actual, potential, or possible concerns reflected by the patient's responses to his condition, and use this to formulate your nursing diagnosis.

Nursing diagnosis

In 1990, the North American Nursing Diagnosis Association (NANDA) defined the nursing diagnosis as "a clinical judgment about individual, family, or community responses to actual or potential health problems or life processes. Nursing diagnoses provide the basis for the selection of nursing interventions to achieve outcomes for which the nurse is accountable."

Identifying the problem

After clustering significant assessment data and analyzing the pattern, your next step is to label the patient's actual and potential health problems. NANDA has developed a taxonomic scheme to help you do this.

Identify, diagnose, and validate

In forming a nursing diagnosis, you'll identify the patient's problem, write a diagnostic statement, and validate the diagnosis. You'll establish several nursing diagnoses for each patient. Arrange the diagnoses according to priority so that you address the patient's most crucial problems first.

The NANDA taxonomy helps you form a clear and accurate nursing diagnosis.

You've got to hand it to NANDA!

Writing the diagnostic statement

The diagnostic statement consists of a nursing diagnosis and the etiology (cause) related to it. For example, a diagnostic statement for a patient who's too weak to bathe himself properly might be *Bathing or hygiene self-care deficit related to weakness*. A diagnostic statement related to an actual problem might be *Impaired gas exchange related to pulmonary edema*. A statement related to a potential problem might be *Risk for injury related to unsteady gait*.

Stress present, balance absent

The etiology is a stressor or something that brings about a response, effect, or change. A stressor results from the presence of a stress agent or the absence of an equilibrium factor. Causative agents may include birth defects, inherited factors, diseases, injuries, signs or symptoms, psychosocial factors, iatrogenic factors, developmental phases, lifestyle, or situational or environmental factors.

Validating each diagnosis

Next, validate the diagnosis. Review clustered data. Are they consistent? Does the patient verify the diagnosis?

Prioritizing the diagnoses

After you've established several nursing diagnoses, categorize them in order of priority. Obviously, life-threatening problems must be addressed first, followed by health-threatening concerns. Also, consider how the patient perceives his health problem; his priority problem may differ from yours.

Consider that the patient may perceive his problem differently from the way you do.

Maslow's hierarchy

One system of categorizing diagnoses uses Maslow's hierarchy of needs, which classifies human needs based on the idea that lower-level, physiologic needs must be met before higher-level, abstract needs. For example, if a patient has shortness of breath, he probably isn't interested in discussing his relationships. (See *Maslow's hierarchy of needs.*)

Maslow's hierarchy of needs

To formulate nursing diagnoses, you must know your patient's needs and values. Of course, physiologic needs—represented by the base of the pyramid in the diagram below—must be met first.

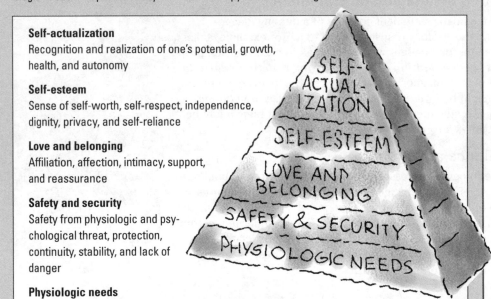

Self-actualization
Recognition and realization of one's potential, growth, health, and autonomy

Self-esteem
Sense of self-worth, self-respect, independence, dignity, privacy, and self-reliance

Love and belonging
Affiliation, affection, intimacy, support, and reassurance

Safety and security
Safety from physiologic and psychological threat, protection, continuity, stability, and lack of danger

Physiologic needs
Oxygen, food, elimination, temperature control, sex, movement, rest, and comfort

Planning

After you establish the nursing diagnoses, you'll develop a written care plan. A written care plan serves as a communication tool among health care team members that helps ensure continuity of care. The plan consists of two parts: patient outcomes, or expected outcomes, which describe behaviors or results to be achieved within a specified time; and nursing interventions needed to achieve those outcomes.

Measure and observe

Be sure to state both parts of the care plan in measurable, observable terms and dates. The statement, "The patient will perceive himself with greater self-worth," is too vague, lacks a time frame, and offers no means to observe the patient's self-perception. A patient outcome such as, "The patient will describe himself in a positive way within 1 week," provides an observable means to evaluate the patient's behavior and a time frame for the behavioral change. (See *Ensuring a successful care plan*.)

Ensuring a successful care plan

Your care plan must rest on a solid foundation of carefully chosen nursing diagnoses. It also must fit your patient's needs, age, developmental level, culture, strengths and weaknesses, and willingness and ability to take part in his care. Your plan should help the patient attain the highest functional level possible while posing minimal risk and not creating new problems. If complete recovery isn't possible, your plan should help the patient cope physically and emotionally with his impaired or declining health.

Using the following guidelines will help ensure that your care plan is effective.

Be realistic.
Avoid setting a goal that's too difficult for the patient to achieve. The patient may become discouraged, depressed, and apathetic if he can't achieve expected outcomes.

Tailor your approach.
Individualize your outcome statements and nursing interventions. Keep in mind that each patient is unique; no two patient problems are exactly alike.

Avoid vague terms.
Use precise, quantitative terms rather than vague ones. For example, if your patient is restless, describe his specific behavior, such as "pulls at restraints" rather than "patient uncooperative." To indicate that the patient's vital signs are stable, document specific measurements, such as "heart rate less than 100 beats/minute" rather than "heart rate stable."

Intervention options

Before you implement a care plan, review your intervention options and then weigh their potential to succeed. Determine if you can obtain the necessary equipment and resources. If not, take steps to get what you need or change the intervention accordingly. Observe the patient's willingness to participate in the various interventions, and be prepared to postpone or modify interventions if necessary.

Implementation

The implementation phase is when you put your care plan into action. Implementation encompasses all nursing interventions directed at solving the patient's problems and meeting health care needs. While you coordinate implementation, you also seek help from the patient, the patient's family, and other caregivers.

Monitor and gauge

After implementing the care plan, continue to monitor the patient to gauge the effectiveness of interventions and adjust them as the patient's condition changes. Documentation of outcomes achieved should be reflected in the care plan. Expect to review, revise, and update the entire care plan regularly, according to facility policy. Keep in mind that the care plan is usually a permanent part of the patient's medical record.

Evaluation

After enough time has elapsed for the care plan to effect desired changes, you're ready for evaluation, the final step in the nursing process. During evaluation, you must decide if the interventions carried out have enabled the patient to achieve the desired outcomes.

Start with the finish

Begin by reviewing the patient outcomes stated for each nursing diagnosis. Then observe your patient's behavioral changes, and judge how well they meet the outcomes related to them. Does the patient's behavior match the outcome or fall short of it?

Consider the evaluation to be positive if the patient's behavior has changed as expected, if the outcomes have been accomplished, or if progress has occurred. Failure to meet these criteria constitutes a negative evaluation and requires new interventions.

Evaluating the care plan's effectiveness is the final step in the nursing process.

Process success

The evaluation phase also allows you to judge the effectiveness of the nursing process as a whole. If the process has been applied successfully, the patient's health status will improve. Either his health problems will have been solved or progress will have been made toward achieving their resolution. He'll also be able to perform self-care measures with a sense of independence and confidence, and you'll feel assured that you've fulfilled your professional responsibility.

Quick quiz

1. When obtaining a health history from a patient, ask first about:
- A.   biographic data.
- B.   his chief complaint.
- C.   health insurance coverage.
- D.   family history.

Answer: A. Take care of the biographic data first; otherwise, you might get involved in the patient history and forget to ask basic questions.

2. The first technique in your physical assessment sequence is:
- A.   palpation.
- B.   auscultation.
- C.   inspection.
- D.   percussion.

Answer: C. The assessment of each body system begins with inspection. It's the most commonly used technique, and it can reveal more than any other technique.

3. When palpating the abdomen, begin by palpating:
- A.   lightly.
- B.   firmly.
- C.   deeply.
- D.   the most tender area.

Answer: A. Light palpation is always done first to detect surface characteristics. Tender areas should always be palpated last.

4. Expected outcomes are defined as:
    A. goals the patient should reach as a result of planned nursing interventions.
    B. what the patient and family ask you to accomplish.
    C. goals a little higher than what the patient can realistically reach to help motivate him.
    D. goals set by the medical team for each patient.

Answer: A. Expected outcomes are realistic, measurable goals and their target dates.

5. A good way to come up with interventions is by:
    A. asking the doctor.
    B. asking the patient what has worked for him before.
    C. reviewing past medical records.
    D. interviewing family members.

Answer: B. You can also ask other nurses, check nursing journals, pick interventions from standardized care plans, or brainstorm.

Scoring

☆☆☆ If you answered all five items correctly, bravo! You're a process pro.

☆☆ If you answered three or four items correctly, way to go! You've got the nursing process pretty down pat.

☆ If you answered fewer than three items correctly, chin up! Process this chapter one more time and try again.

Fluids and electrolytes

Just the facts

In this chapter, you'll learn:

♦ how fluids are distributed throughout the body

♦ what certain fluid- and electrolyte-related terms mean

♦ how fluids and electrolytes move through the body

♦ types of I.V. fluids and how they're used

♦ complications associated with I.V. therapy

♦ how to provide nursing care to a patient receiving I.V. therapy.

A look at fluids

Where would we be without body fluids? Nowhere. Fluids are vital to all forms of life: They help maintain body temperature and cell shape, and they help transport nutrients, gases, and wastes. Let's take a close look at fluids and the way the body balances them.

Making gains = losses

The skin, the lungs, the kidneys—just about all major organs—work together to maintain a proper balance of fluid. To maintain proper balance, the amount of fluid gained throughout the day must equal the amount lost. Some of those losses can be measured (sensible losses); others can't (insensible losses).

We work together with other organs to maintain fluid balance.

Fluid compartments

This illustration shows the primary fluid compartments in the body: intracellular and extracellular, the latter of which is further divided into interstitial and intravascular. Capillary walls and cell membranes separate intracellular fluids from extracellular fluids.

Intracellular

Interstitial

Intravascular

Following the fluid

The body holds fluid in two basic areas, or compartments—inside the cells and outside the cells. Fluid found inside the cells is called intracellular fluid (ICF); fluid found outside them, extracellular fluid (ECF). Capillary walls and cell membranes separate the intracellular and extracellular compartments. (See *Fluid compartments*.) To maintain proper fluid balance, the distribution of fluid between the two compartments must remain relatively constant.

ECF can be broken down further into interstitial fluid, which surrounds the cells, and intravascular fluid or plasma, which is the liquid portion of blood. In an adult, interstitial fluid accounts for about 75% of the ECF. Plasma accounts for the remaining 25%.

A look at electrolytes

Electrolytes work with fluids to maintain health and well-being. They're found in various concentrations, depending on whether they're inside or outside the cells. (See *Understanding electrolytes*.) Electrolytes are crucial for nearly all cellular reactions and functions. Let's take a look at what electrolytes are, how they function, and what upsets their balance.

Memory jogger

To help you remember which fluid belongs to which compartment, keep in mind that IN-TER means between (as in interval — between two events) and INTRA means within or inside (as in intravenous — inside a vein).

Understanding electrolytes

Electrolytes help regulate water distribution, govern acid-base balance, and transmit nerve impulses. They also contribute to energy generation and blood clotting. This table summarizes what the body's major electrolytes do. Check the illustration to see how electrolytes are distributed in and around the cell.

Potassium (K)
• Main intracellular fluid (ICF) cation
• Regulates cell excitability
• Permeates cell membranes, thereby affecting the cell's electrical status
• Helps to control ICF osmolality and, consequently, ICF osmotic pressure

Magnesium (Mg)
• A leading ICF cation
• Contributes to many enzymatic and metabolic processes, particularly protein synthesis
• Modifies nerve impulse transmission and skeletal muscle response (Unbalanced Mg concentrations dramatically affect neuromuscular processes.)

Phosphorus (P)
• Main ICF anion
• Promotes energy storage and carbohydrate, protein, and fat metabolism
• Acts as a hydrogen buffer

Sodium (Na)
• Main extracellular fluid (ECF) cation
• Helps govern normal ECF osmolality (A shift in Na concentrations triggers a fluid volume change to restore normal solute and water ratios.)
• Helps maintain acid-base balance
• Activates nerve and muscle cells
• Influences water distribution (with chloride)

Chloride (Cl)
• Main ECF anion
• Helps maintain normal ECF osmolality
• Affects body pH
• Plays a vital role in maintaining acid-base

balance; combines with hydrogen ions to produce hydrochloric acid

Calcium (Ca)
• A major cation in teeth and bones; found in fairly equal concentrations in ICF and ECF
• Also found in cell membranes, where it helps cells adhere to one another and maintain their shape
• Acts as an enzyme activator within cells (Muscles must have Ca to contract.)
• Aids coagulation
• Affects cell membrane permeability and firing level

Bicarbonate (HCO_3^-)
• Present in ECF
• Primary funcion is regulating acid-base balance

Electrolytes influence water distribution to the cells.

Anions and cations

Electrolytes are substances that, when in solution, separate (or dissociate) into electrically charged particles called ions. Some ions are positively charged; others, negatively charged. Anions are electrolytes that generate a negative charge; cations are electrolytes that produce a positive charge. An electrical charge makes cells function normally. Chloride, phosphorus, and bicarbonate are anions; sodium, potassium, calcium, and magnesium are cations.

Memory jogger

To remind yourself about the difference between anions and cations, remember that the T in "cation" looks like the positive symbol, "+."

Electrolyte balance

Sodium and chloride, the major electrolytes in ECF, exert most of their effects outside the cell. Calcium and bicarbonate are two other electrolytes found in ECF. Potassium, phosphate, and magnesium are among the most abundant electrolytes inside the cell.

Although electrolytes are concentrated in one compartment or another, they aren't locked or frozen in these areas. Like fluids, electrolytes move about trying to maintain balance and electroneutrality.

Fluid and electrolyte movement

Just as the heart beats constantly, fluids and solutes move constantly within the body. That movement allows the body to maintain homeostasis, the constant state of balance the body seeks.

Within the cells

Solutes within the body's intracellular, interstitial, and intravascular compartments move through the membranes separating those compartments in different ways. The membranes are semipermeable, meaning that they allow some solutes to pass through, but not others. Following are the different ways fluids and solutes move through membranes at the cellular level.

Diffusion goes with the flow

In diffusion, solutes move from an area of higher concentration to an area of lower concentration, which eventually results in an equal distribution of solutes within the two areas. Diffusion is a form of passive transport because no energy is required to make it happen; it just happens. Like fish swimming downstream, the solutes simply go with the flow. (See *Diffusion*.)

If I could just get past that semipermeable membrane, I'd be in with the in crowd. Maybe I'll meet George Clooney!

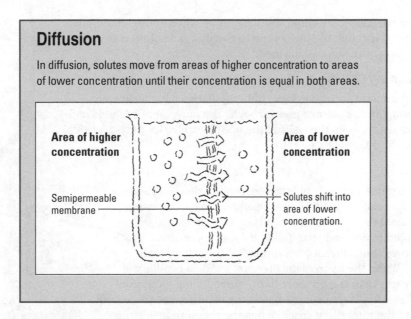

Diffusion

In diffusion, solutes move from areas of higher concentration to areas of lower concentration until their concentration is equal in both areas.

Area of higher concentration

Area of lower concentration

Semipermeable membrane

Solutes shift into area of lower concentration.

Actively transporting

In active transport, solutes move from an area of lower concentration to an area of higher concentration. Like fish swimming upstream, active transport requires energy to make it happen.

The energy required for a solute to move against a concentration gradient comes from a substance called adenosine triphosphate (ATP). Stored in all cells, ATP supplies energy for solute movement in and out of cells.

Some solutes, such as sodium and potassium, use ATP to move in and out of cells in a form of active transport called the sodium-potassium pump. With the help of this pump, sodium ions move from ICF (an area of lower concentration) to ECF (an area of higher concentration). With potassium, the reverse happens: A large amount of potassium in intracellular fluid causes an electrical potential at the cell membrane. As ions rapidly shift in and out of the cell, electrical impulses are conducted. These impulses are essential for maintaining life.

Other solutes that require active transport to cross cell membranes include calcium ions, hydrogen ions, amino acids, and certain sugars.

Osmosis lets fluids through

Osmosis refers to the passive movement of fluid across a membrane from an area of lower solute concentration and comparatively more fluid into an area of higher solute concentration and comparatively less fluid. Osmosis stops when enough fluid has moved through the membrane to equalize the solute concentration on both sides of the membrane. (See *Osmosis*.)

Within the vascular system

Within the vascular system, only capillaries have walls thin enough to let solutes pass through. The movement of fluids and solutes through the walls of the body's capillaries plays a critical role in fluid balance.

The pressure is on

The movement of fluids through capillaries — a process called capillary filtration — results from blood pushing against the walls of the capillary. That pressure, called hydrostatic (or "fluid-pushing") pressure, forces fluids and solutes through the capillary wall.

When the hydrostatic pressure inside a capillary is greater than the pressure in the surrounding interstitial space, fluids and solutes inside the capillary are forced out into the interstitial space. When the pressure inside the capillary is less than the pressure outside of it, fluids and solutes move back into the capillary.

Keeping the fluid in

A process called reabsorption prevents too much fluid from leaving the capillaries no matter how much hydrostatic pressure ex-

> Osmosis is all about balance — making sure the number of solutes on one side equals the number on the other.

Osmosis

In osmosis, fluid moves passively from areas with more fluid (and fewer solutes) to areas with less fluid (and more solutes). Remember that in osmosis fluid moves, whereas in diffusion solutes move.

Area of lower solute concentration equals higher fluid concentration.

Semipermeable membrane

Fluid

Solute

Area of higher solute concentration equals lower fluid concentration.

ists within the capillaries. When fluid filters through a capillary, the protein albumin remains behind in the diminishing volume of water. Albumin is a large molecule that usually can't pass through capillary membranes. As the concentration of albumin inside a capillary increases, fluid begins to move back into the capillaries through osmosis.

Think of albumin as a "water magnet." The osmotic, or pulling, force of albumin in the intravascular space is referred to as the plasma colloid osmotic pressure. The plasma colloid osmotic pressure in capillaries averages about 25 mm Hg. (See *Albumin*.)

You're free to leave the capillaries

As long as capillary blood pressure (the hydrostatic pressure) exceeds plasma colloid osmotic pressure, water and solutes can leave the capillaries and enter the interstitial fluid. When capillary blood pressure falls below plasma colloid osmotic pressure, water and diffusible solutes return to the capillaries.

Normally, blood pressure in a capillary exceeds plasma colloid osmotic pressure in the arteriole end and falls below it in the venule end. As a result, capillary filtration occurs along the first half of the vessel; reabsorption, along the second half. As long as capillary blood pressure and plasma albumin levels remain normal, the amount of water that moves into the vessel equals the amount that moves out.

Occasionally, extra fluid filters out of the capillary. When that happens, the excess fluid shifts into the lymphatic vessels located just outside the capillaries and eventually returns to the heart for recirculation.

Maintaining the balance

Various elements and processes in the body work together to maintain fluid and electrolyte balance. Because one problem can affect the entire fluid-electrolyte maintenance system, it's important to keep all problems in check. Here's a closer look at what makes this balancing act possible.

Kidneys

The kidneys play a vital role in fluid and electrolyte balance. If the kidneys don't work properly, the body has great difficulty controlling fluid balance. The workhorse of the kidney is the nephron, which forms urine. The body puts the nephrons through their paces every day.

Albumin

Albumin, a large protein molecule, acts like a magnet to attract water and hold it inside the blood vessel.

Albumin

Water

Blood vessel

Whew, that capillary was a lot of fun. Let's go see what's happening in the interstitial fluid.

A nephron consists of a glomerulus and a tubule. The tubule, sometimes convoluted, ends in a collecting duct. The glomerulus is a cluster of capillaries that filters blood. Like a vascular cradle, Bowman's capsule surrounds the glomerulus.

Capillary blood pressure forces fluid through the capillary walls and into Bowman's capsule at the proximal end of the tubule. Along the length of the tubule, water and electrolytes are either excreted or retained according to the body's needs. If the body needs more fluid, for instance, it retains more. If it needs less fluid, less is reabsorbed and more is excreted. Electrolytes, such as sodium and potassium, are either filtered or reabsorbed throughout the same area. The resulting filtrate, which eventually becomes urine, flows through the tubule into the collecting ducts and eventually into the bladder as urine.

Come on, you nephrons, show me what you're made of! One, two, three....

Superabsorbent

Nephrons filter about 125 ml of blood every minute, or about 180 L/day. That rate, called the glomerular filtration rate, leads to the production of 1 to 2 L of urine per day. The nephrons reabsorb the remaining 178 L or more of fluid, an amount equivalent to more than 30 oil changes for the family car!

A strict conservationist

If the body loses even 1% to 2% of its fluid, the kidneys take steps to conserve water. Perhaps the most important step involves reabsorbing more water from the filtrate, which produces a more concentrated urine.

The kidneys must continue to excrete at least 20 ml of urine every hour (500 ml/day) to eliminate body wastes. A urine excretion rate that's less than 20 ml/hour usually indicates renal pathology. The minimum excretion rate varies with age.

The kidneys respond to fluid excesses by excreting a more dilute urine, which rids the body of fluid and conserves electrolytes.

I dilute urine to conserve electrolytes and get rid of excess fluid. I'm so smart!

Other organs and glands

In addition to the kidneys, other organs and glands are essential to maintaining fluid and electrolyte balance. Sodium, potassium, chloride, and water are lost from the GI tract; however, electrolytes and fluid are also absorbed from the GI tract.

The parathyroid glands also play a role in electrolyte balance, specifically the balance of calcium and phosphorus. The thyroid gland is also involved by balancing the body's calcium level.

Antidiuretic hormone

Several hormones affect fluid balance, among them a water retainer called antidiuretic hormone (ADH). (You may also hear this hormone called vasopressin.) The hypothalamus produces ADH, but the posterior pituitary gland stores and releases it. If you can remember what ADH stands for, you can remember its job: to restore blood volume by reducing diuresis and increasing water retention.

> The body holds water when fluid levels drop and releases it when they rise.

Sensitive to changes

Increased serum osmolality or decreased blood volume can stimulate the release of ADH, which in turn increases the kidneys' reabsorption of water. The increased reabsorption of water results in more concentrated urine.

Likewise, decreased serum osmolality or increased blood volume inhibits the release of ADH and causes less water to be reabsorbed, making the urine less concentrated. The amount of ADH released varies throughout the day, depending on the body's needs.

This up-and-down cycle of ADH release keeps fluid levels in balance all day long. Like a dam on a river, the body holds water when fluid levels drop and releases it when fluid levels rise.

Renin and angiotensin

To help maintain a balance of sodium and water in the body as well as to maintain a healthy blood volume and blood pressure, special cells (juxtaglomerular cells) near each glomerulus secrete an enzyme called renin. Through a complex series of steps, renin leads to the production of angiotensin II, a powerful vasoconstrictor.

Angiotensin II causes peripheral vasoconstriction and stimulates the production of aldosterone. Both actions raise blood pressure. (See *Aldosterone production*, page 38.)

As soon as the blood pressure reaches a normal level, the body stops releasing renin and this feedback cycle of renin to angiotensin to aldosterone stops.

> The amount of renin secreted depends on blood flow and serum sodium levels.

The ups and downs of renin

The amount of renin secreted depends on blood flow and the level of sodium in the bloodstream. If blood flow to the kidneys diminishes, as happens in a patient who's hemorrhaging, or if the amount of sodium reaching the glomerulus drops, the juxta-

Aldosterone production

The illustration shows the steps involved in the production of aldosterone (a hormone that helps to regulate fluid balance) through the renin-angiotensin-aldosterone system.

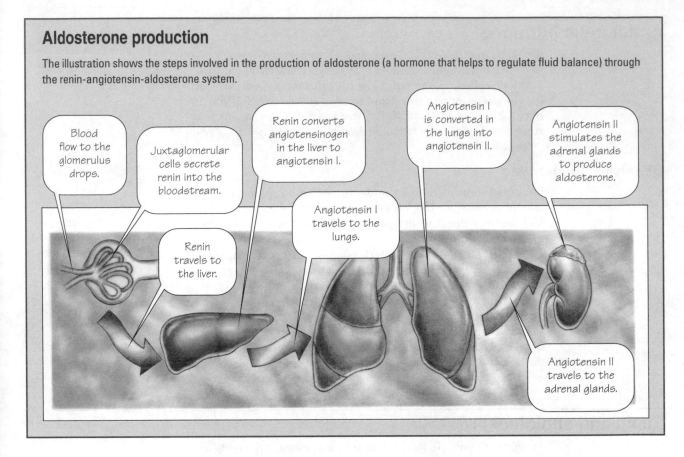

Blood flow to the glomerulus drops.

Juxtaglomerular cells secrete renin into the bloodstream.

Renin travels to the liver.

Renin converts angiotensinogen in the liver to angiotensin I.

Angiotensin I travels to the lungs.

Angiotensin I is converted in the lungs into angiotensin II.

Angiotensin II stimulates the adrenal glands to produce aldosterone.

Angiotensin II travels to the adrenal glands.

glomerular cells secrete more renin. The renin causes vasoconstriction and a subsequent increase in blood pressure.

Conversely, if blood flow to the kidneys increases, or if the amount of sodium reaching the glomerulus increases, juxtaglomerular cells secrete less renin. A drop-off in renin secretion reduces vasoconstriction and helps to normalize blood pressure.

Aldosterone

The hormone aldosterone also plays a role in maintaining blood pressure and fluid and electrolyte balance. Secreted by the adrenal cortex, aldosterone regulates the reabsorption of sodium and water within the nephron.

Triggering active transport

When blood volume drops, aldosterone initiates the active transport of sodium from the distal tubules and the collecting ducts into the bloodstream. That active transport forces sodium back into the bloodstream. When sodium is forced into the bloodstream, more water is reabsorbed and blood volume expands.

Atrial natriuretic peptide

The renin-angiotensin system isn't the only factor at work balancing fluids in the body. A cardiac hormone called atrial natriuretic peptide (ANP) also helps keep that balance. Stored in the cells of the atria, ANP is released when atrial pressure increases. The hormone opposes the renin-angiotensin system by decreasing blood pressure and reducing intravascular blood volume.

This powerful hormone:
- suppresses serum renin levels
- decreases aldosterone release from the adrenal glands
- increases glomerular filtration, which increases urine excretion of sodium and water
- decreases ADH release from the posterior pituitary gland
- reduces vascular resistance by causing vasodilation.

ANP is released when atrial pressure increases — and it's one powerful hormone!

Thirst

Perhaps the simplest mechanism for maintaining fluid balance is the thirst mechanism. Thirst occurs as a result of even small losses of fluid. Losing body fluids or eating highly salty foods leads to an increase in ECF osmolality. This increase leads to the drying of mucous membranes in the mouth, which in turn stimulates the thirst center in the hypothalamus.

Quenching that thirst

Usually, when a person is thirsty, he drinks fluid. The ingested fluid is absorbed from the intestine into the bloodstream, where it moves freely between fluid compartments. This movement leads to an increase in the amount of fluid in the body and a decrease in the concentration of solutes, thus balancing fluid levels throughout the body.

Fluid and electrolyte imbalances

Fluid and electrolyte balance is essential for health. Many factors, such as illness, injury, surgery, and treatments, can disrupt a patient's fluid and electrolyte balance. Even a patient with a minor illness is at risk for fluid and electrolyte imbalance. (See *Understanding electrolyte imbalance.*)

> I get pretty dry when water in the body isn't adequately replaced. I sure could go for a tall glass of water.

Dehydration

The body loses water all the time. A person responds to the thirst reflex by drinking fluids and eating foods that contain water. However, if water isn't adequately replaced, the body's cells can lose water. This causes dehydration, or fluid volume deficit. Dehydration refers to a fluid loss of 1% or more of body weight.

Signs and symptoms of dehydration include:
- dizziness
- irritability
- delirium
- extreme thirst
- dry skin and mucous membranes
- poor skin turgor
- increased heart rate
- falling blood pressure
- decreased urine output
- seizures and coma (in severe dehydration).

Laboratory values may include a serum sodium level above 150 mEq/L and serum osmolality above 305 mOsm/kg.

Treatment of dehydration involves determining its cause (such as diarrhea or decreased fluid intake) and replacing lost fluids—either orally or I.V. Most patients receive hypotonic, low-sodium fluids such as dextrose 5% in water (D_5W).

Hypervolemia

Hypervolemia refers to an excess of isotonic fluid (water and sodium) in ECF. The body has compensatory mechanisms to deal with hypervolemia. However, if these fail, signs and symptoms develop.

Hypervolemia can occur if a person consumes more fluid than needed, if fluid output is impaired, or if too much sodium is retained. Conditions that may lead to hypervolemia include kidney failure, cirrhosis, heart failure, and steroid therapy.

Depending on the severity of hypervolemia, signs and symptoms may include:
- edema
- distended neck and hand veins
- heart failure
- initially, rising blood pressure and cardiac output; later, falling values.

> If the body's compensatory mechanisms fail, so can I. Gulp!

(Text continues on page 45.)

Understanding electrolyte imbalance

The following chart summarizes the causes, signs and symptoms (with defining characteristic in italics), and nursing care related to electrolyte imbalance. For all imbalances, treatment goals include diagnosis and correction of the underlying cause, restoring normal electrolyte levels, and preventing complications and recurrence of the imbalance.

Cause	Signs and symptoms	Nursing care
Hypocalcemia • Hypoparathyroidism, infusion of citrated blood, acute pancreatitis, hyperphosphatemia, inadequate dietary intake of vitamin D, or continuous or long-term use of laxatives • Magnesium deficiency, medullary thyroid carcinoma, low serum albumin levels, or alkalosis • Use of aminoglycosides, caffeine, calcitonin, corticosteroids, loop diuretics, nicotine, phosphates, radiographic contrast media, or aluminum-containing antacids	• *Calcium level below 4.5 mEq/L* • Tingling around the mouth and in the fingertips and feet, numbness, painful muscle spasms, and tetany • Positive Trousseau's and Chvostek's signs • Bronchospasm, laryngospasm, and airway obstruction • Seizures • Changes in cardiac conduction • Depression, impaired memory, confusion, and hallucinations • Dry or scaling skin, brittle nails, dry hair, and cataracts • Skeletal fractures resulting from osteoporosis	• Identify patients at risk for hypocalcemia • Assess the patient for signs and symptoms of hypocalcemia, especially changes in cardiovascular and neurologic status and in vital signs. • Administer I.V. calcium as prescribed. • Administer a phosphate-binding antacid. • Review the procedure for eliciting Trousseau's and Chvostek's signs. • Take seizure or emergency precautions as needed. • Encourage a patient with osteoporosis to exercise regularly. • Encourage the patient to increase his intake of foods that are rich in calcium and vitamin D. • Teach the patient and his family how to prevent, recognize, and treat hypocalcemia.
Hypercalcemia • Malignant neoplasms, metastatic bone cancer, hyperparathyroidism, immobilization and loss of bone mineral, or thiazide diuretic use • High calcium intake • Hyperthyroidism or hypothyroidism	• *Calcium level above 5.5 mEq/L* • Muscle weakness and lack of coordination • Anorexia, constipation, abdominal pain, nausea, vomiting, peptic ulcers, and abdominal distention • Confusion, impaired memory, slurred speech, and coma • Polyuria and renal colic • Cardiac arrest	• Identify patients at risk for hypercalcemia. • If the patient is receiving digoxin, assess him for signs of digoxin toxicity. • Assess the patient for signs and symptoms of hypercalcemia. • Encourage ambulation. • Move the patient carefully to prevent fractures. • Take safety or seizure precautions as needed. • Have emergency equipment available. • Administer phosphate to inhibit GI absorption of calcium. • Administer a loop diuretic to promote calcium excretion. • Force fluids with a high acid-ash concentration, such as cranberry juice, to dilute and absorb calcium. • Reduce dietary calcium. • Teach the patient and his family how to prevent, recognize, and treat hypercalcemia, especially if the patient has metastatic cancer.

(continued)

Understanding electrolyte imbalance (continued)

Cause	Signs and symptoms	Nursing care
Hypokalemia • GI losses from diarrhea, laxative abuse, prolonged gastric suctioning, prolonged vomiting, ileostomy, or colostomy • Renal losses related to diuretic use, renal tubular acidosis, renal stenosis, or hyperaldosteronism • Use of certain antibiotics, including penicillin G sodium, carbenicillin, or amphotericin B • Steroid therapy • Severe perspiration • Hyperalimentation, alkalosis, or excessive blood insulin levels • Poor nutrition	• *Potassium level under 3.5 mEq/L* • Fatigue, muscle weakness, and paresthesia • Prolonged cardiac repolarization, decreased strength of myocardial contraction, orthostatic hypotension, reduced sensitivity to digoxin, increased resistance to antiarrythmics, and cardiac arrest • Flat ST segment and Q wave on electrocardiogram (ECG) • Decreased bowel motility • Suppressed insulin release and aldosterone secretion • Inability to concentrate urine and increased renal phosphate excretion • Respiratory muscle weakness • Metabolic alkalosis, low urine osmolality, slightly elevated glucose level, and myoglobinuria	• Identify patients at risk for hypokalemia. • Assess the patient's diet for a lack of potassium. • Assess the patient for signs and symptoms of hypokalemia. • Administer a potassium replacement as prescribed. • Encourage intake of high-potassium foods, such as bananas, dried fruit, and orange juice. • Monitor the patient for complications. • Have emergency equipment available for cardiopulmonary resuscitation and cardiac defibrillation. • Teach the patient and his family how to prevent, recognize, and treat hypokalemia.
Hyperkalemia • Decreased renal excretion related to oliguric renal failure, potassium-sparing diuretic use, or adrenal steroid deficiency • High potassium intake related to the improper use of oral supplements, excessive use of salt substitutes, or rapid infusion of potassium solutions • Acidosis, tissue damage, or malignant cell lysis after chemotherapy	• *Potassium level above 5 mEq/L* • Cardiac conduction disturbances, ventricular arrhythmias, prolonged depolarization, decreased strength of contraction, and cardiac arrest • Tall tented T wave, prolonged QRS complex and PR interval on ECG • Muscle weakness and paralysis • Nausea, vomiting, diarrhea, intestinal colic, uremic enteritis, decreased bowel sounds, abdominal distention, and paralytic ileus	• Identify patients at risk for hyperkalemia. • Assess the patient's diet for excess use of salt substitutes. • Assess the patient for signs and symptoms of hyperkalemia. • Assess arterial blood gas studies for metabolic alkalosis. • Take precautions when drawing blood samples. A falsely elevated potassium level can result from hemolysis or prolonged tourniquet application. • Have emergency equipment available. • Administer calcium gluconate to decrease myocardial irritability. • Administer insulin and I.V. glucose to move potassium back into cells. • Administer sodium polystyrene sulfonate (Kayexalate) with 70% sorbitol to exchange sodium ions for potassium ions in the intestine.

Understanding electrolyte imbalance *(continued)*

Cause	Signs and symptoms	Nursing care
Hyperkalemia *(continued)*		• Perform hemodialysis or peritoneal dialysis to remove excess potassium. • Teach the patient and his family how to prevent, recognize, and treat hyperkalemia.
Hypomagnesemia • Alcoholism, protein-calorie malnutrition, I.V. therapy without magnesium replacement, gastric suctioning, malabsorption syndromes, laxative abuse, bulimia, anorexia, intestinal bypass for obesity, diarrhea, or colonic neoplasms • Hyperaldosteronism or renal disease that impairs magnesium reabsorption • Use of osmotic diuretics or antibiotics (such as ticarcillin, gentamicin, carbenicillin, cyclosporine, and cisplatin) • Overdose of vitamin D or calcium, burns, pancreatitis, sepsis, hypothermia, exchange transfusion, hyperalimentation, or diabetic ketoacidosis	• *Magnesium level under 1.5 mEq/L* • Muscle weakness, tremors, tetany, and clonic or focal seizures • Laryngeal stridor • Decreased blood pressure, ventricular fibrillation, tachyarrhythmias, and increased susceptibility to digoxin toxicity • Apathy, depression, agitation, confusion, delirium, and hallucinations • Nausea, vomiting, and anorexia • Decreased calcium level • Positive Chvostek's and Trousseau's signs	• Identify patients at risk for hypomagnesemia. • Assess the patient for signs and symptoms of hypomagnesemia. • Administer I.V. magnesium as prescribed. • Encourage the patient to consume magnesium-rich foods. • If the patient is confused or agitated, take safety precautions. • Take seizure precautions as needed. • Have emergency equipment available. Calcium gluconate is used to treat tetany. • Teach the patient and his family how to prevent, recognize, and treat hypomagnesemia.
Hypermagnesemia • Renal failure, excessive antacid use (especially in a patient with renal failure), adrenal insufficiency, or diuretic abuse • Excessive magnesium replacement or excessive use of milk of magnesia or other magnesium-containing laxative	• *Magnesium level above 2.5 mEq/L* • Peripheral vasodilation with decreased blood pressure, facial flushing and sensations of warmth and thirst • Lethargy or drowsiness, apnea, and coma • Loss of deep tendon reflexes, paresis, and paralysis • Cardiac arrest	• Identify patients at risk for hypermagnesemia. • Review all medications for a patient with renal failure. • Assess the patient for signs and symptoms of hypermagnesemia. • Assess reflexes; if absent, notify the doctor. • Administer calcium gluconate. • Have emergency equipment available. • Prepare the patient for hemodialysis if prescribed. • If the patient is taking an antacid, a laxative, or another drug that contains magnesium, instruct him to stop. • Teach the patient and his family how to prevent, recognize, and treat hypermagnesemia.

(continued)

Understanding electrolyte imbalance (continued)

Cause	Signs and symptoms	Nursing care
Hyponatremia *Dilutional* • Excessive water gain caused by inappropriate administration of I.V. solutions, syndrome of inappropriate antidiuretic hormone secretion, oxytocin use for labor induction, water intoxication, heart failure, renal failure, or cirrhosis	• *Sodium level under 136 mEq/L* • Confusion • Nausea, vomiting • Weight gain • Edema • Muscle spasms, convulsions	• Identify patients at risk for hyponatremia. • Assess fluid intake and output. • Assess the patient for signs and symptoms of hyponatremia. • If the patient has dilutional hyponatremia, restrict his fluid intake. • If the patient has true hyponatremia, administer isotonic I.V. fluids • Teach the patient and his family dietary measures that ensure appropriate fluid and sodium intake.
True • Excessive sodium loss due to GI losses, excessive sweating, diuretic use, adrenal insufficiency, burns, lithium use, or starvation	• *Sodium level under 136 mEq/L* • Orthostatic hypotension • Tachycardia • Dry mucous membranes • Weight loss • Nausea, vomiting • Oliguria	• If the patient is receiving lithium, teach him how to prevent alterations in his sodium levels. • If the patient has adrenal insufficiency, teach him how to prevent hyponatremia. • Teach the patient and his family how to prevent, recognize, and treat hyponatremia.
Hypernatremia • Sodium gain that exceeds water gain related to salt intoxication (resulting from sodium bicarbonate use in cardiac arrest), hyperaldosteronism, or use of diuretics, vasopressin, corticosteroids, or some antihypertensives • Water loss that exceeds sodium loss related to profuse sweating, diarrhea, polyuria resulting from diabetes insipidus or diabetes mellitus, high-protein tube feedings, inadequate water intake, or insensible water loss	• *Sodium level above 145 mEq/L* • Thirst; rough, dry tongue; dry sticky mucous membranes; flushed skin, oliguria; and low-grade fever that returns to normal when sodium levels return to normal • Restlessness, disorientation, hallucinations, lethargy, seizures, and coma • Muscle weakness and irritability • Serum osmolality above 295 mOsm/kg and urine specific gravity above 1.015	• Identify patients at risk for hypernatremia. • Assess the patient for fluid losses and gains. • Assess the patient for signs and symptoms of hypernatremia. • Consult with a nutritionist to determine the amount of free water needed with tube feedings. • Encourage the patient to increase his fluid intake but decrease his sodium intake. • If the patient is agitated or is experiencing a seizure, take safety precautions. • Teach the patient and his family how to prevent, recognize, and treat hypernatremia.

Understanding electrolyte imbalance (continued)

Cause	Signs and symptoms	Nursing care
Hypophosphatemia • Glucose administration or insulin release, nutritional recovery syndrome, overzealous feeding with simple carbohydrates, respiratory alkalosis, alcohol withdrawal, diabetic ketoacidosis, or starvation • Malabsorption syndromes, diarrhea, vomiting, aldosteronism, diuretic therapy, or use of drugs that bind with phosphate, such as aluminum hydroxide (Amphojel) or magnesium salts (milk of magnesia)	• *Phosphorus level below 2.5 mg/ dl or 0.97 mmol/L* • Irritability, apprehension, confusion, decreased level of consciousness, seizures, and coma • Weakness, numbness, and paresthesia • Congestive cardiomyopathy • Respiratory muscle weakness • Hemolytic anemia • Impaired granulocyte function, elevated creatine kinase level, hyperglycemia, and metabolic acidosis	• Identify patients at risk for hypophosphatemia. • Assess the patient for signs and symptoms of hypophosphatemia, especially neurologic and hematologic ones. • Administer phosphate supplements as prescribed. • Note calcium and phosphorus levels because calcium and phosphorus have an inverse relationship. • Gradually introduce hyperalimentation as prescribed. • Teach the patient and his family how to prevent, recognize, and treat hypophosphatemia.
Hyperphosphatemia • Renal disease • Hypoparathyroidism or hyperthyroidism • Excessive vitamin D intake • Muscle necrosis, excessive phosphate intake, or chemotherapy	• *Phosphorus level above 4.5 mg/ dl or 1.45 mmol/L* • Soft-tissue calcification (chronic hyperphosphatemia) • Hypocalcemia, possible with tetany • Increased red blood cell count	• Identify patients at risk for hyperphosphatemia. • Assess the patient for signs and symptoms of hyperphosphatemia and hypocalcemia, including tetany and muscle twitching. • Advise the patient to avoid foods and medications that contain phosphorus. • Administer phosphorus-binding antacids. • Prepare the patient for possible dialysis. • Teach the patient and his family how to prevent, recognize and treat hyperphosphatemia.

Laboratory tests may reveal a serum sodium level above 135 mEq/L and serum osmolality above 275 mOsm/kg.

Treatment involves determining the cause and treating the underlying condition. Typically, patients require fluid and sodium restrictions and diuretic therapy.

Water intoxication

Water intoxication occurs when excess fluid moves from the ECF to the ICF. Excessive low-sodium fluid in the ECF is hypotonic to cells; cells are hypertonic to the fluid. As a result, fluids shift into the cells, which have comparatively less fluid and more solutes.

That fluid shift occurs to balance the concentrations of fluid between the two spaces.

Water intoxication may occur in a patient with syndrome of inappropriate antidiuretic hormone (SIADH) — which can result from central nervous system or pulmonary disorders, head trauma, tumors, or use of certain drugs. Other causes of water intoxication include:
- rapid infusion of hypotonic solutions
- excessive use of tap water as a nasogastric tube irrigant or enema
- psychogenic polydipsia, a psychological disturbance in which

a person drinks large amounts of fluid even when they aren't needed.

Water intoxication may occur in a patient with SIADH.

I.V. fluid replacement

To maintain health, the balance of fluids and electrolytes in the intracellular and extracellular spaces must remain relatively constant. Whenever a person experiences an illness or a condition that prevents normal fluid intake or causes excessive fluid loss, I.V. fluid replacement may be necessary.

Quick and predictable

I.V. therapy that provides the patient with life-sustaining fluids, electrolytes, and medications offers the advantages of immediate and predictable therapeutic effects. The I.V. route is, therefore, the preferred route — especially for administering fluids, electrolytes, and drugs in an emergency.

This route also allows for fluid intake when a patient has GI malabsorption. I.V. therapy permits accurate dosage titration for analgesics and other medications. Potential disadvantages associated with I.V. therapy include drug and solution incompatibility, adverse reactions, infection, and other complications.

Float like a butterfly, sting like a bee — I offer immediate and predictable therapy for fluid imbalance.

Types of solutions

Solutions used for I.V. fluid replacement fall into the broad categories of crystalloids (which may be isotonic, hypotonic, or hypertonic) and colloids (which are always hypertonic).

Crystalloids

Crystalloids are solutions with small molecules that flow easily from the bloodstream into cells and tissues. Isotonic crystalloids contain about the same concentration of osmotically active particles as ECF, so fluid doesn't shift between the extracellular and intracellular areas.

Hypotonic crystalloids are less concentrated than ECF, so they move from the bloodstream into the cell, causing the cell to swell. In contrast, hypertonic crystalloids are more highly concentrated than ECF, so fluid is pulled into the bloodstream from the cell, causing the cell to shrink. (See *Comparing fluid tonicity*.)

Isotonic solutions

Isotonic solutions, such as D_5W, have an osmolality (or concentration) of 275 to 295 mOsm/kg. The dextrose metabolizes quickly, however, acting like a hypotonic solution and leaving water behind. Large amounts of the solution may cause hyperglycemia.

More isotonic solutions

Normal saline solution, another isotonic solution, contains only the electrolytes sodium and chloride. Other isotonic fluids are more similar to ECF. For instance, Ringer's solution contains sodium, potassium, calcium, and chloride. Lactated Ringer's

Crystalloids are solutions with small molecules that flow easily from the bloodstream into cells and tissues.

Comparing fluid tonicity

The illustrations below show the effects of different types of I.V. fluids on fluid movement and cell size.

Isotonic
Isotonic fluids, such as normal saline solution, have a concentration of dissolved particles, or tonicity, equal to that of intracellular fluid (ICF). Osmotic pressure is therefore the same inside and outside the cells, so they neither shrink nor swell with fluid movement.

Hypertonic
Hypertonic fluid has a tonicity greater than that of ICF, so osmotic pressure is unequal inside and outside the cells. Dehydration or a rapidly infused hypertonic fluid, such as 3% saline or 50% dextrose, draws water out of the cells into the more highly concentrated extracellular fluid (ECF).

Hypotonic
Hypotonic fluids, such as half-normal saline solution, have a tonicity less than that of ICF, so osmotic pressure draws water into the cells from the ECF. Severe electrolyte losses or inappropriate use of I.V. fluids can make body fluids hypotonic.

Normal cell

Cell shrinks

Cell swells

solution contains those electrolytes plus lactate, which the liver converts to bicarbonate.

Hypotonic fluids

Hypotonic fluids are those fluids that have an osmolality less than 275 mOsm/kg. Examples of hypotonic fluids include:
- half-normal saline solution
- 0.33% sodium chloride solution
- dextrose 2.5% in water.

It makes a cell swell

Hypotonic solutions should be given cautiously because fluid then moves from the extracellular space into cells, causing them to swell. That fluid shift can cause cardiovascular collapse from vascular fluid depletion. It can also cause increased intracranial pressure (ICP) from fluid shifting into brain cells.

Hypotonic solutions shouldn't be given to a patient at risk for increased ICP—for example, those who have had a stroke, head trauma, or neurosurgery. Signs of increased ICP include a change in the patient's level of consciousness, motor or sensory deficits, and changes in the size, shape, or response to light in the pupils. Hypotonic solutions also shouldn't be used for patients who suffer from abnormal fluid shifts into the interstitial space or the body cavities—for example, as a result of liver disease, a burn, or trauma.

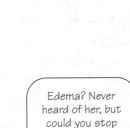

Yes, I'm swell, but — ummph — not so good. Enough with the hypotonic solutions, thank you!

Hypertonic solutions

Hypertonic solutions are those that have an osmolality greater than 295 mOsm/kg. Examples include:
- dextrose 5% in half-normal saline solution
- dextrose 5% in normal saline solution
- dextrose 5% in lactated Ringer's solution
- dextrose 10% in water.

The incredible shrinking cell

A hypertonic solution draws fluids from the intracellular space, causing cells to shrink and the extracellular space to expand. Patients with cardiac or renal disease may be unable to tolerate extra fluid. Watch for fluid overload and pulmonary edema.

Because hypertonic solutions draw fluids from cells, patients at risk for cellular dehydration (patients with diabetic ketoacidosis, for example) shouldn't receive them.

Edema? Never heard of her, but could you stop the hypertonic solutions, please?

Colloids

The doctor may prescribe a colloid (plasma expander) if your patient's blood volume doesn't improve with crystalloids. Examples of colloids that may be given include:

• albumin (available in 5% solutions, which are osmotically equal to plasma, and 25% solutions, which draw about four times their volume in interstitial fluid into the circulation within 15 minutes of administration)
• plasma protein fraction
• dextran
• hetastarch.

I'm with him. No more hypertonics!

Flowing into the stream

Colloids pull fluid into the bloodstream. The effects of colloids last several days if the lining of the capillaries is normal. The patient needs to be closely monitored during a colloid infusion for increased blood pressure, dyspnea, and bounding pulse, which are all signs of hypervolemia.

If neither crystalloids nor colloids are effective in treating the imbalance, the patient may require a blood transfusion or other treatment.

Delivery methods

The choice of I.V. therapy delivery is based on the purpose of the therapy and its duration; the patient's diagnosis, age, and health history; and the condition of the patient's veins. I.V. solutions can be delivered through a peripheral or a central vein. Catheters are chosen based on the therapy and the site to be used. Here's a look at how to choose a site—peripheral or central—and which equipment you'll need for each.

Don't gamble with thrombophlebitis. Be sure to avoid veins in the foot when choosing an I.V. site.

Peripheral lines

Peripheral I.V. therapy is administered for short-term or intermittent therapy through a vein in the arm, hand, leg, or foot. Potential I.V. sites include the metacarpal, cephalic, basilic, median cubital, and greater saphenous veins. Using veins in the leg or foot is unusual because of the risk of thrombophlebitis.

Central lines

Central venous therapy involves administering solutions through a catheter placed in a central vein, typically the subclavian or internal jugular vein, less commonly the femoral vein.

Central venous therapy is used for patients who have inadequate peripheral veins, need access for blood sampling, require a large volume of fluid, need a hypertonic solution to be diluted by rapid blood flow in a larger vein, need to receive vessel-irritating drugs, or need a high-calorie nutritional supplement. Types of central venous catheters include the traditional multilumen catheter for short-term therapy and a peripherally inserted central catheter or a vascular access port (such as a Broviac or Hickman catheter) for long-term therapy.

Complications of I.V. therapy

Caring for a patient with an I.V. line requires careful monitoring as well as a clear understanding of the possible complications, what to do if they arise, and how to deal with flow issues.

Infiltration

During infiltration, fluid may leak from the vein into surrounding tissue. This occurs when the access device dislodges from the vein. Look for coolness at the site, pain, swelling, leaking, and lack of blood return. Also look for a sluggish flow that continues even if a tourniquet is applied above the site. If you see infiltration, stop the infusion, elevate the extremity, and apply warm soaks.

Go small

To prevent infiltration, use the smallest catheter that will accomplish the infusion; avoid placement in joint areas; and anchor the catheter in place.

Infection

I.V. therapy involves puncturing the skin, one of the body's barrier to infection. Look for purulent drainage at the site, tenderness, erythema, warmth, or hardness on palpation. Signs and symptoms that the infection has become systemic include fever, chills, and an elevated white blood cell count.

Vital vitals monitoring

Nursing actions for an infected I.V. site include monitoring vital signs and notifying the doctor. Swab the site for culture, and remove the catheter as ordered. Always maintain sterile technique to prevent this complication.

Phlebitis and thrombophlebitis

Phlebitis is inflammation of the vein; thrombophlebitis is an irritation of the vein with the formation of a clot and is usually more painful than phlebitis. Either poor insertion technique or the pH or osmolality of the infusing solution or medication can cause these complications. Look for pain, redness, swelling, or induration at the site; a red line streaking along the vein; fever; or a sluggish flow of the solution.

Prevention begins with big veins

When phlebitis or thrombophlebitis occurs, remove the I.V. line, monitor the patient's vital signs, notify the doctor, and apply warm soaks to the site. To prevent these complications, choose large-bore veins and change the catheter every 72 hours when infusing a medication or solution with high osmolality.

Extravasation

Extravasation, similar to infiltration, is the leakage of fluid into surrounding tissues. It results when medications, such as dopamine, calcium solutions, and chemotherapeutic agents, seep through veins and produce blistering and, eventually, necrosis. Initially, the patient may experience discomfort, burning, or pain at the site. Also, look for skin tightness, blanching, and lack of blood return. Delayed reactions include inflammation and pain within 3 to 5 days and ulcers or necrosis within 2 weeks.

Review policy

When administering medications that may extravasate, know your facility's policy. Nursing actions include stopping the infusion, notifying the doctor, infiltrating the site with an antidote as ordered (this is usually done through the I.V. line before removing the catheter), applying ice early and warm soaks later, and elevating the extremity. Assess the circulation and nerve function of the limb.

Air embolism

An air embolism occurs when air enters the vein. It can cause a decrease in blood pressure, an increase in the pulse rate, respiratory distress, an increase in ICP, and a loss of consciousness.

Clamp off the I.V. line

If the patient develops an air embolism, notify the doctor and clamp off the I.V. line. Place the patient on his left side, and lower his head to allow the air to enter the right atrium, where it can disperse more safely by way of the pulmonary artery. Monitor the patient and administer oxygen. To avoid this serious complication in

Look for skin tightness, blanching, and lack of blood return if you suspect extravasation.

the future, prime all tubing completely, tighten all connections securely, and use an air detection device on an I.V. pump.

How you intervene

Nursing care for the patient with an I.V. line includes the following actions.

Check, measure, monitor...

• Check the I.V. order for completeness and accuracy. Most I.V. orders expire after 24 hours. A complete order should specify the amount and type of solution, specific additives and their concentrations, and the rate and duration of the infusion. If the order is incomplete or confusing, clarify the order before proceeding.
• Measure intake and output carefully at scheduled intervals. The kidneys attempt to restore fluid balance during dehydration by reducing urine production. Urine output less than 30 ml/ hour signals retention of metabolic wastes. Notify the doctor if your patient's urine output falls below 30 ml/hour.
• Monitor daily weights to document fluid retention or loss. A 2% increase or decrease in body weight is significant. A 2.2-lb (1-kg) change corresponds to 1 qt (1 L) of fluid gained or lost.
• Always carefully monitor the infusion of solutions that contain medication, because rapid infusion and circulation of the drug can be dangerous.

Most I.V. orders expire after 24 hours.

...and all the rest

• Note the pH of the I.V. solution. The pH can alter the effect and stability of drugs mixed in the I.V. bag. Consult medication literature or the doctor if you have questions.
• Change the site, dressing, and tubing as often as facility policy requires. Solutions should be changed at least every 24 hours.
• When changing I.V. tubing, be sure not to move or dislodge the I.V. catheter. If you have trouble disconnecting the used tubing, use a hemostat to hold the I.V. hub while twisting the tubing. Don't clamp the hemostat shut because doing so may crack the hub.
• Always report needle-stick injuries. Exposure to a patient's blood increases the risk of infection with blood-borne viruses, such as human immunodeficiency virus (HIV), hepatitis B virus, hepatitis C virus, and cytomegalovirus. About 1 out of 300 people with occupational needle-stick injuries become HIV-seropositive.
• Always follow standard precautions when inserting, caring for, or discontinuing an I.V. line.

Focus on the patient

• Always listen to your patient carefully. Subtle statements such as "I just don't feel right" may be your clue to the beginning of an allergic reaction. (See *Teaching about I.V. therapy*.)

• Keep in mind that a candidate for home I.V. therapy must have a family member or friend who can safely and competently administer the I.V. fluids as well as a backup helper, a suitable home environment, a telephone, available transportation, adequate reading skills, and the ability to prepare, handle, store, and dispose of equipment properly. Procedures for caring for the I.V. line are the same at home as in a health care facility, except at home the patient uses clean technique instead of sterile technique.

Education edge

Teaching about I.V. therapy

Make sure you cover the following points with your patient and then evaluate his learning:

• what to expect before, during, and after the I.V. procedure

• signs and symptoms of complications and when to report them

• activity or diet restrictions

• how to care for an I.V. line at home.

Quick quiz

1. Hydrostatic pressure, which pushes fluid out of the capillaries, is opposed by colloid osmotic pressure, which involves:

    A.   reduced renin secretion.
    B.   the pulling power of albumin to reabsorb water.
    C.   an increase in ADH secretion.
    D.   aldosterone production.

Answer: B. Albumin in capillaries draws water toward it, a process called reabsorption.

2. When a person's blood pressure drops, the kidneys respond by:

    A.   secreting renin.
    B.   producing aldosterone.
    C.   slowing the release of ADH.
    D.   increasing urine output.

Answer: A. Juxtaglomerular cells in the kidneys secrete renin in response to low blood flow or a low sodium level. The eventual effect of renin secretion is an increase in blood pressure.

3. The main extracellular cation is:

    A.   calcium.
    B.   potassium.
    C.   magnesium.
    D.   sodium.

Answer: D. Sodium is the main extracellular cation. Among other things, it helps regulate fluid balance in the body.

4. Hypertonic solutions cause fluids to move from the:
   A.   interstitial space to the intracellular space.
   B.   intracellular space to the extracellular space.
   C.   extracellular space to the intracellular space.
   D.   extracellular space to the interstitial space.

Answer: B. Hypertonic solutions, because of their increased osmolality, draw fluids out of the cells and into the extracellular space.

5. Extravasation of I.V. fluid is associated with administration of which of the following?
   A.   Hypertonic fluid
   B. D_5W
   C.   An antineoplastic
   D.   Normal saline solution

Answer: C. Antineoplastics are highly irritating to the veins and are typically administered using a steel needle. Extravasation is common in those situations.

Scoring

☆☆☆   If you answered all five items correctly, great job! Your fluid and electrolyte knowledge is flowing smoothly.

☆☆   If you answered three or four items correctly, nice going! You'll have fluid and electrolyte imbalances on the run in no time.

☆   If you answered fewer than three items correctly, relax! With a little more active transport of this chapter, it will all balance out.

Perioperative care

Just the facts

In this chapter, you'll learn:

♦ perioperative nursing measures

♦ the effects of anesthesia

♦ how to prevent or manage postoperative complications

♦ how to plan for the patient's discharge.

A look at perioperative care

Many technological advances have made operations quicker, safer, and more effective. Even so, surgery remains one of the most stressful experiences a patient can undergo. Before the patient enters the operating room, you must fully address his psychological and physiologic needs. If prepared properly with careful teaching, a surgical patient will experience less pain, fewer postoperative complications, and shorter hospitalization.

Preoperative care

Careful, considerate preoperative care will help prevent future complications for the patient and ease anxiety felt by the patient and his family.

> Good preoperative care can help prevent future complications.

What to look for

A thorough preoperative assessment helps systematically identify and correct problems before surgery and establishes a baseline for postoperative comparison. When performing this assess-

History lesson

Finding out about the patient's history is very important. Ask about allergies to drugs, food, and environment. Find out if anyone in the family has experienced problems with anesthesia. Ask if the patient takes any medications regularly (including herbal preparations). Find out how often these medications are taken and if any were taken before admission.

Coughing exercises

Question the patient about alcohol and drug use. A patient using recreational drugs has a higher tolerance for anesthesia and pain medications. A patient in substance withdrawal may exhibit behavioral changes and be more difficult to manage in the operating room and postoperatively. Determine the frequency of substance use to assess if the patient may begin substance withdrawal postoperatively.

Ask female patients about pregnancy. Depending on the facility, it isn't uncommon to check pregnancy status of all females age 10 and older. Be considerate when asking adolescent girls about being sexually active and pregnancy in the presence of family members.

Finally, ask patients if they:
• have any loose teeth
• wear dentures or a partial plate
• wear glasses or contact lenses
• use a hearing aid
• are wearing jewelry
• have joint implants, metal implants, or a pacemaker
• have body piercings.

ment, focus on problem areas suggested by the patient's history and on any body system that will be directly affected by the surgery. (See *History lesson*.) Consider your findings in relation to the specific age-group norms. Don't forget to include the patient's psychological status in your assessment because depression and anxiety can significantly interfere with recovery from surgery.

Patient teaching

Your teaching can help the patient cope with the physical and psychological stress of surgery. Preadmission and preoperative teaching are more important than ever in these days of shorter hospital stays and same-day surgeries.

Evaluate, adapt, and consider

Evaluate the patient's understanding and dispel any lingering doubts or misconceptions about surgery or hospitalization. Adapt your teaching to fit the patient's age, understanding, and cultural background. Also, consider the needs of the patient's family or caregivers.

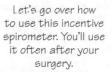

Let's talk about your surgery. What doubts or concerns do you have?

What to teach

Be sure to include the following in your preoperative patient teaching:
• diagnostic tests
• concerns about anesthesia
• diet
• operating room procedure
• I.V. therapy
• what to expect on the postanesthesia care unit (PACU)
• pain control.

Prepare for postoperative

Before surgery, teach the patient early postoperative mobility and ambulation techniques and leg exercises. In addition, teach coughing and deep-breathing exercises, including how to use an incentive spirometer. Make it clear that the patient will have to repeat these maneuvers several times after surgery. (See *Teaching coughing and deep-breathing exercises*, page 58.)

Tell the patient that postoperative exercises help prevent such complications as:
• atelectasis
• hypostatic pneumonia
• thrombophlebitis
• constipation
• abdominal distention
• venous pooling.

Have the patient perform postoperative exercises to assess whether further teaching is necessary and to support the teaching plan.

Let's go over how to use this incentive spirometer. You'll use it often after your surgery.

Getting ready

To prepare the patient for surgery, you may have to perform skin and bowel preparations and administer drugs.

Education edge

Teaching coughing and deep-breathing exercises

The exercises described below will speed your patient's recovery and reduce his risk of respiratory complications.

Coughing exercises

Patients who risk developing excess secretions should practice coughing exercises before surgery. However, patients about to undergo ear or eye surgery or repair of hiatal or large abdominal hernias won't need to practice coughing. Also, patients undergoing neurosurgery shouldn't cough postoperatively because intracranial pressure will rise.

• If the patient's condition permits, instruct him to sit on the edge of his bed. Provide a stool if his feet don't touch the floor. Tell him to bend his legs and lean slightly forward.

• If the patient is scheduled for chest or abdominal surgery, teach him how to splint his incision before he coughs.

• Instruct the patient to take a slow, deep breath; he should breathe in through his nose and concentrate on fully expanding his chest. Then he should breathe out through his mouth, and concentrate on feeling his chest sink downward and inward. Then he should take a second breath in the same manner.

• Next, tell him to take a third deep breath and hold it. He should then cough two or three times in a row (once isn't enough). This will clear his breathing passages. Encourage him to concentrate on feeling his diaphragm force out all the air in his chest. Then he should take three to five normal breaths, exhale slowly, and relax.

• Have the patient repeat this exercise at least once. After surgery, he'll need to perform it at least every 2 hours to help keep his lungs free from secretions. Reassure the patient that his stitches are very strong and won't split during coughing.

Deep-breathing exercises

Advise the patient that performing deep-breathing exercises several times per hour helps keep lungs fully expanded. To deep-breathe correctly, he must use diaphragm and abdominal muscles, not just his chest muscles. Tell the patient to practice the following exercise two or three times per day before surgery, as follows:

• Have him lie on his back in a comfortable position with one hand placed on his chest and the other over his upper abdomen, as shown in the illustration. Instruct him to relax, and bend his legs slightly.

• Instruct him to exhale normally. He should then close his mouth and inhale deeply through his nose, concentrating on feeling his abdomen rise. His chest shouldn't expand. Have him hold his breath and slowly count to five.

• Next, have the patient purse his lips as though about to whistle, then exhale completely through his mouth, without letting his cheeks puff out. His ribs should sink downward and inward.

• After resting several seconds, the patient should repeat the exercise five to ten times. He should also do this exercise while lying on his side, sitting, standing, or while turning in bed.

Skin preparation

In most facilities, skin preparation is carried out during the intra-operative phase. However, making sure the skin is as free from microorganisms as possible reduces the risk of infection at the incision site. The patient may be asked to bathe, shower, or scrub a local skin area with an antiseptic the evening before or the morning of surgery. The doctor will usually specify the site for a local skin scrub if indicated.

Make it big, real big

To reduce the number of microorganisms in areas near the incision site, prepare a much larger area than the expected incision site. Doing so also helps prevent contamination during surgical draping. Document skin preparation, including the area prepared and any unexpected outcomes.

Bowel preparation

The extent of bowel preparation depends on the type and site of surgery. A patient scheduled for several days of postoperative bed rest who hasn't had a recent bowel movement may receive a mild laxative or sodium phosphate enema. On the other hand, a patient scheduled for GI, pelvic, perianal, or rectal surgery will undergo more extensive intestinal preparation.

After 3, make the call

If enemas are ordered until the bowel is clear and the third enema still hasn't removed all stool, notify the doctor because repeated enemas may cause fluid and electrolyte imbalances. Elderly patients, children, and patients who are allowed nothing by mouth and haven't received I.V. fluids are at particularly high risk for these imbalances.

Preoperative drugs

The doctor may order preoperative or preanesthesia drugs to:
- ease anxiety
- permit a smoother induction of anesthesia
- decrease the amount of anesthesia needed
- create amnesia for the events preceding surgery
- minimize the flow of pharyngeal and respiratory secretions.

Document skin preparation, including the area prepared and unexpected outcomes.

Fluid and electrolyte balance can be a problem for me — not to mention a two-wheeler. Whoa!

And the drugs are...

Expect to administer ordered drugs 45 to 75 minutes before induction of anesthesia. Teach the patient about ordered drugs, their desired effects, and their possible adverse effects. These drugs include:
- anticholinergics (vagolytic or drying agents)
- sedatives
- antianxiety drugs
- narcotic analgesics
- neuroleptanalgesic agents
- histamine-2 receptor antagonists.

Final check

Before surgery, follow these important steps:
- Make sure the patient has had no solid food for 6 hours and no water for 2 hours before surgery.
- Make sure the chart contains all necessary information, such as signed surgical consent, diagnostic test results, health history, and physical examination. Patient allergies should be easily visible.
- Tell the patient to remove jewelry (including body piercings), makeup, and nail polish. Ask the patient to shower with antimicrobial soap, if ordered, and to perform mouth care. Warn against swallowing water.
- Instruct him to remove dentures or partial plates. Note on the chart if he has dental crowns, caps, or braces. Also have him remove contact lenses, glasses, or prostheses (such as an artificial eye). You may remove his hearing aid to make sure it doesn't become lost. However, if the patient wishes to keep his hearing aid in place, inform operating room and PACU staff of this decision.
- Have the patient void and put on a surgical cap and gown.
- Take and record vital signs.
- Administer preoperative medication as ordered.

The patient should have no solid food for 6 hours and no water for 2 hours before surgery.

Intraoperative care

The intraoperative period begins with the transfer of the patient to the operating room bed and ends with the admission to the PACU. No matter what kind of surgery your patient needs, he'll receive an anesthetic during this time.

No matter what surgery your patient needs, he'll receive an anesthetic during the intraoperative phase.

Anesthesia

To induce loss of the pain sensation, the anesthesiologist or nurse-anesthetist will use some form of anesthesia. (See *Types of anesthesia.*)

What the OR nurse does

Operating room responsibilities are divided between the scrub nurse and the circulating nurse. The scrub nurse scrubs before the operation, sets up the sterile table, prepares sutures and special equipment, and provides help to the surgeon and his assistants throughout the operation. The circulating nurse manages the operating room and monitors cleanliness, humidity, lighting, and safety of equipment. She also coordinates activities of operating room personnel and monitors aseptic practices.

Other nursing responsibilities during the intraoperative period may include positioning the patient, preparing the incision site, and draping the patient.

Types of anesthesia

The three types of anesthesia are general, regional, and balanced. The chart below describes each type.

Type	Description
General	• Blocks awareness centers in the brain • Produces unconsciousness, body relaxation, and loss of sensation • Is administered by inhalation or I.V. infusion
Regional	• Inhibits excitatory processes in nerve endings or fibers • Provides analgesia over a specific body area • Doesn't produce unconsciousness • Can be applied topically or be injected (nerve infiltration or epidural or spinal administration)
Balanced	• Combines narcotics, sedative-hypnotics, nitrous oxide, and muscle relaxants • Induces rapid anesthesia with minimal cardiac depression and decreased postoperative adverse effects (such as nausea and pain) • Produces sleep and analgesia, eliminating certain reflexes and providing good muscle relaxation

Postoperative care

The patient's recovery from the anesthetic is monitored in the PACU. His ongoing recovery is managed on either an intensive care unit or medical-surgical unit. The postoperative period extends from the time the patient leaves the operating room until the last follow-up visit with the surgeon.

What the PACU nurse does

This postoperative period begins when the patient arrives in the PACU, accompanied by the anesthesiologist or nurse-anesthetist. The PACU nurse's main goal is to meet the patient's physical and emotional needs, thereby minimizing the development of postoperative complications. Such factors as pain, lack of oxygen, and sudden movement may threaten his physiologic equilibrium.

Thanks to the use of short-acting anesthetics, the average PACU stay lasts less than 1 hour. The patient is assessed every 10 to 15 minutes initially and then as his condition warrants.

Thanks to technological advances, the average PACU stay is less than 1 hour.

Discharge

Whether the patient is discharged from the PACU to the medical-surgical unit, the intensive care unit, or to the short-procedure unit, safety remains the major consideration. Postoperative complications should be resolved or stabilized. In addition, the patient should:
• demonstrate quiet and unlabored respirations
• be awake or easily aroused to answer simple questions
• have stable vital signs with patent airway and spontaneous respirations
• have a gag reflex
• feel minimal pain
• have return of movement and partial return of sensation to all anesthetized areas if a regional anesthetic was administered.

If the patient had major surgery or has a concurrent serious illness or if complications occurred during or immediately after surgery, he may be discharged to the intensive care unit. Appropriate documentation should accompany the patient on discharge, according to facility policy.

Medical-surgical unit

When assessing the patient after he returns to the medical-surgical unit, be systematic yet sensitive to his needs. Compare your findings with intraoperative and preoperative assessment findings, and report significant changes immediately.

Have a system

Follow a systematic approach to your physical assessment in order to make easier comparisons. Facilities typically have protocols for assessing patients postoperatively. Some facilities require assessments every 15 minutes until the patient stabilizes, every hour for the next 4 hours, and then every 4 hours after that.

Immediately report significant differences in your findings and those from the preoperative and intraoperative assessments.

Assessing respiratory status

Encourage deep breathing to promote elimination of the anesthetic and optimal gas exchange and acid-base balance. Encourage coughing if the patient has secretions. Excessive sedation from analgesics or a general anesthetic can cause respiratory depression. Respiratory depression can also occur if reversal agents wear off. (See *Assessing for respiratory distress*, page 64.)

Make sure the patient has a patent airway and check his respiratory rate, rhythm, and depth. Additional assessment measures include:
• observing for tracheal deviation from the midline
• noting chest symmetry, lung expansion, or use of accessory muscles
• assessing the patient's level of consciousness by testing his ability to follow commands
• taking the patient's apical pulse rate for 1 minute, and assessing the rate and quality of radial and pedal pulses, noting any dependent edema
• obtaining the patient's blood pressure (Systolic pressure shouldn't vary more than 15% from the preoperative reading except in patients who experience preoperative hypotension.)
• taking the patient's temperature, which may be low (due to slowing of basal metabolism associated with anesthesia or cold operating room or I.V. solution) or high (due to the body's response to the trauma of surgery).

Systolic pressure shouldn't vary more than 15% from the preoperative reading.

Assessing for respiratory distress

Cyanosis is a major indicator of respiratory distress. Circumoral, nail bed, or sublingual cyanosis indicates an arterial oxygen saturation level of less than 80%. Earlobe cyanosis, usually accompanying chronic obstructive pulmonary disease, may be exacerbated by anesthesia. Also, assess for other signs of respiratory distress, including:

• nasal flaring
• inspiratory or expiratory grunts
• changes in posture to ease breathing
• progressive disorientation.

    You may use a pulse oximeter to supplement your assessment. This monitor will help you determine life-threatening levels of oxygen saturation (70% or less).

Examining surgical wounds closely can help minimize complications.

Examining the surgical wound

When examining the surgical wound, follow the doctor's orders. Don't remove dressings from a surgical wound without permission. Removing dressings too quickly may be contraindicated. Some dressings provide pressure to the wound; others keep skin grafts intact. If the dressing is stained by drainage, estimate the quantity and note its color and odor. If the patient has a drainage device, record the amount and color of drainage. Make sure the device is secure and free from kinks. If the patient has an ileostomy or colostomy, describe output. If the wound isn't dressed, note the wound's location and describe its length, width, and type (horizontal, transverse, or puncture). Describe the sutures, staples, or adhesive strips used to close the wound and assess approximation of wound edges.

Assessing the abdomen

When assessing the abdomen, first observe for changes in abdominal contour. Abdominal dressings, tubes, or other devices may distort this contour. To detect asymmetry, view the abdomen from the foot of the patient's bed. Also, observe for Cullen's sign, a bluish hue around the umbilicus that commonly accompanies intra-abdominal or peritoneal bleeding.

Auscultation station

Auscultate bowel sounds for at least 1 minute in each of the four quadrants. You probably won't be able to detect bowel sounds for 6 hours or more after surgery because general anesthetics slow peristalsis. If the doctor handled the patient's intestines during surgery, bowel sounds will be absent even longer.

Patent patient

If the patient has a nasogastric tube, regularly check its patency. Confirm proper tube placement by instilling air with a bulb syringe while you auscultate over the epigastric area, checking pH of gastric aspirate (normal pH is from 1 to 4), or by X-ray. Document findings for a baseline assessment and for future reference.

General anesthetics slow peristalsis, so bowel sounds may be absent for at least 6 hours after surgery.

Providing comfort

The postsurgical patient may be unable to assume a comfortable position because of incisional pain, activity restrictions, immobilization devices, or an array of tubes and monitoring lines. Assess the patient's pain by using the pain scale (1 to 10) and offer analgesics as ordered. Although most patients will tell you when they experience severe pain, some may suffer silently. Increased pulse rate and blood pressure may provide the only clues to their condition.

Support, promote, and discuss

Although emotional support can do much to relieve pain, it doesn't replace adequate analgesia. Physical measures, such as positioning, back rubs, and creating a comfortable environment in the patient's room, can also promote comfort and enhance the effectiveness of analgesics. Discuss specific measures the patient can take to prevent or reduce incisional pain. (See *Tips for reducing incisional pain,* page 66.) Encourage the patient to request analgesics or use patient-controlled analgesia before pain is severe.

Physical measures, such as creating a comfortable environment, can promote comfort and enhance the analgesic effect.

Recording intake and output

Measure postoperative intake of food and fluids, including ice chips, I.V. fluids, blood products, and irrigation fluid. Measure postoperative output of urine, tube drainage, and wound drainage.

Education edge

Tips for reducing incisional pain

Teach the postoperative patient the following techniques to reduce pain when he moves, coughs, or breathes deeply.

Proper movement
Instruct the patient to use the bed's side rails for support when he moves and turns. He should move slowly and smoothly, without sudden jerks. Advise him to wait to move until after his pain medication has taken effect, whenever possible.

The patient should frequently move parts of his body not affected by surgery to prevent them from becoming stiff and sore. Make sure the patient is medicated so that he can move comfortably. If moving alone proves difficult for the patient, urge him to ask a staff member to help.

Splinting the incision
Following chest or abdominal surgery, splinting the incision may help the patient reduce pain when he coughs or moves.

Splinting with the hands
Have the patient place one hand above and the other hand below his incision, as shown, then press gently and breathe normally when he moves.

Splinting with a pillow
Alternatively, the patient may place a small pillow over his incision. As he holds the pillow in place with his hands and arms, he should press gently, as shown, breathe normally, and move to a sitting or standing position.

Acting like an adult

An adult should have a minimum urine output of 0.5 to 1 ml/kg/hour. Report an output of less than 240 ml per shift. After surgery, the patient may have difficulty voiding; this occurs when medications, such as atropine, depress parasympathetic stimulation. In order to assess for catheterization, monitor the patient's intake and palpate his bladder or use a bladder scanner regularly.

Because some anesthetics slow peristalsis, the patient may not defecate until his bowel sounds return.

Ordinary output

When documenting output, note the source of output; its quantity, color, and consistency; and the duration over which the output occurred. Notify the doctor of significant changes, such as a change in the color and consistency of nasogastric contents from dark green to "coffee grounds" or a larger volume of output than expected.

Postoperative complications

After surgery, take steps to avoid complications. Be ready to recognize and manage them if they occur.

Reducing the risk of complications

To avoid extending the patient's hospital stay and to speed his recovery, perform the following measures to prevent postoperative complications.

Turn and reposition the patient

Turn and reposition the patient every 2 hours to promote circulation and reduce the risk of skin breakdown, especially over bony prominences. When the patient is in a lateral recumbent position, tuck pillows under bony prominences to reduce friction and promote comfort. Each time you turn the patient, carefully inspect the skin to detect redness or other signs of breakdown.

Don't turn 'em all

Keep in mind that turning and repositioning may be contraindicated in some patients such as those who have undergone neurologic or musculoskeletal surgery that demands immobilization postoperatively.

Encourage coughing and deep breathing

Deep breathing promotes lung expansion, which helps clear anesthetics from the body. Coughing and deep breathing also lower the risk of pulmonary and fat emboli and of hypostatic pneumonia associated with secretion buildup in the airways.

Encourage the patient to deep-breathe and cough every hour while he's awake. (Deep breathing doesn't increase intracranial pressure.) Also, show him how to use an incentive spirometer. (See *Using spirometers.*)

Monitor nutrition and fluids

Adequate nutrition and fluid intake is essential to ensure proper hydration, promote healing, and provide energy to match the increased basal metabolism associated with surgery. If the patient has a protein deficiency or compromised immune function preoperatively, expect to deliver supplemental protein via parenteral nutrition to promote healing. If he has renal failure, this treatment would be contraindicated because his inability to break down protein could lead to dangerously high blood urea nitrogen levels.

Supplemental protein is contraindicated in patients with renal failure.

Promote exercise and ambulation

Early postoperative exercise and ambulation can significantly reduce the risk of thromboembolism. They can also improve ventilation and brighten the patient's outlook.

Passive, okay; active, better

Perform passive range-of-motion (ROM) exercises — better yet, encourage active ROM exercises — to prevent joint contractures and muscle atrophy and to promote circulation. These exercises can also help you assess the patient's strength and tolerance.

Tolerance test

Before encouraging ambulation, have the patient dangle his legs over the side of the bed and perform deep-breathing exercises. How well the patient tolerates this step is usually a key predictor of out-of-bed tolerance. Document frequency of movement, the patient's tolerance, use of analgesics, and any other relevant information.

Despite your best efforts, complications sometimes occur.

Detecting and managing complications

Despite your best efforts, complications sometimes occur. These may include atelectasis, pneumonia, and pulmonary embolism and thrombophlebitis. By knowing how to recognize and manage them, you can limit their effects. (See *Detecting and managing postoperative complications,* pages 70 and 71.)

Using spirometers

Although all spirometers encourage slow, sustained maximal inspiration, they can be divided into two types: flow incentive and volume incentive. A flow incentive spirometer measures the patient's inspiratory effort (flow rate) in cubic centimeters per second (cc/second). A volume incentive spirometer goes one step further. From the patient's flow rate, it calculates the volume of air the patient inhales. Because of this extra step, many volume incentive spirometers are larger, more complicated, and more expensive than flow incentive spirometers.

Volume incentive

For the patient using a volume incentive spirometer, the doctor or respiratory therapist will order a "goal volume" (in cubic centimeters) for the patient to reach. This will be the amount of air the patient should inspire when he takes a deep breath.

One type of volume incentive spirometer includes a display of the goal volume. As the patient inhales, the volume of air he takes into his lungs is also shown, climbing a scale until he reaches or surpasses the goal volume. This not only helps him fully expand his lungs, but also provides immediate feedback as to how well he's doing.

The patient usually does this exercise five times each day. Between exercises he should rest. Each morning, he should reset the goal-volume-achieved display so he can try to do even better.

With another smaller and easier-to-use volume incentive spirometer, the patient inhales slowly and deeply as a piston inside a cylinder rises to meet the preset volume. The number of exercises the patient should do each day remains the same.

Flow incentive

Flow incentive spirometers have no preset volume. These spirometers usually have three cylinders, each containing a colored ball. As the patient inhales, the balls rise, one at a time. The patient's flow rate is measured in cc/second. For example, when the first ball rises, the flow rate may be 600 cc/second; the second ball, 900 cc/second; and the third ball, 1,200 cc/second. The number of exercises the patient should do each day is the same as with volume incentive spirometers.

Which type is best for your patient?

That depends. For low-risk patients, a flow incentive spirometer is probably better. Lightweight and durable, it can be left at

Volume incentive spirometer

Volume scale lights

Mouthpiece

Flow tube

Flow incentive spirometer

Mouthpiece

Balls

Flow tube

the bedside for the patient to use even when you aren't there to supervise.

However, the patient who faces high risk of developing atelectasis may require a volume incentive spirometer. Because it measures lung inflation more precisely, this type of spirometer helps you determine whether your patient is inhaling adequately.

What do I do?

Detecting and managing postoperative complications

The chart below will help you recognize some postoperative complications and intervene appropriately.

Complication	What to look for	What to do
Septicemia and septic shock	*For septicemia* • Fever, chills, rash, abdominal distention, prostration, pain, headache, nausea, or diarrhea	*For septicemia* • Obtain specimens (blood, wound, and urine) for culture and sensitivity tests. • Administer antibiotics as ordered. • Monitor vital signs and level of consciousness to detect septic shock.
	For septic shock • Early stages: warm, dry, flushed skin; slightly altered mental status; increased pulse and respiratory rates; decreased or normal blood pressure; and reduced urine output • Late stage: pale, moist, cold skin; significant decrease in mentation, pulse and respiratory rates, blood pressure, and urine output	*For septic shock* • Administer I.V. antibiotics as ordered. • Monitor serum peak and trough levels. • Administer I.V. fluids and blood or blood products.
Paralytic ileus	• Severe abdominal distention and possibly vomiting • Severe constipation, or passage of flatus and small, liquid stools	• Encourage ambulation and keep the patient on nothing by mouth status. • Insert a nasogastric tube as ordered; keep the tube patent and functioning properly. • Monitor for nausea and vomiting. If nausea occurs, administer an antiemetic to prevent vomiting.
Urine retention	• Absence of voided urine • Distended bladder above the level of the symphysis pubis on palpation • Discomfort or pain, restlessness, anxiety, diaphoresis, or hypertension	• Help the patient ambulate as soon as possible after surgery unless contraindicated. • Assist the patient to a normal voiding position and, if possible, leave him alone. • Turn on the water so the patient can hear it, and pour warm water over his perineum. • Prepare for urinary catheterization if the patient can't void despite other interventions.
Wound infection, dehiscence, and evisceration	*For wound infection* • Increased tenderness, deep pain, and edema at wound site • Increased pulse rate and temperature • Elevated white blood cell count	*For wound infection* • Obtain a wound culture and sensitivity test as ordered. • Administer antibiotics as ordered. • Irrigate the wound with an appropriate solution as ordered, and monitor wound drainage.

Detecting and managing postoperative complications *(continued)*

Complication	What to look for	What to do
Wound infection, dehiscence, and evisceration *(continued)*	*For dehiscence* • Gushes of serosanguineous fluid from the wound • Patient reports a "popping sensation" after retching or coughing *For evisceration* • Protruding contents; visible coils of intestine	*For dehiscence or evisceration* • Stay with the patient; have a colleague notify the doctor. • If an abdominal wound dehisces, help the patient to low Fowler's position, with knees bent in. This will decrease abdominal tension. • Cover the extruding wound contents with warm, sterile normal saline soaks. • Monitor the patient's vital signs.
Altered body image	• Comments from the patient that indicate depression or insecurity • Inability to look at or talk about his incision or stoma	• Encourage verbalization and offer support. • Refer to appropriate support group and counseling. • Encourage participation in care.
Postoperative psychosis	• Change in behavior from baseline	• Reorient the patient frequently to person, place, and time. • Place a clock and calendar in his room where he can see them. • Keep changes in his environment to a minimum. • Provide familiar objects close by. • Encourage family participation in postoperative care. • Use sedatives and restraints only if necessary.

Discharge planning

Begin planning for the patient's discharge at your first contact with him. Include his family or other caregivers in your planning to ensure proper home care. The discharge plan should include:

- medication
- diet
- activity
- home care procedures and referrals
- potential complications
- return appointments.

Problem potential

Recognizing potential problems early on will help your discharge plan succeed. The initial nursing history and preoperative assessment as well as subsequent assessments can provide useful information. Tailor the contents of your plan to the patient's individual needs. Assess the strengths and limitations of the patient and his family. Consider several factors, including:

• physiologic factors — general physical and functional abilities, current medications, and general nutritional status

• psychological factors — self-concept, motivation, and learning abilities

• social factors — duration of care needed, types of services available, and family involvement in the patient's care.

Can I get that in writing?

Provide written materials, when appropriate, as a reference for the patient at home. Assess your patient's reading level and always make sure that readings are reinforced by personal teaching. Include information on:

• *medications.* Teach the patient the purpose of drug therapy, proper dosages and routes, special instructions, potential adverse effects, and when to notify the doctor. Try to establish a medication schedule that fits in with the patient's lifestyle.

• *diet.* Teach the patient and, if appropriate, the family member or caregiver who will prepare his meals. Recommend a good diet book. Refer the patient to a dietitian if appropriate.

• *activity.* After surgery, the patient is commonly advised not to lift a heavy weight such as a basket of laundry. Restrictions usually last 4 to 6 weeks after surgery. Let him know when he can return to work, drive, and resume sexual activity.

• *home care procedures.* After the patient watches you demonstrate a procedure, have him (or his caregiver) perform a return demonstration. If the patient needs to rent or purchase special equipment, such as a hospital bed or walker, give him a list of suppliers in the area.

Dressing for success

• *wound care.* Teach the patient about changing his wound dressing. Tell him to keep the incision clean and dry, and teach proper hand-washing technique.

• *potential complications.* Make sure the patient can recognize signs and symptoms of wound infection and other potential complications, and provide this information in writing. Advise the patient to call the doctor with any questions.

• *return appointments.* Stress the importance of the follow-up appointment in your teaching, and make sure the patient has the doctor's office telephone number. If the patient has no means of transportation, refer him to an appropriate community resource.

Provide written materials for your patient to refer to at home. Make sure that any readings you give out are reinforced by teaching.

• *referrals.* Reassess whether the patient needs referral to a home care agency or other community resource. In some hospitals, the responsibility for making referrals falls to a home care coordinator, discharge planning nurse, or case manager.

Quick quiz

1. What is the value of a thorough preoperative assessment?

A. To identify and correct problems before surgery and establish a baseline for postoperative comparison

B. To save time doing an assessment after the patient returns from surgery

C. To provide the doctor with information that may have been missed during the preadmission assessment

D. To ensure that postoperative complications don't occur

Answer: A. A thorough preoperative assessment helps systematically identify and correct problems before surgery and establish a baseline for postoperative comparison. During the assessment, the nurse should focus on problem areas suggested by the history and body systems that will be directly affected by surgery.

2. In teaching about pain management, the nurse will discuss:

A. the need to use pain medication only when absolutely necessary.

B. that pain medication will be ordered according to the patient's needs.

C. how the method of pain medication administration can't be altered after surgery.

D. the use of a patient controlled device that will deliver medication to the patient whenever he wants it.

Answer: B. The patient should be aware that pain medication will be ordered according to his needs. Because each patient responds differently to pain and medication, dosage and administration is individualized.

3. What is balanced anesthesia?

A. Medication that enhances certain reflexes and provides good muscle tone

B. The use of narcotic medication preoperatively, intraoperatively, and postoperatively

C. A combination of narcotics, sedative-hypnotics, nitrous oxide, and muscle relaxants

D. The use of both local and general anesthesia

Answer: C. Balanced anesthesia is a combination of narcotics, sedative-hypnotics, nitrous oxide, and muscle relaxants.

4. The patient is sent to the PACU after surgery:
  A. to be monitored while recovering from anesthesia.
  B. to remain near the surgeon immediately after surgery.
  C. to allow the medical-surgical unit time to prepare for transfer.
  D. to provide time for the patient to cope with the effects of surgery.

Answer: A. The patient is sent to the PACU to be monitored while recovering from anesthesia.

5. To help prevent postoperative complications, the nurse should:
  A. have the patient rest quietly for the first 24 hours with minimal exertion.
  B. have the patient splint his incision and take deep, rapid breaths before moving.
  C. encourage the patient to begin exercising as soon as possible after surgery.
  D. encourage the patient to drink increased fluids beginning immediately after surgery.

Answer: C. Early postoperative exercises and ambulation can significantly improve circulation, ventilation, and psychological outlook.

6. Discharge planning begins:
  A. on the day of admission.
  B. the day after surgery.
  C. the day of discharge.
  D. the day of surgery.

Answer: A. Although the day of admission may also be the day of surgery, planning for the patient's discharge should begin on admission and first contact with the patient.

Scoring

☆☆☆ If you answered all six items correctly, wowee! You're perioperative perfection!

☆☆ If you answered four or five items correctly, gadzooks! You're perilously close to perfect in perioperative care!

☆ If you answered fewer than four items correctly, perk up! Follow this perioperative teaching plan: Review the chapter, and try again!

Pain management

Just the facts

In this chapter, you'll learn:

♦ the types of pain and theories that explain them

♦ how opioid and nonopioid analgesics control pain

♦ interventions to help alleviate pain.

A look at pain

Pain is whatever the patient says it is and occurs whenever she says it does.

Pain is a complex, subjective phenomenon that involves biological, psychological, cultural, and social factors. To put it succinctly, pain is whatever the patient says it is, and it occurs whenever she says it does. The only true authority on any given pain is the person experiencing it. Therefore, health care professionals must understand and rely on the patient's description of her pain when developing a pain management plan.

Each patient reacts to pain differently because pain thresholds and tolerances vary. Pain threshold is a physiologic attribute that denotes the intensity of the stimulus needed to sense pain. Pain tolerance is a psychological attribute that describes the amount of stimulus (duration and intensity) that the patient can endure before stating that she's in pain.

Theories about pain

Three theories attempt to explain the mechanisms of pain:

 specificity

 pattern

 gate control.

Let's get specific

The specificity theory maintains that individual specialized peripheral nerve fibers are responsible for pain transmission. This biologically oriented theory doesn't explain pain tolerance, nor does it allow for social, cultural, or empirical factors that influence pain.

Pain pattern

The pattern theory suggests that excessive stimulation of all nerve endings produces a unique pattern interpreted by the cerebral cortex as pain. Although this theory addresses the brain's ability to determine the amount, intensity, and type of sensory input, it doesn't address nonbiological influences on pain perception and transmission.

Opening the gate

The gate control theory asserts that some sort of gate mechanism in the spinal cord allows nerve fibers to receive pain sensations. (See *Understanding the gate control theory*.) This theory has encouraged a more holistic approach to pain management and research by taking into account the nonbiological components of pain. Pain management techniques, such as cutaneous stimulation, distraction, and acupuncture are, in part, based on this theory.

Types of pain

There are two fundamental pain types: acute and chronic.

Acute pain

Acute pain commonly accompanies tissue damage from injury or disease. It varies from mild to severe in intensity and typically lasts for a brief period (less than 6 months). Acute pain is considered a protective mechanism, alerting the individual to tissue damage or organ disease. A patient can get relief from acute pain, and the pain itself dissipates as the underlying disorder heals.

Relief and healing

Treatment goals for acute pain include relieving pain and healing the underlying injury or disease responsible for the pain. Palliative treatment may include surgery, drug therapy, application of heat or cold, or psychological and behavioral techniques to control pain.

A closer look

Understanding the gate control theory

Intensive research into the pathophysiology of pain has yielded several theories about pain perception, including the Melzack-Wall gate control theory. According to this theory, pain and thermal impulses travel along small-diameter, slow-conducting afferent nerve fibers to the spinal cord's dorsal horns. There, they terminate in an area of gray matter called the *substantia gelatinosa*.

Open or close the gate

When sensory stimulation reaches a critical level, a theoretical "gate" in the substantia gelatinosa opens, allowing nearby transmission cells to send the pain impulse to the brain along the interspinal neurons to the spinothalamic tract, and then to the thalamus and cerebral cortex (see illustration below, left). The small size of the fibers enhances pain transmission.

In contrast, large-diameter fibers inhibit pain transmission. Stimulation of these large, fast-conducting afferent nerve fibers counters the input of the smaller fibers, thereby closing the theoretical gate in the substantia gelatinosa and blocking the pain transmission (see illustration below, right).

Keys to the gate

Descending (efferent) impulses along various tracts from the brain and brain stem can enhance or reduce pain transmission at the gate. For example, triggering specific brain processes, such as attention, emotions, and memory of pain, can intensify pain by opening the gate.

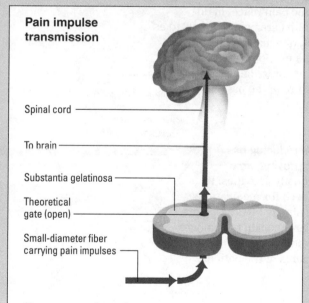

Pain impulse transmission

Spinal cord

To brain

Substantia gelatinosa

Theoretical gate (open)

Small-diameter fiber carrying pain impulses

How we perceive pain

This diagram shows how pain impulses traveling along a small-diameter nerve fiber pass through an open gate in the substantia gelatinosa, and then travel to the brain for interpretation.

Blocked pain transmission

Spinal cord

To brain

Substantia gelatinosa

Theoretical gate (closed)

Small-diameter fiber carrying pain impulses

Large-diameter fiber carrying non-pain impulses

How pain transmission is blocked

Impulses carried by a large-diameter fiber can close the gate to small-fiber impulses, blocking the transmission of pain.

Chronic pain

The cause of chronic pain isn't always clear. Chronic pain can stem from prolonged disease or dysfunction, as in cancer and arthritis, or it can be associated with a mental disorder such as posttraumatic stress syndrome. It can be intermittent, limited, or persistent and usually lasts 6 months or longer. This type of pain is strongly influenced by the patient's emotions and environment.

There are three categories of chronic pain:

☝ chronic nonmalignant pain, such as the pain associated with nonprogressive or healed tissue injury

✌ chronic malignant pain, such as the pain associated with cancer or other progressive disorders

🖐 chronic intractable pain, such as the pain that increases as the patient's ability to cope deteriorates.

Patients with chronic pain react in different ways, making it difficult for us to assess their pain.

Not the pain next door

Chronic pain isn't always localized, which makes it difficult at times for the patient to clearly describe what he's feeling. Furthermore, a patient with chronic pain reacts in different ways, making it difficult for health care professionals to assess the pain. One patient may cry out, one may groan, and still another may simply withdraw. Changes in appetite, sleeping patterns, or other behavior (such as anxiety or irritability) can be important clues into the nature of the patient's pain.

Have a stable day

Treatment for chronic pain focuses on reducing or eliminating the patient's pain while improving, or at least stabilizing, his ability to conduct daily activities. It also attempts to reduce the patient's need for medications. In mild chronic pain, treatment might simply involve ice massage and exercise. However, severe chronic pain typically requires a multidisciplinary program to address the physiological, psychological, and social components of the patient's condition.

In mild chronic pain, treatment might include exercise. How does that feel?

Better, thanks!

Assessing pain

The only way to get an accurate understanding of the patient's pain is to ask him. Begin by asking the patient to describe his pain. Where does it hurt? What exactly does it feel like? When does it start, how long does it last, and how often does it recur? What provokes it? What makes it feel better? There are a variety of assessment tools that can help. Encourage the patient to use one to obtain a more accurate and consistent description of pain intensity and relief—two important measurements. (See *Pain assessment tools*.)

Where does it hurt?

Find out how the patient responds to pain. Does his pain interfere with eating? Sleeping? Working? His sex life? His relationships? Ask the patient to point to the area where he feels pain, keeping in mind that:
- localized pain is felt only at its origin
- projected pain travels along the nerve pathways
- radiated pain extends in several directions from the point of origin
- referred pain occurs in places remote from the site of origin.

Nature's source

Factors that influence the nature of a patient's pain include duration, severity, and source. The source may be:
- cutaneous, originating in the skin or subcutaneous tissue
- deep somatic, which includes nerve, bone, muscle, and supporting tissue
- visceral, which includes the body organs.

Watch for physiologic responses to pain (nausea, vomiting, changes in vital signs) and behavioral responses to pain (facial expression, movement and positioning, what the patient says or doesn't say). Also note psychological responses, such as anger, depression, and irritability.

All about attitude

Assess the patient's attitude about pain. Ask him how he usually handles pain. Does he tell others when he hurts, or does he try to hide it? Does his family understand his pain and try to help him deal with it? Does he accept their help?

Pain assessment tools

Several easy-to-use tools can help you better understand the patient's pain:
- A *rating scale* is a quick method of determining the patient's perception of pain intensity. Ask him to rate his pain on a scale from 1 to 10, with 1 representing pain-free and 10 representing the most pain imaginable.
- A *face rating scale* uses illustrations of five or more faces with expressions that range from happy to very unhappy. The patient chooses the face that represents how he feels at the moment. It's particularly useful with a young child or a patient with language difficulty.
- A *body diagram* allows the patient to draw the location and radiation of pain on an illustration of the body.
- A *questionnaire* provides the patient with key questions about the pain's location, intensity, quality, onset, and factors that relieve and aggravate pain.

Managing pain

Pain management can involve drug therapy with opioid or nonopioid analgesics, including patient-controlled analgesia (PCA) and adjuvant analgesics; neurosurgery; transcutaneous electrical nerve stimulation (TENS); and cognitive-behavioral strategies.

> Agonists are the drugs of choice for severe chronic pain.

Opioid analgesics

Opioid analgesics are prescribed to relieve moderate to severe pain. They include opiates and opioids. Opiates are natural opium alkaloids and their derivatives; opioids are synthetic compounds but can also include opiates. Morphine is the prototype for both types of opioid analgesics.

The agony and the ecstasy

Opioid analgesics are classified as agonists or agonist-antagonists. Agonists are drugs that produce analgesia by binding to central nervous system (CNS) opiate receptors. These drugs are the drugs of choice for severe chronic pain. They include:
- codeine
- hydromorphone
- levorphanol
- meperidine
- methadone
- morphine
- propoxyphene.

Up the anti

Agonist-antagonists also produce analgesia by binding to CNS receptors. However, they're of limited use for patients with chronic pain because many have a ceiling effect or upper dosing limit. As the dosage increases, they also can cause hallucinations and other psychotomimetic effects and, in opioid-dependent patients, can produce withdrawal symptoms. This class of drugs includes:
- buprenorphine
- butorphanol
- nalbuphine
- pentazocine.

> I.V. administration for severe pain is preferred because it acts quickly and permits precise dosing.

Any route you choose

Most opioid analgesics can be given orally, I.M., I.V., epidurally, or intrathecally. For most patients, oral administration is preferred.

I.M. administration, though effective, can result in erratic absorption, especially in debilitated patients.

For severe pain, such as the pain caused by an angina attack, I.V. administration may be preferred because it acts quickly and permits precise dosage control. Be aware that sudden profound respiratory depression and hypotension can occur with this route. Continuous I.V. infusion using a PCA system allows lower dosing. (See *Understanding patient-controlled analgesia*, page 82.)

> Opioids are safe for many patients; however, possibly severe adverse effects make caution the key to effective treatment.

Caution is the key

Opioids can produce severe adverse effects; therefore, caution is the key. They're contraindicated in patients with severe respiratory depression and should be used cautiously in patients with:
• chronic obstructive pulmonary disease
• hepatic or renal impairment because they're metabolized by the liver and excreted by the kidneys
• head injuries or any condition that raises intracranial pressure (ICP) because they increase ICP and can induce miosis (which can mask pupil dilation, an indicator of increased ICP).

But wait, there's more...

Other possible adverse effects include drowsiness, dizziness, nausea, vomiting, itching, constipation, and urine retention. Prolonged use can lead to increased tolerance and physiologic and psychological dependence.

I'll pencil you in

Analgesic schedules are commonly used in the management of chronic pain. The schedule may call for a single medication or a combination—for example, an opioid and a nonsteroidal anti-inflammatory drug (NSAID). To maximize pain control, a sustained-release opioid analgesic, such as morphine sulfate and fentanyl patches, may be used on a set schedule with a short-acting opioid as needed to control breakthrough, or acute, pain.

> Gulp. If the patient's respiratory rate decreases to 10 breaths per minute or less, you need to act — please!

Monitoring

Before giving an opioid analgesic, make sure the patient isn't already taking a CNS depressant such as a barbiturate. Concurrent use of another CNS depressant enhances drowsiness, sedation, and disorientation.

During administration, check the patient's vital signs and watch for respiratory depression. If his respiratory rate declines to 10 breaths/minute or less, call his name, touch him, and tell him to breathe deeply. If he can't be aroused or if he's confused or

Understanding patient-controlled analgesia

A patient-controlled analgesia (PCA) system provides optimal opioid dosing while maintaining a constant serum concentration of the drug.

How it works

A PCA system consists of a syringe injection pump piggybacked into an I.V. or subcutaneous infusion port. When the patient presses a button, he receives a preset bolus dose of medication. The doctor programs the bolus dose and the "lock-out" time between boluses, thus preventing overdose. The device automatically records the number of times the patient presses the button, helping the doctor adjust the dosage.

In some cases, the PCA system allows a reduction in drug dosage, possibly because the patient feels more control over his pain relief and knows that, if he's in pain, analgesia is quickly available. This tends to reduce the patient's level of stress and anxiety, which can exacerbate pain.

Programmable dosage and time regulator

Opioid-filled syringe

Handheld button

restless, notify the doctor and prepare to administer oxygen. If ordered, administer an opioid antagonist such as naloxone.

Countering adverse effects

Opioids may have several adverse effects. To prevent or manage them, follow these recommendations:

• If the patient experiences persistent nausea and vomiting during therapy, ask the doctor about changing medications and give the patient an antiemetic, such as chlorpromazine, as ordered.
• To help prevent constipation, administer a stool softener together with a mild laxative. Also, provide a high-fiber diet, and encourage fluids, as ordered. Regular exercise may also promote motility.
• Encourage the patient to practice coughing and deep-breathing. These exercises promote ventilation and prevent pooling of secretions, which can cause respiratory difficulty.
• Because opioid analgesics can cause postural hypotension, take measures to avoid accidents. For example, keep the bed's side rails raised. If the patient is able to move around, help him in and out of bed and walk with him to provide support if necessary.

Evaluate for effect

Evaluate the effectiveness of the drug. Is the patient experiencing relief? Does his dosage need to be increased because of persistent or worsening pain? Is he developing a tolerance to the drug? Remember that the patient should receive the smallest effective dose over the shortest period. At the same time, a dosage that's too low to be effective is pointless. Opioid analgesics are safe and effective; they simply require close monitoring to ensure the most effective dosage. Physical and psychological dependence are rare. In fact, psychological dependence occurs in less than 1% of hospitalized patients.

Don't worry. Psychological dependence on these drugs occurs in less than 1% of hospitalized patients.

Patient teaching

Teach the patient about his drug therapy and ways to avoid or resolve adverse effects. Tell him to:
• take the prescribed drug before the pain becomes intense to maximize its effectiveness and talk with the doctor if the drug seems less effective over time.
• not increase the dose or frequency of administration and take a missed dose as soon as he remembers, while maintaining the interval between doses.
• skip the missed dose if it's just about time for the next dose to avoid serious complications of a double dose.
• refrain from drinking alcohol while taking the drug to avoid pronounced CNS depression.
• talk with his doctor if he decides to stop taking the drug because the doctor can suggest an appropriate gradual dosage reduction to avoid withdrawal symptoms.

• avoid postural hypotension by getting up slowly when getting out of bed or a chair.
• eat a high-fiber diet, drink plenty of fluids, and take a stool softener, if prescribed.

Watch out for O.D.

Teach the patient's family the signs of overdose: cold, clammy skin; confusion; severe drowsiness or restlessness; slow or irregular breathing; pinpoint pupils; or unconsciousness. Tell them to notify the doctor immediately if they notice these signs. Teach them how to maintain the patient's respiration in an emergency until help arrives.

Nonopioid analgesics

Nonopioid analgesics are prescribed to manage mild to moderate pain. When used with an opioid analgesic, they help relieve moderate to severe pain and also allow lower dosing of the opioid agent. These drugs include acetaminophen and NSAIDs, such as aspirin, ibuprofen, indomethacin, naproxen, naproxen sodium, phenylbutazone, and sulindac.

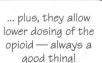

When opioid and nonopioid analgesics are used together, they relieve moderate to severe pain...

Special effects

NSAIDs and acetaminophen produce antipyretic and analgesic effects. In addition, as their name suggests, NSAIDs have an anti-inflammatory effect. Because these drugs all differ in chemical structure, they vary in their onset of action, duration of effect, and method of metabolism and excretion.

In most cases, the analgesic regimen includes a nonopioid drug even if the patient's pain is severe enough to warrant treatment with an opioid. They're commonly used to treat postoperative and postpartum pain, headache, myalgia, arthralgia, dysmenorrhea, and cancer pain.

Not so special effects

The chief adverse effects of NSAIDs include:
• inhibited platelet aggregation (rebounds when drug is stopped)
• GI irritation
• hepatotoxicity
• nephrotoxicity
• headache
• liver damage (in long-term, high-dose use).

NSAIDs shouldn't be used in patients with aspirin sensitivity, especially those with allergies, asthma, and aspirin-induced nasal polyps, due to the increased risk of bronchoconstriction or anaphylaxis. Also, NSAIDs are con-

... plus, they allow lower dosing of the opioid — always a good thing!

traindicated in patients with thrombocytopenia, and should be used cautiously in neutropenic patients because antipyretic activity may mask the only sign of infection. Some NSAIDs are contraindicated in patients with renal dysfunction, hypertension, GI inflammation, or ulcers.

Just call me in the morning

Aspirin increases prothrombin and bleeding times; consequently, it's contraindicated in a patient with hemophilia or other bleeding disorders. Don't administer aspirin with anticoagulants or other ulcer-causing drugs such as corticosteroids. Avoid aspirin use in a patient scheduled for surgery within 1 week.

Acetaminophen may be used in place of aspirin and other NSAIDs in patients with peptic ulcer or a bleeding disorder. High doses of acetaminophen may lead to hepatic damage, however.

Monitoring

Before administering nonopioid analgesics, check the patient's history for a previous hypersensitivity reaction, which may indicate hypersensitivity to a related drug in this group. If the patient is already taking an NSAID, ask him if he has experienced GI irritation. If he has, the doctor may choose to reduce the dosage or discontinue the drug.

If the patient is undergoing long-term therapy, report any abnormalities in renal and liver function studies. Also, monitor hematologic studies and evaluate complaints of nausea or gastric burning. Watch for signs of iron deficiency anemia, such as pallor, unusual fatigue, and weakness.

Patient teaching

For a patient taking an NSAID, teach him the signs and symptoms of overdose, hypersensitivity, and GI bleeding, such as rash, dyspnea, confusion, blurred vision, nausea, bloody vomitus, and black, tarry stools. Tell him to report any of these signs to his doctor immediately.

If the patient is taking acetaminophen, teach him that nausea, vomiting, abdominal cramps, or diarrhea may indicate an overdose and that he should notify his doctor immediately.

Understanding adverse effects

To help the patient respond to adverse effects, teach him to:

Just say "no" to NSAIDs — at least for the long term in high doses — or I'm done for!

Sacre bleu! Not the nonopioid analgesics!

I think he's abnormal. What do you think?

• take his medication with food or a full glass of water to minimize the GI upset that can accompany the use of NSAIDs
• remain standing for 15 to 30 minutes after taking his medication if he experiences esophageal irritation
• notify the doctor if he experiences gastric burning or pain
• take special care to avoid injury that could cause bleeding because NSAIDs can increase bleeding time
• talk to the doctor about persistent tinnitus (a reversible, dose-related adverse effect)
• exercise caution when driving or using machinery when taking ibuprofen, naproxen, or sulindac (which may cause dizziness)
• get periodic blood tests to detect possible nephritis or hepatotoxicity.

Tell the patient to be careful when driving. Of course, discontinuing the drug won't make him a better driver. Whoa!

Adjuvant analgesics

Adjuvant analgesics are drugs that have other primary indications but are used as analgesics in some circumstances. Adjuvants may be given in combination with opioids or used alone to treat chronic pain. Patients receiving adjuvant analgesics should be reevaluated periodically to monitor their pain level and check for adverse reactions.

A real potpourri

Drugs used as adjuvant analgesics include certain anticonvulsants, local and topical anesthetics, muscle relaxants, tricyclic antidepressants, selective serotonin reuptake inhibitors, benzodiazepines, psychostimulants, and cholinergic blockers. (See *Understanding adjuvant analgesics*.)

Neurosurgery

Neurosurgery is an extreme form of pain management and is rarely needed. However, there are a number of procedures, such as rhizotomy and cordotomy, that can control pain by surgically modifying critical points in the nervous system. (See *Surgical interventions for pain*, page 88.)

TENS

TENS relieves acute and chronic pain by using a mild electrical current that stimulates nerve fibers to block the transmission of pain impulses to the brain. The current is delivered through elec-

Understanding adjuvant analgesics

Adjuvant analgesics are drugs that have other primary indications but are used as analgesics in some circumstances. The major types are discussed here.

Anticonvulsants

Anticonvulsants may be used to treat neuropathic pain (pain generated by peripheral nerves). Carbamazepine and gabapentin are the anticonvulsants most commonly used as adjuvant analgesics; others include clonazepam, phenytoin, and valproic acid.

Local anesthetics

Local anesthetics may be used to help manage neuropathic pain or as an alternative to general anesthesia. These drugs include:
• amide drugs, such as bupivacaine, etidocaine, lidocaine, mepivacaine, prilocaine, and ropivacaine
• ester drugs, such as benzocaine, cocaine, chloroprocaine, procaine, and tetracaine.

Topical anesthetics

Topical anesthetics are applied directly to the skin or mucous membranes to prevent or relieve minor pain. These agents include:
• amide drugs, such as dibucaine and lidocaine
• ester drugs, such as benzocaine, cocaine, dyclonine, pramoxine, and tetracaine.
    This drug category also includes topical combinations of local anesthetics, such as:
• Aerocaine—a mixture of benzocaine and benzethonium
• Cetacaine—a mixture of benzocaine, butamben, dyclonine, lidocaine, and tetracaine
• EMLA (eutectic mixture of local anesthetics), which contains lidocaine and prilocaine.

Muscle relaxants

Muscle relaxants can be classified as:
• neuromuscular agents (such as metocurine and tubocurarine), used primarily as adjuncts to general anesthesia (and secondarily to induce muscle relaxation and promote relaxation in patients on mechanical ventilation)

• antispasmodic agents, used to relieve spasticity associated with central nervous system disorders (such as baclofen, dantrolene, and diazepam)
• agents used for short-term pain relief and muscle spasms (such as carisoprodol, chlorzoxazone, cyclobenzaprine, methocarbamol, and tizanididine).

Tricyclic antidepressants (TCAs)

Of the various types of antidepressants, TCAs have the longest history in managing pain — particularly neuropathic pain. TCAs include amitriptyline, amoxapine, clomipramine, desipramine, doxepin, imipramine, maprotiline, nortriptyline, and protriptyline.

Selective serotonin reuptake inhibitors (SSRIs)

A well-known class of antidepressants, SSRIs are being investigated for pain relief as well. These agents include fluoxetine, paroxetine, and sertraline.

Benzodiazepines

Benzodiazepines are used primarily to ease anxiety. Although they aren't effective in treating acute pain, they have some value in easing muscle spasms. Benzodiazepines include alprazolam, diazepam, lorazepam, midazolam, and oxazepam.

Psychostimulants

Psychostimulants are used mainly to treat such disorders as Parkinson's disease and attention deficit hyperactivity disorder. In pain management, they may be used adjunctively to manage acute or chronic pain disorders. Psychostimulants include caffeine, dextroamphetamine, and methylphenidate.

Cholinergic blockers

Cholinergic blockers are used to treat spastic or hyperactive conditions of the GI tract. They relax muscles and decrease GI secretions. Major cholinergic blockers are the belladonna alkaloids, which include belladonna and scopolamine hydrobromide.

Surgical interventions for pain

Surgery is typically considered to manage pain only when pharmacologic therapies fail. More and more, however, these techniques are being used earlier with excellent effect. Surgical procedures used to treat pain include neurectomy, rhizotomy, cordotomy, cryoanalgesia, and radio-frequency lesioning.

Neurectomy

Neurectomy involves the resection or partial or total excision of a spinal or cranial nerve. This procedure is relatively quick and only requires local or regional anesthesia. Unfortunately, loss of motor sensation is a possible adverse effect, and pain relief may only be temporary. Peripheral neurectomy is considered when all standard pain management therapies have failed.

Rhizotomy

Rhizotomy involves cutting a nerve to relieve pain. Rhizotomy of the dorsal nerve root may produce analgesia for localized severe pain, such as on the trunk, abdomen, or limb. Motor function is usually unaffected if one dorsal nerve root for the area is left intact.

Cordotomy

Cordotomy can be performed as an open surgery or percutaneously. A unilateral cordotomy is performed to relieve somatic pain on one side of the body. A bilateral cordotomy is performed to relieve visceral pain on both sides of the body.

Cryoanalgesia

Cryoanalgesia deactivates a nerve using a cooled probe that causes temporary nerve injury. Nerve function returns over time and the procedure can be repeated. Cryoanalgesia can provide effective pain relief for the patient with pain from a surgical scar, a neuroma trapped in scar tissue, and occipital neuralgia.

Radio-frequency lesioning

Radio-frequency lesioning may affect the nerve from the heat generated, the magnetic field created by the radio waves, or both. Nerve function is stopped for a prolonged period. If it does return, the procedure can be repeated. The most frequent use of this technology is to treat pain related to the facet joint and lumbar sympathetic and peripheral nerves. Because it's a focused therapy, it's used when specific nerves can be targeted.

trodes placed on the skin at points determined to be related to the pain. TENS is used to treat:

- chronic back pain
- postoperative pain
- dental pain
- labor pain
- pain from peripheral neuropathy or nerve injury
- postherpetic neuralgia
- reflex sympathetic dystrophy
- musculoskeletal trauma
- arthritis
- phantom limb pain.

Can't touch this

Although TENS therapy presents few risks, the electrodes should never be placed over the carotid sinus nerves or over laryngeal or pharyngeal muscles. Similarly, the electrodes should never be placed on the eyes or over the uterus of a pregnant patient because this treatment's safety during pregnancy has yet to be determined.

TENS is contraindicated if the patient has a pacemaker. The current may also interfere with electrocardiography or cardiac monitoring. Furthermore, TENS shouldn't be used when the etiology of the pain is unknown because it might mask a new pathology.

Safety of TENS treatment for pregnant patients has yet to be determined.

Patient preparation

Make sure that the skin beneath the electrode sites is intact. Clean it with an alcohol wipe and dry well. Shave the area if necessary. Next, if electrodes aren't pregelled, apply a small amount of electrode gel to the bottom of each to improve conductivity. Place the electrodes on the skin. If they aren't self-adhering, secure them with tape, leaving at least 2″ (5 cm) of space between the electrodes.

Turn that off

Make sure the controls on the control box are turned to the OFF position. Attach the leadwires to the electrodes, and plug them into the control box. Set the pulse width and rate as recommended. Turn on the unit, and adjust the intensity to the prescribed setting or to the setting most comfortable for the patient. Now secure the unit to the patient. After the prescribed duration of treatment, turn the unit off and remove the electrodes. Wash and dry the patient's skin. Then clean the unit and replace the battery pack.

If you must relocate electrodes, first turn off the TENS unit.

Monitoring

Assess the patient for signs of excessive or inadequate stimulation. Muscle twitching may indicate overstimulation, whereas an inability to feel any tingling sensation may mean that the current is too low. If the patient complains of pain or intolerable paresthesia, check the settings, connections, and electrode placements. Adjust the settings if necessary. If you must relocate the electrodes during treatment, first turn off the TENS unit. Evaluate the patient's response to each TENS treatment and compare the results. Also, use your baseline assessment to evaluate the effectiveness of the procedure.

Patient teaching

If the patient will use the TENS unit at home, have him demonstrate the procedure, including electrode placement, the setting of the unit's controls, electrode removal, and proper care of the equipment. Explain that he should strictly follow the prescribed settings and electrode placements.

Warn against using high voltage, which can increase pain, or using the unit to treat pain for which he doesn't know the cause. Also, tell the patient to notify the doctor if pain worsens or develops at another site.

It's electric

If skin irritation occurs, instruct the patient to keep the area clean and apply a soothing lotion. However, if skin breakdown occurs, he should notify the doctor. Make sure the patient understands that he should remove the unit before bathing or swimming to avoid possible electrocution.

Cognitive-behavioral techniques have the added benefit of being virtually risk-free. Those are pretty good odds!

Cognitive-behavioral techniques

Behavior modification and relaxation techniques may be used to help the patient reduce the suffering associated with pain. These techniques include biofeedback, distraction, guided imagery, hypnosis, and meditation. These "mind-over-pain" techniques allow the patient to exercise a degree of control over his pain. In addition, they have the added benefit of being virtually risk-free with few contraindications. Even so, if the patient has a significant psychiatric problem, a psychotherapist should teach him the relaxation techniques.

Patient preparation

Because all of these techniques require concentration, try to choose a time when the patient isn't feeling pain or when pain is at it's lowest ebb. However, if pain is persistent, begin with short, simple exercises and build on the patient's abilities.

First, relaxxxxx...

Choose a quiet location and dim the lights. Have the patient remove or loosen restrictive clothing. To help the patient lessen muscle tension, tell him to alternately tighten and relax a specific group of muscles — for example, muscles in his neck — while concentrating on tension and relaxation. Repeat the exercise for all muscles groups. If a particular muscle group is painful, move on to the next group.

Good feedback

Biofeedback requires the use of a special machine that allows the patient to see how his body reacts to his efforts. When the patient is connected to the machine, he performs the relaxation technique that he finds most beneficial. The equipment provides feedback regarding his progress with tones, lights, or a digital readout. In this way, the patient can determine which techniques work best to promote relaxation and reduce pain.

Forgetting to feel the pain

Distraction is a technique that involves focusing on music, a book or magazine, or the television or a movie instead of pain and related health issues. If the patient listens to music, suggest that he use a headset to help him focus on the music or imagery produced by the music. Keeping time to the beat or increasing the volume can help if the pain worsens. Other distraction strategies include singing, rhythmic breathing, and meditation.

Keeping time to the beat or increasing the volume can help if pain worsens. One, two, three, one, two, three...

I have a dream

In *guided imagery*, the patient concentrates on visualizing the calm and peaceful images described by the leader, either you or a recording. Many recordings are available, so the patient should experiment to find imagery that helps him most. Quiet and peaceful nature imagery — for example, the smell of spring grass, the sound of rolling ocean surf, or the burbling of a forest brook — seems to be most effective.

Look into my eyes

Hypnosis is performed by a qualified therapist. During the session, the therapist may use a variety of techniques, such as symptom suppression, which helps block the patient's awareness of pain, or symptom substitution, which encourages a positive interpretation of pain.

Acting differently

In *behavior modification* therapy, the patient is encouraged to identify behaviors that reinforce or exacerbate pain, suffering, and disability, such as being overly dependent on others or using a cane when it isn't medically indicated. With the therapist's help, the patient defines specific goals, such as reducing his dependence on others, and then uses positive and negative reinforcement to shed old behaviors and promote new, beneficial patterns of behavior.

Monitoring

Remember to be consistent when working with the patient, and make sure that all staff members are aware of the patient's choices for cognitive pain reduction. If the patient becomes frustrated with his progress with any of these techniques, calmly have him stop and try again later. End each session on a positive note by pointing out improvements; even small improvements show progress.

> Even small improvements show progress. You're doing great!

Patient teaching

If the patient has overwhelming psychosocial problems, recommend that he seek therapy. Provide him with referrals to appropriate professionals. Any gains in pain management may be quickly lost unless he deals with these factors.

For all others, help develop a plan for using the cognitive-behavioral strategies at home. A plan will increase the likelihood that the patient will continue to benefit from these strategies after he's home again.

Nursing care of the patient in pain

> Around-the-clock pain medication helps avoid major peaks and valleys of pain and relief.

These nursing interventions are appropriate for a patient in pain:
• Assess the pain's location and ask the patient to rate the pain using a pain scale.
• Ask the patient to describe the pain's quality and pattern, including any precipitating or relieving factors.

Making faces

• Monitor the patient's vital signs and note subjective responses to pain, such as facial grimacing and guarding the affected part of the body.
• Administer pain medication around-the-clock, as ordered. This schedule is preferred to as-needed dosing because it avoids major peaks and valleys of pain and relief. Teach the patient the importance of taking the prescribed analgesics before the pain becomes severe.
• Provide comfort measures, such as back massage, positioning, linen changes, and oral or skin care.
• Teach noninvasive techniques to control pain, such as relaxation, guided imagery, distraction, and cutaneous stimulation.
• Explain the role of sleep and the importance of being well rested.

Quick quiz

1. The person who knows the most about the patient's pain is the:
- A. doctor.
- B. nurse.
- C. patient.
- D. physical therapist.

Answer: C. The person who experiences the pain is the only true authority on that pain.

2. What does the pain threshold reflect?
- A. The frequency of pain that the patient experiences in 24 hours
- B. The duration or intensity of pain the patient can tolerate before openly expressing pain
- C. The location of the pain and the areas to which it radiates
- D. The intensity of stimulus the patient needs to sense pain

Answer: D. A person's pain threshold is a physiologic component that reflects the intensity of stimulus needed to cause painful sensation.

3. The best type of pain assessment tool to use with an adult who has difficulty communicating due to stroke is the:
- A. 1-to-10 number scale.
- B. face rating scale.
- C. body diagram.
- D. questionnaire.

Answer: B. The face rating scale would be best for this patient because he can simply point to the face that illustrates how he's feeling.

4. What should you monitor in a patient taking high doses of acetaminophen over a prolonged period?
- A. Prothrombin time
- B. GI irritation
- C. Liver function
- D. Kidney function

Answer: C. Prolonged use of high doses of acetaminophen increases the risk of liver damage.

5. What makes techniques, such as relaxation, distraction, and guided imagery, effective tools in managing pain?

A.   Drug interaction
B.   Electrical stimulation
C.   Surgical intervention
D.   Power of the mind

Answer: D. The power of the mind makes cognitive-behavioral pain control techniques effective.

Scoring

☆☆☆ If you answered all five items correctly, bravo! You've got this pain topic under control.

☆☆ If you answered three or four items correctly, nicely done! We'd say you just missed a perfect TENS on this quiz.

☆ If you answered fewer than three items correctly, don't suffer needlessly. A quick review will alleviate your pain.

Neurologic disorders

Just the facts

In this chapter, you'll learn:

♦ neurologic structures and functions

♦ components of a neurologic assessment

♦ relevant diagnostic tests and nursing diagnoses

♦ common neurologic disorders and treatments.

Complex and infinitely diverse, the nervous system is the body's internal communication network. It coordinates all body functions and all adaptations to changes in the body's internal and external environments. Consequently, a patient suffering illness or injury can develop related neurologic impairments.

Anatomy and physiology

The nervous system is divided into the central nervous system (CNS), the peripheral nervous system, and the autonomic nervous system. Through complex and coordinated interactions, these three parts integrate all physical, intellectual, and emotional activities.

Central nervous system

The CNS includes the brain and the spinal cord, the two structures that collect and interpret voluntary and involuntary motor and sensory stimuli. (See *The CNS*, page 96.)

Brain

The brain consists of the cerebrum (cerebral cortex), the brain stem, and the cerebellum. It collects, integrates, and interprets all

Me and the spinal cord make up the central nervous system. It's a good thing we get along!

A closer look

The CNS

This illustration shows a cross section of the brain and spinal cord, which together make up the central nervous system (CNS). The brain joins the spinal cord at the base of the skull and ends near the second lumbar vertebra. Note the H-shaped mass of gray matter in the spinal cord.

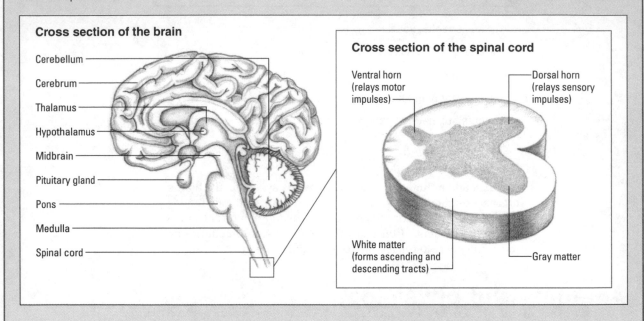

Cross section of the brain

- Cerebellum
- Cerebrum
- Thalamus
- Hypothalamus
- Midbrain
- Pituitary gland
- Pons
- Medulla
- Spinal cord

Cross section of the spinal cord

Ventral horn (relays motor impulses)

Dorsal horn (relays sensory impulses)

White matter (forms ascending and descending tracts)

Gray matter

stimuli; in addition, it initiates and monitors voluntary and involuntary motor activity.

I think; therefore, I am

The cerebrum gives us the ability to think and reason. Within the skull, it's enclosed in three membrane layers called *meninges*. If blood or fluid accumulates between these layers, pressure builds inside the skull and compromises brain function.

The cerebrum has four lobes and two hemispheres. The right hemisphere controls the left side of the body, and the left hemisphere controls the right side of the body. Each lobe controls specific functions. (See *The lobes of the cerebrum.*)

A closer look

The lobes of the cerebrum

The cerebrum's four lobes—the parietal, occipital, temporal, and frontal lobes—are discerned by anatomic landmarks and functional differences. The name of each lobe is derived from the overlying cranial bone. This illustration shows the locations of the cerebral lobes and explains their functions. It also shows the location of the cerebellum.

Parietal lobe
Sensations, awareness of body shape

Occipital lobe
Visual stimuli

Temporal lobe
Hearing, language and comprehension, storage and recall of memories

Cerebellum
Not part of cerebrum, but controls balance and coordination

Sensory cortex
Sensory impulses

Motor cortex
Movement

Frontal lobe
Personality, judgment, abstract reasoning, social behavior, language expression, movement

Regulatory affairs

A part of the cerebrum called the *diencephalon* contains the thalamus and hypothalamus. The thalamus relays sensory impulses. The hypothalamus regulates many body functions, including temperature control, pituitary hormone production, and water balance.

Motoring up the path

The brain stem is beneath the diencephalon and is divided into the midbrain, pons, and medulla. The brain stem contains the nuclei for cranial nerves III through XII. It relays messages between the cerebrum and diencephalon and the

Darn! My hypothalamus must be on the fritz again!

spinal cord; it also regulates automatic body functions, such as heart rate, breathing, swallowing, and coughing.

At the back of the brain

At the back of the brain, the cerebellum consists of two hemispheres. It facilitates smooth, coordinated muscle movement and equilibrium.

Spinal cord

The spinal cord is the primary path for nerve impulses traveling between peripheral areas of the body and the brain. It also contains the sensory-to-motor pathway known as the *reflex arc*. A reflex arc is the route followed by nerve impulses to and from the CNS in the production of a reflex action. (See *Understanding the reflex arc*.)

Where it is and what it's got

The spinal cord extends from the upper border of the first cervical vertebra to the lower border of the first lumbar vertebra. It's encased by meninges, the same membrane structure as the brain, and is protected by the bony vertebrae of the spine. The spinal cord is made up of an H-shaped mass of gray matter, divided into the dorsal (posterior) and ventral (anterior) horns. White matter surrounds the horns.

What matter, white matter?

Dorsal white matter contains ascending tracts that transmit impulses up the spinal cord to higher sensory centers. Ventral white matter contains descending motor tracts that transmit motor impulses down from the higher motor centers to the spinal cord.

Mapping the nerves

Sensory (afferent) nerve fibers originate in the nerve roots along the spine — cervical, thoracic, lumbar, or sacral — and supply specific areas of the skin. These areas, known as *dermatomes*, provide a nerve "map" of the body and help when testing sensation to determine the location of a lesion.

Peripheral nervous system

The peripheral nervous system includes the peripheral and cranial nerves. Peripheral sensory nerves transmit stimuli from sensory receptors in the skin, muscles, sensory organs, and viscera to the

A closer look

Understanding the reflex arc

Spinal nerves have sensory and motor portions and control deep tendon and superficial reflexes. A simple reflex arc requires a sensory (afferent) neuron and a motor (efferent) neuron. The knee-jerk or patellar reflex illustrates the sequence of events in a normal reflex arc.

First, a sensory receptor detects the mechanical stimulus produced by the reflex hammer striking the patellar tendon. The sensory neuron carries the impulse along its axon by way of the spinal nerve to the dorsal root, where it enters the spinal column.

Next, in the anterior horn of the spinal cord, shown here, the sensory neuron joins with a motor neuron, which carries the impulse along its axon by way of a spinal nerve to the muscle. The motor neuron transmits the impulse to the muscle fibers through stimulation of the motor end plate. This triggers the muscle contraction that extends the leg. *Don't stand directly in front of a patient when testing this reflex!*

Patellar reflex arc

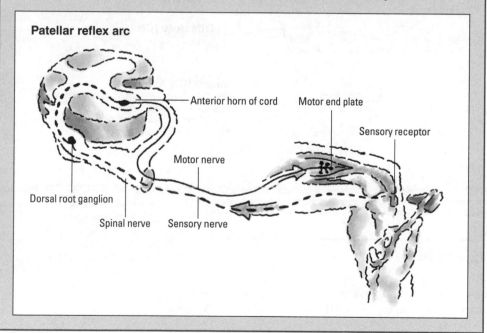

dorsal horn of the spinal cord. The upper motor neurons of the brain and the lower motor neurons of cell bodies in the ventral horn of the spinal cord carry impulses that affect movement. The 12 pairs of cranial nerves are the primary motor and sensory paths in the brain, head, and neck. (See *Identifying cranial nerves,* page 100.)

Identifying cranial nerves

Each cranial nerve (CN) has sensory function, motor function, or both. Although each cranial nerve has a name, it's also identified by Roman numerals, which are written this way: CN I, CN II, CN III, and so forth. The illustration here shows the location and functions of each cranial nerve.

Oculomotor (CN III)
Most eye movement, pupillary constriction, upper eyelid elevation

Facial (CN VII)
Expressions in forehead, eye, and mouth; taste

Trochlear (CN IV)
Down and in eye movement

Optic (CN II)
Vision

Acoustic (CN VIII)
Hearing, balance

Abducent (CN VI)
Lateral eye movement

Olfactory (CN I)
Smell

Trigeminal (CN V)
Chewing, corneal reflex, face and scalp sensations

Glossopharyngeal (CN IX)
Swallowing, salivating, taste

Vagus (CN X)
Swallowing, gag reflex, talking; sensations of throat, larynx, and abdominal viscera; activities of thoracic and abdominal viscera, such as heart rate and peristalsis

Hypoglossal (CN XII)
Tongue movement

Accessory (CN XI)
Shoulder movement, head rotation

Autonomic nervous system

The autonomic nervous system contains motor neurons that regulate visceral organs and innervate (supply nerves to) smooth and cardiac muscles and the glands. This nervous system has two parts:

the sympathetic portion, which controls fight-or-flight responses

the parasympathetic portion, which maintains baseline body functions.

My friends and I make up the autonomic nervous system and help control visceral organs as well as some muscles and glands.

Assessing neurologic function

Conducting an assessment for possible neurologic impairment includes a thorough health history and an investigation of physical signs of impairment.

History

Begin by asking the patient why he's seeking care at this time. Gather details about his current health, previous health, family health, and lifestyle. Also, perform a systems review. It's best to include members of the patient's family in the assessment process, if they're available, or a close friend. If the patient does have neurologic impairment, he may have trouble remembering or remembering accurately. Family or friends can help corroborate or correct the details.

Document in the patient's own words his chief complaint.

Current health status

Discover the patient's chief complaint by asking such questions as, "Why have you come to the hospital?" or "What has been bothering you lately?" Using his words, document his reasons for seeking care. If he's suffering a neurologic disorder, you can expect reports of headaches, motor disturbances (including weakness, paresis, and paralysis), seizures, sensory deviations, or an altered level of consciousness (LOC).

Ask and you will *perceive*

Encourage the patient, or a family member, to elaborate on his current condition by asking such questions as:
• Do you have headaches? If so, how often? What precipitates them?
• Do you feel dizzy from time to time? If so, how often and what seems to precipitate the episodes?
• Do you ever feel a tingling or prickling sensation or numbness? If so, where?
• Have you ever had seizures or tremors? How about weakness or paralysis in your arms or legs?
• Do you have trouble urinating? Walking?
• How's your memory and ability to concentrate?
• Have you had trouble speaking or understanding others?
• Do you have trouble reading or writing?

Previous health status

Many chronic diseases can affect the neurologic system, so ask the patient what medications, if any, he's taking as well as questions about his past health. Specifically, ask if he has had any:

- major illnesses
- recurrent minor illnesses
- accidents
- injuries
- surgical procedures
- allergies.

Chronic diseases can affect the neurologic system, so investigate any health conditions or medications the patient is taking.

Family health status

Information about the patient's family may reveal a hereditary disorder. Ask if anyone in his family has had diabetes, cardiac or renal disease, high blood pressure, cancer, a bleeding disorder, a mental disorder, or a stroke.

Lifestyle patterns

The patient's cultural and social background will affect decisions about his care, so ask questions about these facets of his life. Also, note the patient's education level, occupation, drug use, and hobbies. As you gather this information, assess the patient's self-image as well.

Physical examination

A complete neurologic examination is so long and detailed that — as a medical-surgical nurse — you'll probably never perform one in its entirety. Instead, you'll rely on a brief neurologic assessment, called a "neuro-check," which involves frequent evaluations of key neurologic status indicators, including:

- LOC
- pupil size and response
- verbal responsiveness
- extremity strength and movement
- vital signs.

When baseline values are established, regular reevaluation of these indicators will reveal trends in the patient's neurologic function and help detect the transient changes that may signal pending problems.

Because a complete neurologic assessment is so long, med-surg nurses will more commonly conduct a neuro-check.

In more detail

If the initial assessment suggests that the patient has an existing neurologic problem, a more detailed assessment is warranted. Always examine the patient's neurologic system in an orderly fashion. Begin with the highest levels of neurologic function and proceed to the lowest, covering these five areas:

 mental status (cerebral function)

 cranial nerve function

 sensory function

 motor function

reflexes.

When it comes to neurologic assessment, evaluate my highest functions first!

Mental status

Develop a sense of the patient's mental status as you talk with him during the health history. Listen and watch for clues to his orientation and memory. If you have doubts about his mental status, perform a brief screening examination. (See *Quick check of mental status*, page 104.)

Stop, look, and listen

Assessing mental status involves evaluating the patient's LOC, appearance, behavior, speech, cognitive function, and constructional ability.

• *Level of consciousness.* A change in LOC is the earliest and most sensitive indicator that neurologic status has changed. The Glasgow Coma Scale is one objective way to assess the patient's LOC. (See *Using the Glasgow Coma Scale*, page 105.)

• *Appearance and behavior.* Note the patient's behavior, dress, and grooming. Even subtle changes in behavior can signal the onset of chronic disease or an acute change involving the frontal lobe.

• *Speech.* Listen to how well the patient expresses himself. His ability to follow instructions and cooperate with the examination will provide clues about his level of comprehension.

• *Cognitive function.* Evaluate the patient's memory, orientation, attention span, thought content, ability to perform calculations, capacity for abstract thought, judgment, and emotional status.

• *Constructional ability.* Assess the patient's ability to perform simple tasks and use common objects.

An alteration in the patient's LOC is the earliest sign of a change in his neurologic status.

Quick check of mental status

You can get a quick idea of how well the patient organizes his thoughts by asking the questions below. An incorrect answer to any question may indicate the need for a more thorough examination of mental status. Be sure you know the correct answers before asking the questions.

Question	Function screened
What's your name?	Orientation to person
What's today's date?	Orientation to time
What year is it?	Orientation to time
Where are you now?	Orientation to place
How old are you?	Memory
Where were you born?	Remote memory
What did you have for breakfast?	Recent memory
Who's the U.S. president?	General knowledge
Can you count backward from 20 to 1?	Attention and calculation skills
Why are you here?	Judgment

Cranial nerves

Cranial nerve assessment provides valuable information about the status of the CNS, particularly the brain stem.

Getting on your nerves

Due to their location, the optic, oculomotor, trochlear, and abducens nerves are more vulnerable to an increase in intracranial pressure (ICP) than other cranial nerves. For this reason, assessment and screening focuses on these four nerves. However, if the patient's history or symptoms indicate a potential cranial nerve disorder, or a complete nervous system assessment is ordered, assess all cranial nerves.

Using the Glasgow Coma Scale

The Glasgow Coma Scale provides an easy way to describe a patient's baseline mental status and to help detect and interpret changes from baseline findings. To use the scale, test the patient's ability to respond to verbal, motor, and sensory stimulation and grade your findings according to the scale. If a patient is alert, can follow simple commands, and is oriented to person, place, and time, his score will total 15 points, the highest possible score. A low score in one or more categories may signal an impending neurologic crisis. A score of 7 or less indicates severe neurologic damage.

Test	Score	Patient's response
Eye opening response		
Spontaneously	4	Opens eyes spontaneously
To speech	3	Opens eyes when told to
To pain	2	Opens eyes only on painful stimulus
None	1	Doesn't open eyes in response to stimulus
Motor response		
Obeys	6	Shows two fingers when asked
Localizes	5	Reaches toward painful stimulus and tries to remove it
Withdraws	4	Moves away from painful stimulus
Abnormal flexion	3	Assumes a decorticate posture (below)

Abnormal extension	2	Assumes a decerebrate posture (below)

None	1	No response; just lies flaccid (an ominous sign)
Verbal response		
Oriented	5	Tells correct date
Confused	4	Tells incorrect year
Inappropriate words	3	Replies randomly with incorrect words
Incomprehensible	2	Moans or screams
No response	1	No response

Total score ☐

Sensory function

Sensory function assessment helps reveal problems related to:
• stimuli detection by sensory receptors
• sensory impulse transmission to the spinal cord by afferent nerves
• sensory impulse transmission to the brain by sensory tracts in the spinal cord.

Few and light

Typically, screening consists of evaluating light-touch sensation in all extremities and comparing arms and legs for symmetry of sensation. Some experts also recommend evaluating the patient's sense of pain and vibration in the hands and feet and his ability to recognize objects by touch (stereognosis). Because the sensory system becomes fatigued with repeated stimulation, complete sensory system testing in all dermatomes tends to yield unreliable results. Usually, a few screening procedures are sufficient to reveal dysfunction.

Wait! I'm receiving a sensory impulse... I think it's telling me to... um... oh, yes! Lift, lift!

Motor function

Assessing the motor system includes inspecting the muscles and testing muscle tone and strength. Cerebellar testing is also done because the cerebellum plays a role in smooth-muscle movements, such as tics, tremors, or fasciculations.

Tone up

Muscle tone represents muscular resistance to passive stretching. To test arm muscle tone, move the shoulder through passive range-of-motion (ROM) exercises. You should feel a slight resistance. Then let the arm drop to the patient's side. It should fall easily.

   To test muscle tone in a leg, guide the hip through passive ROM exercises; then let the leg fall to the bed. If it falls into an externally rotated position, this is an abnormal finding.

Strength and symmetry

To perform a general examination of muscle strength, observe the patient's gait and motor activities. To evaluate muscle strength, ask the patient to move major muscles and muscle groups against resistance. For instance, to test shoulder girdle strength, have him extend his arms with his palms up and maintain this position for 30 seconds.

Let the arm drop to the patient's side, which should fall easily — the arm, that is — not the patient!

If he can't maintain this position, test further by pushing down on his outstretched arms. If he lifts both arms equally, look for pronation of the hand and downward drift of the arm on the weaker side.

Heel to toe for the cerebellum

Cerebellar function is evaluated by testing the patient's balance and coordination. Ask the patient to walk heel to toe, and observe his balance. Then perform Romberg's test. (See *Romberg's test.*)

Reflexes

Reflex assessment is usually performed as part of a comprehensive neurologic assessment. It evaluates deep tendon and superficial reflexes to determine:
• the integrity of the sensory receptor organ
• how effective afferent nerves are in relaying sensory impulses to the spinal cord
• how effectively the lower motor neurons transmit impulses to the muscles
• how well the muscles respond to the motor impulses.

Deep or superficial?

Deep tendon reflexes (muscle-stretch reflexes) occur when deep muscles stretch in response to a sudden stimulus. Superficial reflexes (cutaneous reflexes) can be elicited by light, rapid tactile stimulation, such as stroking or scratching the skin. Sometimes called *primitive reflexes*, pathologic superficial reflexes usually occur in early infancy and then disappear as time passes. When present in adults, they usually indicate an underlying neurologic disease.

Diagnostic tests

Nervous system evaluation typically includes imaging studies, angiography, and electrophysiologic studies. Keep in mind that while these tests may be routine for you, they can be frightening for the patient. It's important to carefully prepare the patient for each procedure because stress and anxiety can affect test results.

Imaging studies

The most common imaging studies used to detect neurologic disorders include:
• computed tomography (CT) scan

Romberg's test

Observe the patient's balance as he stands with his eyes open, feet together, and arms at his sides. Then ask him to close his eyes. Hold your arms out on either side of him to protect him if he sways. If he falls to one side, the result of Romberg's test is positive.

- isotope brain scan
- magnetic resonance imaging (MRI)
- positron emission tomography (PET)
- skull and spinal X-rays.

Computed tomography scan

CT scanning combines radiology and computer analysis of tissue density (determined by contrast dye absorption) to study intracranial structures. Although CT doesn't show blood vessels as well as an angiogram, it carries less risk of complications and causes less trauma than cerebral angiography.

A scan for all seasons

A CT scan of the spine helps the doctor to assess spinal disorders, such as a herniated disk, spinal cord tumors, and spinal stenosis. A CT scan of the brain can help detect:
- brain contusion
- brain calcifications
- cerebral atrophy
- hydrocephalus
- inflammation
- space-occupying lesions (tumors, hematomas, abscesses)
- vascular anomalies (arteriovenous malformations [AVMs], infarctions, blood clots, hemorrhage).

Nursing considerations

- Confirm that the patient isn't allergic to iodine or shellfish. (A patient with these allergies may have an adverse reaction to the contrast medium.)
- If the test calls for a contrast medium, explain that an I.V. catheter will be inserted for injection of the contrast medium.
- Explain to the patient that he may feel flushed or notice a metallic taste in his mouth when the contrast medium is injected (if used).
- Tell him that the CT scanner will circle around him for 10 to 30 minutes (depending on the procedure and type of equipment) and that he must lie still during the test.

Good to go

- Encourage the patient to resume normal activities and a regular diet after the test.
- Explain that the contrast medium may discolor his urine for 24 hours, and suggest that he drink more fluids to help flush this medium out of his system.

A CT scan may not show blood vessels as well as an angiogram, but it sure is nicer on me!

Encourage the patient to drink more fluids to help flush the contrast medium out of his system.

Isotope brain scan

In this procedure, a scanning device monitors the brain's uptake of a radioactive isotope, such as technetium-99m pertechnetate. Damaged brain tissue absorbs more of the isotope than healthy tissue (probably due to an abnormally permeable blood-brain barrier). While the brain scan can locate cerebral lesions and determine their size, it doesn't reveal the cause — for example, whether it's caused by a tumor, cerebral edema, an infarction, a hematoma, or an abscess.

Make sure that the patient doesn't have allergies to iodine or shellfish to minimize the risk of an adverse reaction to the contrast medium.

Nursing considerations

• Withhold medications, as ordered.
• Confirm that the patient isn't allergic to iodine or shellfish. (A patient with these allergies may have an adverse reaction to the contrast medium.)
• Explain that an I.V. catheter will be inserted for injection of the contrast medium.
• Tell him that he'll be asked to change position several times during the procedure while a technician takes pictures of his brain.
• Unless contraindicated, suggest that he drink more fluids to help flush the contrast medium out of his system.

Magnetic resonance imaging

MRI generates detailed pictures of body structures. The test may involve the use of a contrast medium such as gadolinium.

Feeling superior

Compared with conventional X-rays and CT scans, MRI provides superior contrast of soft tissues, sharply differentiating healthy, benign, and cancerous tissue and clearly revealing blood vessels. In addition, MRI permits imaging in multiple planes, including sagittal and coronal views in regions where bones normally hamper visualization. MRI is especially useful for studying the CNS because it can detect the structural and biochemical abnormalities associated with such conditions as transient ischemic attacks (TIAs), tumors, multiple sclerosis (MS), cerebral edema, and hydrocephalus.

Diagnostic procedures can be frightening. Take time to discuss each test with the patient and explain how long each test could take.

Nursing considerations

• Explain to the patient that the procedure can take up to 1½ hours and that he'll have to remain still for intervals of 5 to 20 minutes.

• Have the patient remove all metallic items, such as hair clips, bobby pins, jewelry (including body piercing jewelry), watches, eyeglasses, hearing aids, or dentures.
• Explain that the test is painless, but the machinery may seem loud and frightening and the tunnel confining. Tell the patient that he'll receive earplugs for the noise.
• Provide sedation, as ordered, to promote relaxation during the test.
• Encourage the patient to resume normal activities, as ordered.

Positron emission tomography

PET provides colorimetric information about the brain's metabolic activity by detecting how quickly tissues consume radioactive isotopes. This technology can help reveal cerebral dysfunction associated with tumors, seizures, TIAs, head trauma, some mental illnesses, Alzheimer's disease, Parkinson's disease, and MS. In addition, a PET scan can help evaluate the effect of drug therapy and neurosurgery.

Inject, scan, and translate

In PET, a technician administers a radioactive gas or an I.V. injection of glucose (or another biochemical substance) tagged with isotopes, which act as tracers. The isotopes emit positrons that combine with negatively charged electrons in tissue cells to create gamma rays. After the scanner registers the gamma rays, a computer translates the information into patterns that reflect cerebral blood flow, blood volume, and neuron and neurotransmitter metabolism.

A PET scan may not involve these guys, but it helps reveal cerebral dysfunction related to many disorders and evaluates the effect of drug therapy and surgery.

Nursing considerations

• Assure the patient that the test won't expose him to dangerous levels of radiation.
• Explain that the test may require insertion of an I.V. catheter.
• Encourage the patient to resume normal activities, as ordered.

Skull and spinal X-rays

Typically, the skull X-ray is taken from two angles: anteroposterior (AP) and lateral. The doctor may also order other angles, including Waters' view to examine the frontal and maxillary sinuses, facial bones, and eye orbits and Towne's view to examine the occipital bone. Skull X-rays help detect:
• fractures
• bony tumors or unusual calcifications
• pineal displacement (indicates a space-occupying lesion)

- skull or sella turcica erosion (indicates a space-occupying lesion)
- vascular abnormalities.

Is your spine fine?

If the doctor suspects spinal disease or an injury to the cervical, thoracic, lumbar, or sacral vertebral segments, he may order AP and lateral spinal X-rays. Depending on the patient's condition, he may also order special angles such as the open-mouth view (to confirm odontoid fracture). Spinal X-rays help detect:
- spinal fracture
- displacement and subluxation (partial dislocation)
- destructive lesions (such as primary and metastatic bone tumors)
- arthritic changes or spondylolisthesis
- structural abnormalities (such as kyphosis, scoliosis, and lordosis)
- congenital abnormalities.

Nursing considerations

- Reassure the patient that X-rays are painless.
- Administer an analgesic before the procedure, as ordered, if the patient has existing pain so he'll be more comfortable.
- Remove a cervical collar if cervical X-rays reveal that no fracture is present and the doctor permits it.
- Encourage the patient to resume normal activities, as ordered.

The X-rays won't cause any pain.

Angiographic studies

Angiographic studies include cerebral angiography and digital subtraction angiography (DSA).

Cerebral angiography

For cerebral angiography, the doctor injects a radiopaque contrast medium, usually into the brachial artery (through retrograde brachial injection) or the femoral artery (through catheterization). This procedure highlights cerebral vessels, making it easier to:
- detect stenosis or occlusion associated with thrombi or spasms
- identify aneurysms and AVMs
- locate vessel displacement associated with tumors, abscesses, cerebral edema, hematoma, or herniation
- assess collateral circulation.

Nursing considerations

• Explain the procedure to the patient and answer his questions.
• Confirm that he isn't allergic to iodine or shellfish. (A patient with these allergies may have an adverse reaction to the contrast medium.)
• Tell him that he'll need to lie still during the procedure.

Feel the burn

• Explain that he'll probably feel a flushed sensation in his face as the dye is injected.
• Maintain bed rest, as ordered, and monitor his vital signs.
• Monitor the catheter injection site for signs of bleeding.
• As ordered, keep a sandbag over the injection site.
• Monitor the patient's peripheral pulse in the arm or leg used for catheter insertion (mark the site).
• Unless contraindicated, encourage the patient to drink more fluids to help flush the dye from his system.
• Monitor the patient for neurologic changes and such complications as hemiparesis, hemiplegia, aphasia, and impaired LOC.
• Monitor for an adverse reaction to the contrast medium, which may include restlessness, tachypnea and respiratory distress, tachycardia, facial flushing, urticaria, and nausea and vomiting.

Digital subtraction angiography

Like cerebral angiography, DSA highlights cerebral blood vessels. Using a special type of computerized fluoroscopy, a technician takes an image of the selected area, which is then stored in the computer's memory. After administering a contrast medium, the technician takes several more images. By manipulating the two sets of images, the computer produces high-resolution images for interpretation. Although arterial DSA requires more contrast medium than cerebral angiography, because it's injected I.V., DSA doesn't increase the patient's risk of stroke and can be performed on an outpatient basis.

Nursing considerations

• Confirm that the patient isn't allergic to iodine or shellfish. (A patient with these allergies may have an adverse reaction to the contrast medium.)
• Restrict the patient's consumption of solid foods for 4 hours before the test.
• Explain that the test requires insertion of an I.V. catheter.
• Tell him that he must remain still during the test.
• Explain that he'll probably feel a flush or have a metallic taste in his mouth as the contrast medium is injected.

DSA highlights blood vessels like cerebral angiography, but can be performed on an outpatient basis.

• Tell the patient to alert the doctor immediately if he feels discomfort or shortness of breath.
• After the catheter is removed, encourage the patient to resume his normal activities.
• Encourage him to drink more fluids for the rest of the day to help flush the contrast medium out of his system.

Electrophysiologic studies

Electrophysiologic studies are commonly performed and include EEG and electromyography.

Electroencephalography

By recording the brain's continuous electrical activity, EEG can help identify seizure disorders, head injuries, intracranial lesions (such as abscesses and tumors), TIAs, stroke, or brain death. In EEG, electrodes attached to standard areas of the patient's scalp record a portion of the brain's activity. These electrical impulses are transmitted to an electroencephalogram, which magnifies them 1 million times and records them as brain waves on moving strips of paper.

> EEG records my electrical activity. I guess that means... I'm electric! Do do do do do do do do do....

Nursing considerations

• Tell the patient that during the EEG, he'll be positioned comfortably in a reclining chair or on a bed.
• Explain that a technician will apply paste and attach electrodes to areas of skin on the patient's head and neck after these areas have been lightly abraded to ensure good contact.
• Explain that he must remain still throughout the test.
• Discuss any specific activity that the patient will be asked to perform, such as hyperventilating for 3 minutes or sleeping, depending on the purpose of the EEG.
• Use acetone to remove any remaining paste from the patient's skin.
• Encourage him to resume his normal activities, as ordered.

> Help reduce the patient's anxiety by discussing the procedure thoroughly ahead of time.

Electromyography

Electromyography records a muscle's electrical impulses to help distinguish lower motor neuron disorders from muscle disorders—for example, amyotrophic lateral sclerosis (ALS) from muscular dystrophy. It also helps evaluate neuromuscular disorders such as myasthenia gravis. In this test, a needle electrode is inserted percutaneously into a muscle.

The muscle's electrical discharge is then displayed and measured on an oscilloscope screen.

Nursing considerations

- Tell the patient that the test may take 1 hour to complete and that he may be asked to sit or lie down during the procedure.
- Warn him that he'll probably feel some discomfort when the doctor inserts a needle attached to an electrode into his muscle and when a mild electrical charge is delivered to the muscle.
- Explain that he must remain still during the test except when asked to contract or relax a muscle.
- Explain that an amplifier may emit crackling noises whenever his muscle moves.
- Encourage him to resume his normal activities, as ordered.

Treatments

The most common treatments for neurologic disorders are drug therapy and surgery.

Drug therapy

Drug therapy is a common and important treatment for neurologic disorders. When caring for a patient undergoing drug therapy, you'll need to be alert for severe adverse reactions and for interactions with other drugs. Some drugs, such as barbiturates, also carry a high risk of toxicity.

Keep in mind that drug therapy's success hinges on the patient's strict adherence to his medication schedule. Compliance is especially critical for drugs that require steady-state blood levels for therapeutic effectiveness, such as anticonvulsants, or for drugs used prophylactically such as beta-adrenergic blockers. (See *Drugs used to treat neurologic disorders*.)

Surgery

Surgery is commonly the only viable intervention when a neurologic disorder is life-threatening. Surgical procedures typically used to treat neurologic disorders include cerebellar stimulator implantation, cerebral aneurysm repair, craniotomy, and intracranial hematoma aspiration. As a medical-surgical nurse, you should prepare to handle the patient's preoperative assessment and preparation and postoperative care.

Med-surg nurses prepare patients for surgery — physically and emotionally.

Drugs used to treat neurologic disorders

This chart lists the most common classes of drugs used to treat neurologic disorders and includes several examples of each.

Drug classification	Examples
Adrenergic blockers	Dihydroergotamine mesylate, ergotamine tartrate
Anticonvulsants	Carbamazepine, clonazepam, diazepam, ethosuximide, fosphenytoin, gabapentin, lamotrigine, phenobarbital, phenytoin, primidone, valproate
Antiparkinson agents	Benztropine, carbidopa-levodopa, levodopa, pergolide, pramipexole, ropinirole, selegiline, tolcapone, trihexyphenidyl
Calcium channel blockers	Nimodipine
Corticosteroids	Dexamethasone, prednisone
Diuretics	Mannitol
Opioid analgesics	Codeine, meperidine, morphine
Skeletal muscle relaxants	Baclofen, dantrolene
Vasodilators	Clopidogrel, dipyridamole

Questions, concerns, fears

When confronted with surgery, the patient and his family usually have questions, concerns, and fears that require compassionate attention. Keep in mind that a patient requiring surgery to address a neurologic disorder may be left with deficits that can be frustrating and embarrassing for him and his family. A positive, caring attitude and support can help them cope with their ordeal.

Cerebellar stimulator implantation

Cerebellar stimulator implantation positions two electrodes in the patient's cerebellum. The electrodes are connected to a power source and pulse generator, which may be internal or external. The generator sends electrical impulses to

Let's talk about what questions or concerns you have about surgery.

the electrodes, which stimulate nerve fibers in the cerebellar cortex. These electrical impulses help regulate uncoordinated neuromuscular activity. Although this procedure was originally developed to prevent seizures in patients who were unresponsive to drug therapy, it usually improves neuromuscular control in patients with cerebral palsy.

Slow bennies

Benefits for the patient may include a reduction in spasticity and abnormal movements, improved muscle and sphincter control, clearer speech, and a decreased number of seizures. However, not every patient experiences improvement and it can be slow in coming, commonly taking months or years to manifest.

Patient preparation
• Describe the implantation procedure in understandable terms.
• Explain that the patient will receive general anesthesia and that an anesthesiologist will meet with him before the procedure to describe the medication he'll receive.

The razor's edge

• Tell the patient that his head will be shaved and positioned in a special headrest for the operation.
• Explain that the surgeon will make four incisions for implanting the electrodes and system components, two on the head, one on the neck, and one on the abdomen.
• Discuss postoperative care, including medication, activity and fluid restrictions, progressive ambulation, and antibiotic therapy.
• Assure the patient and his family that he'll be closely monitored to evaluate the device's effectiveness.

Monitoring and aftercare
• Assess the patient's neurologic status and vital signs every hour for the first 24 hours, then every 2 hours for the next few days.
• Watch for signs of complications, such as increased ICP, infection, and fluid imbalance.
• Provide I.V. fluids as ordered if the patient experiences excessive nausea and vomiting due to cerebellar manipulation.
• Observe for seizures or spasticity, and record occurrences to help the doctor evaluate the device's effectiveness.
• Keep the patient on bed rest until the 2nd postoperative day. Elevate his head 15 to 30 degrees, and turn him every 2 hours.
• Slowly increase the patient's activities, but make sure he avoids overexertion. Excessive activity can cause pooling of serous fluid or cerebrospinal fluid (CSF) in the subcutaneous pocket that holds part of the unit, which can damage the equipment.

I.V. fluids may help the patient who experiences excessive nausea and vomiting after cerebellar manipulation.

• Check the patient's dressings regularly for excessive bleeding or drainage, and change them as necessary. Assess suture lines for signs of infection and provide wound care.
• Administer antibiotics and analgesics, as ordered, but don't give the patient sedatives for sleep; they may skew neurologic findings.

Home care instructions

• Explain that the patient can gradually resume his normal routine, but caution against excessive physical activity.
• Teach the patient and his family how to change a dressing and recommend that they change it about once every 2 days until the surgeon removes the sutures (usually 2 weeks after surgery). Teach them how to care for the wound and suture lines as well.
• Describe the signs of infection, such as fever and swelling or redness along the sutures or subcutaneous pocket, and explain the importance of reporting any sign promptly.
• Explain the need to record the time, type, and duration of seizures to help the doctor evaluate the effectiveness of the cerebellar stimulator.
• Impress upon the patient that follow-up appointments are important to check on the patient's health and the operation of the device.

Cerebral aneurysm repair

Surgical intervention is the only sure method for preventing rupture or rebleeding of a cerebral aneurysm. First, a craniotomy is performed to expose the aneurysm. Then, there are several corrective techniques the surgeon may use, depending on the shape and location of the aneurysm. He can clamp the affected artery, wrap the aneurysm wall with a biological or synthetic material, or clip or ligate the aneurysm. (See *Aneurysm clip*, page 118.)

Patient preparation

• Tell the patient and his family that he'll be monitored in the intensive care unit (ICU) before and after surgery, where he'll be observed for signs of vasospasm, bleeding, and elevated intracranial pressure.
• Explain that he'll return to the medical-surgical unit for further care when his condition is stable.

Monitoring and aftercare

• Gradually increase the patient's level of activity, as ordered.
• Monitor the incision for signs of infection or drainage.
• Monitor the patient's neurologic status and vital signs, and report acute changes immediately. Watch for increased ICP: pupil changes, weakness in extremities, headache, and a change in LOC.

Surgery is the only sure way to prevent rupture or rebleeding of a cerebral aneurysm. I'm sold!

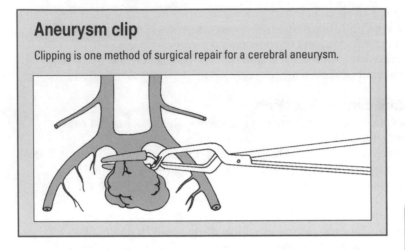

Aneurysm clip

Clipping is one method of surgical repair for a cerebral aneurysm.

After surgery, help the patient and family cope with residual neurologic deficits.

• Provide the patient and his family with emotional support as they cope with residual neurologic deficits.

Home care instructions
• Teach the patient or family member proper wound care techniques and how to evaluate the incision regularly for redness, warmth, or tenderness, and to report any occurrence to the doctor immediately.

Dazed and confused
• Remind the patient to continue taking prescribed anticonvulsant medications to minimize the risk of seizures. Depending on the type of surgery performed, he may need to continue anticonvulsant therapy for up to 12 months after surgery. Also, tell him to notify his doctor of any adverse drug reactions such as excessive drowsiness or confusion.
• Emphasize the importance of returning for scheduled follow-up examinations and tests.
• Refer the patient and his family for appropriate home care or support groups.

Craniotomy

Craniotomy involves creation of a surgical incision into the skull to expose the brain for various treatments, such as ventricular shunting, excision of a tumor or abscess, hematoma aspiration, and aneurysm clipping. Craniotomy has many potential complications, including infection, hemorrhage, respiratory compromise, and increased ICP. The degree of risk depends on the patient's condition and the surgery's complexity.

Patient preparation

• Answer questions the family may have about the procedure to help reduce confusion and anxiety and help them cope.
• Explain that the patient's head will be shaved.
• Discuss the recovery period so the patient understands what to expect. Explain that he'll awaken with a dressing on his head to protect the incision and may have a surgical drain as well.
• Tell him to expect a headache and facial swelling for 2 to 3 days after surgery, and reassure him that he'll receive pain medication.
• Perform and document a baseline neurologic assessment.
• Explain that the patient will go to the ICU after surgery for close monitoring.

Monitoring and aftercare

• Gradually increase the patient's level of activity, as ordered.
• Monitor the incision site for signs of infection or drainage.
• Monitor the patient's neurologic status and vital signs, and report any acute change immediately. Watch for signs of increased ICP, such as pupil changes, weakness in extremities, headache, and change in LOC.
• Provide the patient and his family with emotional support as they cope with residual neurologic deficits.

Home care Instructions

• Teach the patient or family member proper wound care techniques and how to evaluate the incision regularly for redness, warmth, or tenderness and report occurrences to the doctor.
• Remind the patient to continue taking prescribed anticonvulsant medications to minimize the risk of seizures. Depending on the type of surgery performed, he may need to continue anticonvulsant therapy for up to 12 months after surgery. Also, remind him to report any adverse drug reactions, such as excessive drowsiness or confusion.
• Emphasize the importance of returning for scheduled follow-up examinations and tests.
• Refer the patient and his family for home care or support groups as appropriate.

Intracranial hematoma aspiration

In intracranial hematoma aspiration, an epidural, subdural, or intracerebral hematoma is aspirated with a small suction tip. This suction tip is inserted through burr holes in the skull (for a fluid hematoma) or through a craniotomy (for a solid clot or a liquid one that can't be aspirated through burr holes).

Okay, here I am. Do what you gotta do — shunt, excise, aspirate, clip — whatever.

Depending on surgery type, the patient may need to continue anticonvulsants for up to 12 months after surgery.

What do I do?

Emergency intracranial hematoma aspiration

An intracranial hematoma (epidural, subdural, or intracerebral) commonly requires immediate, lifesaving surgery to lower intracranial pressure. Even if the patient's life isn't in immediate danger, timely surgery remains the only viable option for preventing irreversible damage from cerebral or brain stem ischemia.

When emergency aspiration is necessary, tailor your patient preparation to the time available. Start with a brief, succinct description of the procedure. As time allows, cover these additional points:

• Clarify the surgeon's explanation, if necessary, and ask the patient if he has any questions. Provide clear, concise answers.

• Tell the patient that his head will be shaved for the procedure.

• Explain that after surgery, he'll awaken with a dressing on his head to protect the incision and may have a surgical drain in place.

• Tell him he'll probably have a headache and swollen face for 2 to 3 days after surgery.

• Reassure him that he'll receive pain medication.

• Explain that he'll be in the intensive care unit after surgery for close monitoring.

• Perform a baseline neurologic assessment.

It's complicated

Patients undergoing hematoma aspiration risk severe infection and seizures as well as physiologic problems associated with immobility during the prolonged recovery period. Even if hematoma removal proves successful, associated head injuries and other complications, such as cerebral edema, can produce permanent neurologic deficits, coma, or even death. (See *Emergency intracranial hematoma aspiration*.)

What you can do

Patient preparation, monitoring and aftercare, and home care instructions are the same as those for cerebral aneurysm repair.

Hematoma aspiration carries significant risks — during and after the procedure. What are you thinking?

I'm thinking that I'm not going to think about that.

Nursing diagnoses

When caring for patients with neurologic disorders, certain nursing diagnoses are commonly used. When developing your care plan, keep in mind interventions to prevent the three most common complications in patients with neurologic disorders: respiratory infection, urinary tract infection (UTI), and infected pressure ulcers.

Impaired physical mobility

Impaired physical mobility can occur in ALS, cerebral palsy, stroke, MS, muscular dystrophy, myasthenia gravis, Parkinson's disease, poliomyelitis, or spinal cord injury.

Include interventions in your care plan to prevent common neurologic disorder complications: respiratory, urinary tract, and pressure ulcer infection.

Expected outcomes

• The patient will show no evidence of complications, such as contractures, venous stasis, thrombus formation or skin breakdown.
• The patient will achieve the highest level of mobility possible.
• The patient will maintain muscle strength and joint ROM.

Nursing interventions and rationales

• Have the patient perform ROM exercises at least once every shift, unless contraindicated. Progress from passive to active exercises, as tolerated. This prevents joint contractures and muscular atrophy.
• Turn and position the dependent patient every 2 hours. Establish a turning schedule, post this schedule at the bedside, and monitor the frequency of turning. Turning prevents skin breakdown by relieving pressure.
• Place joints in functional positions (use hand splints if needed and available), use a trochanter roll along the thigh, abduct the thighs, use high-top sneakers, and put a small pillow under the patient's head. These measures maintain joints in a functional position and prevent musculoskeletal deformities.
• Identify the patient's level of functioning using a functional mobility scale. Communicate the patient's skill level to all staff members to provide continuity and preserve a specific level of independence.
• Encourage mobility independence by helping the patient use a trapeze and side rails to reposition himself; use his good leg to move his affected leg; and perform self-care activities, such as feeding and dressing, to increase muscle tone and build self-esteem.

Declaration of independence

• If one-sided weakness or paralysis is present, place items within reach of the patient's unaffected arm to promote independence.

• Monitor and record evidence of immobility complications (such as contractures, venous stasis, thrombus, pneumonia, and UTI) each day. The patient with a history of a neuromuscular disorder or dysfunction may be prone to complications.
• Promote progressive mobilization to the degree possible in light of the patient's condition (bed mobility to chair mobility to ambulation) to maintain muscle tone and prevent complications.
• Refer the patient to physical and occupational therapists for development of a mobility regimen to help rehabilitate the patient's musculoskeletal deficits. Request written mobility plans and use these as references.
• Teach the patient and his family about ROM exercises, transfers, skin inspection, and the mobility regimen to prepare the patient for discharge.
• Demonstrate the mobility regimen, and have the patient and his caregivers do a return demonstration and note the dates of both. This ensures continuity of care and correct completion.
• Help identify resources that will help the patient carry out the mobility regimen, such as Strokesurvivors International, the United Cerebral Palsy Associations, and the National Multiple Sclerosis Society, to help provide a comprehensive approach to rehabilitation.

Impaired physical mobility relates to a whole host of neurologic disorders.

Impaired skin integrity

Impaired skin integrity is a potential (and common) problem for anyone with a lower than normal level of activity. However, it can be deadly for a patient who can't turn or move by himself. Infected pressure ulcers are one of the primary causes of death in a patient with neurologic disease. Even when not infected, pressure ulcers still cause prolonged distress and adversely affect the patient's ability to function and his quality of life.

Expected outcomes
• The patient will maintain intact skin integrity.
• The patient won't develop complications, should skin breakdown occur.
• The patient will maintain the optimal nutrition needed to prevent skin breakdown.

Nursing interventions and rationales
• Turn and move the patient at least every 2 hours if he's unable to do so. Teach wheelchair patients to shift position sev-

Infected pressure ulcers are one of the primary causes of death for patients with neurologic disease.

eral times each hour; provide help if needed. Pressure reduces skin circulation very quickly, which is a precursor to breakdown.

Steering clear of breakdowns

- Use appropriate support surfaces, such as 4″ convoluted foam mattresses or gelmats. If the patient develops pressure ulcers, consult established guidelines and protocols to determine the proper supportive surfaces for the patient. Repositioning and proper support surfaces reduce pressure on skin and help prevent skin breakdown.
- Consult with an enterostomal therapist and published guidelines to determine preventive measures and interventions.
- Encourage optimal food and fluid intake to maintain skin health.

Impaired urinary elimination

Impaired urinary elimination is another of the major complications affecting patients with neurologic disorders. Many of these patients have bladder spasticity or are unable to empty their bladders fully or properly. UTIs are common and can lead to prolonged hospitalization or even death.

Expected outcomes

- The patient will empty his bladder completely and regularly.
- The patient won't develop a UTI.

Nursing interventions and rationales

- Use appropriate strategies for assessing adequacy of output and bladder emptying. Although regular emptying is essential to urinary tract health, the patient may be unable to do so or may be unable to sense whether or not he's completely emptying his bladder.
- Encourage the patient to drink plenty of fluids each day. Fluid intake is essential to the production of urine to clean the urinary tract and bladder.
- If the patient can't empty his bladder alone, use the least invasive strategies to improve bladder emptying. Start with such techniques as Credé's maneuver, in which the patient bends forward and presses on the bladder while urinating. Intermittent self-catheterization is more invasive, but less likely to cause infection than an indwelling urinary catheter.
- If the patient voids adequately but is incontinent, a condom catheter will help keep his skin dry, while being less

To help the patient improve bladder emptying, start with the least invasive techniques.

Running the water always worked for me.

likely than intermittent or indwelling urinary catheterization to cause infection.

Impaired gas exchange

Impaired gas exchange relates to the third most common complication for patients with neurologic disorders: respiratory infection.

Expected outcomes

• The patient won't develop a respiratory infection.
• The patient will maintain optimal oxygen saturation levels.

Nursing interventions and rationales

• If the patient is immobile or has impaired respiratory muscle function, encourage the use of incentive spirometry, deep breathing, and coughing several times per day. Deep breathing and coughing help prevent atelectasis, which can become a respiratory infection as secretions accumulate.
• Encourage fluid intake. Fluids keep respiratory secretions thin and easy to cough up.
• Discourage smoking and exposure to second-hand smoke that impair respiration and the body's ability to clear the lungs.
• Encourage adequate rest, exercise, and nutrition, which will help maintain the strength of respiratory muscles.

Toss me a line, would ya? Encourage fluid intake to keep respiratory secretions thin and easy to cough up.

Common neurologic disorders

Below are several common neurologic disorders, along with their causes, pathophysiology, signs and symptoms, diagnostic test findings, treatments, and nursing interventions.

Alzheimer's disease

Alzheimer's disease is a progressive neurologic disorder that affects the brain and results in cognitive impairments, such as impaired thinking, memory loss, and bizarre behavior. Alzheimer's disease is the most common form of dementia and the fourth leading cause of death in adults.

What causes it

The cause of Alzheimer's disease isn't known; however, several factors appear to have some association with the disease. These include:
- deficiencies in the neurotransmitters acetylcholine, somatostatin, substance P, and norepinephrine
- repeated head trauma
- abnormalities on chromosomes 14 or 21
- deposits of beta amyloid protein.

You don't have to be a brain to know that *atrophic* doesn't sound good!

Pathophysiology

The brain tissue of patients with Alzheimer's disease has three distinguishing features:

 neurofibrillatory tangles (fibrous proteins)

 amyloid plaques (composed of degenerating axons and dendrites)

granulovacuolar degeneration.

Autopsy commonly reveals an atrophic brain that can weigh 1,000 g or less. Normal brain weight is 1,380 g. (See *Brain tissue changes in Alzheimer's disease*, page 126.)

What to look for

The onset of Alzheimer's disease is insidious. Initial changes are almost imperceptible, but gradually progress to serious problems. Initial signs and symptoms include:
- forgetfulness and short-term memory loss
- difficulty learning and remembering new information
- deterioration in personal hygiene and appearance
- inability to concentrate.
    Later signs and symptoms include:
- difficulty with abstract thinking and activities that require judgment
- progressive difficulty communicating
- severe deterioration in memory, language, and motor function
- repetitive actions or perseveration (a key sign)
- nocturnal wakening, disorientation, and personality changes, such as restlessness and irritability.

Perseveration, or inappropriate repetition of a thought or act, is a key sign of Alzheimer's disease.

What tests tell you

- Psychometric testing and neurologic examination can help establish the diagnosis.

A closer look

Brain tissue changes in Alzheimer's disease

The brain tissue of patients with Alzheimer's disease exhibits three characteristic features:

• *neurofibrillatory tangles,* which are bundles of filaments (in neurons) that twist abnormally around one another. They're most numerous in areas of the brain associated with memory and learning, fear and aggression, and thinking.

• *amyloid plaques,* also known as senile plaques, are deposits found outside neurons in the extracellular space of the cerebral cortex and hippocampus. Amyloid plaques contain a core of beta amyloid protein surrounded by abnormal nerve endings, or neurites.

• *granulovacuolar degeneration,* or degeneration of neurons in the hippocampus, is a process in which fluid-filled spaces called *vacuoles* enlarge the cell body, resulting in neuron malfunction or death.

• A PET scan measures the metabolic activity of the cerebral cortex and may help confirm an early diagnosis.
• EEG, CT scan, and MRI may help diagnose later stages of Alzheimer's disease.
• Additional tests may help rule out other causes of dementia, such as vitamin B_{12} deficiency and hypothyroidism.

How it's treated

While there's no known cure for Alzheimer's disease, donepezil, tacrine, and rivastigmine have proven partially effective in improving mental performance. Drug therapy is also used to treat behavioral symptoms, such as aggression, paranoia, depression, and delusions. These drugs include:
• antipsychotics, such as haloperidol, olanzapine, quetiapine, and risperidone
• anxiolytics, such as alprazolam, buspirone, diazepam, and lorazepam
• antidepressants, such as amitriptyline, bupropion, fluoxetine, and paroxetine.

What to do

Care focuses on supporting the patient's remaining abilities and compensating for those he has lost. These interventions can help.
• Establish an effective communication system with the patient and his family to help them adjust to his altered cognitive abilities.

Returning to a safe haven

• Protect the patient from injury by providing a safe, structured environment.
• Encourage the patient to exercise, as ordered, to help maintain mobility.
• Refer family members to appropriate social service agencies that can help the family assess its needs.
• Evaluate the patient. He should be free from injury; have an established, adequate sleep pattern; and have adequate nutrition.
• Assess the patient's family to determine if they have sufficient support systems to help them cope with this crisis.
• Encourage the patient and his family to express their feelings of loss. (See *Alzheimer's disease teaching tips*.)

Amyotrophic lateral sclerosis

ALS causes progressive physical degeneration while leaving the patient's mental status intact. Thus, the patient is keenly aware of each new physical change. The most common motor neuron disease of muscular atrophy, ALS results in degeneration of upper motor neurons in the medulla oblongata and lower motor neurons in the spinal cord.

Onset typically occurs between ages 40 and 70, and most patients die within 3 to 10 years, usually due to aspiration pneumonia or respiratory failure.

What causes it

The cause of ALS isn't known; however, factors associated with ALS include:
• autosomal dominant inheritance
• a slow-acting virus
• a nutritional deficiency in motor neurons related to a disturbance in enzyme metabolism
• metabolic interference in nucleic acid production by the nerve fibers
• an autoimmune disorder.

Precipitating factors for acute deterioration include trauma, viral infections, and physical exhaustion.

Education edge

Alzheimer's disease teaching tips

• Teach the patient and his family about Alzheimer's disease—what's known, what's suspected, and the degenerative nature of the disorder. Listen to their concerns and answer all questions honestly and with compassion.
• Refer the family to local and national support groups for additional information and coping strategies. Family members commonly find a degree of solace in knowing that other families are going through the same devastating experience. To locate support groups in your area, contact the Alzheimer's Disease and Related Disorders Association.
• Encourage the family to allow the patient as much independence as possible while keeping him safe.
• Explain how proper diet, regular daily routines, and normal sleep patterns can help.

Pathophysiology

In ALS, motor neurons located in the anterior horns of the spinal column and motor nuclei located in the lower brain stem die. As they die, the muscles they served begin to atrophy. The loss of motor neurons may occur in the upper and lower motor neuron systems. Signs and symptoms vary according to the motor neurons affected because specific neurons activate specific muscle fibers.

What to look for

The patient with ALS develops fasciculations (twitching, involuntary muscle contractions) accompanied by atrophy and weakness, especially in the muscles of the forearms and hands. Other signs and symptoms include:
• impaired speech
• difficulty chewing and swallowing
• difficulty breathing
• depression
• choking
• excessive drooling.

What tests tell you

• Electromyography and muscle biopsy help determine if the disease is affecting the nerves rather than the muscles.
• In one-third of all patients with ALS, CSF examination reveals an increased protein level.

How it's treated

No effective treatment exists for ALS. Management focuses on controlling symptoms and providing the patient and his family with the emotional, psychological, and physical support they need.

What to do

ALS poses a real challenge to the coping skills of the patient and his family. Care begins with a complete neurologic assessment, which functions as a baseline for future evaluations. Collectively, these assessments will reveal the progression of ALS over time.

Consider these additional interventions to ease the impact of the disease and help the patient and his family cope more effectively.
• Implement a rehabilitation program that maintains as much independence for the patient for as long as possible.

Loss of motor neurons may occur in the upper and lower motor neuron systems. Gulp — is anyone safe these days?!

On the road again

• Help the patient obtain equipment that will help him move about, such as a walker or a wheelchair. Arrange for a visiting nurse to oversee home care and provide ongoing support, and to teach the family about the illness.

• Depending on the patient's muscular ability, help with bathing, personal hygiene, and transfers from wheelchair to bed, as needed. Encourage a regular bowel and bladder routine.

• Provide meticulous skin care if the patient is bedridden, to prevent skin breakdown. Also, turn him often, keep his skin clean and dry, and use sheepskins or pressure-relieving devices to preserve skin integrity.

• If the patient has trouble swallowing, give him soft, solid foods and position him upright during meals. He'll need gastrostomy and nasogastric (NG) tube feedings when he's no longer able to swallow.

Making informed decisions

• Provide the patient and his family with emotional support and the information they need to make informed decisions regarding end-of-life care and help them prepare for the eventual death of the patient. Encourage all concerned to start the grieving process. The patient with ALS may benefit from a hospice program.

• Evaluate the patient. Intervene as need to maintain adequate respiratory function with a patent airway, clear lungs, and acceptable results from pulmonary function studies. Help maintain a system of communication and as much physical mobility as possible for as long as possible. Note whether the patient expresses feelings of loss. (See *ALS teaching tips*.)

Arteriovenous malformation

In AVM, a tangled array of dilated vessels forms an abnormal network of communication between the arterial and venous systems. AVMs are usually located in the cerebral hemispheres. Spontaneous bleeding from these lesions into the subarachnoid space or brain tissue causes the patient's signs and symptoms.

AVMs range in size from a few millimeters to large malformations extending from the cerebral cortex to the ventricles. Most are present at birth; however, symptoms rarely occur before ages 10 to 30. AVMs are more common in men than in women.

What causes it

• Congenital defects in capillary development
• Traumatic injury (a possible cause)

Education edge

ALS teaching tips

• Teach one or more family members the proper way to suction the patient. This will help the patient cope with the increasing accumulation of secretions and dysphagia.

• Explain that he must eat slowly at mealtime and always sit upright. If he develops swallowing difficulties, refer him to the dysphagia team for further evaluation and treatment.

• If the patient is still able to feed himself, teach him (and a family member) how to administer gastrostomy feedings.

• When verbal communication becomes too difficult, teach the patient an alternate method of communicating with those around him.

Pathophysiology

AVMs lack the structural characteristics typical of normal blood vessels. The vessels of an AVM are very thin; when more than one artery feeds into the AVM, it appears dilated and torturous. Because vessels are thin, there's a risk that an aneurysm will develop. If the AVM is large enough, shunting can deprive surrounding tissue of adequate blood flow. In addition, the thin-walled vessels may ooze small amounts of blood or they may rupture, causing hemorrhage into the brain or subarachnoid space.

AVMs range in size from a few milliliters to large malformations.

What to look for

* Seizures that are initially focal but become generalized
* Headache that doesn't respond to treatment

Mind games

* Transient episodes of syncope, dizziness, motor weakness, or sensory deficits
* Tingling, aphasia, dysarthria, visual deficits (usually hemianopsia)
* Mental confusion
* Intellectual impairment

What tests tell you

* Cerebral angiography provides the most definitive diagnostic information by localizing the AVM and enabling visualization of large feeding arteries and large drainage veins.
* A CT scan can help differentiate an AVM from a clot or tumor, especially when a contrast medium is used.
* EEG may help localize the AVM.
* Brain scan immediately after isotope injection will reveal an uptake in the AVM.
* MRI-magnetic resonance angiography (especially with gadolinium) may provide information that supports a diagnosis of AVM.

How it's treated

The choice of treatment depends on the size and location of the AVM, the feeder vessels supplying it, and the age and general health of the patient. Possible methods include embolization, proton-beam radiation, Nd:YAG laser surgery, surgical excision, and a combination of embolization and surgery.

Cerebral angiography provides the most definitive diagnostic information for an AVM.

What to do

If hemorrhage hasn't occurred, focus efforts on preventing bleeding. Control hypertension and seizure activity, and reduce activities and eliminate stressors that raise the patient's systemic blood pressure. Before surgery, treatment will be very similar to treatment for cerebral aneurysm.

- Maintain a quiet, therapeutic environment.
- Monitor and control associated hypertension with drug therapy, as ordered.
- Conduct an ongoing neurologic assessment.
- Monitor the patient's vital signs frequently.
- Assess and monitor characteristics of headache, seizure activity, or bruit, as needed.
- Provide emotional support.
- Evaluate the patient's LOC, body temperature, heart rate, respiratory rate, and blood pressure.
- Assess whether he continues to experience pain or seizures.
- Note whether the patient has expressed feelings of loss to members of the staff, his friends, or his family. Similarly, note whether his family or friends have expressed their understanding of the disease process, treatment options, and outcome. (See *AVM teaching tips*.)

Bell's palsy

Bell's palsy blocks conduction of impulses along the facial nerve (CN VII), which is the nerve responsible for motor innervation of the facial muscles. This block results from an inflammatory reaction around the nerve (usually at the internal auditory meatus).

Bell's palsy affects all age-groups, but occurs most commonly in patients under age 60. Onset is rapid and, in 80% to 90% of all patients, it subsides spontaneously, with complete recovery in 1 to 8 weeks. Recovery can take longer in elderly patients. If patients experience only partial recovery, contractures may develop on the paralyzed side of the face. Bell's palsy may recur on the same or opposite side of the face.

What causes it

- Infection
- Hemorrhage
- Tumor
- Meningitis
- Local traumatic injury

In 80% to 90% of patients, Bell's palsy subsides spontaneously in 1 to 8 weeks.

Pathophysiology

Inflammation around CN VII where it leaves bony tissue blocks conduction along the nerve. As a consequence, CN VII can't adequately stimulate the muscle fibers, and unilateral or bilateral facial weakness or paralysis is the result.

What to look for

• Unilateral facial weakness or paralysis, with aching at the jaw angle
• Drooping mouth, causing drooling on the affected side
• Distorted taste perception over the affected anterior portion of the tongue
• Markedly impaired ability to close the eye on the weak side
• Incomplete eye closure and Bell's phenomenon (eye rolling upward as eye is closed)
• Inability to raise the eyebrow, smile, show the teeth, or puff out the cheek on the affected side

What tests tell you

Electromyography helps predict recovery by distinguishing temporary conduction defects from a pathologic interruption of nerve fibers.

How it's treated

Prednisone, an oral corticosteroid, reduces facial nerve edema and improves nerve conduction and blood flow. Specific antiviral agents can also be helpful. After the 14th day of prednisone therapy, electrotherapy may help prevent atrophy of facial muscles.

What to do

• Apply moist heat to the affected side of the face to reduce pain, taking care not to burn the skin.
• Massage the patient's face with a gentle upward motion two to three times daily for 5 to 10 minutes, and teach him how to perform this massage.
• Apply a facial sling to improve lip alignment.

Residual effects

• Give the patient frequent and complete mouth care. Remove residual food that collects between the cheeks and gums.
• Provide support, and reassure the patient that recovery is likely within 1 to 8 weeks.

• Assess the effectiveness of pain medications and whether they provide adequate relief.
• Assess the patient's nutritional status. Bell's palsy shouldn't interfere with the patient's ability to maintain adequate nutrition.
• Note whether the patient has expressed feelings of loss or fear to staff, friends, or family. (See *Bell's palsy teaching tips*.)

Cerebral aneurysm

Cerebral aneurysm, a localized dilation of a cerebral artery, results from a weakness in the arterial wall. (See *Common sites of cerebral aneurysm*, page 134.) The incidence is slightly higher in women than in men, especially those in their late 40s to mid-50s, but cerebral aneurysm may occur at any age.

Prognosis is uncertain because cerebral aneurysms can rupture and cause subarachnoid hemorrhage; one-half of all patients suffering subarachnoid hemorrhages die immediately. However, with new and better treatment, the prognosis is improving.

What causes it

Cerebral aneurysm results from congenital vascular disease, infection, or atherosclerosis.

Pathophysiology

Blood flow exerts pressure against a congenitally weak area of arterial wall, causing it to stretch and thin, somewhat like an overblown balloon. At this point, the risk of rupture is high. A rupture is followed by a subarachnoid hemorrhage, in which blood spills into the space normally occupied by CSF. In some cases, blood also spills into brain tissue, where a clot can damage brain tissue or cause a life-threatening increase in ICP.

What to look for

Most patients are asymptomatic until the time of bleeding. Premonitory symptoms resulting from oozing of blood into the subarachnoid space include:
• headache, intermittent nausea
• nuchal rigidity
• stiff back and legs.
    Rupture usually occurs abruptly and may cause:
• sudden severe headache
• nausea and projectile vomiting
• altered LOC, including deep coma

Education edge

Bell's palsy teaching tips

• Advise the patient to protect the eye on the affected side by covering it with an eye patch, especially when outdoors. The eyelid must be taped shut at night using a small piece of hypoallergenic tape. Tell him to keep warm and to avoid exposure to dust and wind. If exposure is unavoidable, instruct him to cover his face.
• To prevent excessive weight loss, teach the patient how to cope with eating and drinking difficulties. Tell him to chew on the unaffected side of his mouth. Provide a nutritionally balanced diet of soft foods. Eliminate hot foods and fluids (soups, sauces, and purees, for example). Arrange for privacy at mealtimes to minimize embarrassment.
• When the patient is ready, teach him to exercise facial muscles by grimacing in front of a mirror.

Common sites of cerebral aneurysm

A cerebral aneurysm usually arises at arterial bifurcations in the circle of Willis and its branches. The shaded areas in the illustration below indicate the most common sites for aneurysm.

Anterior communicating artery

Left anterior cerebral artery

Circle of Willis

Left posterior communicating artery

Right middle cerebral artery

Right posterior cerebral artery

Basilar artery

Right vertebral artery

Most patients with a cerebral aneurysm are asymptomatic until the time of bleeding.

• meningeal irritation, resulting in nuchal rigidity, back and leg pain, fever, restlessness, irritability, seizures, photophobia, and blurred vision
• hemiparesis, hemisensory defects, dysphagia, and visual defects
• diplopia, ptosis, dilated pupils, and an inability to rotate the eye.

What tests tell you

• Angiography can confirm an unruptured cerebral aneurysm. Unfortunately, diagnosis usually follows the rupture.
• A CT scan may help detect subarachnoid hemorrhage.
• MRI may detect vasospasm.

How it's treated

To reduce the risk of rebleeding, the doctor may attempt to repair the aneurysm. Usually, surgical repair (by clipping, ligating, or wrapping the aneurysm neck with muscle) takes place within several days after the initial bleed.

More conservative

The patient may receive conservative treatment if surgical correction poses too great a risk (common with elderly patients and those with heart, lung, or other serious diseases), the aneurysm is in a particularly dangerous location, or vasospasm necessitates a delay in surgery.

Commonly, treatment for the patient who isn't a good candidate for surgery includes bed rest in a quiet, darkened room for as long as 4 to 6 weeks. The patient must avoid stimulants, including coffee, and aspirin. He may receive codeine or another analgesic, hydralazine or another antihypertensive (if he's hypertensive), corticosteroids to reduce edema, and phenobarbital or another sedative. Nimodipine may be prescribed to limit possible neurologic deficits. If the patient is hypotensive, he may receive dopamine to ensure adequate brain perfusion.

If surgery is too risky, a more conservative treatment for cerebral aneurysm, such as drug therapy, may be pursued.

What to do

An accurate neurologic assessment, good patient care, patient and family teaching, and psychological support can speed recovery and reduce complications. The medical-surgical nurse assumes care for the patient recovering from an aneurysm repair when he's transferred from the ICU. Focus patient care and teaching on the patient's needs and neurologic deficits, if any.
• Assess neurologic status to screen for changes in the patients condition.
• Administer medications, as ordered.
• Maintain adequate nutrition.
• Promote activity based on the patient's ability.
• Provide support to the patient and his family, especially if neurologic deficits have occurred.
• Refer the patient to appropriate health care team members, such as a social services representative and home care organization.
• Check for a patent airway, normal breath sounds, consistent LOC with no additional neurologic deficits, and adequate hydration and nutrition. (See *Cerebral aneurysm teaching tips*.)

Epilepsy

Patients with epilepsy are susceptible to recurrent seizures—paroxysmal events associated with abnormal electrical discharge of neurons in the brain. These discharges may be focal or diffuse, and the sites of the discharges determine the clinical manifestations that occur during the attack.

Seizures are among the most commonly observed neurologic dysfunctions in children and can occur with widely varying CNS conditions. The onset of seizures in adults should lead health care providers to suspect brain tumor or head injury.

What causes it

Epilepsy is idiopathic (cause unknown) in about one-half of all cases. For the other half, possible causes include:
- genetic disorders or degenerative disease, such as phenylketonuria or tuberous sclerosis
- birth trauma (inadequate oxygen supply to the brain, blood incompatibility, or hemorrhage)
- infectious diseases (meningitis, encephalitis, or brain abscess)
- ingestion of toxins (mercury, lead, or carbon monoxide)
- brain tumors, head injury or trauma
- stroke (hemorrhage, thrombosis, or embolism).

> One-half of all cases of epilepsy are idiopathic, which means the cause isn't known.

Pathophysiology

Although the cause of epilepsy remains unclear, it's thought that a group of neurons may lose afferent stimulation (ability to transmit impulses from the periphery toward the CNS) and function as an epileptogenic focus. These neurons are hypersensitive and easily activated. In response to changes in the cellular environment, the neurons become hyperactive and fire abnormally.

Fighting fire with fire

Upon stimulation, the epileptogenic focus fires and spreads electrical current toward the synapse and surrounding cells. These cells fire in turn, and the impulse cascades to one side of the brain (a partial seizure), both sides of the brain (a generalized seizure), or toward the cortical, subcortical, or brain stem areas. A continuous seizure state known as *status epilepticus* can cause respiratory distress and even death. (See *Treating status epilepticus.*)

What to look for

The hallmark of epilepsy is recurring seizures. There are generally six types of seizure:

    simple partial

complex partial

 absence

 myoclonic

 generalized tonic-clonic

 atonic.

Simple partial seizure
- Sensory symptoms (flashing lights, smells, auditory hallucinations)
- Autonomic symptoms (sweating, flushing, pupil dilation)
- Psychic symptoms (dream states, anger, fear)

Complex partial seizure
- Altered LOC
- Amnesia

Sensory symptoms, such as flashing lights, may indicate the onset of a simple partial seizure.

What do I do?

Treating status epilepticus

Status epilepticus is a continuous seizure that must be interrupted using emergency measures. It can occur during all types of seizures. For example, generalized tonic-clonic status epilepticus is a continuous generalized tonic-clonic seizure without an intervening return to consciousness.

Always an emergency

Status epilepticus is accompanied by respiratory distress and can be life-threatening. It can result from withdrawal of antiepileptic medications, hypoxic or metabolic encephalopathy, acute head trauma, or septicemia secondary to encephalitis or meningitis.

Acting fast

Typically, emergency treatment consists of diazepam, lorazepam, fosphenytoin, or phenobarbital; 50% dextrose I.V. when seizures are secondary to hypoglycemia; and thiamine I.V. in patients with chronic alcoholism or those undergoing withdrawal.

Absence seizure

• A brief change in LOC indicated by blinking or rolling of the eyes, a blank stare, and slight mouth movements

Myoclonic seizure

• Brief involuntary muscular jerks of the body or extremities

Generalized tonic-clonic seizure

• Typically beginning with a loud cry
• Change in LOC
• Body stiffening, alternating between muscle spasm and relaxation
• Tongue biting, incontinence, labored breathing, apnea, cyanosis
• Upon wakening, possible confusion and difficulty talking
• Drowsiness, fatigue, headache, muscle soreness, weakness

Atonic seizure

• General loss of postural tone
• Temporary loss of consciousness

What tests tell you

Primary diagnostic tests include:
• CT scan and MRI, which provide density readings of the brain and may indicate structural abnormalities
• EEG, which may show paroxysmal abnormalities that confirm the diagnosis of epilepsy by providing evidence of the continuing tendency to have seizures. (A negative EEG doesn't rule out epilepsy because the paroxysmal abnormalities occur intermittently.)

Other informative tests include:
• serum glucose, electrolyte, drug, and calcium levels
• lumbar puncture
• brain scan
• PET scan
• cerebral angiography.

Confusion and difficulty talking upon wakening is a sign of generalized tonic-clonic seizure — and my typical morning!

How it's treated

Typically, treatment consists of drug therapy. The most commonly prescribed drugs are phenytoin, carbamazepine, phenobarbital, and primidone for generalized tonic-clonic seizures and complex partial seizures. Valproic acid, clonazepam, and ethosuximide are commonly prescribed for absence seizures.

If drug therapy fails, the doctor may choose to surgically remove a demonstrated focal lesion in an attempt to bring an end to

Education edge

Epilepsy teaching tips

• Encourage the patient and his family to express their feelings about the patient's condition. Answer their questions honestly, and help them cope by dispelling some of the myths about epilepsy.
• Assure the patient and his family that following a prescribed regimen of medication will help in controlling seizures and maintaining a normal lifestyle.
• Stress the need for compliance with the prescribed drug schedule.
• Assure the patient that antiepileptics are safe when taken as ordered. Reinforce dosage instructions, and find methods to help the patient remember to take his medication. Caution him to monitor the amount of medication left so he doesn't run out of it. It shouldn't be discontinued abruptly. He shouldn't take nonprescription drugs or herbs without consulting the doctor.
• Describe the signs that may indicate an adverse reaction, such as drowsiness, lethargy, hyperactivity, confusion, and vision and sleep disturbances. Tell the patient to report these signs to his doctor immediately as they may indicate the need for a dosage adjustment.
• Phenytoin therapy may lead to hyperplasia of the gums, which can be relieved by conscientious oral hygiene.

• Emphasize the importance of having antiepileptic blood levels checked at regular intervals, even if the seizures are under control. Also, warn the patient against drinking alcoholic beverages.

Generalized tonic-clonic seizures
Generalized tonic-clonic seizures may necessitate first aid. Teach the patient's family how to give such aid correctly. Include these teaching points:
• Teach the family to provide safety measures if a seizure occurs by helping the patient to a lying position, loosening any tight clothing, and placing something flat and soft, such as a pillow, jacket, or hand, under his head. Advise them to clear the area of hard objects and not to force anything into the patient's mouth if his teeth are clenched. However, if his mouth is open, they can place a soft object (such as a folded cloth) between his teeth to protect his tongue.
• Know which social agencies in the patient's community can help. Refer the patient to the Epilepsy Foundation of America for general information and to the state motor vehicle department for information about his driver's license.

seizures. Emergency treatment for status epilepticus usually consists of diazepam, lorazepam, fosphenytoin, or phenobarbital; 50% dextrose I.V. (when seizures are secondary to hypoglycemia); and thiamine I.V. (in chronic alcoholism or withdrawal). Rectal preparations of diazepam and oral solutions of diazepam and lorazepam are concentrated and fast-acting.

What to do

• Monitor the patient for signs and symptoms of medication toxicity, such as nystagmus, ataxia, lethargy, dizziness, drowsiness, slurred speech, irritability, nausea, and vomiting.
• Administer phenytoin according to guidelines (not more than 50 mg/minute), and monitor the patient's vital signs often.

Oral solutions of diazepam and lorazepam are concentrated and fast-acting.

• Evaluate the patient to determine the effectiveness of the medication; seizure activity should decrease or stop. Note whether the patient has expressed his feelings regarding his illness to his friends or family. (See *Epilepsy teaching tips*, page 139.)

Guillain-Barré syndrome

An acute, rapidly progressive, and potentially fatal form of polyneuritis, Guillain-Barré syndrome causes muscle weakness and mild distal sensory loss. About 95% of patients experience spontaneous and complete recovery, although mild motor or reflex deficits in the feet and legs may persist.

What causes it

The precise cause of this syndrome is unknown, but it may be a cell-mediated immunologic attack on peripheral nerves in response to a virus. Precipitating factors may include:
• mild febrile or viral illness
• surgery
• rabies or swine influenza vaccination
• Hodgkin's disease or some other cancer
• systemic lupus erythematosus.

Pathophysiology

The major pathologic manifestation of Guillain-Barré syndrome is segmental demyelination of the peripheral nerves, which prevents normal transmission of electrical impulses. Because this syndrome causes inflammation and degenerative changes in the posterior (sensory) and anterior (motor) nerve roots, signs of sensory and motor loss occur simultaneously. Additionally, autonomic nerve transmission may be impaired. (See *Phases of Guillain-Barré syndrome*.)

Signs of sensory and motor loss occur simultaneously in Guillain-Barré syndrome.

What to look for

• Symmetrical muscle weakness, usually appearing in the legs first (ascending type) and then extending to the arms and facial nerves within 24 to 72 hours
• Facial diplegia, possibly with ophthalmoplegia (ocular paralysis)
• Dysphagia, dysarthria
• Hypotonia, areflexia

What tests tell you

• Protein levels in CSF begin to rise several days after onset of signs and symptoms and peak in 4 to 6 weeks. White blood cell count in the CSF remains normal but, in severe disease, CSF pressure may rise above normal.

Juvenile offenders

• Complete blood count (CBC) shows leukocytosis and immature forms early in the illness, but blood studies soon return to normal.
• Electromyography may show repeated firing of the same motor unit instead of widespread sectional stimulation. Nerve conduction velocities are slowed soon after paralysis develops.

How it's treated

At the onset of symptoms, the patient should be hospitalized. Monitor respiratory function several times daily because the ascending pathology can lead to respiratory failure. Mechanical ventilation may be necessary. The other key treatment is plasmapheresis, which temporarily reduces circulating antibodies. Patients need less ventilator support if plasmapheresis begins within 2 weeks of onset. High-dose immune globulins and steroids are also used.

What to do

• Watch for ascending motor loss. Commonly, sensation isn't lost; in fact, the patient may be hypersensitive to pain and touch.
• Monitor the patient's vital signs and LOC.
• Assess respiratory function. Watch for signs of increasing partial pressure of arterial carbon dioxide ($Paco_2$), such as confusion and tachypnea. Auscultate breath sounds, turn and position the patient, and encourage coughing and deep breathing. If respiratory failure becomes imminent, establish an emergency airway and assist with endotracheal intubation.
• Provide meticulous skin care to prevent skin breakdown.
• Perform passive ROM exercises within the patient's pain limits, perhaps using a Hubbard tank to prevent contractures. When the patient's condition stabilizes, change to gentle stretching and active assistance exercises.
• Evaluate the patient's gag reflex. If he has no gag reflex, administer NG feedings, as ordered. If it's present, simply elevate the head of the bed before the patient eats.
• As the patient regains strength and can tolerate a vertical position, be alert for hypotension; prevent it with slow position changes.

Phases of Guillain-Barré syndrome

The clinical course of Guillain-Barré syndrome has three phases:

acute phase, which begins when the first definitive symptom develops and ends 1 to 3 weeks later, when no further deterioration is noted

plateau phase, which lasts for several days to 2 weeks

recovery phase, which is believed to coincide with remyelination and axonal process regrowth and can last from 4 months to 3 years.

Monitor respiratory function to avoid respiratory failure.

• Inspect the patient's legs regularly for signs of thrombophlebitis, a common complication of Guillain-Barré syndrome. To prevent thrombophlebitis, apply antiembolism stockings and a sequential compression device and give prophylactic anticoagulants, as ordered.

• Provide eye and mouth care every 4 hours if the patient has facial paralysis.

• Watch for urine retention. Measure and record intake and output every 8 hours, and offer the bedpan every 3 to 4 hours. Encourage adequate fluid intake (2 qt [2 L] day), unless contraindicated. If urine retention develops, the patient may need to use Credé's maneuver to urinate. Catheterize the patient, if ordered.

Bulking up

• To prevent or relieve constipation, offer prune juice and a high-bulk diet. If necessary, give daily or alternate-day suppositories (glycerin or bisacodyl), or enemas, as ordered.

• Refer the patient for physical therapy, as needed.

• Evaluate the patient for adequate respiratory function with a patent airway and clear lungs, adequate nutritional status, and optimal activity level.

• Note whether the patient has expressed his feelings about his illness to members of the staff, his friends, or his family. (See *Guillain-Barré syndrome teaching tips.*)

Headache

Muscle contraction and vascular abnormalities cause 90% of headaches. Occasionally, however, a headache indicates an underlying intracranial, systemic, or psychological disorder.

Throbbing, vascular headaches—migraine headaches—affect up to 10% of Americans. Migraines usually begin in childhood or adolescence and recur throughout adulthood. Migraine headaches tend to run in families and are more common in women than in men.

What causes it

Most chronic headaches result from muscle tension caused by:

• emotional stress or fatigue
• menstruation
• environmental stimuli (noise, crowds, bright lights).
    However, there are other possible causes, including:
• glaucoma
• inflammation of the eyes or of the nasal or paranasal sinus mucosa

Education edge

Guillain-Barré syndrome teaching tips

• Before discharge, prepare a home care plan and review it thoroughly with the patient and his family.

• Reinforce the physical and occupational therapist's teaching about how to transfer from bed to wheelchair and from wheelchair to toilet or tub as well as how to walk short distances with a walker or a cane.

• Teach the family how to help the patient eat, compensate for facial weakness, and prevent skin breakdown.

• Stress the need for a regular bowel and bladder routine. Explain Credé's maneuver, if complete urinary emptying is a problem.

• Provide the patient and his family with appropriate referrals to support organizations and public service agencies in the area.

- diseases of the scalp, teeth, extracranial arteries, or external or middle ear
- vasodilators (nitrates, alcohol, histamine)
- systemic disease
- hypertension
- head trauma or tumor
- intracranial bleeding, abscess, or aneurysm.

Pathophysiology

Headache pain may emanate from the pain-sensitive structures of the skin, scalp, muscles, arteries, and veins; from cranial nerves V, VII, IX, and X; or from cervical nerves 1, 2, and 3. Intracranial mechanisms of headache include traction or displacement of arteries, venous sinuses, or venous tributaries and inflammation or direct pressure on the cranial nerves with afferent pain fibers.

    The cause of migraine headaches isn't known, but researchers associate the disorder with constriction and dilation of intracranial and extracranial arteries.

What to look for

Signs and symptoms depend on the type or cause of the headache: migraine headache, muscle contraction and traction-inflammatory vascular headache, intracranial bleeding, or tumor.

Migraine headache

- Unilateral pulsating pain, which becomes more generalized over time
- Premonitory aura of scintillating scotoma, hemianopsia, unilateral paresthesia, or a speech disorder
- Irritability, anorexia, nausea, vomiting, photophobia

Muscle contraction and traction-inflammatory vascular headache

- Dull, persistent ache or severe, unrelenting pain
- Tender spots on the head or neck
- Feeling of tightness around the head with a characteristic "hatband" distribution

Intracranial bleeding

- Neurologic deficits, such as paresthesia and muscle weakness
- Pain unrelieved by narcotics

Tumor

- Pain that's most severe when the patient wakes

90% of headaches stem from muscle contraction or vascular abnormalities. However, occasionally, a headache indicates an underlying disorder.

Research associates migraines with constriction and dilation of intracranial and extracranial arteries.

What tests tell you

Skull X-rays (including cervical spine and sinus), EEG, CT scan (performed before lumbar puncture to rule out increased ICP), brain scan, and lumbar puncture may help determine the cause.

How it's treated

Depending on the type of headache, analgesics ranging from aspirin to codeine or meperidine may provide symptomatic relief. A tranquilizer, such as diazepam, may help during acute attacks, as could identification and elimination of causative factors and, possibly, psychotherapy for headaches caused by emotional stress. Chronic tension headaches may require muscle relaxants.

Taking a coffee break

For migraine headache, ergotamine alone or with caffeine provides the most effective treatment. Sumatriptan, which binds with serotonin receptors, is also effective in aborting migraine headaches. These drugs and others, such as metoclopramide or naproxen, work best when taken early in the course of an attack. Antiemetics, such as promethazine, may be prescribed to control nausea and vomiting. Drugs that can help prevent migraine headache include propranolol; calcium channel blockers, such as verapamil and diltiazem; and antiseizure medications such as divalproex.

What to do

Unless the headache is caused by a serious underlying disorder, hospitalization is rarely required. In these rare cases, direct your attention to treating the primary problem. The patient with migraine usually needs to be hospitalized only if nausea and vomiting are severe enough to induce dehydration and possible shock.

Finding a sea of tranquility

Evaluate the patient to determine the effectiveness of prescribed analgesics, tranquilizers, or muscle relaxants and document your findings. Help the patient understand the possible causes and remedies for the headaches. (See *Headache teaching tips*.)

Huntington's disease

Huntington's disease (Huntington's chorea) is a hereditary disease that causes degeneration in the cerebral cortex and basal ganglia. This degeneration leads to chronic progressive chorea and mental deterioration that ends in dementia.

Education edge

Headache teaching tips

• Help the patient understand the reason for headaches so that he can avoid exacerbating factors. Use his history and diagnosis as a guide.
• Advise him to lie down in a dark, quiet room during an attack and to place ice packs on his forehead or a cold cloth over his eyes, or use other measures that are helpful for him.
• Instruct the patient to take prescribed medication at the onset of migraine symptoms, prevent dehydration by drinking plenty of fluids after nausea and vomiting subside, and use other headache-relief measures.

What causes it

The cause of Huntington's disease isn't known. However, it's transmitted as an autosomal dominant trait.

Pathophysiology

Huntington's disease involves a disturbance in neurotransmitter substances, primarily gamma aminobutyric acid (GABA) and dopamine. GABA neurons in the basal ganglia, frontal cortex, and cerebellum are destroyed and replaced with glial cells. The deficiency of GABA (an inhibitory neurotransmitter) causes an excess of dopamine and abnormal neurotransmission along the affected pathways.

What to look for

• Severe choreic movements (involuntary, rapid, usually violent, and purposeless movements), initially unilateral and more prominent in the face and arms than in the legs
• Dementia, typically mild at first and then growing more severe until it disrupts the personality
• Loss of musculoskeletal control

What tests tell you

• PET scan and deoxyribonucleic acid analysis can detect Huntington's disease.
• CT scan and MRI reveal brain atrophy.

How it's treated

Huntington's disease has no known cure. Therefore, treatment focuses on supporting and protecting the patient and treating symptoms. Tranquilizers and drugs, such as chlorpromazine, haloperidol, and imipramine, can help control choreic movement and alleviate discomfort and depression. However, they can't stop mental deterioration. In addition, tranquilizers increase rigidity. To control choreic movements without rigidity, the doctor may order choline.

What to do

• Attend to the patient's basic needs, such as hygiene, skin care, bowel and bladder care, and nutrition. Increase support as his mental and physical deterioration becomes more pronounced.
• Provide emotional support. The patient and his family can feel overwhelming despondency due to the degenerative and irreversible course of the disease. An extremely depressed patient

may attempt suicide. Be alert for signs, and make sure the patient's environment is free from instruments that could permit self-inflicted injury.

Maintaining high levels

- Evaluate the patient's mobility and level of function. Plan interventions that help him maintain the highest level of mobility and independence possible for as long as possible.
- Keep the patient free from injury.
- Help the family identify resources that can help them cope with the patient's illness. (See *Huntington's disease teaching tips.*)

Meningitis

In meningitis, infection (bacterial or otherwise) causes inflammation of the brain and spinal meninges that can involve all three meningeal membranes: dura mater, arachnoid, and pia mater.

What causes it

- Bacteremia, especially due to pneumonia, empyema, osteomyelitis, or endocarditis
- Other infections, such as sinusitis, otitis media, encephalitis, or myelitis
- Brain abscess, usually caused by *Neisseria meningitidis*, *Haemophilus influenzae*, *Streptococcus pneumoniae*, or *Escherichia coli*
- Head injury, such as skull fracture, penetrating head wound, or neurosurgery
- Virus or other organism (aseptic meningitis)

What to look for

- Fever, chills, malaise
- Headache, vomiting
- Signs of meningeal irritation, such as nuchal rigidity, positive Brudzinski's and Kernig's signs, exaggerated and symmetrical deep tendon reflexes, or opisthotonos
- Seizures
- Delirium, deep stupor, and coma (See *Important signs of meningitis.*)

What tests tell you

Typically, CSF testing and positive Brudzinski's and Kernig's signs establish the diagnosis:

Education edge

Huntington's disease teaching tips

- Talk with the patient and family about the disease. Listen to their concerns and fears, and provide clear answers to questions.
- Keep in mind the patient's dysarthria and allow him time to express his thoughts.
- Teach the family appropriate patient care measures, and help them assume a greater role as the patient's condition deteriorates.
- Explain that children have a 50% chance of inheriting the disease and that genetic counseling is a good idea before starting a family.
- Refer the patient and family to organizations that can help them cope with the disease, such as a visiting nurse service, social services, psychiatric counseling, and long-term care facilities.

Important signs of meningitis

A positive response to these tests helps establish a diagnosis of meningitis.

Brudzinski's sign

Place the patient in a dorsal recumbent position, and then put your hands behind his neck and bend it forward. Pain and resistance may indicate neck injury or arthritis. However, if the patient also flexes the hips and knees, chances are that he has meningeal irritation and inflammation, a sign of meningitis.

Kernig's sign

Place the patient in a supine position. Flex his leg at the hip and knee, and then straighten the knee. Pain or resistance suggests meningitis.

• Look for elevated CSF pressure, high CSF protein levels and, possibly, low glucose levels.
• CSF culture and sensitivity tests usually identify the infecting organism unless it's a virus.

How it's treated

Treatment includes antibiotic therapy and vigorous supportive care. Usually, the patient receives I.V. antibiotics for 2 or more weeks, followed by oral antibiotics. Other prescribed drugs may include:

• digoxin to control arrhythmias
• mannitol to decrease cerebral edema
• an anticonvulsant or a sedative to reduce restlessness
• acetaminophen to relieve headache and fever.

Oh no! Culture and sensitivity tests usually give me away.

Recognizing aseptic meningitis

Aseptic meningitis, a benign syndrome, is characterized by headache, fever, vomiting, and meningeal symptoms. It results from infection by enteroviruses (most common), arboviruses, herpes simplex virus, mumps virus, or lymphocytic choriomeningitis virus.

First, a fever

Aseptic meningitis begins suddenly with a fever up to 104° F (40° C), alterations in level of consciousness (drowsiness, confusion, stupor), and neck or spine stiffness (slight at first) when bending forward. Other signs and symptoms include headache, nausea, vomiting, abdominal pain, poorly defined chest pain, and sore throat.

What virus is this anyway?

Patient history of recent illness and knowledge of seasonal epidemics are essential in differentiating among the many forms of aseptic meningitis. Negative bacteriologic cultures and cerebrospinal fluid (CSF) analysis that show pleocytosis and increased protein levels suggest the diagnosis. Isolation of the virus from the CSF confirms it.

Begin with bed rest

Supportive measures include bed rest, maintenance of fluid and electrolyte balance, analgesics for pain, and exercises to combat residual weakness. Isolation isn't necessary. Careful handling of excretions and good hand-washing technique prevent spreading the disease.

Positive cultures

Supportive measures include bed rest and measures to prevent dehydration. If nasal cultures are positive, isolation is necessary. Any coexisting conditions, such as endocarditis and pneumonia, are treated as well.

If nasal cultures are positive, isolation is necessary.

What to do

• Assess the patient's neurologic function often and watch for deterioration. Be especially alert for a temperature increase up to 102° F (38.9° C), deteriorating LOC, onset of seizures, and altered respirations, all of which may signal an impending crisis.

Finding fluid equilibrium

• Monitor the patient's fluid balance. Make sure he consumes enough fluids to prevent dehydration, but avoids fluid overload to decrease the risk of cerebral edema. Measure his central venous pressure, and record intake and output accurately.

• Position the patient carefully to prevent joint stiffness and neck pain. Turn him often, according to a planned positioning schedule. Help with ROM exercises.
• Maintain adequate nutrition and elimination.
• Maintain a quiet, comfortable environment. If necessary, darkening the room can help reduce photophobia.
• Relieve headache with a nonnarcotic analgesic, such as acetaminophen, as ordered. (Narcotics interfere with accurate neurologic assessment.)
• Use strict aseptic technique when treating the patient with a head wound or skull fracture. (See *Recognizing aseptic meningitis.*)
• Provide reassurance and support. The patient may be frightened by his illness and the need for frequent lumbar punctures. If he's disoriented or confused, calm and reorient him as often as needed. Reassure the family that the delirium and changes in behavior caused by meningitis usually disappear during recovery. However, if a severe neurologic deficit appears permanent, refer the patient to a rehabilitation program as soon as the acute phase of the illness has passed.
• Evaluate the patient's progress. If treatment is succeeding, the patient will be pain-free and his LOC will be normal. He'll maintain adequate hydration and nutrition and his blood pressure, heart rate, and respiratory rate will remain within normal limits. (See *Meningitis teaching tips.*)

Education edge

Meningitis teaching tips

• Teach the patient and his family about the illness and expected recovery. The family may need to receive prophylactic antibiotics.
• Teach the patient and his family how to help prevent meningitis by seeking proper medical treatment for chronic sinusitis or other chronic infections.

Multiple sclerosis

MS is a major cause of chronic disability in young adults. It results from progressive demyelination of the white matter of the brain and spinal cord and is characterized by exacerbations and remissions. The prognosis varies. MS may progress rapidly, disabling patients by early adulthood or causing death within months of onset. Fortunately, however, 70% of all patients lead active, productive lives with long periods of remission.

What causes it

The exact cause is unclear; however, current theories suggest that it may be caused by an autoimmune response to a slow-acting or latent viral infection or by environmental or genetic factors.

Pathophysiology

In MS, axon demyelination and nerve fiber loss occur in patches throughout the CNS, inducing widely disseminated and varied neurologic dysfunction.

Fortunately, 70% of patients with MS lead active, productive lives with long periods of remission.

What to look for

Accurate diagnosis requires evidence of multiple neurologic exacerbations and remissions. Signs and symptoms, which can vary considerably, include:
• vision disturbances, such as optic neuritis, diplopia, ophthalmoplegia, and blurred vision
• sensory impairment such as paresthesia
• muscle dysfunction, such as weakness, paralysis ranging from monoplegia to quadriplegia, spasticity, hyperreflexia, intention tremor, and gait ataxia
• urinary disturbances, such as incontinence, frequency, urgency, and frequent infections

Highs and lows

• emotional lability, such as mood swings, irritability, and euphoria
• associated signs, such as poorly articulated speech and dysphagia.

Because diagnosing MS is difficult, some patients undergo years of testing and close observation.

What tests tell you

Because of the difficulty inherent in establishing a diagnosis, some patients may undergo years of periodic testing and close observation. These tests may help diagnose MS:
• In one-third of all patients, EEG shows nonspecific abnormalities.
• Lumbar puncture reveals CSF with elevated gamma globulin fraction of immunoglobulin G, but normal total protein levels. An elevated CSF gamma globulin level is significant only when serum gamma globulin levels are normal. It reflects hyperactivity of the immune system due to chronic demyelination. Oligoclonal bands of immunoglobulin can be detected when CSF gamma globulin is examined by electrophoresis.

Evoking a reaction

• Evoked potential studies demonstrate slowed conduction of nerve impulses in 80% of patients.
• A CT scan may reveal lesions within the brain's white matter.
• MRI is the most sensitive method of detecting lesions and is also used to evaluate disease progression. Lesions are present in more than 90% of all patients undergoing this test.

How it's treated

The aim of treatment is to shorten exacerbations and relieve neurologic deficits to help the patient maintain as normal a lifestyle as possible. Drug therapy and other measures can achieve these goals.

Medicate, don't exacerbate

Methylprednisolone is commonly prescribed during acute exacerbations to reduce CNS inflammation. Other typically used corticosteroids include dexamethasone, prednisone, betamethasone, and prednisolone. For relapsing MS, glatiramer acetate may be prescribed to reduce the frequency of attacks. Interferon beta-1a or interferon beta-1b may be effective in reducing disability progression and in decreasing the frequency of exacerbations.

In conjunction with corticosteroids, the doctor may prescribe:
- fluoxetine to combat depression
- baclofen or dantrolene to relieve spasticity
- oxybutynin to relieve urine retention and minimize frequency and urgency.

Support to cut short

During acute exacerbation, treatment routinely calls for:
- bed rest
- physical therapy and massages
- measures to prevent fatigue
- meticulous skin care to prevent pressure ulcers
- bowel and bladder training (if necessary)
- antibiotic treatment of bladder infection
- counseling.

What to do

Treatment focuses on maintaining mobility, ensuring proper nutrition, and controlling pain during exacerbations.
- Form a care plan based on the patient's abilities and symptoms.
- Help with physical therapy and provide massages, relaxing baths, and other measures that promote comfort.
- Assist with active, resistive, and stretching exercises to maintain muscle tone and joint mobility, reduce spasticity, improve coordination, and boost morale.
- Encourage emotional stability by helping the patient establish a daily routine that maintains optimal functioning. Let the patient's tolerance regulate the level of daily activity. Encourage daily physical exercise and regular rest periods to prevent fatigue.
- Watch for drug therapy adverse effects. (See *MS teaching tips*.)

Myasthenia gravis

Myasthenia gravis produces sporadic but progressive weakness and abnormal fatigue in striated (skeletal) muscles. This weakness and fatigue are exacerbated by exercise and repeated movement but improved by anticholinesterase drugs. Usually, myasthenia gravis affects muscles innervated by the cranial nerves (face, lips, tongue, neck, and throat), but it can affect any muscle group.

Education edge

MS teaching tips

- Teach the patient and family about the chronic course of the disease. Explain that exacerbations are unpredictable and will require physical and emotional adjustments.
- Emphasize the need to avoid stress, infections, and fatigue and to maintain independence by finding new ways to perform daily activities.
- Explain the value of a well-balanced, nutritious diet that contains sufficient fiber.
- Evaluate the need for bowel and bladder training and provide instruction, as needed.
- Encourage adequate fluid intake and regular urination.
- Teach the patient the correct use of suppositories to help establish a regular bowel schedule.
- Refer the patient and family to the National Multiple Sclerosis Society for more information.

Hard to predict

Myasthenia gravis has an unpredictable course that includes periods of exacerbation and remission. There's no known cure. Drug treatment has improved the prognosis and allows patients to lead relatively normal lives, except during exacerbations. However, if the disease involves the respiratory system, it can be life-threatening. Myasthenia gravis affects 2 to 20 people per 100,000. It's most common in women between ages 18 and 25 and in men between ages 50 and 60.

What causes it

The cause of myasthenia gravis isn't known; however, it commonly accompanies autoimmune and thyroid disorders. In fact, 15% of all patients with myasthenia gravis have thymomas.

Pathophysiology

The patient's blood cells and thymus gland produce antibodies that block, destroy, or weaken the neuroreceptors that transmit nerve impulses, causing a failure in transmission of nerve impulses at the neuromuscular junction. (See *What happens in myasthenia gravis.*)

> In myasthenia gravis, we produce antibodies that ultimately cause nerve impulse transmission failure. We wish we knew why we do that!

What to look for

Common signs of myasthenia gravis include:
• gradual, progressive skeletal muscle weakness and fatigue that worsens during the day
• weak eye closure, ptosis, and diplopia
• blank, masklike facial expression
• difficulty chewing and swallowing
• a hanging jaw
• bobbing motion of the head
• symptoms of respiratory failure if respiratory muscles are involved.

What tests tell you

• The Tensilon test confirms the diagnosis by temporarily improving muscle function after an I.V. injection of edrophonium or neostigmine. Long-standing ocular muscle dysfunction, however, may not respond. This test also differentiates a myasthenic crisis from a cholinergic crisis.
• Electromyography helps differentiate nerve disorders from muscle disorders.
• Nerve conduction studies test for receptor antibodies.

A closer look

What happens in myasthenia gravis

During normal neuromuscular transmission, a motor nerve impulse travels to a motor nerve terminal, stimulating the release of a chemical neurotransmitter called acetylcholine (ACh). When ACh diffuses across the synapse, receptor sites in the motor end plate react and depolarize the muscle fiber. The depolarization spreads through the muscle fiber, causing muscle contraction.

Those darned antibodies

In myasthenia gravis, antibodies attach to the ACh receptor sites. They block, destroy, and weaken these sites, leaving them insensitive to ACh, thereby blocking neuromuscular transmission.

Axon

Vesicle containing ACh

Neuromuscular junction

Release site

ACh receptor site

Muscle

Motor end plate

Junctional fold

Thymectomy may lead to remission in adult-onset myasthenia gravis.

How it's treated

Treatment is symptomatic. Anticholinesterase drugs, such as neostigmine and pyridostigmine, counteract fatigue and muscle weakness and enable about 80% of normal muscle function. However, these measures become less effective as the disease worsens. Corticosteroids may help to relieve symptoms. A patient may undergo plasmapheresis. One with thymomas requires thymectomy, which may lead to remission in adult-onset myasthenia gravis.

In a crisis

Acute exacerbations that cause severe respiratory distress necessitate emergency treatment. Tracheotomy, positive-pressure ventilation, and vigorous suctioning to remove secretions usually yield improvement in a matter of days. Anticholinesterase drugs aren't effective during myasthenic crisis, so they're discontinued until respiratory function begins to improve. A crisis requires immediate hospitalization and vigorous respiratory support.

What to do

• Establish an accurate neurologic and respiratory baseline. Help remove secretions as they accumulate. Be alert for signs of an impending crisis (increased muscle weakness, respiratory distress, and difficulty talking or chewing).
• For the best results, administer drugs at evenly spaced intervals and on time, as ordered. Be prepared to give atropine for anticholinesterase overdose or toxicity.
• Plan periods of exercise, meals, patient care, and daily activities to take advantage of peaks in the patient's energy level.
• Provide soft, solid foods instead of liquids to reduce the risk of choking. Always sit the patient up to eat.
• Encourage the patient to take a roll in deciding about his care.
• Evaluate the patient. Look for normal vital signs, evidence of adequate hydration and normal elimination, skin that's free from sores or problems, and an optimal capacity for activity.
• Encourage the patient and his family to discuss their feelings, especially feelings of frustration, grief, or loss. Listen and provide emotional support. (See *Myasthenia gravis teaching tips*.)

Parkinson's disease

Parkinson's disease, a slowly progressive and degenerative disorder, is one of the most common neurologic disorders in the United States. Parkinson's disease may appear at any age; however, it's rare in people under age 30 and risk increases with age. Parkinson's disease most commonly affects men, and strikes 1 out of every 100 people over age 60.

What causes it

In most instances, the cause of Parkinson's disease isn't known. However, some cases result from exposure to toxins, such as manganese dust and carbon monoxide, that destroy cells in the substantia nigra of the brain.

Education edge

Myasthenia gravis teaching tips

• Help the patient plan daily activities to coincide with energy peaks. Stress the need for frequent rest periods throughout the day. Emphasize that periodic remissions, exacerbations, and day-to-day fluctuations are common.
• Teach the patient how to recognize adverse effects and signs of toxicity of anticholinesterase drugs (headaches, weakness, sweating, abdominal cramps, nausea, vomiting, diarrhea, excessive salivation, bronchospasm) and corticosteroids. Warn him to avoid strenuous exercise, stress, infection, and unnecessary exposure to the sun or cold weather. Caution him to avoid taking other medications without consulting his primary health care provider.
• Refer the patient to the Myasthenia Gravis Foundation for more information.

Pathophysiology

Parkinson's disease affects the extrapyramidal system, which influences the initiation, modulation, and completion of movement. The extrapyramidal system includes the corpus striatum, globus pallidus, and substantia nigra.

In Parkinson's disease, a dopamine deficiency occurs in the basal ganglia, the dopamine-releasing pathway that connects the substantia nigra to the corpus striatum. Reduction of dopamine in the corpus striatum upsets the normal balance between the dopamine (inhibitory) and acetylcholine (excitatory) neurotransmitters. Symptoms occur when affected brain cells can no longer perform their normal inhibitory function within the CNS.

My cells can't be expected to perform under these conditions! Where's the dopamine?!

What to look for

Signs and symptoms include:
• insidious tremor that begins in the fingers (unilateral pill-roll tremor), increases during stress or anxiety, and decreases with purposeful movement and sleep
• muscle rigidity that resists passive muscle stretching; it may be uniform (lead-pipe rigidity) or jerky (cogwheel rigidity)
• difficulty walking (gait lacks normal parallel motion and may be retropulsive or propulsive)
• bradykinesia or slowing of muscle movements
• high-pitched monotone voice
• drooling
• masklike facial expression, poor blink reflex, and wide-open eyes
• loss of postural control (body bent forward while walking)
• slowed, monotonous, slurred speech that may become severely dysarthric
• dysphagia
• oculogyric crises (eyes are fixed upward, with involuntary tonic movements) and, occasionally, blepharospasm.

What tests tell you

Laboratory test results rarely identify Parkinson's disease. Consequently, diagnosis depends on the patient's age, health history, and presence of characteristic signs of disease. However, urinalysis may reveal decreased dopamine levels, and CT scan or MRI may help rule out other disorders such as an intracranial tumor.

So, is it Parkinson's disease?

Hmmm? Oh, lab results rarely identify Parkinson's disease. I'm looking at my vacation schedule.

How it's treated

There's no known cure for Parkinson's disease. Treatment focuses on relieving symptoms and maintaining as high a level of function as possible for as long as possible. Drug therapy and physical therapy are the modes of treatment. In severe disease, stereotactic neurosurgery may be used.

Typical drug therapy includes levodopa, a dopamine replacement that's most effective in the early stages. Levodopa can cause significant adverse reactions, so it's frequently prescribed with carbidopa, which halts peripheral dopamine synthesis. If levodopa proves ineffective or too toxic, alternative drug therapy may include:
• dopamine agonists, such as pergolide, pramipexole, or ropinirole
• anticholinergics such as trihexyphenidyl
• antihistamines such as diphenhydramine
• amantadine, an antiviral agent
• selegiline, an enzyme inhibitor.

A class by itself

A new class of drugs, catechol-O-methyltransferase (COMT) inhibitors (tolcapone), which are taken with levodopa, are achieving some measure of success in prolonging relief from symptoms. These drugs block the enzyme that breaks down levodopa before it enters the brain. This enhances and prolongs the effect of levodopa. In younger patients, dopamine agonists may be used before COMT inhibitors. Unfortunately, prolonged use of any drug tends to reduce its effectiveness.

In stereo

If drug therapy fails, stereotactic neurosurgery may offer a viable alternative. This procedure interrupts the function of the subthalamic nucleus, the pallidum, or the ventrolateral nucleus of the thalamus to prevent involuntary movement. This treatment is most effective in younger and otherwise healthy patients who have unilateral tremor or muscle rigidity. Neurosurgery is a palliative measure that can only relieve symptoms, not reverse the disease.

One deep brain

In some cases, deep brain stimulation is used to stop uncontrolled movements. The surgeon places electrodes in the thalamus or globus pallidus. Leads connect the electrodes to a device that the patient can activate when symptoms occur.

Get physical

Physical therapy complements drug treatment and neurosurgery to maintain normal muscle tone and function. Typically, physical

Here's to COMT inhibitors. I'll take all the help I can get!

therapy includes active and passive ROM exercises, routine daily activities, walking, and baths and massage to help relax muscles.

What to do

• If the patient has had surgery, monitor his LOC and vital signs closely for hemorrhage or increased ICP.

• Encourage independence. A patient with excessive tremor may have better control if he sits in a chair and uses the chair's arms to steady himself. Remember that fatigue can exacerbate symptoms and, in turn, increase the patient's dependence on others.

• Establish a regular bowel routine by encouraging the patient to drink 2 qt (2 L) of liquid daily and eat high-fiber foods. An elevated toilet seat can make it easier to transition from standing to sitting.

• Encourage the patient to remain as active as possible. The disease progresses more slowly in those who stay active.

• Encourage the patient and his family to ask questions. Listen to their concerns and provide succinct, accurate answers.

• Evaluate the patient. Optimal oxygen saturation levels will indicate adequate respiratory function. He should have normal urinary function and be free from UTI. In addition, he should perform normal daily activities within the limits imposed by his condition. The patient and his family should understand Parkinson's disease and its treatment. (See *Parkinson's disease teaching tips*.)

Stroke

Stroke is the sudden interruption of circulation in one or more of the blood vessels supplying the brain. During a stroke, brain tissue fails to receive adequate oxygenation, resulting in serious tissue damage or necrosis. The speed with which circulation is restored determines the patient's chances for complete recovery.

Not the back stroke

Strokes are classified by their course of progression. The least severe type, called *TIA*, results from a temporary interruption of blood flow. (See *Understanding TIA*, page 158.) A progressive stroke, or stroke-in-evolution (thrombus-in-evolution), begins with a slight neurologic deficit that worsens over a day or two. In a complete stroke, the patient experiences maximum neurologic impairment immediately.

Factor this in

Stroke is the third most common cause of death in the United States and the most common cause of neurologic disability. Risk factors include a history of TIAs, atherosclerosis, hypertension, arrhythmias, lack of exercise, use of hormonal contraceptives, smoking, and a family history of cerebrovascular disease.

Education edge

Parkinson's disease teaching tips

• Teach the patient and family about the disease, its possible progressive stages, therapeutic management, and prevention of complications and injuries.

• Instruct the patient on his drug therapy and the relationship of drug administration to diet and food intake if he's taking levodopa. Caution him that drugs for Parkinson's disease commonly interact with medications taken for many other conditions.

• Encourage exercise, maximal independence in activities of daily living, and physical and occupational therapy to maintain muscle strength.

• Refer the patient and family to the National Parkinson Foundation or the United Parkinson Foundation for more information.

What causes it

Major causes of stroke include:
• thrombosis of the cerebral arteries that supply the brain or the intracranial vessels, occluding blood flow
• embolism from a thrombus outside the brain—for example, in the heart, aorta, or common carotid artery
• hemorrhage from an intracranial artery or vein, possibly due to hypertension, ruptured aneurysm, AVM, trauma, hemorrhagic disorder, or septic embolism.

Pathophysiology

Thrombosis, embolus, and hemorrhage act in different ways.
• Thrombosis causes congestion and edema in the affected vessel and ischemia in the tissues supplied by the vessel.
• Embolus cuts off circulation in the cerebral vasculature by lodging in a narrow portion of the artery, causing necrosis and edema. If the embolus is septic and the infection extends beyond the vessel wall, an aneurysm may form, which increases the risk of a sudden rupture and cerebral hemorrhage.

Thrombosis, embolus, and hemorrhage are the major causes of stroke, the third most common cause of death in the United States.

Understanding TIA

A transient ischemic attack (TIA) is a recurrent episode of neurologic deficit, lasting from seconds to hours, that clears within 12 to 24 hours. It's usually considered a warning sign of an impending thrombotic stroke. In fact, TIAs have been reported in 50% to 80% of patients who have had a cerebral infarction from thrombosis. The age of onset varies, but incidence rises dramatically after age 50 and is highest among blacks and men.

Interrupting blood flow
In a TIA, microemboli released from a thrombus may temporarily interrupt blood flow, especially in the small distal branches of the brain's arterial tree. Small spasms in those arterioles may precede the TIA and also impair blood flow.

A transient experience
The most distinctive characteristics of TIAs are the transient duration of neurologic deficits and the complete return of normal function. The signs and symptoms of a TIA correlate with the location of the affected artery. They include double vision, unilateral blindness, staggering or uncoordinated gait, unilateral weakness or numbness, falling because of weakness in the legs, dizziness, and speech deficits, such as slurring and thickness.

Preventing a complete stroke
During an active TIA, treatment aims to prevent a complete stroke and consists of aspirin or anticoagulants to minimize the risk of thrombosis. After or between attacks, preventive treatment includes carotid endarterectomy or cerebral microvascular bypass.

• In hemorrhage, an artery in the brain bursts, rapidly reducing the blood supply to tissues served by the artery. Blood accumulates deep within the brain, causing even greater damage by further compromising neural tissue.

What to look for

When assessing signs of stroke, "sudden" is the key word. Signs typically include the sudden onset of:
• headache with no known cause
• numbness or weakness of the face, arm, or leg, especially on one side of the body
• confusion, trouble speaking or understanding
• trouble seeing or walking, dizziness, loss of coordination.

When assessing for stroke, remember three S's: Signs of stroke are sudden.

What tests tell you

• MRI or a CT scan shows evidence of thrombotic or hemorrhagic stroke, tumor, or hydrocephalus.
• Brain scan reveals ischemia, but may not be positive for up to 2 weeks after the stroke.
• In hemorrhagic stroke, lumbar puncture may reveal blood in the CSF.
• Carotid ultrasound may detect a blockage, stenosis, or reduced blood flow.
• Ophthalmoscopy may detect signs of hypertension and atherosclerosis in retinal arteries.
• Angiography can help pinpoint the site of occlusion or rupture.
• EEG may help localize the area of damage.
• Other laboratory studies, such as urinalysis, coagulation studies, CBC, serum osmolality, and electrolyte, glucose, lipid profile, antinuclear antibody, creatinine, and blood urea nitrogen levels, help establish a baseline.

How it's treated

Medical management of stroke commonly includes physical rehabilitation, diet and drug regimens to help reduce risk factors, possibly surgery, and care measures to help the patient adapt to specific deficits, such as motor impairment and paralysis.

Medical management of stroke includes a drug regimen to help reduce risk factors.

Surgery possibilities

Depending on the stroke's cause and extent, the patient may undergo craniotomy to remove a hematoma, endarterectomy to remove atherosclerotic plaques from an arterial wall, or extracranial bypass to circumvent a blocked artery. Ventricular shunts may be needed to drain CSF.

Take two

Drug therapy for stroke includes:
• aspirin or ticlopidine as an antiplatelet agent to prevent recurrent stroke (but not in hemorrhagic stroke)
• benzodiazepines, such as lorazepam and diazepam, to treat seizures
• anticonvulsants to treat or prevent seizures after the patient's condition has stabilized
• thrombolytics, such as alteplase for emergency treatment of embolic stroke (typically within 3 hours of onset), or aspirin or heparin for patients with embolic or thrombotic stroke who aren't candidates for alteplase
• stool softeners, such as dioctyl sodium sulfosuccinate, to prevent straining, which increases ICP
• antihypertensives and antiarrhythmics to reduce risks associated with recurrent stroke
• corticosteroids, such as dexamethasone, to minimize associated cerebral edema
• analgesics to relieve headache following a hemorrhagic stroke.

What to do

• Maintain a patent airway and oxygenation. Loosen constricting clothes. Watch the patient's cheeks. If one side "balloons" with respiration, that's the side the stroke affected. If unconscious, the patient may aspirate saliva; keep him in a lateral position to promote drainage, or suction as needed. Insert an artificial airway and start mechanical ventilation or supplemental oxygen if needed.
• Check the patient's vital signs and neurologic status. Record observations and report any significant changes, such as changes in pupil dilation, signs of increased ICP, and nuchal rigidity or flaccidity. Monitor blood pressure, LOC, motor function (voluntary and involuntary movements), senses, speech, skin color, and temperature. A subsequent stroke may be imminent if blood pressure rises suddenly, the pulse is rapid and bounding, and the patient complains of a sudden headache.

Checking for color changes

• Watch for signs and symptoms of pulmonary emboli, such as chest pain, shortness of breath, dusky color, tachycardia, fever, and changed sensorium. If the patient is unresponsive, monitor his arterial blood gas levels often, and alert the doctor to increased $Paco_2$ or decreased partial pressure of arterial oxygen.
• Maintain fluid and electrolyte balance. If the patient can drink fluids, offer them as often as fluid limitations permit. Give I.V. fluids as ordered; yet, never give a large volume rapidly as this can

Watch the patient's cheeks. If one side balloons with respiration, that's the affected side.

increase ICP. Offer the bedpan or help the patient to the bathroom every 2 hours. If incontinent, the patient may need an indwelling urinary catheter. This increases the risk of infection.
- Ensure adequate nutrition. Check for gag reflex before offering small amounts of semisolid foods. Place the food tray within the patient's visual field. If the patient can't eat, insert an NG tube.
- Manage GI problems. Be alert for signs of straining as this increases ICP. Modify the patient's diet and administer a stool softener, as ordered. If the patient is nauseous, position him on his side to prevent aspiration of vomit. Provide antacids to reduce the risk of ulcer formation.
- Clean and irrigate the patient's mouth or dentures to remove food particles.

Keeping a watchful eye

- Provide meticulous eye care. Remove secretions with a gauze pad and sterile normal saline solution. Instill eyedrops, as ordered. If he's unable to close his eye, cover it with a patch.
- Position the patient. High-top sneakers, splints, or a footboard will help prevent footdrop and contracture. To prevent pressure ulcers, reposition the patient often or use a special mattress. Turn the patient at least once every 2 hours to prevent pneumonia. Raise the hand on the affected side to control dependent edema.
- Help the patient exercise. Perform ROM exercises for the affected and unaffected sides. Show him how to use his unaffected limbs to exercise his affected limbs.
- Administer medications, as ordered, and monitor the patient for adverse reactions.

Speak no evil

- Maintain communication with the patient. If he's aphasic, set up a simple method of communicating. Remember that an unresponsive patient may be able to hear. Don't say anything in his presence that you wouldn't want him to hear.
- Provide emotional support and establish a rapport. Spend time with the patient. Set realistic short-term goals and get the patient's family involved in his care when possible.
- Evaluate the patient. Look for a patent airway, normal breath sounds, adequate mobility, stable or improving LOC, and proper nutrition. Encourage the patient and his family as they cope with the disorder. (See *Stroke teaching tips*.)

Education edge

Stroke teaching tips

- Teach the patient to comb his hair, dress, and wash, if needed. Obtain appliances, such as walkers, grab bars for the bathtub and toilet, and ramps, as needed.
- Encourage the patient to begin speech therapy, and follow through with the speech pathologist's suggestions.
- Involve the patient's family in all aspects of rehabilitation.
- If aspirin has been prescribed to minimize the risk of embolic stroke, tell the patient to watch for GI bleeding related to ulcer formation. Make sure the patient realizes that he can't substitute acetaminophen for aspirin.
- Warn the patient and family to report symptoms of stroke, such as severe headache, drowsiness, confusion, and dizziness. Emphasize the importance of regular follow-up visits.

Quick quiz

1. The most common cause of dementia is:
   A.   Alzheimer's disease.
   B.   stroke.
   C.   Parkinson's disease.
   D.   aging.

Answer: A. Alzheimer's disease is the most common cause of dementia and the fourth leading cause of death in adults.

2. Brudzinski's sign and Kernig's sign are two tests that help diagnose:
   A.   stroke.
   B.   seizure disorder.
   C.   meningitis.
   D.   Parkinson's disease.

Answer: C. A positive response to one or both tests indicates meningeal irritation.

3. MS is characterized by:
   A.   progressive demyelination in the CNS.
   B.   impaired cerebral circulation.
   C.   deficiency of the neurotransmitter dopamine.
   D.   deterioration of the spinal column.

Answer: A. Patches of demyelination cause widespread neurologic dysfunction.

4. Drug therapy for seizure disorder typically includes:
   A.   antibiotics.
   B.   anticonvulsants.
   C.   antihypertensives.
   D.   antiparkinson agents.

Answer: B. Anticonvulsants are commonly prescribed to control seizures. Adhering to the prescribed drug treatment plan and obtaining follow-up care to evaluate drug effectiveness are very important in controlling seizure activity.

Scoring

☆☆☆   If you answered all four items correctly, YOWZA! Your neurons are firing at hyperspeed!

 ☆☆   If you answered three items correctly, what an achievement! Hope you didn't strain a cranial nerve.

  ☆   If you answered fewer than three items correctly, never fear. A review will restore your knowledge of neurologic disorders.

Eye disorders

Just the facts

In this chapter, you'll learn:

♦ tools and techniques to evaluate the eyes

♦ relevant diagnostic tests

♦ commonly used nursing diagnoses

♦ common eye disorders and treatments.

About 70% of all sensory information reaches the brain through the eyes. Disorders in vision can interfere with a patient's ability to function independently, perceive the world, and enjoy beauty.

No matter where you practice nursing, you're likely to encounter patients with eye problems. Some patients may report an eye problem as their chief complaint; others may tell you of a problem while you're evaluating another complaint or performing routine care.

Some patients may seek care for an eye problem, and others may tell you of a problem during routine care.

Anatomy and physiology

The eye is the sensory organ of sight. It's a hollow ball filled with fluid (vitreous humor) and consists of three layers:

fibrous outer layer—sclera, bulbar conjunctiva, and cornea

vascular middle layer—iris, ciliary body, and choroid

inner layer—retina.

Lens and liquids

Between the iris and retina lies the lens, suspended by ligaments from the ciliary body. The vitreous and aqueous humors are separated by the lens. The vitreous humor lies behind the lens, and the aqueous humor, in front of the lens.

A close look at the eye

This cross section details important anatomic structures of the eye.

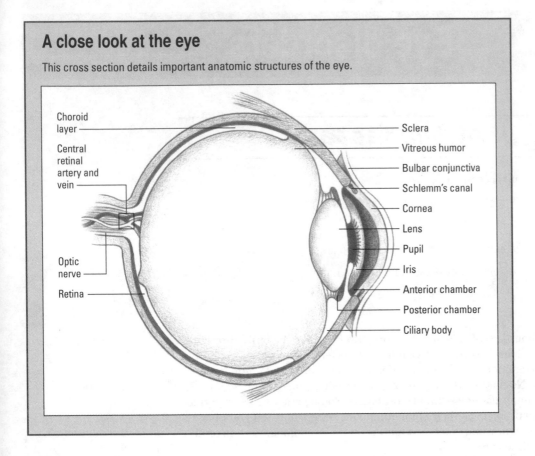

Choroid layer
Central retinal artery and vein
Optic nerve
Retina

Sclera
Vitreous humor
Bulbar conjunctiva
Schlemm's canal
Cornea
Lens
Pupil
Iris
Anterior chamber
Posterior chamber
Ciliary body

Eyelids, lashes, and the lacrimal apparatus protect the eye.

Muscles for movement

Six extraocular muscles, innervated by the cranial nerves, control the movement of the eyes. The coordinated actions of those muscles allow the eyes to move in tandem, ensuring clear vision.

Lashes and lacrimals

Outside the eye, the bony orbits protect it from trauma. Eyelids (palpebrae), lashes, and the lacrimal apparatus protect the eye from injury, dust, and foreign bodies. (See *A close look at the eye.*)

Sclera, bulbar conjunctiva, and cornea

The sclera is the white coating on the outside of the eyeball. Together with the vitreous humor on the inside, the sclera helps maintain the retina's placement and the eyeball's nearly spherical shape. The bulbar conjunctiva is a thin, transparent membrane that lines the eyelid and covers and protects the anterior portion of the white sclera. The cornea is a smooth, avascular, transparent tissue that refracts (bends) light rays entering the eye. It's coated with a tear film, which keeps the eye moist, and merges with the sclera at the corneal limbus.

Here's mud in your eye

The cornea, located in front of the iris, is fed by the ophthalmic branch of cranial nerve V (trigeminal nerve). Stimulation of this nerve initiates a protective blink called the *corneal reflex.*

Iris and pupil

The iris is a circular, contractile diaphragm that contains smooth and radial muscles and is perforated in the center by the pupil. Varying amounts of pigment granules within the iris's smooth muscle fibers give it color. Its posterior portion contains involuntary muscles that control pupil size to regulate the amount of light entering the eye.

Grand opening

The pupil, the iris's central opening, is normally round and equal in size to the opposite pupil. The pupil permits light to enter the eyes. Depending on the patient's age, pupil diameter can range from 3 to 5 mm.

Ciliary body and choroid

Suspensory ligaments attached to the ciliary body control the lens's shape for close and distant vision. The pigmented, vascular choroid supplies the outer retina's blood supply, then drains blood through its remaining vasculature.

Lens and vitreous chamber

Located behind the iris at the pupillary opening, the lens consists of avascular, transparent fibrils in an elastic membrane called the *lens capsule.* The lens refracts and focuses light onto the retina. The vitreous chamber located behind the lens occupies four-fifths of the eyeball. This chamber is filled with vitreous humor, the gelatinous substance that, along with the sclera, maintains the shape of the eyeball.

Posterior and anterior chambers

The posterior chamber, located directly in front of the lens, is filled with a watery fluid called *aqueous humor.* As it flows through the pupil into the anterior chamber, this fluid bathes the

Is that your corneal reflex, or are you just happy to see me?

The lens of the eye refracts and focuses light onto the retina.

lens capsule. The amount of aqueous humor in the anterior chamber varies to maintain pressure in the eye. Fluid drains from the anterior chamber through collecting channels (trabecular meshwork) into Schlemm's canal.

Retina

The retina is the innermost layer of the eyeball. It receives visual stimuli and transmits images to the brain for processing. Vision of any kind depends on the retina and its structures. The retina contains the retinal vessels, the optic disk, the physiologic cup, rods and cones, the macula, and the fovea centralis.

I have a great relationship with my retinas. We're constantly communicating.

Retinal vessels

There are four sets of retinal vessels. Each of the four sets contains a transparent arteriole and vein that nourish the inner areas of the retina. As these vessels leave the optic disk, they become progressively thinner, intertwining as they extend to the periphery of the retina.

Optic disk and physiologic cup

The optic disk is a well-defined, round or oval area measuring less than 1/8″ (0.3 cm) within the retina's nasal portion. It's the opening through which the ganglion nerve fibers (axons) exit the retina to form the optic nerve. This area is called the *blind spot* because no light-sensitive cells (photoreceptors) are located there. The physiologic cup is a light-colored depression within the temporal side of the optic disk where blood vessels enter the retina. It covers one-fourth to one-third of the disk.

Rods and cones

Photoreceptor neurons called *rods and cones* make vision possible. Rods respond to low-intensity light and shades of gray. Cones respond to bright light and are responsible for sharp, color vision.

Nothing is black and white, just many shades of gray.

Here comes the sun. Wow, check it out, man. Psychedelic!

Macula and fovea centralis

Located near the center of the retina lateral to the optic disk, the macula is slightly darker than the rest of the retina. The macula provides the sharpest vision, used for reading and recognizing faces, for example. The fovea centralis, a slight depression within the macula, contains the heaviest concentration of cones and is the area that provides clearest vision and color perception.

Assessment

Now that you're familiar with the anatomy and physiology of the eyes, you're ready to assess them.

History

To obtain an accurate and complete patient history, adjust questions to the patient's specific complaint and compare the answers with the results of the physical assessment.

Current health status

To obtain an accurate history of the eyes, first ask the patient questions about his vision, including:
• Do you have problems with your eyes?
• Do you wear or have you ever worn corrective lenses? If so, for how long? Are they glasses or hard or soft contact lenses?
• For what eye condition do you wear corrective lenses? Do you wear them all the time or just for certain activities, such as reading or driving?

Previous health status

To gather information about the patient's past eye health, ask these questions:
• Have you ever had blurred vision? Have you ever seen spots, floaters, or halos around lights?
• Have you ever had eye surgery or an eye injury?
• Do you have a history of high blood pressure or diabetes?
• Are you taking prescription medications for your eyes or other conditions? If so, which medications and how often?

Family health status

Next, question the patient about possible familial eye disorders. Ask if anyone in the patient's family has ever been treated for myopia, cataracts, glaucoma, or loss of vision.

Lifestyle patterns

To explore the patient's daily habits that might affect his eyes, ask these questions:
• Does your occupation require intensive use of your eyes, such as long-term reading or prolonged use of a video display terminal?

Ask your patient whether he has ever had blurred vision.

• Does the air where you work or live contain anything that causes you to have eye problems?
• Do you wear goggles when working with power tools, chain saws, or table saws, or when engaging in sports that might irritate or endanger the eye, such as swimming, fencing, or playing racquetball?

Do you wear goggles when playing sports such as racquetball?

Physical examination

An eye assessment involves inspecting the conjunctivae, assessing the pupils, assessing eye muscle function, and examining intraocular structures with an ophthalmoscope.

Inspecting the conjunctivae

To inspect the conjunctivae, ask the patient to look up. Gently pull the lower eyelid down to inspect the bulbar conjunctiva. It should be clear and shiny. Note excessive redness or exudate. Also observe the sclera's color, which should be white to buff. In black patients, you may see flecks of tan.

Pink palpebrae

To examine the palpebral conjunctiva (the membrane that lines the eyelids), have the patient look down. Then lift the upper lid, holding the upper lashes against the eyebrow with your finger. The palpebral conjunctiva should be uniformly pink.

Assessing the pupils

Each pupil should be equal in size, round, and about one-fourth the size of the iris in normal room light. Unequal pupils generally indicate neurologic damage, iritis, glaucoma, or therapy with certain drugs.

Be direct

Test the pupils for direct and consensual response. In a slightly darkened room, hold a penlight about 20″ (51 cm) from the patient's eyes, and direct the light at one eye from the side. Note the reaction of the pupil you're testing (direct response) and the opposite pupil (consensual response). They should both react the same way. Also note sluggishness or inequality in the response. A pupil that doesn't react to light (a "fixed" pupil) can be an ominous neurologic sign. Repeat the test with the other pupil.

Direct the light at one eye from the side, and note the reaction of the pupil you're testing and of the opposite pupil.

Cardinal positions of gaze

This diagram shows the six cardinal positions of gaze.

RIGHT SUPERIOR

LEFT SUPERIOR

RIGHT LATERAL

LEFT LATERAL

RIGHT INFERIOR

LEFT INFERIOR

So accommodating

To test the pupils for accommodation, place your finger approximately 4″ (10 cm) from the bridge of the patient's nose. Ask the patient to look at a fixed object in the distance and then to look at your finger. His pupils should constrict and his eyes converge as he focuses on your finger.

Assessing eye muscle function

Testing the six cardinal positions of gaze evaluates the function of each of the six extraocular muscles and the cranial nerves responsible for their movement (cranial nerves III, IV, and VI).

Roving eyes

To perform the test, ask the patient to remain still while you hold a pencil or other small object directly in front of his nose at a distance of about 18″ (46 cm). Ask him to follow the object with his eyes without moving his head. Then move the object to each of the six cardinal positions, returning to the midpoint after each movement. The patient's eyes should remain parallel as they move. (See *Cardinal positions of gaze*.)

Examining intraocular structures

The ophthalmoscope allows you to directly observe internal structures of the eye. To see those structures properly, you should ad-

Follow this cardinal with your eyes without moving your head.

just the lens disc several times during your examination. Use the black, positive numbers on the disc to focus on near objects, such as the patient's cornea and lens. Use the red, negative numbers to focus on distant objects such as the retina. (See *Seeing eye to eye*.)

Looking at the lens

First, set the ophthalmoscope's lens disc to zero and hold the ophthalmoscope about 4″ (10 cm) from the patient's eye. Direct the light through the pupil to elicit the red reflex, a reflection of light off the choroid.

Now, move the ophthalmoscope closer to the eye. Adjust the lens disc so you can focus on the eye's anterior chamber and lens. If the lens is opaque, indicating cataracts, you may not be able to complete the examination.

Rotating to the retinal structures

To examine the retinal structures, start with the dial turned to zero. Rotate the lens-power disc to keep the retinal structures in focus. The first retinal structures you'll see are the blood vessels. Rotating the dial into the negative numbers will bring the blood vessels into focus. The arteries will look thinner and brighter than the veins.

Follow one of the vessels along its path toward the nose until you reach the optic disk, where all vessels in the eye originate. Examine arteriovenous crossings for arteriovenous nicking (localized constrictions in the retinal vessels), which might be a sign of hypertension.

Diggin' the disk and depression

The optic disk is a creamy pink to yellow-orange structure with clear borders and a round-to-oval shape. The disk may fill or exceed your field of vision. If you don't see it, follow a blood vessel toward the center until you do. The nasal border of the disk may be somewhat blurred.

Riveted on the retina

Completely scan the retina by following four blood vessels from the optic disk to different peripheral areas. As you scan, note lesions or hemorrhages. (See *A close look at the retina*.)

Movin' in on the macula

Finally, move the light laterally from the optic disk to locate the macula, the part of the eye most sensitive to light. It appears as a darker structure, free from blood vessels. If you locate it, ask the patient to shift his gaze into the light.

Seeing eye to eye

This illustration shows the correct position for the examiner and the patient when an ophthalmoscope is used to examine the internal structures of the eye.

Constrictions in the retinal vessels may be a sign of hypertension. Ack!

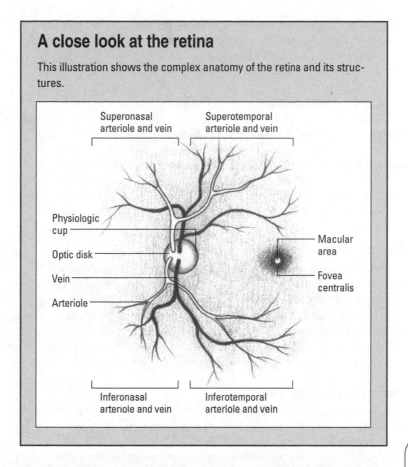

A close look at the retina

This illustration shows the complex anatomy of the retina and its structures.

Superonasal arteriole and vein

Superotemporal arteriole and vein

Physiologic cup

Optic disk

Vein

Arteriole

Macular area

Fovea centralis

Inferonasal arteriole and vein

Inferotemporal arteriole and vein

Diagnostic tests

Tests to determine the presence of eye disorders include direct evaluation as well as radiologic and imaging studies.

Direct evaluation

Refraction, slit-lamp examination, and tonometry allow direct evaluation of various eye structures and functions.

Refraction

Defined as the bending of light rays by the cornea, aqueous humor, lens, and vitreous humor in the eye, refraction enables images to focus on the retina and directly affects visual acuity. This test is done routinely during a complete eye examination

Refraction helps determine the degree of correction to provide in eyeglasses or contact lenses.

or whenever a patient complains of a change in vision. It defines the degree of impairment (refractive error) and determines the degree of correction required to improve visual acuity with glasses or contact lenses.

Nursing considerations

Tell the patient:
• The test is painless and safe; it takes 10 to 20 minutes.
• Eyedrops may be instilled to dilate the pupils and inhibit accommodation by the lens. Ask whether he has had a hypersensitivity reaction to eyedrops, has angle-closure glaucoma, or has an intraocular lens implant. Dilating eyedrops shouldn't be administered to anyone with those conditions.

Slit-lamp examination

The slit lamp is an instrument equipped with a special lighting system and a binocular microscope. This tool allows the doctor to visualize in detail the anterior segment of the eye, which includes the eyelids, eyelashes, conjunctiva, sclera, cornea, tear film, anterior chamber, iris, lens, and anterior portion of the vitreous humor (vitreous face). If abnormalities are noted, special devices may be attached to the slit lamp to allow more detailed investigation.

Nursing considerations

• Patients wearing contact lenses should remove them before the test, unless the test is being performed to evaluate the fit of the contact lenses.
• Don't administer dilating eyedrops to the patient who has angle-closure glaucoma, is hypersensitive to mydriatics, or has an intraocular lens implant.
• When instilling dilating drops, tell the patient that his near vision will be blurred for 40 minutes to 2 hours. Advise him to wear dark glasses in bright sunlight until his pupils return to normal diameter.

Tonometry

Tonometry allows noninvasive measurement of intraocular pressure (IOP) to detect glaucoma, a common cause of blindness, at an early stage in the disease. In the early stages of glaucoma, increased IOP causes the eyeball to harden and become more resistant to extraocular pressure. Indentation tonometry tests this resistance by measuring how deeply a known weight depresses the cornea; applanation tonometry provides the same information by measuring the amount of force required to flatten a known corneal area.

Tell the patient taking dilating eyedrops to wear dark glasses in bright sunlight.

Nursing considerations

• Because an anesthetic is instilled before the test, tell the patient not to rub his eyes for at least 20 minutes after the test, to prevent corneal abrasion.
• If the patient wears contact lenses, tell him not to reinsert them for at least 30 minutes after the test.
• If the tonometer moved across the cornea during the test, tell the patient that he may feel a slight scratching sensation in the eye when the anesthetic wears off. This sensation could be the result of a corneal abrasion and should disappear within 24 hours. However, it may need to be treated with prophylactic antibiotic drops.

Radiologic and imaging studies

Radiologic and imaging studies include fluorescein angiography, ocular ultrasonography, and orbital computed tomography (CT).

Fluorescein angiography

Fluorescein angiography records the appearance of blood vessels inside the eye through rapid-sequence photographs of the fundus (posterior inner part of the eye). The photographs, which are taken with a special camera, follow the I.V. injection of sodium fluorescein. This contrast medium enhances the visibility of microvascular structures of the retina and choroid, allowing evaluation of the entire retinal vascular bed, including retinal circulation.

Nursing considerations

• Check the patient's history for an intraocular lens implant, glaucoma, and hypersensitivity reactions, especially reactions to contrast media and dilating eyedrops.
• If miotic eyedrops are ordered, tell the patient with glaucoma not to use them on the day of the test.
• Observe the patient for hypersensitivity reactions to the dye, such as vomiting, dry mouth, metallic taste, sudden increased salivation, sneezing, light-headedness, fainting, and hives. Rarely, anaphylactic shock may result.
• Explain to the patient that eyedrops will be instilled to dilate his pupils and that a dye will be injected into his arm. Remind him to maintain his position and fixation as the dye is injected. Tell him that he may briefly experience nausea and a feeling of warmth. Reassure him as necessary.
• Remind the patient that his skin and urine will be a yellow color for 24 to 48 hours after the test and that his near vision will be blurred for up to 12 hours.

Show me that beautiful retinal circulation. Work it, work it!

Ocular ultrasonography

Ocular ultrasonography involves the transmission of high-frequency sound waves through the eye and the measurement of their reflection from ocular structures. Illustrating the eyes' structures through ultrasound especially helps to evaluate a fundus clouded by an opaque medium such as a cataract. In such a patient, this test can identify pathologies that are normally undetectable through ophthalmoscopy. Ocular ultrasonography may also be performed before such surgery as cataract removal or implantation of an intraocular lens.

Ocular ultrasonography may identify pathologies that ophthalmoscopy might miss.

Nursing considerations

• Tell the patient that a small transducer will be placed on his closed eyelid and that the transducer will transmit high-frequency sound waves that are reflected by the structures in the eye.
• Inform him that he may be asked to move his eyes or change his gaze during the procedure and that his cooperation is required to ensure accurate determination of test results.
• After the test, remove the water-soluble jelly that was placed on the patient's eyelids.

Orbital computed tomography

Orbital CT allows visualization of abnormalities not readily seen on standard X-rays, such as delineating their size, position, and relationship to adjoining structures. Contrast media may be used in CT to define ocular tissues and help confirm a suspected circulatory disorder, hemangioma, or subdural hematoma. Application of CT to ophthalmology extends beyond the evaluation of the orbital and adjoining structures; it also permits precise diagnosis of many intracranial lesions that affect vision.

Nursing considerations

• If a contrast medium will be administered, withhold food and fluids from the patient for 4 hours before the test. Check his history for hypersensitivity reactions to iodine, shellfish, or radiographic dyes.
• Tell the patient that he'll be positioned on an X-ray table and that the head of the table will be moved into the scanner, which will rotate around his head and make loud, clacking sounds.
• If a contrast medium will be used for the procedure, tell the patient that he may feel flushed and warm and may experience a transient headache, a salty taste, and nausea or vomiting after injection of the medium. Reassure him that these reactions to the contrast medium are typical.

Tell the patient that he'll lie on an X-ray table that will move into the scanner, which will rotate around his head and make loud, clacking sounds.

Treatments

For eye disorders, treatments consist of drug therapy and surgery.

Drug therapy

Topical medications are commonly used to treat eye disorders; however, the doctor may also prescribe systemic medications. These medications include anti-infectives, anti-inflammatories, miotics, mydriatics, vasoconstrictors, and other medications. Proper patient teaching and instillation of topical agents are essential. (See *Instilling eye ointment and eyedrops.*)

Surgery

Surgical treatments for eye disorders include cataract removal, iridectomy, laser surgery, scleral buckling, and trabeculectomy.

Cataract removal

Cataracts can be removed using one of two techniques: intracapsular cataract extraction (ICCE) and extracapsular cataract extraction (ECCE).

Intra isn't in

In ICCE, the entire lens is removed, most commonly with a cryoprobe. However, this technique isn't widely used today.

Nothing extra in *extra* extraction

In ECCE, the patient's anterior capsule, cortex, and nucleus are removed, leaving the posterior capsule intact. ECCE represents the primary treatment for congenital and traumatic cataracts.

In with the implant

Immediately after removal of the natural lens, many patients receive an intraocular lens implant. An implant is especially well suited for elderly patients who are unable to use eyeglasses or contact lenses (because of arthritis or tremors, for example).

Patient preparation

Tell the patient:
• that wearing an eye patch after surgery is temporarily necessary to prevent traumatic injury and infection

Education edge

Instilling eye ointment and eyedrops

To teach about instilling eye ointment, instruct the patient to:
• Hold the tube for several minutes to warm the ointment.
• Squeeze a small amount of ointment ¼″ to ½″ (0.5 to 1.5 cm) inside the lower lid.
• Gently close the eye and roll the eyeball in all directions with the eye closed.
• Wait 10 minutes before instilling other ointments.

To teach about instilling eyedrops, instruct the patient to:
• Tilt his head back and pull down on his lower lid.
• Drop the medication into the conjunctival sac.
• Apply pressure to the inner canthus for 1 minute after administration.
• Wait 5 minutes before instilling a second drop or other eye solutions.

• to be sure to get assistance when getting out of bed
• to sleep on the unaffected side to reduce IOP.

Monitoring and aftercare

After the patient returns from surgery, follow these important steps:
• Notify the doctor if the patient has severe pain. Also, report if IOP has increased.
• Because of the change in the patient's depth perception, assist him with ambulation and observe other safety precautions.
• Make sure the patient wears the eye patch for 24 hours, except when instilling eyedrops as ordered, and have him wear an eye shield, especially when sleeping.
• Instruct the patient to continue wearing the shield at night or whenever he sleeps for several weeks, as ordered.

Home care instructions

Teach the patient or a family member:
• how to administer eyedrops or ointments
• to contact the doctor immediately if sudden eye pain, red or watery eyes, photophobia, or sudden vision changes occur
• to avoid activities that raise IOP, including heavy lifting, straining during defecation, and vigorous coughing and sneezing
• not to exercise strenuously for 6 to 10 weeks
• to wear dark glasses to relieve the glare that he might experience
• that changes in his vision can present safety hazards if he wears eyeglasses
• to use up-and-down head movements to judge distances in order to compensate for loss of depth perception
• how to insert, remove, and care for contact lenses, if appropriate, or how to arrange to visit a doctor routinely for removal, cleaning, and reinsertion of extended-wear lenses
• when he should remove the eye patch and when to begin his eyedrops.

Iridectomy

Performed by laser or standard surgery, an iridectomy reduces IOP by facilitating the drainage of aqueous humor. This procedure makes a hole in the iris, creating an opening through which the aqueous humor can flow to bypass the pupil. An iridectomy is commonly performed to treat acute angle-closure glaucoma.

Wearing an eye patch will prevent injury and infection after surgery — and you can pretend you're a pirate. Aaargh!

Another angle

Because glaucoma is a bilateral disorder, preventive iridectomy is commonly performed on the unaffected eye. It may also be indicated for a patient with an anatomically narrow angle between the cornea and iris. An iridectomy is also used for chronic angle-closure glaucoma, with excision of tissue for biopsy or treatment, and sometimes with other eye surgeries, such as cataract removal, keratoplasty, and glaucoma-filtering procedures.

Patient preparation

Make it clear to the patient that an iridectomy doesn't restore vision loss caused by glaucoma but that it may prevent further loss.

Monitoring and aftercare

After an iridectomy:
• Watch for hyphema (hemorrhaging into the anterior chamber of the eye) with sudden, sharp eye pain or the presence of a small half-moon-shape blood speck in the anterior chamber when checked with a flashlight. If either occurs, have the patient rest quietly in bed, with his head elevated, and notify the doctor.
• Administer a topical corticosteroid to decrease inflammation and medication to dilate the pupil.
• Administer a stool softener to prevent constipation and straining during bowel movements, which increases venous pressure in the head, neck, and eyes leading to elevated IOP or strain on the suture line or blood vessels in the affected area.

Make sure the patient understands that iridectomy won't restore lost vision but may prevent further loss.

Home care instructions

Teach the patient:
• to report sudden, sharp eye pain immediately, because it may indicate increased IOP
• to refrain from strenuous activity for 3 weeks
• to refrain from coughing, sneezing, and vigorous nose blowing, which raise venous pressure
• to move slowly, keep his head raised, and sleep with two pillows under his head.

Laser surgery

Laser surgery is the treatment of choice for a wide variety of ophthalmic disorders because it's relatively painless and especially useful for elderly patients, who may be poor surgical risks. Depending on the type of laser, the finely focused, high-energy beam shines at a specific wavelength and color to produce various effects. Laser surgery can be used to treat retinal tears, diabetic retinopathy, macular degeneration, and glaucoma.

Laser surgery is especially useful for elderly patients.

Patient preparation

Advise the patient:
• He'll be awake and seated at a slit lamp–like instrument for the procedure.
• His chin will be supported and a special contact lens will prevent him from closing his eye.
• Laser use requires safety precautions, including the use of eye protection for everyone in the room. Reflection of the laser beam from a smooth surface, such as a refractor, to a surface such as a disposable drape can start a fire.

Monitoring and aftercare

After the procedure, the patient may occasionally have eye pain. Apply ice packs as needed to help decrease the pain. The patient may be discharged after this office procedure.

Home care instructions

Instruct the patient to receive follow-up care as scheduled. Tell the patient that ice packs may ease eye discomfort.

Scleral buckling

Used to repair retinal detachment, scleral buckling involves applying external pressure to the separated retinal layers, bringing the choroid into contact with the retina. Indenting (or buckling) brings the layers together so that an adhesion can form. It also prevents vitreous fluid from seeping between the detached layers of the retina and leading to further detachment and possible blindness. (See *Scleral buckling for retinal detachment.*)

Another method of reattaching the retina is pneumatic retinopexy. This procedure involves sealing the tear or hole with cryotherapy and introducing gas to provide a tamponade of the retina.

Scleral buckling also prevents me from seeping between layers of the retina.

Patient preparation

Depending on the patient's age and the surgeon's preference, advise him whether he'll receive a local or general anesthetic.

Monitoring and aftercare

After scleral buckling:
• Notify the doctor immediately if you observe eye discharge or if the patient experiences fever or sudden, sharp, or severe eye pain.

Scleral buckling for retinal detachment

In scleral buckling, cryothermy (cold therapy), photocoagulation (laser therapy), or diathermy (heat therapy) creates a sterile inflammatory reaction that seals the retinal hole and causes the retina to readhere to the choroid. The surgeon then places a silicone plate or sponge—called an *explant*—over the site of reattachment and holds it in place with a silicone band. The pressure exerted on the explant indents (buckles) the eyeball and gently pushes the choroid and retina closer together.

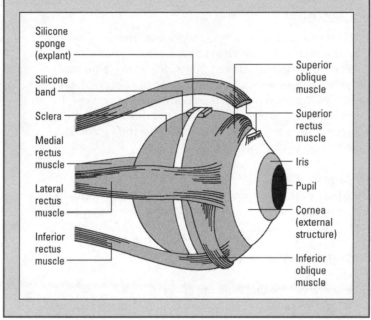

- As ordered, administer mydriatic and cycloplegic eyedrops to keep the pupil dilated, an antibiotic to prevent infection, and a corticosteroid to reduce inflammation.
- For swelling of the eyelids, apply ice packs.
- Because the patient will probably have binocular patches in place for several days, institute safety precautions while he's hospitalized. Raise the side rails of his bed, and help him when he walks.
- Advise the patient to avoid activities that increase IOP, such as hard coughing or sneezing, or straining during defecation. If the he's nauseated, administer an antiemetic, because vomiting increases IOP.

Home care instructions

Instruct the patient:
- to notify the doctor of signs of recurring detachment, including floating spots, flashing lights, and progressive shadow
- to report fever, persistent excruciating eye pain, or drainage
- to avoid activity that risks eye injury
- to avoid heavy lifting, straining, or any strenuous activity that increases IOP
- how to use prescribed dilating, antibiotic, or corticosteroid drops.

Tell the patient to avoid strenuous activity that increases IOP.

Trabeculectomy

Trabeculectomy is a surgical filtering procedure that removes part of the trabecular meshwork to allow aqueous humor to bypass blocked outflow channels and flow safely away from the eye. This procedure creates a filtering bleb or opening under the conjunctiva. An iridectomy is then performed to prevent the iris from prolapsing into the new opening and obstructing the flow of aqueous humor. A trabeculectomy helps treat glaucoma that doesn't respond to drug therapy.

Patient preparation

Inform the patient that this procedure will probably prevent further vision impairment but that it won't restore vision that's already lost.

Monitoring and aftercare

After a trabeculectomy:
- Report excessive bleeding from the affected area.
- Observe for nausea and administer an antiemetic, because vomiting can raise IOP.
- Administer eyedrops (usually a miotic such as pilocarpine).
- Immediately instill a cycloplegic such as atropine. If ordered, give a corticosteroid to reduce iritis, an analgesic to relieve pain, and a beta-adrenergic blocker to reduce pressure.
- Continue previously prescribed eyedrops — a miotic such as pilocarpine or a beta-adrenergic blocker — in the unaffected eye.
- Remind the patient that he should avoid all activities that increase IOP, including hard coughing or sneezing as well as straining during defecation.

Trabeculectomy will probably prevent further vision problems but won't restore the vision you've already lost.

Home care instructions

Instruct the patient:
- to immediately report sudden onset of severe eye pain, photophobia, excessive lacrimation, inflammation, or vision loss
- that glaucoma isn't curable but can be controlled and that he must take prescribed drugs regularly to treat this condition
- to avoid constrictive clothing, coughing, sneezing, or straining because they can increase IOP
- that changes in his vision can present safety hazards and that to overcome the loss of peripheral vision, he should turn his head fully to view objects at his side.

Nursing diagnoses

When caring for patients with eye disorders, you'll find that several nursing diagnoses may be used over and over. These diagnoses are listed here along with nursing interventions and rationales.

Disturbed sensory perception (visual) is about environmental stimuli deprivation.

Disturbed sensory perception (visual)

Related to a vision impairment, *Disturbed sensory perception (visual)* represents the patient's deprivation of environmental stimuli. It's associated with near-sightedness, far-sightedness, diabetes mellitus, cataracts, detached retina, glaucoma, hemianopsia, macular degeneration, optic nerve damage, and blindness.

Expected outcomes

- Patient performs self-care activities safely and within limits.
- Patient uses adaptive and assistive devices.

Nursing interventions and rationales

- Allow the patient to express his feelings about his vision loss. Allowing him to voice his fears aids acceptance of vision loss.
- Remove excess furniture or equipment from the patient's room, and orient him to his surroundings. If appropriate, allow him to direct the arrangement of the room. This provides for the patient's safety while allowing him to maintain an optimal level of independence.

Don't read the fine print

- Modify the patient's environment to maximize any vision the patient may have. Place objects within his visual field, and make sure he's aware of them. Provide large-print books. Modifying the environment helps the patient meet his self-care needs.

• Always introduce yourself or announce your presence when entering the patient's room, and let him know when you're leaving. Familiarizing the patient with the caregiver aids reality orientation.
• Provide nonvisual sensory stimulation to help compensate for the patient's vision loss through talking books, audiotapes, or the radio. Nonvisual sensory stimulation helps the patient adjust to his vision loss.
• Teach the patient about adaptive devices, such as eyeglasses, magnifying glasses, and contact lenses. A knowledgeable patient will be better able to cope with vision loss.
• Refer the patient to appropriate support groups, community resources, or organizations such as the American Foundation for the Blind. Postdischarge support will help the patient and his family cope better with vision loss.

Teach the patient about adaptive devices to help him cope better with his vision loss.

Risk for infection

Related to eye surgery, *Risk for infection* represents the patient's risk of contracting an infection.

Expected outcomes

• Patient has a normal temperature.
• Patient develops no infection postoperatively.
• Patient states that he understands postoperative care and the symptoms of infection.

Nursing interventions and rationales

• Minimize the patient's risk of infection by washing your hands before and after providing care and by wearing gloves when providing direct care. Hand washing is the single best way to avoid spreading pathogens, and gloves offer protection when handling wound dressings or carrying out various treatments.
• Monitor the patient's temperature. Report elevations immediately. An elevated temperature lasting longer than 24 hours after surgery may indicate ocular infection.
• Use strict aseptic technique when suctioning the lower airway, inserting indwelling urinary catheters, providing wound care, and providing I.V. care. This technique helps prevent the spread of pathogens.
• Educate the patient regarding good hand-washing technique, factors that increase infection risk, and the signs and symptoms of infection. These measures allow the patient to participate in his care and help the patient modify his lifestyle to maintain optimal health.

Hand washing is the best way to minimize infection risk.

Common eye disorders

Cataracts, glaucoma, retinal detachment, and vascular retinopathies are common eye disorders.

Cataracts

A common cause of vision loss, a cataract is a gradually developing opacity of the lens or lens capsule of the eye. Cataracts commonly occur bilaterally, with each progressing independently. Exceptions are traumatic cataracts, which are usually unilateral, and congenital cataracts, which may remain stationary. Cataracts are most prevalent in patients over age 70. Prognosis is usually good. Surgery improves vision in 95% of cases.

Cataracts are most prevalent in patients over age 70, but surgery improves vision in 95% of cases. Phew!

What causes it

• Senile cataracts develop in elderly people, probably because of changes in the chemical state of lens proteins.
• Congenital cataracts occur in neonates as genetic defects or as a result of maternal rubella during the first trimester.
• Traumatic cataracts develop after a foreign body injures the lens with sufficient force to allow aqueous or vitreous humor to enter the lens capsule.
• Complicated cataracts occur secondary to uveitis, glaucoma, retinitis pigmentosa, or detached retina. They may also occur in the course of a systemic disease (such as diabetes, hypoparathyroidism, or atopic dermatitis) or can result from ionizing radiation or infrared rays.
• Toxic cataracts result from drug or chemical toxicity with ergot, dinitrophenol, naphthalene, phenothiazine and, in patients with galactosemia, from galactose.

Pathophysiology

Pathophysiology may vary with each form of cataract. However, cataract development typically goes through these four stages:
• immature—partially opaque lens
• mature—completely opaque lens; significant vision loss
• tumescent—water-filled lens, which may lead to glaucoma
• hypermature—deteriorating lens proteins and peptides that leak through the lens capsule, which may develop into glaucoma if intraocular outflow is obstructed.

What to look for

Signs and symptoms of a cataract include:
• painless, gradual blurring and loss of vision
• with progression, whitened pupil
• appearance of halos around lights
• blinding glare from headlights at night
• glare and poor vision in bright sunlight.

What tests tell you

• Shining a penlight on the pupil reveals the white area behind it (unnoticeable until the cataract is advanced).
• Ophthalmoscopy or slit-lamp examination confirms the diagnosis by revealing a dark area in the normally homogeneous red reflex.

How it's treated

Treatment consists of surgical extraction of the opaque lens and postoperative correction of vision deficits. The current trend is to perform the surgery as a 1-day procedure.

What to do

For information on care of the patient undergoing cataract removal surgery, see "Cataract removal," page 175. For patient teaching topics on cataract removal, see *Teaching the patient with cataracts.*

Education edge

Teaching the patient with cataracts

Provide your patient with information on postoperative care, including:
• Avoid bright sunlight by wearing sunglasses that filter out ultraviolet rays.
• Avoid activities that increase intraocular pressure, such as straining with coughing, bowel movements, or lifting heavy objects.

Glaucoma

The term *glaucoma* refers to a group of disorders characterized by abnormally high IOP that can damage the optic nerve. It occurs in three primary forms: open-angle (primary), acute angle-closure, and congenital. It may also be secondary to other causes. In the United States, glaucoma affects 2% of the population over age 40 and accounts for 12.5% of all new cases of blindness. Its incidence is highest among blacks. Prognosis is good with early treatment.

What causes it

Risk factors for chronic open-angle glaucoma include genetics, hypertension, diabetes mellitus, aging, race (blacks), and severe myopia. Precipitating risk factors for acute angle-closure glaucoma include drug-induced mydriasis (extreme dilation of the pupil) and excitement or stress, which can lead to hypertension. Sec-

Glaucoma accounts for 12.5% of all new cases of blindness in the United States.

ondary glaucoma may result from uveitis, trauma, steroids, diabetes, infections, or surgery.

Pathophysiology

Chronic open-angle glaucoma results from overproduction of aqueous humor or obstruction of its outflow through the trabecular meshwork or Schlemm's canal, causing increased IOP and damage to the optic nerve. (See *How aqueous humor normally flows*, page 186.) In secondary glaucoma, such conditions as trauma and surgery increase the risk of intraocular fluid obstruction caused by edema or other abnormal processes.

Outflow obstruction

Acute angle-closure glaucoma, also called *narrow-angle glaucoma*, results from obstruction to the outflow of aqueous humor from anatomically narrow angles between the anterior iris and the posterior corneal surface. It also results from shallow anterior chambers, a thickened iris that causes angle closure on pupil dilation, or a bulging iris that presses on the trabeculae, closing the angle (peripheral anterior synechiae). Any of these conditions may cause IOP to increase suddenly.

Regardless of the type of glaucoma, it's all about flow.

What to look for

Patients with IOP within the normal range of 8 to 21 mm Hg can develop signs and symptoms of glaucoma, and patients who have abnormally high IOP may have no clinical effects. Nonetheless, each type of glaucoma has specific signs and symptoms.

What's the angle?

Chronic open-angle glaucoma is usually bilateral and slowly progressive. Symptoms don't appear until late in the disease. These symptoms include:
• mild aching in the eyes
• gradual loss of peripheral vision
• seeing halos around lights
• reduced visual acuity, especially at night, that's uncorrectable with glasses.

Rapid onset is acute

The onset of acute angle-closure glaucoma is typically rapid, constituting an ophthalmic emergency. Unless treated promptly, this glaucoma produces permanent loss of or decreased vision in the affected eye. Signs and symptoms include:
• unilateral inflammation and pain
• pressure over the eye

Onset of acute angle-closure glaucoma is typically an ophthalmic emergency.

How aqueous humor normally flows

Aqueous humor, a plasmalike fluid produced by the ciliary epithelium of the ciliary body, flows from the posterior chamber to the anterior chamber through the pupil. Here it flows peripherally and filters through the trabecular meshwork to Schlemm's canal and ultimately into venous circulation.

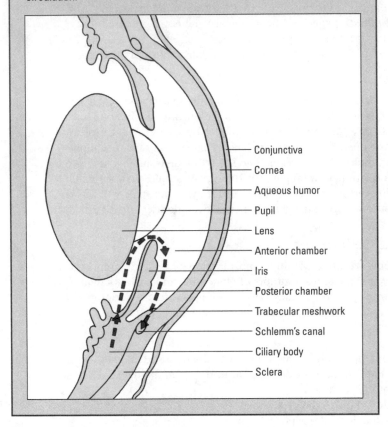

- moderate pupil dilation that's nonreactive to light
- cloudy cornea and blurring and decreased visual acuity
- photophobia and seeing halos around lights
- nausea and vomiting.

What tests tell you

- Tonometry (using an applanation, Schiøtz's, or pneumatic tonometer) measures the IOP and provides a reference baseline.
- Slit-lamp examination is used to assess the anterior structures of the eye, including the cornea, iris, and lens.

• Gonioscopy determines the angle of the eye's anterior chamber, enabling differentiation between chronic open-angle glaucoma and acute angle-closure glaucoma. The angle is normal in chronic open-angle glaucoma; however, in older patients, partial closure of the angle may also occur, so the two forms of glaucoma coexist.
• Ophthalmoscopy provides visualization of the fundus, where cupping and atrophy of the optic disk are apparent in chronic open-angle glaucoma. These changes appear later in uncontrolled chronic angle-closure glaucoma. A pale disk appears in acute angle-closure glaucoma.
• Perimetry establishes peripheral vision loss in chronic open-angle glaucoma. Fundus photography recordings are used to monitor the optic disk for changes.

How it's treated

Treatment for open-angle glaucoma initially decreases IOP through administration of a beta-adrenergic blocker (such as timolol or betaxolol), epinephrine, or a carbonic anhydrase inhibitor (such as acetazolamide). Drug treatment also includes miotic eyedrops, such as pilocarpine, to facilitate outflow of aqueous humor.

When drugs don't work

Patients who are unresponsive to drug therapy may be candidates for argon laser trabeculoplasty or a surgical filtering procedure called *trabeculectomy*, which creates an opening for aqueous outflow.

It's an emergency

In treating acute angle-closure glaucoma as an emergency, drug therapy may lower IOP. When pressure decreases, laser iridotomy or surgical peripheral iridectomy is performed to maintain aqueous flow from the posterior to the anterior chamber. Iridectomy relieves pressure by excising part of the iris to reestablish aqueous humor outflow. A prophylactic iridectomy is performed a few days later on the normal eye.

Drugs STAT

Medical emergency drug therapy includes acetazolamide to lower IOP; pilocarpine to constrict the pupil, forcing the iris away from the trabeculae and allowing fluid to escape; and I.V. mannitol (20%) or oral glycerin (50%) to force fluid from the eye by making the blood hypertonic. Severe pain may necessitate a narcotic analgesic.

What to do

• For the patient with acute angle-closure glaucoma, give medications, as ordered, and prepare him psychologically for laser iridotomy or surgery. (For care of the surgical patient, see "Iridectomy," page 176, and "Trabeculectomy," page 180.)
• Evaluate the patient. He should follow the treatment regimen and obtain frequent IOP tests. He should recognize the symptoms of elevated IOP and know when to seek immediate medical attention. (See *Teaching the patient with glaucoma.*)

Retinal detachment

In retinal detachment, the retinal layers split, creating a subretinal space. This space then fills with fluid, called *subretinal fluid.* Retinal detachment usually involves only one eye but may involve the other eye later. Surgical reattachment is almost always successful. However, prognosis for good vision depends on the affected retinal area.

What causes it

Predisposing factors include high myopia and cataract surgery. The most common causes are degenerative changes in the retina or vitreous humor. Other causes include:
• trauma or inflammation
• systemic diseases such as diabetes mellitus
• rarely, retinopathy of prematurity or tumors.

Pathophysiology

Any retinal tear or hole allows the vitreous humor to seep between the retinal layers, separating the retina from its choroidal blood supply. Retinal detachment may also result from seepage of fluid into the subretinal space or from traction that's placed on the retina by vitreous bands or membranes. (See *Understanding retinal detachment.*)

What to look for

Signs and symptoms of retinal detachment include:
• floaters
• light flashes
• sudden, painless vision loss that may be described as a curtain that eliminates a portion of the visual field.

Education edge

Teaching the patient with glaucoma

• Stress the importance of meticulous compliance with prescribed drug therapy to prevent increased intraocular pressure disk changes and vision loss.
• Inform the patient that lost vision can't be restored but treatment may prevent further loss.
• Stress the importance of glaucoma screening for early detection and prevention. All persons over age 35, especially those with a family history of glaucoma, should have an annual tonometric examination.

Symptoms of retinal detachment include light flashes.

A closer look

Understanding retinal detachment

Traumatic injury or degenerative changes cause retinal detachment by allowing the retina's sensory tissue layers to separate from the retinal pigment epithelium. This permits fluid—for example, from the vitreous—to seep into the space between the retinal pigment epithelium and the rods and cones of the tissue layers.

   The pressure that results from the fluid entering the space balloons the retina into the vitreous cavity away from choroidal circulation. Separated from its blood supply, the retina can't function. Without prompt repair, the detached retina can cause permanent vision loss.

Rod and cone layer

Retina separated from choroid

Vitreous humor in subretinal space

Retinal pigment epithelium

Choroid

What tests tell you

• Ophthalmoscopic examination through a well-dilated pupil confirms the diagnosis. In severe detachment, examination reveals folds in the retina and a ballooning out of the area.
• Indirect ophthalmoscopy is also used to search the retina for tears and holes.
• Ocular ultrasonography may be necessary if the lens is opaque or the vitreous humor is cloudy.

How it's treated

Depending on the location and severity of the detachment, treatment may include:
• Restricting eye movements through bed rest and sedation. If the patient's macula is threatened, positioning his head so the tear or

hole is below the rest of the eye may be required before surgical intervention.
• A hole in the peripheral retina can be treated with cryotherapy; a hole in the posterior portion, with laser therapy.
• Retinal detachment rarely heals spontaneously. Surgery—including scleral buckling, pneumatic retinopexy, or vitrectomy (or a combination of these procedures)—can reattach the retina.

What to do

• Provide emotional support because the patient may be understandably distraught about his loss of vision.
• Position the patient face down if gas has been injected to maintain pressure on the retina.
• Evaluate the patient. With successful treatment, he'll experience restored vision without impairment. He should follow up as directed. (See *Teaching the patient with retinal detachment.*)

Vascular retinopathies

Vascular retinopathies are noninflammatory disorders that result from disruption of the eye's blood supply. The four distinct types of vascular retinopathy are central retinal artery occlusion, central retinal vein occlusion, hypertensive retinopathy, and diabetic retinopathy.

Backup on the central artery

Central retinal artery occlusion typically causes permanent blindness. However, some patients experience resolution within hours of treatment and regain partial vision.

What causes it

Central retinal artery occlusion may be idiopathic (no known cause) or result from:
• embolism, atherosclerosis, or infection (such as syphilis or rheumatic fever)
• conditions that retard blood flow, such as temporal arteritis, massive hemorrhage, or carotid occlusion by atheromatous plaques.

In the same vein

Vascular retinopathy may result from prolonged hypertensive disease and from diabetes. Central retinal vein occlusion can result from:
• trauma or external compression of the retinal vein

Education edge

Teaching the patient with retinal detachment

• Explain to the patient undergoing laser surgery that he may have blurred vision for several days afterward.
• Show the patient having scleral buckling surgery how to instill eyedrops properly. After surgery, remind him to lie in the position recommended by the doctor.
• Instruct the patient to rest and to avoid driving, bending, heavy lifting, and other activities that affect intraocular pressure for several days after eye surgery. Discourage activities that could cause the patient to bump the eye.
• Review early symptoms of retinal detachment, and emphasize the need for immediate treatment.

• diabetes, phlebitis, thrombosis, atherosclerosis, glaucoma, polycythemia vera, or sickling hemoglobinopathies.

Pathophysiology

Central retinal artery occlusion and central retinal vein occlusion
occur when a retinal vessel becomes obstructed. The diminished
blood flow causes vision deficits.

Diabetes dysfunction

Diabetic retinopathy results from the microcirculatory changes
that occur with diabetes. These changes occur more rapidly when
diabetes is poorly controlled. Diabetic retinopathy may be nonproliferative or proliferative; proliferative diabetic retinopathy produces fragile new blood vessels (neovascularization) on the disk
and elsewhere in the fundus.

Hypertension havoc

Hypertensive retinopathy results from prolonged hypertension,
which produces retinal vasospasm and consequent damage to and
narrowing of the arteriolar lumen.

Artery or
vein — it's
still all about
flow — or lack
of it. Oh, aye!

What to look for

Signs and symptoms of vascular retinopathies depend on the
cause:
• *central retinal artery occlusion* — sudden painless, unilateral
loss of vision (partial or complete) that may follow transient
episodes of unilateral loss of vision.
• *central retinal vein occlusion* — reduced visual acuity, allowing
perception of only hand movement and light; painless except
when it results in secondary neovascular glaucoma (uncontrolled
proliferation of blood vessels)
• *diabetic retinopathy* — in nonproliferative form, possibly no
signs or symptoms or loss of central visual acuity and diminished
night vision from fluid leakage into the macular region; in proliferative form, sudden vision loss from vitreous hemorrhage or
macular distortion or retinal detachment from scar tissue formation
• *hypertensive retinopathy* — signs and symptoms dependent
on the location of retinopathy (for example, blurred vision if located near the macula).

Symptoms and
tests for vascular
retinopathies
depend on the
type.

What tests tell you

Tests depend on the type of vascular retinopathy. (See *Diagnostic tests for vascular retinopathies*, page 192.)

Diagnostic tests for vascular retinopathies

In vascular retinopathies, diagnostic tests vary depending on the type of retinopathy, such as central retinal artery occlusion, central retinal vein occlusion, diabetic retinopathy, or hypertensive retinopathy.

Central retinal artery occlusion
• Ophthalmoscopy (direct or indirect) shows blockage of retinal arterioles during transient attack.
• Retinal examination within 2 hours of onset shows clumps or segmentation in artery. Later, a milky white retina is seen around the disk because of swelling and necrosis of ganglion cells caused by reduced blood supply. Also, a cherry red spot in macula is seen that subsides after several weeks.
• Color Doppler tests evaluate carotid occlusion without the need for arteriography.

Central retinal vein occlusion
• Ophthalmoscopy (direct or indirect) shows flame-shaped hemorrhages, retinal vein engorgement, white patches among hemorrhages, and edema around the disk.
• Color Doppler tests confirm or rule out occlusion of blood vessels.

Diabetic retinopathy
• Indirect ophthalmoscopic examination shows retinal changes, such as microaneurysms (earliest change), retinal hemorrhages and edema, venous dilation and beading, lipid exudates, fibrous bands in the vitreous, and growth of new blood vessels. Infarcts of the nerve fiber layer are observed.
• Fluorescein angiography shows leakage of fluorescein from weak-walled vessels and "lights up" microaneurysms, differentiating them from true hemorrhages.

Hypertensive retinopathy
• Ophthalmoscopy (direct or indirect) in early stages shows hard, shiny deposits; flame-shaped hemorrhages; silver wire appearance of narrowed arterioles; and nicking of veins where arteries cross them (arteriovenous nicking). In late stages, cotton wool patches, lipid exudates, retinal edema, papilledema due to ischemia and capillary insufficiency, hemorrhages, and microaneurysms in both eyes are seen.

How it's treated

Treatment depends on the cause of the retinopathy:
• *central retinal artery occlusion* — no known treatment, although the doctor may attempt to release the occlusion into the peripheral circulation. To reduce IOP, therapy includes acetazolamide, eyeball massage using a Goldman-type gonioscope and, possibly, anterior chamber paracentesis. The patient may receive inhalation therapy of carbogen (95% oxygen and 5% carbon dioxide) to improve retinal oxygenation. The patient may receive inhalation treatments hourly for 48 hours, so he should be hospitalized for careful monitoring.
• *central retinal vein occlusion* — anticoagulant administration. The doctor may also recommend laser photocoagulation for patients with widespread capillary nonperfusion to reduce the risk of neovascular glaucoma.
• *diabetic retinopathy* — includes controlling the patient's blood glucose levels and laser photocoagulation to cauterize weak, leaking blood vessels. If a vitreous hemorrhage occurs when one of these weak blood vessels breaks and it isn't absorbed in 3 to 6 months, vitrectomy may be performed to restore partial vision.

• *hypertensive retinopathy* — controlling the patient's blood pressure.

What to do

• Arrange for immediate ophthalmologic evaluation when a patient complains of sudden, unilateral loss of vision. Blindness may be permanent if treatment is delayed.
• Administer acetazolamide I.M. or I.V. as ordered. During inhalation therapy, monitor vital signs carefully and discontinue if blood pressure fluctuates markedly or if the patient becomes arrhythmic or disoriented. Monitor the patient's blood pressure if he complains of occipital headache or blurred vision.

Removing obstacles

• Maintain a safe environment for a patient with vision impairment, and teach him how to make his home safer (by removing obstacles and throw rugs, for instance).
• Evaluate the patient. After successful therapy, the patient with a chronic illness should receive follow-up care as directed and comply with the treatment regimen. The patient with diabetes should understand the need for a stable blood glucose level. The patient with hypertension should keep his blood pressure in a safe range.
• If vision worsens, the patient should seek immediate medical attention and follow safety precautions to prevent injury. (See *Teaching the patient with vascular retinopathy.*)

Education edge

Teaching the patient with vascular retinopathy

• Encourage patients with diabetes to comply with prescribed diet, exercise, and medication regimens to prevent diabetic retinopathy.
• Advise patients with diabetes to receive regular ophthalmologic examinations.
• For patients with hypertensive retinopathy, stress the importance of complying with antihypertensive therapy.

Quick quiz

1. Cone receptors are mainly responsible for sensing:
A.   light.
B.   shades of gray.
C.   shapes.
D.   color.

Answer: D. Cones aid in color recognition and are located in the fovea centralis.

2.   A gradually developing opacity of the lens can be found when the patient has:
A.   cataracts.
B.   glaucoma.
C.   corneal abrasion.
D.   vascular retinopathy.

Answer: A. A gradually developing opacity of the lens is a characteristic of cataracts.

3.   A patient complains of unilateral eye inflammation and pain, pressure over his eye, blurred and decreased visual acuity, seeing halos around lights, and nausea and vomiting. He most likely has:
   A.   acute angle-closure glaucoma.
   B.   chronic open-angle glaucoma.
   C.   cataracts.
   D.   retinal detachment.

Answer: A. Eye inflammation and pain, pressure of the eye, blurred and decreased visual acuity, seeing halos around lights, and nausea and vomiting are characteristics of acute angle-closure glaucoma.

4.   The most common cause of retinal detachment is:
   A.   diabetes mellitus.
   B.   brain tumors.
   C.   degenerative changes in the retina or vitreous.
   D.   trauma.

Answer: C. Degenerative changes are the most common cause of retinal detachment.

5.   What *isn't* true about chronic open-angle glaucoma?
   A.   It results from overproduction of aqueous humor or obstruction of its outflow through the trabecular meshwork.
   B.   It's usually familial.
   C.   It results from obstruction to the outflow of aqueous humor from anatomically narrow angles between the anterior iris and the posterior corneal surface.
   D.   It affects 90% of patients with glaucoma.

Answer: C. Acute angle-closure glaucoma—not chronic open-angle glaucoma—results from obstruction to the outflow of aqueous humor from narrow angles between the anterior iris and the posterior corneal surface.

Scoring

☆☆☆   If you answered all five items correctly, gadzooks! Your understanding of eye disorders is 20/20.

☆☆   If you answered three or four items correctly, good job! You have a keen insight on eye disorders.

☆   If you answered fewer than three items correctly, no tears! Focus in on the chapter and try again.

Ear, nose, and throat disorders

Just the facts

In this chapter, you'll learn:

♦ structures and functions of the ear, nose, and throat

♦ how to assess the ear, nose, and throat

♦ nursing diagnoses appropriate for ear, nose, and throat disorders

♦ common ear, nose and throat disorders.

Because ear, nose, and throat (ENT) conditions can cause pain and severely impair a patient's ability to communicate, they require careful nursing assessment and, in many cases, recommendations for follow-up treatment. For example, you may need to refer a patient with a hearing loss to an audiologist for further evaluation or refer a patient with rhinitis to a doctor for hypersensitivity testing.

Anatomy and physiology

To perform an accurate physical assessment, you'll need to understand the anatomy and physiology of the ears, nose, and throat. Let's look at each of them.

Ear

The ear, a sensory organ, enables hearing and maintains equilibrium. It's divided into three main parts — the external ear, the middle ear, and the inner ear.

External and eardrum

The external ear is made up of the skin-covered cartilaginous auricle (pinna) and the external auditory canal. The tympanic

A close look at the ear

Use this illustration to review the structures of the ear.

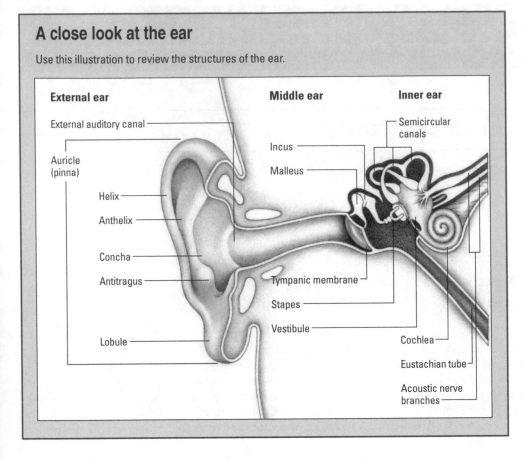

External ear

- External auditory canal
- Auricle (pinna)
- Helix
- Anthelix
- Concha
- Antitragus
- Lobule

Middle ear

- Incus
- Malleus
- Tympanic membrane
- Stapes
- Vestibule

Inner ear

- Semicircular canals
- Cochlea
- Eustachian tube
- Acoustic nerve branches

Sound waves strike the tympanic membrane, which starts all those good vibrations. Can you dig it?

membrane (eardrum) separates the external ear from the middle ear at the proximal portion of the auditory canal.

Three in the middle

The middle ear, a small, air-filled cavity in the temporal bone, contains three small bones—the malleus, the incus, and the stapes.

The inner labyrinth

This cavity leads to the inner ear, a bony and membranous labyrinth, which contains the vestibule, the semicircular canals (the vestibular apparatus), and the cochlea. (See *A close look at the ear.*)

How we hear here

The auricle picks up sound waves and channels them into the auditory canal. There, the waves strike the tympanic membrane, which vibrates and causes the handle of the malleus to vibrate too. These vibrations travel from the malleus, to the incus, to the stapes, through the oval window and the fluid in the cochlea, to the round window.

Hearing hair

The membrane covering the round window shakes the delicate hair cells in the organ of Corti, which stimulates the sensory endings of the cochlear branch of the acoustic nerve (cranial nerve VIII). The nerve sends the impulses to the auditory area of the temporal lobe in the brain, which then interprets the sound.

Nose, sinuses, and mouth

Not only is the nose the sensory organ for smell, but it also warms, filters, and humidifies inhaled air. The sinuses are hollow, air-filled cavities that lie within the facial bones. They include the frontal, sphenoidal, ethmoidal, and maxillary sinuses. The same mucous membrane lines the sinuses and the nasal cavity. Consequently, the same viruses and bacteria that cause upper respiratory tract infections also infect the sinuses. In addition to aiding voice resonance, the sinuses may also warm, humidify, and filter inhaled air, although this role hasn't been firmly established. (See *A close look at the nose and mouth*, page 198.)

Open wide

The lips surround the mouth anteriorly. The soft palate and uvula (a small, cone-shaped muscle lined with mucous membrane that hangs from the soft palate) border it posteriorly. The mandibular bone, which is covered with loose, mobile tissue, forms the floor of the mouth; the hard and soft palates form the roof of the mouth.

Throat

Located in the anterior part of the neck, the throat includes the pharynx, epiglottis, and larynx (voice box). Food travels through the pharynx to the esophagus. Air travels through it to the larynx. The epiglottis diverts material away from the glottis during swallowing and helps prevent aspiration.

High jinx in the larynx

By vibrating exhaled air through the vocal cords, the larynx produces sound. Changes in vocal cord length and air pressure affect the voice's pitch and intensity. The larynx also stimulates the vital cough reflex when a foreign body touches its sensitive mucosa. The most important function of the larynx is to act as a passage for air between the pharynx and the trachea.

Sure, smelling is important, but the nose also helps warm inhaled air, which is pretty important right about now!

A close look at the nose and mouth

These illustrations show the anatomic structures of the nose and mouth.

Nose and mouth

- Superior turbinate
- Middle turbinate
- Kiesselbach's area
- Inferior turbinate
- Hard palate
- Soft palate
- Tongue
- Adenoids
- Mandible

Mouth and oropharynx

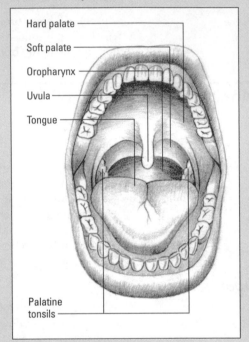

- Hard palate
- Soft palate
- Oropharynx
- Uvula
- Tongue
- Palatine tonsils

Assessment

Now that you're familiar with the anatomy and physiology of the ears, nose, and throat, you're ready to assess them.

History

Before the interview, determine whether the patient hears well. If not, look directly at him and speak clearly.

Current health status

Document in the patient's own words his chief complaint. Ask relevant questions, such as:

If your patient doesn't hear well, look directly at him and speak clearly.

• Have you recently noticed a difference in hearing in one or both ears?
• Do you have ear pain? Is it unilateral or bilateral?
• Do you have frequent headaches, nasal discharge, or postnasal drip?
• Do you experience frequent or prolonged nosebleeds, difficulty swallowing or chewing, or hoarseness or changes in the sound of your voice?

Previous health status

To gather information about the patient's past ENT health, inquire about previous hospitalization, drug therapy, or surgery for an ENT disorder or other relevant condition. Also, be sure to ask these questions:
• Have you ever had an ear injury? Do you suffer from frequent ear infections?
• Are you or have you experienced ringing or crackling in your ears?
• Have you had drainage from your ears or problems with balance, dizziness, or vertigo?
• Do you have sinus infections or tenderness, allergies that cause breathing difficulty, or sensations that your throat is closing?

Family health status

Next, question the patient about possible familial ENT disorders. Ask whether anyone in the patient's family has ever had hearing, sinus, or nasal problems?

Lifestyle patterns

To explore the patient's daily habits that might affect the eyes, ask these questions:
• Do you work around loud equipment, such as printing presses, air guns, or airplanes? If so, do you wear ear protectors?
• Do you smoke, chew tobacco, use cocaine, or drink alcohol? If so, to what extent?

Physical examination

You'll primarily use inspection and palpation to assess the ears, nose, and throat. If appropriate, you'll also perform an otoscopic examination.

If your patient drinks alcohol, find out how much and how often.

Inspecting and palpating the ears

Examine ear color and size. The ears should be similarly shaped, colored the same as the face, and sized in proportion to the head. Look for drainage, nodules, and lesions. Cerumen is usually present and varies from gray-yellow to light brown and black.

Palpate pinna to process; then pull for pain

Palpate the external ear, including the pinna and the tragus, and the mastoid process to discover areas of tenderness, swelling, nodules, or lesions. Then gently pull the helix of the ear backward to determine whether the patient feels pain or tenderness.

Performing an otoscopic examination

Before examining the auditory canal and the tympanic membrane, become familiar with the function of the otoscope. (See *Using an otoscope.*)

Ears don't have to be identical but should be a similar shape, the same color as the face, and in proportion to the head.

Assessing the nose

Inspect the nose for midline position and proportion to other facial features. To assess nasal symmetry, ask the patient to tilt his head back; then observe the position of the nasal septum. The septum should be aligned with the bridge of the nose. With the head in the same position, use a nasal speculum to inspect the inferior and middle turbinates, the nasal septum, and the nasal mucosa. Note the color of the mucosa, evidence of bleeding, and the color and character of drainage. The nasal mucosa is normally redder than the oral mucosa. Identify abnormalities such as polyps.

Palpate for pain and patency

Next, palpate the nose, checking for painful or tender areas, swelling, and deformities. Evaluate nostril patency by gently occluding one nostril with your finger and having the patient exhale through the other.

Assessing the sinuses

To assess the paranasal sinuses, inspect, palpate, and percuss the frontal and maxillary sinuses. (The ethmoidal and sphenoidal sinuses lie above the middle and superior turbinates of the lateral nasal walls and can't be assessed.) To assess the frontal and maxillary sinuses, first inspect the external skin surfaces above and to the side of the nose for inflammation or edema. Then palpate and percuss the sinuses. (See *Palpating the maxillary sinuses*, page 202.) If the nose and sinuses require more extensive assessment, use the techniques of direct inspection and transillumination.

Using an otoscope

Here's how to use an otoscope to examine the ears.

Inserting the speculum

Before inserting the speculum into the patient's ear, straighten the ear canal by grasping the auricle and pulling it up and back, as shown at right.

Positioning the scope

To examine the ear's external canal, hold the otoscope with the handle parallel to the patient's head, as shown at right. Bracing your hand firmly against his head keeps you from hitting the canal with the speculum.

Viewing the structures

Gently insert the speculum to inspect the canal and tympanic membrane. When the otoscope is positioned properly, you should see the tympanic membrane structures, as shown below. The tympanic membrane should be pearl gray, glistening, and transparent. The annulus should be white and denser than the rest of the membrane.

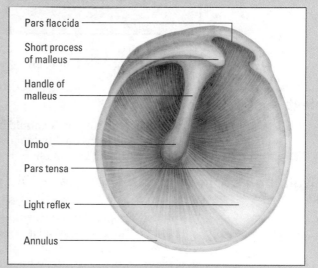

Pars flaccida

Short process of malleus

Handle of malleus

Umbo

Pars tensa

Light reflex

Annulus

Assessing the mouth and throat

Inspection and palpation are used to assess the mouth and throat. First, inspect the patient's lips. They should be pink, moist, symmetrical, and without lesions. Use a tongue blade and a bright light to inspect the oral mucosa. Have the patient open his mouth; then place the tongue blade on top of his tongue. The oral mucosa should be pink, smooth, moist, and free from lesions and unusual odors.

Past the teeth, past the gums

Next, observe the gums (gingivae). They should be pink and moist and should have clearly defined margins at each tooth. Inspect the teeth, noting

Aren't you going to check my ethmoidal sinuses?

That's a trick question, isn't it?

Palpating the maxillary sinuses

To palpate the maxillary sinuses, gently press your thumbs on each side of the nose just below the cheekbones, as shown. The illustration also shows the location of the frontal sinuses.

Oh, boy. I'm gonna need a big tongue blade for this assessment!

their number and condition, and whether any are missing or crowded.

Next stop, the tongue

Next, inspect the tongue. It should be midline, moist, pink, and free from lesions. It should move easily in all directions, and it should lie straight to the front at rest.

Uvula and oropharynx and tonsils — Oh, my!

Inspect the back of the throat (oropharynx) by asking the patient to open his mouth while you shine the penlight on the uvula and palate. You may need to insert a tongue blade into the mouth to depress the tongue. The uvula and oropharynx should be pink and moist, without inflammation or exudates. The tonsils should be pink and shouldn't be hypertrophied. Ask the patient to say "Ahhh." Observe for movement of the soft palate and uvula.

Palpation station

Finally, palpate the lips, tongue, and oropharynx. Note lumps, lesions, ulcers, or edema of the lips or tongue. Assess the patient's gag reflex by gently touching the back of the pharynx with a cotton-tipped applicator or the tongue blade. This should produce a bilateral response.

Diagnostic tests

Tests to determine the presence of ENT disorders should cause your patient little discomfort. These tests include auditory screening tests, audiometric tests, and cultures.

Auditory screening tests

Several tests can help you screen for hearing loss. The first test, the voice test, is a crude method and must be used with other auditory screening tests. Two other screening tests, the Weber and Rinne tests, help detect conductive or sensorineural hearing loss.

Voice test

For the voice test, have the patient occlude one ear with his finger. Test the other ear by standing behind the patient at a distance of 1' to 2' (30 to 60 cm) and whispering a word or phrase. A patient with normal acuity should be able to repeat what was whispered.

Weber test

The Weber test evaluates bone conduction. Perform the test by placing a vibrating tuning fork on top of the patient's head at midline or in the middle of the patient's forehead. The patient should perceive the sound equally in both ears.

Lateral means loss

If the patient has a conductive hearing loss, the sound will lateralize to the ear with the conductive loss because the sound is being conducted directly through the bone to the ear. With a sensorineural hearing loss in one ear, the sound will lateralize to the unimpaired ear because nerve damage in the impaired ear prevents hearing.

Normal is negative

Document a normal Weber test by recording a negative lateralization of sound—that is, sound heard with equal volume in both ears.

Rinne test

The Rinne test compares bone conduction to air conduction in both ears. To administer this test, strike the tuning fork against your hand and place it over the patient's mastoid process. Ask him to tell you when the tone stops, and note this time in seconds. Next, move the still-vibrating tuning fork to the opening of his ear without touching the ear. Ask him to tell you when the tone stops. Note the time in seconds. (See *Positioning the tuning fork*, page 204.)

The voice test should be used only with other auditory screening tests.

Ask the patient to tell you when the tone stops, and note each time in seconds.

Positioning the tuning fork

These illustrations show how to hold a tuning fork to test a patient's hearing.

Weber test
With the tuning fork vibrating lightly, position the tip on the patient's forehead at the midline, as shown, or place the tuning fork on the top of the patient's head.

Rinne test
Strike the tuning fork against your hand, and then hold it behind the patient's ear, as shown. When your patient tells you the tone has stopped, move the still-vibrating tuning fork to the opening of his ear.

To hear air is normal

The patient should hear the air-conducted tone for twice as long as he hears the bone-conducted tone. If he doesn't hear the air-conducted tone longer than he hears the bone-conducted tone, he has a conductive hearing loss in the affected ear.

Audiometric tests

Audiometric tests include acoustic immittance tests and pure tone audiometry. Audiologists perform these tests to confirm hearing loss.

Acoustic immittance tests

Immittance tests help diagnose middle ear disorders, lesions in the seventh (facial) or eighth (acoustic) cranial nerve, and eustachian tube dysfunction. They also can help verify a labyrinthine fistula and identify nonorganic hearing loss. Acoustic immittance tests evaluate middle ear function by measuring sound energy's flow into the ear (admittance) and the opposition to that flow (im-

Immittance tests measure the flow of sound into the ear and the resistance to that flow.

pedance). Acoustic immittance tests include tympanometry and acoustic reflex testing.

Membrane resistance

Tympanometry is the indirect measurement of mobility (compliance) and impedance (resistance of the tympanic membrane and ossicles of the middle ear). It's performed by subjecting the external auditory canal and tympanic membrane to positive and negative air pressure.

That's intense

Acoustic reflex testing measures the change in admittance produced by contraction of the stapedial muscle as it responds to an intense sound. A stimulation in one ear causes reaction in both ears.

Nursing considerations

Instruct the patient:
• not to move, speak, or swallow while admittance is being measured
• not to startle during the loud tone, reflex-eliciting measurement
• to report discomfort or dizziness (which occurs rarely)
• that the probe forms an airtight seal in the ear canal and may cause discomfort but that it won't harm the ear.

Pure tone audiometry

Performed with an audiometer in a soundproof booth, pure tone audiometry provides a record of the thresholds (the lowest intensity levels) at which a patient can hear a set of test tones through earphones or a bone conduction (sound) vibrator. Comparison of air and bone conduction thresholds can help identify a conductive, sensorineural, or mixed hearing loss but won't indicate the cause of the loss.

Nursing considerations

• Make sure the patient has had no exposure to unusually loud noises in the past 16 hours.
• For bone conduction testing, remove the earphones and place the vibrator on the mastoid process of the better ear (the auricle shouldn't touch the vibrator).
• It's important that the ear canals be free from cerumen before audiologic testing begins.

Make sure the patient hasn't been exposed to unusually loud noises in the past 16 hours.

Cultures

Nasopharyngeal and throat cultures can identify various pathogens related to ENT disorders.

Nasopharyngeal culture

Nasopharyngeal culture is used to isolate and identify pathogens in nasopharyngeal secretions. After a specimen is obtained, it's streaked onto a culture plate and organisms present are left to grow. Cultured pathogens may then require sensitivity testing to determine appropriate antibiotic therapy.

Nursing considerations

• Ask the patient to cough before you begin collecting the specimen. Then have him sit with his head tilted back.
• Using a penlight and a tongue blade, inspect the nasopharyngeal area.
• Next, gently pass the swab through the nostril and into the nasopharynx, keeping the swab near the septum and floor of the nose. Rotate the swab quickly and remove it.
• Take care not to injure the nasal mucosa and cause bleeding.

Throat culture

A throat culture primarily isolates and identifies group A beta-hemolytic streptococci *(Streptococcus pyogenes)*, allowing early treatment of pharyngitis and prevention of aftereffects, such as rheumatic heart disease and glomerulonephritis. A throat culture also screens for carriers of *Neisseria meningitidis*.

Swab it

This test involves swabbing the throat, streaking a culture plate, and allowing the organisms to grow so that pathogens can be isolated and identified.

Nursing considerations

Before beginning ordered antibiotic therapy, obtain the throat specimen by implementing this procedure:
• With the patient in a sitting position, tell him to tilt his head back and close his eyes. With the throat well illuminated, check for inflamed areas using a tongue blade.
• Swab the tonsillar areas from side to side, including inflamed or purulent sites. Don't touch the tongue, cheeks, or teeth with the swab.

Say good-bye to that streptococci and live to play another day...

• Immediately place the swab in the culture tube. If you're using a commercial sterile collection and transport system, crush the ampule and force the swab into the medium to keep the swab moist.

Treatments

Here's practical information about the most common drugs and surgical procedures used to treat ENT disorders.

Drug therapy

> The route of administration for ENT drug therapy depends on the disorder.

Drugs used to treat ENT disorders include antihistamines and decongestants as well as anti-infective agents (otic route). The route of administration depends on the disorder:
• nasal — for relief of seasonal or perennial rhinitis and nasal congestion
• systemic — for relief of inflammation and nasal congestion and to treat infection
• otic — for external ear infections, cerumen removal, pain from otitis media, and inflammation of the external ear (instruct the patient using eardrops to lie on his side with the affected ear up for 15 minutes to promote absorption).

Surgery

Surgical treatment of ENT disorders includes the Caldwell-Luc procedure and tonsillectomy and adenoidectomy.

Caldwell-Luc procedure

The Caldwell-Luc procedure, a surgical approach to the maxillary sinus, permits visualization of the antrum, facilitates sinus drainage, and allows access to infected sinuses when an intranasal approach isn't possible because of suppuration or inflammation. It's usually used to treat chronic sinusitis that doesn't respond to other treatments. This procedure also halts persistent epistaxis, provides a tissue sample for histologic analysis, and supplements other treatments such as ethmoidectomy.

Patient preparation

Explain the procedure to the patient. Be sure to tell him:
• to expect considerable swelling of his cheek and numbness and tingling on his upper lip

• that his maxillary sinus and nose may be packed. The packing in the nose is removed after 24 hours; antral packing, after 48 to 72 hours.

Monitoring and aftercare

Immediately after surgery:
• Check for facial edema, and advise the patient to report adverse reactions such as paresthesia of his upper lip.
• If the patient has packing in place, explain that the doctor will remove it within 48 hours. If he has a drainage tube in place for irrigation, assist with irrigation and tell him that the tube will be removed in 3 to 4 days.
• Assess the patient's mouth frequently for bleeding.
• Remind the patient not to touch the incision with his tongue or finger.
• If the patient wears dentures, instruct him not to insert his upper plate for 2 weeks. Also, caution him not to brush his teeth, but rather to rinse his mouth gently with tepid saline solution or diluted mouthwash.
• Until the incision heals, avoid giving foods that require thorough chewing.

> Until the incision heals, avoid giving foods that require thorough chewing.

Home care instructions

Tell the patient:
• to expect some drainage from his nose for a few days after surgery and to monitor the amount, color, and odor
• to call the doctor if he notices bleeding or a foul smell or if drainage persists for more than 5 days
• not to rub or bump his incision
• to avoid engaging in vigorous activity or blowing his nose forcefully for 2 weeks and to sniff gently if he needs to clear his nostrils.

Tonsillectomy and adenoidectomy

Tonsillectomy is the surgical removal of the palatine tonsils. Adenoidectomy is the surgical removal of the pharyngeal tonsils. These procedures were once routinely combined in an adenotonsillectomy to treat enlarged tonsils and adenoids. However, these procedures aren't as common today. Instead, antibiotics are given to treat tonsils and adenoids enlarged by bacterial infection.

Still surgery sometimes

Even so, either or both of these surgeries may be used to resolve tonsillar tissue enlargement that obstructs the upper airway, causing hypoxia or sleep apnea. These procedures may also be used to relieve peritonsillar abscess, chronic tonsillitis, and recurrent otitis media.

Patient preparation

If a patient is scheduled for an adenoidectomy, evaluate whether he has nasal speech or difficulty articulating. If you note these problems, arrange for evaluation by a speech therapist.

Monitoring and aftercare

• Monitor vital signs closely for 24 hours, and watch for hemorrhage. Use a flashlight to check the throat and assess for bleeding. Remember, blood can seep down the back of the patient's throat. Pay special attention to frequent swallowing; it may indicate excessive bleeding.
• Take care not to dislodge clots: Make sure the patient doesn't place straws or other utensils in his mouth. When ordered, start him on soft foods.
• Expect some vomiting; even coffee-ground vomitus is the normal result of swallowed blood. However, notify the doctor if you see bright red blood; this indicates that vomiting has induced bleeding at the operative site.
• If the patient complains of a sore throat, provide cool compresses or an ice collar.

Home care instructions

Instruct the patient:
• to immediately report bleeding and that the risk of bleeding is greatest 7 to 10 days after surgery, when the membrane formed at the operative site begins to slough off
• to consume only liquids and soft foods for 1 to 2 weeks to avoid dislodging clots or precipitating bleeding
• to practice good oral hygiene by gently brushing his teeth but avoiding vigorous brushing, gargling, and irritating mouthwashes for several weeks
• to rest and avoid vigorous activity for 7 to 10 days after discharge
• to avoid exposure to persons with colds or other contagious illnesses for at least 2 weeks.

Nursing diagnoses

When caring for the patient with an ENT disorder, several nursing diagnoses can be used repeatedly. These commonly used diagnoses appear here, along with appropriate nursing interventions and rationales.

Impaired swallowing

Related to pain and inflammation, *Impaired swallowing* may be associated with such conditions as pharyngitis, tonsillitis, and laryngitis.

Expected outcomes

- Patient can swallow.
- Patient maintains adequate hydration.
- Patient exhibits effective airway clearance.

Nursing interventions and rationales

- Elevate the head of the bed 90 degrees after food or fluid intake and at least 45 degrees at all other times to promote swallowing and prevent aspiration.
- Position the patient on his side while recumbent to decrease the risk of aspiration. Have suction equipment available in case aspiration occurs.
- Assess swallowing function frequently, especially before meals, to prevent aspiration.
- Administer pain medication before meals to enhance swallowing ability.
- Provide a liquid to soft diet and consult with the dietitian, as necessary, to promote less painful swallowing.
- Provide mouth care frequently to remove secretions and enhance comfort and appetite.
- If the patient can't swallow fluids, notify the doctor and administer I.V. fluids, as ordered, to maintain hydration.

Position the patient on her side when recumbent to decrease aspiration risk.

Disturbed sensory perception (auditory)

Related to altered auditory reception or transmission, *Disturbed sensory perception (auditory)* may be associated with such conditions as otitis media, mastoiditis, otosclerosis, Ménière's disease, and labyrinthitis.

Expected outcomes

• Patient understands that progressive hearing loss is caused by the disease.
• Patient can communicate.

Nursing interventions and rationales

• Assess the patient's degree of hearing impairment, and determine the best way to communicate with him (for example, using gestures, lip reading, or written words) to ensure adequate patient care.
• When talking to a hearing-impaired person, speak clearly and slowly in a normal to deep voice and offer concise explanations of procedures to include the patient in his own care.
• Provide sensory stimulation by using tactile and visual stimuli to help compensate for hearing loss.
• Encourage the patient to express feelings of concern and loss for his hearing deficit, and be available to answer questions. This helps him accept his loss, clears up misconceptions, and reduces anxiety.
• Encourage the patient to use his hearing aid as directed to enhance auditory function.
• Upon discharge, teach him to watch for visual cues in the environment, such as traffic lights and flashing lights on emergency vehicles, to avoid injury.

When talking to a hearing-impaired person, speak clearly and slowly in a normal to deep voice.

Ineffective airway clearance

Related to nasopharyngeal obstruction, *Ineffective airway clearance* may be associated with such conditions as nasal papillomas, adenoid hyperplasia, nasal polyps, pharyngitis, and tonsillitis.

Expected outcomes

• Patient has clear nasal airways.
• Patient sleeps with normal oxygen saturation.
• Patient is free from infection.
• Patient is free from complications.

Nursing interventions and rationales

• Assess respiratory status (including rate, depth, and stridor) at least every 4 hours to detect early signs of compromise.
• Position the patient with the head of his bed elevated 45 to 90 degrees to promote drainage of secretions and aid breathing and chest expansion.

Assess respiratory status at least every 4 hours to detect early signs of compromise.

- Suction upper airways, as needed, to help remove secretions.
- Have emergency equipment at the bedside in case of airway obstruction.
- Encourage the patient to cough and deep-breathe every 2 hours to help loosen secretions in his lungs.
- Encourage the patient to drink at least 3 qt (3 L) of fluid per day to ensure adequate hydration and loosen secretions.

Common ENT disorders

Hearing loss, laryngitis, otitis externa, otitis media, and sinusitis are common ENT disorders.

I said, "Impaired hearing is the most common disability in the United States."

Hearing loss

Impaired hearing, the most common disability in the United States, results from a mechanical or nervous system impediment to the transmission of sound waves. Hearing loss is further defined as an inability to perceive the normal range of sounds audible to an individual with normal hearing. Types of hearing loss include congenital hearing loss, sudden deafness, noise-induced hearing loss, and presbycusis.

What causes it

Causes of hearing loss depend on the type. (See *Causes of hearing loss.*)

Pathophysiology

The major forms of hearing loss are classified as:
- *conductive*, in which transmission of sound impulses from the external ear to the junction of the stapes and oval window is interrupted
- *sensorineural*, in which impaired cochlear or acoustic (eighth cranial) nerve function prevents transmission of sound impulses within the inner ear or brain
- *mixed*, in which conductive and sensorineural transmission dysfunction combine.

What to look for

Although congenital hearing loss may produce no obvious signs of hearing impairment at birth, deficient response to auditory stimuli

Causes of hearing loss

Causes of hearing loss depend on the type: congenital, sudden, noise-induced, or presbycusis.

Congenital hearing loss
• Dominant, autosomal dominant, autosomal recessive, or sex-linked recessive trait
• Maternal exposure to rubella during the first trimester or syphilis during pregnancy
• Prematurity, low birthweight, or serum bilirubin levels above 20 mg/dl
• Use of ototoxic drugs during pregnancy, trauma or prolonged fetal anoxia during delivery, or congenital abnormalities of the ears, nose, or throat

Sudden deafness
• Acute infection, especially mumps (most common cause of unilateral sensorineural hearing loss in children) and other bacterial and viral infections
• Metabolic disorders, such as diabetes mellitus and hypothyroidism

• Vascular disorders, such as hypertension and arteriosclerosis
• Head trauma, brain tumors, or stroke
• Use of ototoxic drugs, such as ethacrynic acid, furosemide, gentamicin, quinine, streptomycin, and tobramycin
• Neurologic disorders, such as multiple sclerosis and neurosyphilis
• Blood dyscrasias, such as leukemia and hypercoagulation

Noise-induced hearing loss
• Prolonged exposure to loud noise (85 to 90 dB)
• Brief exposure to extremely loud noise (greater than 90 dB)

Presbycusis
• Loss of hair cells in the organ of Corti (otologic effect of aging)

The degree of noise-induced hearing loss depends on the duration and intensity of the noise. Heel, Wags, heel!

usually becomes apparent within 2 to 3 days. As the child grows older, hearing loss impairs speech development.

How long and how loud

Noise-induced hearing loss causes sensorineural damage, the extent of which depends on the duration and intensity of the noise. Initially, the patient loses perception of certain frequencies (around 4,000 Hz) but, with continued exposure, he eventually loses perception of all frequencies.

Tinnitus comes first

Presbycusis usually produces tinnitus, with progressive decline in hearing ability and the inability to understand the spoken word.

What tests tell you

Patient, family, and occupational histories and a complete audiologic examination usually provide ample evidence of hearing loss and suggest possible causes or predisposing factors.

Other tests include:
• Weber and Rinne tests as well as specialized audiologic tests that differentiate between conductive and sensorineural hearing loss
• automatic brain stem response test, imaging studies, and electronystagmography.

How it's treated

To treat sudden deafness, the underlying cause must be promptly identified. Educating patients and health care professionals about the many causes of sudden deafness can greatly reduce the incidence of this problem.

Deafness and decibels

For individuals whose hearing loss was induced by noise levels greater than 90 dB for several hours, treatment includes:
• overnight rest, which usually restores normal hearing unless the patient was repeatedly exposed to such noise
• speech and hearing rehabilitation as the patient's hearing deteriorates, because hearing aids are rarely helpful
• a hearing aid for most cases of presbycusis.

What to do

• When talking to a patient with hearing loss who can read lips, stand directly in front of him, with the light on your face, and speak slowly and distinctly.
• Assess the degree of hearing impairment without shouting.
• Approach the patient within his visual range, and get his attention by raising your arm or waving; touching him may unnecessarily startle him.
• Write instructions on a tablet, if necessary, to make sure the patient understands.
• If the patient is learning to use a hearing aid, provide emotional support and encouragement.
• Inform other staff members and hospital personnel of the patient's disability and his established method of communication.

Approach the patient within his visual range, and get his attention by raising your arm or waving.

Seeing clues

• Make sure the patient is in an area where he can observe unit activities and persons approaching, because a patient with hearing loss depends on visual clues.
• Evaluate the patient. Make sure he expresses that his hearing loss has resolved or stabilized, is able to maintain communication with others, exhibits decreased anxiety, and he and his family members understand the importance of wearing protective de-

vices while in a noisy environment. (See *Teaching the patient with hearing loss.*)
• To prevent noise-induced hearing loss, the public must be educated about the dangers of noise exposure and come to insist on the use, as mandated by law, of protective devices, such as earplugs, during occupational exposure to noise.

Laryngitis

Laryngitis is an inflammation of the vocal cords. Acute laryngitis may occur as an isolated infection or as part of a generalized bacterial or viral upper respiratory tract infection. Repeated attacks of acute laryngitis cause inflammatory changes associated with chronic laryngitis.

What causes it

Acute laryngitis results from infection, excessive use of the voice, inhalation of smoke or fumes, or aspiration of caustic chemicals. Chronic laryngitis results from upper respiratory tract disorders (such as sinusitis, bronchitis, nasal polyps, or allergy), mouth breathing, smoking, gastroesophageal reflux, constant exposure to dust or other irritants, or alcohol abuse.

Pathophysiology

Edema of the vocal cords caused by irritation (from an infection or overuse of the voice or other cause) impairs the normal mobility of the vocal cords, causing an abnormal sound.

What to look for

Signs and symptoms of laryngitis include:
• hoarseness (persistent hoarseness in chronic laryngitis)
• pain (especially when swallowing or speaking)
• a dry cough, fever, malaise, dyspnea, throat clearing, restlessness, or laryngeal edema.

What tests tell you

• Indirect laryngoscopy confirms the diagnosis by revealing exudate and red, inflamed, and occasionally hemorrhagic vocal cords, with rounded (not sharp) edges. Bilateral swelling that restricts movement but doesn't cause paralysis also may be apparent.
• Videostroboscopy and electromyography may also be performed.

Education edge

Teaching the patient with hearing loss

• Explain the cause of hearing loss and the medical or surgical treatment options.
• Teach the patient who just received a hearing aid how it works and how to maintain it.
• Emphasize the danger of excessive exposure to noise, and encourage the use of protective devices in a noisy environment.
• Stress the danger of exposure to drugs, chemicals, and infection (especially rubella) for pregnant women.

How it's treated

Treatment of laryngitis includes:
• resting the voice (primary treatment)
• symptomatic care, such as an analgesic and throat lozenges (for viral infection)
• antibiotic therapy (bacterial infection), usually with cefuroxime
• identification and elimination of underlying cause (chronic laryngitis)
• possible hospitalization (in severe acute laryngitis)
• possible tracheotomy if laryngeal edema results in airway obstruction
• drug therapy, which includes antacids, histamine-2 blockers, antibiotics, and systemic steroids.

What to do

• Tell the patient to refrain from talking to avoid straining the vocal cords and allow vocal cord inflammation to decrease.
• If the patient is hospitalized, place a sign over his bed to remind others of talking restrictions and mark the intercom panel so other hospital personnel are aware that the patient can't answer.
• Provide a pad and pencil or a slate for communication.
• Provide an ice collar, a throat irrigant, and cold fluids for comfort.
• Evaluate the patient. Make sure he isn't hoarse or in pain; doesn't have a fever; doesn't need a tracheotomy; understands the need to stop smoking, maintain humidification, and complete his antibiotic therapy; and modifies his environment appropriately to prevent recurrence. (See *Teaching the patient with laryngitis*.)

Otitis externa

Otitis externa, or inflammation of the external ear canal skin and auricle, may be acute or chronic. It usually occurs in hot, humid summer weather and is also called *swimmer's ear*. With treatment, the acute form usually subsides within 7 days, although it may become chronic. Severe chronic otitis externa may reflect underlying diabetes mellitus, hypothyroidism, or nephritis.

What causes it

Causes may include:
• bacteria, such as *Pseudomonas*, *Proteus vulgaris*, streptococci, and *Staphylococcus aureus*
• fungi, such as *Aspergillus niger* and *Candida albicans.*
• dermatologic conditions, such as seborrhea or psoriasis.

Education edge

Teaching the patient with laryngitis

• Suggest that the patient maintain adequate humidification by using a vaporizer or humidifier during the winter, avoiding air conditioning during the summer (because it dehumidifies), using medicated throat lozenges, and avoiding smoking and smoky environments.
• Teach the patient about prescribed medication, including dosage, frequency, and adverse effects.
• Instruct the patient to complete the prescribed antibiotic therapy.
• Obtain a detailed patient history to help determine the cause of chronic laryngitis.
• Encourage modification of predisposing habits.
• Advise the patient to avoid crowds and people with upper respiratory tract infections.

Pathophysiology

Otitis externa usually results when a traumatic injury or an excessively moist ear canal predisposes the area to infection.

What to look for

Acute otitis externa is characterized by moderate to severe pain. The pain increases when manipulating the auricle or tragus, clenching the teeth, opening the mouth, or chewing. If palpating the tragus or auricle causes pain, the problem is otitis externa, not otitis media. Fungal otitis externa may be asymptomatic. However, *A. niger* produces a black or gray, blotting, paperlike growth in the ear canal.

And now for more

Other signs and symptoms of acute infection include:
• fever
• foul-smelling aural discharge
• regional cellulitis
• partial hearing loss
• scaling, itching, inflammation, or tenderness
• a swollen external ear canal and auricle, which can be seen on otoscopy
• periauricular lymphadenopathy (tender nodes in front of the tragus, behind the ear, or in the upper neck).

What tests tell you

• Otoscopic examination can determine the need for microscopic examination.
• Culture and sensitivity tests can identify the causative organism and help determine the appropriate antibiotic treatment.

How it's treated

Treatment for acute otitis externa consists of:
• heat application to the periauricular region (via heat lamp; hot, damp compresses; or heating pad)
• drug therapy, including topical analgesics, such as otic antipyrine and benzocaine; antibiotic eardrops (with or without hydrocortisone) that are instilled after the ear is cleaned and debris removed; and, if fever persists or regional cellulitis develops, a systemic antibiotic
• careful ear cleaning (especially in fungal otitis externa), including application of a keratolytic or 2% salicylic acid in cream containing nystatin (for candidal organisms) or instillation of slightly

Culture and sensitivity tests can identify the causative organism.

acidic eardrops such as 0.5% neomycin (for most fungi and *Pseudomonas* organisms)
• repeated cleaning of the ear canal with baby oil (for *A. niger* organisms).

The tonic for chronic

External ear infections are painful, and the patient with chronic otitis externa may require analgesia. Other treatments include:
• cleaning the ear and removing debris with antibiotic irrigations (primary)
• instilling antibiotic eardrops and applying antibiotic ointment or cream, such as neomycin, bacitracin, or polymyxin B, possibly combined with hydrocortisone (supplemental)
• for mild chronic otitis externa, instilling antibiotic eardrops once or twice weekly and wearing specially fitted earplugs while showering, shampooing, and swimming.

What to do

• Monitor vital signs, particularly temperature. Watch for and record the type and amount of aural drainage.
• Remove debris and gently clean the ear canal with 0.5% neomycin or polymyxin B. Place a wisp of cotton soaked with solution into the patient's ear, and apply a saturated compress directly to the auricle. Afterward, dry the ear gently but thoroughly. (If the patient has severe otitis externa, such cleaning may be delayed until after initial treatment with antibiotic eardrops.)

Traveling in the canal

• To instill eardrops in an adult, pull the pinna back to straighten the canal. To ensure that the drops reach the epithelium, insert a wisp of cotton moistened with eardrops, or have the patient lie on his side with the affected ear up for 15 minutes after instilling drops.
• If the patient has chronic otitis externa, clean the ear thoroughly. Use wet soaks intermittently on oozing or infected skin. If the patient has a chronic fungal infection, clean the ear canal well, and then apply an exfoliative ointment.
• Evaluate the patient. Make sure the patient is afebrile and pain-free, can administer his eardrops properly, and knows which risk factors to avoid. (See *Teaching the patient with otitis externa.*)

Otitis media

Otitis media, or inflammation of the middle ear, may be acute, chronic, or serous. The infection appears suddenly and lasts only

Education edge

Teaching the patient with otitis externa

• Teach the patient how to administer eardrops.
• Suggest that the patient use earplugs to keep water out of his ears when showering, shampooing, and swimming. (Two or three drops of rubbing alcohol or 2% acetic acid should be instilled before and after swimming to toughen the skin of the external ear canal.)
• Instruct the patient to clean his hands after instilling drops to avoid getting them in his eyes.
• Teach him about medications and the importance of taking the entire course of antibiotics.
• Instruct him to avoid risk factors, such as swimming in contaminated water; cleaning the ear canal with a cotton swab; and regularly using earphones, which trap moisture in the ear canal, creating a culture medium for infection.
• Tell the patient to see the doctor immediately if symptoms reappear.

Sites of otitis media

Middle ear inflammation may be suppurative or secretory. In the suppurative form, nasopharyngeal flora reflux through the eustachian tube and colonize in the middle ear. In the secretory form, obstruction of the eustachian tube promotes transudation of sterile serous fluid from blood vessels in the membrane lining the middle ear.

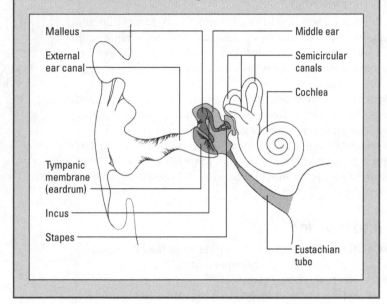

a short time. Its incidence rises during the winter months, paralleling the seasonal rise in bacterial respiratory tract infections. It results from disruption of eustachian tube patency. (See *Sites of otitis media.*)

What causes it

Acute otitis media occurs as a result of pneumococci, beta-hemolytic streptococci, staphylococci, and gram-negative bacteria such as *Haemophilus influenzae.* Chronic otitis media results from inadequate treatment of acute infection as well as infection by resistant strains of bacteria.

Serious about serous

Serous otitis media occurs as a result of:
• viral upper respiratory tract infection, allergy, or residual otitis media
• enlarged lymphoid tissue

• barotrauma (pressure injury caused by an inability to equalize pressures between the environment and the middle ear).
  The causes of chronic serous otitis media are:
• adenoidal tissue overgrowth that obstructs the eustachian tube
• edema resulting from allergic rhinitis or chronic sinus infection
• inadequate treatment of acute suppurative otitis media.

Pathophysiology

With the acute form of otitis media, respiratory tract infection, allergic reaction, or positional changes (such as holding an infant in the supine position during feeding) allow reflux of nasopharyngeal flora through the eustachian tube and colonization in the middle ear.

With prompt treatment, the prognosis for acute otitis media is excellent; however, prolonged accumulation of fluid within the middle ear cavity causes chronic otitis media.

With serous otitis media, obstruction of the eustachian tube results in negative pressure in the middle ear that promotes transudation of sterile serous fluid from blood vessels in the membrane of the middle ear.

Prolonged accumulation of fluid within the middle ear cavity can lead to chronic otitis media.

What to look for

Although the patient with acute otitis media may be asymptomatic, typical signs and symptoms include:
• severe, deep, throbbing pain
• upper respiratory tract infection with a mild to high fever
• hearing loss, usually mild and conductive
• lack of response or inattention to spoken word
• sensation of blockage in the ear, dizziness, nausea, and vomiting
• obscured or distorted bony landmarks of the tympanic membrane (evident on otoscopy)
• bulging of the tympanic membrane with concomitant erythema
• purulent drainage in the ear canal from tympanic membrane rupture.

Serous symptoms

Many patients with serous otitis media are asymptomatic but end up developing severe conductive hearing loss ranging from 15 to 35 dB, depending on the thickness and amount of fluid in the middle ear cavity. Other signs and symptoms include:
• a sensation of fullness in the ear or hearing an echo when speaking
• popping, crackling, and clicking sounds with swallowing and jaw movement
• experiencing a vague feeling of top-heaviness

Is that my cereal crackling or a sign of serous otitis media?

- tympanic membrane retraction, which causes the bony landmarks to appear more prominent (seen on otoscopy)
- clear or amber fluid behind the tympanic membrane seen on otoscopy with possible presence of an air bubble
- blue-black tympanic membrane (seen on otoscopy) if hemorrhage into the middle ear has occurred.

In the long term

Chronic otitis media usually begins in childhood and persists into adulthood. Its effects include:
- decreased or absent tympanic membrane mobility (tympanosclerosis)
- cystlike mass in the middle ear (cholesteatoma)
- erythema and perforation of the eardrum
- painless, purulent discharge (otorrhea)
- conductive hearing loss that varies with the size and type of tympanic membrane perforation and ossicular destruction
- thickening and possible scarring of the tympanic membrane (seen on otoscopy).

What tests tell you

- Otoscopic examination can determine the need for microscopic examination.
- Culture and sensitivity testing can determine the causative organism.
- Pneumatoscopy can show decreased tympanic membrane mobility. However, this procedure is painful because of the bulging, erythematous tympanic membrane that occurs in acute otitis media.

How it's treated

For acute secretory otitis media, the only treatment required may be inflation of the eustachian tube several times per day using Valsalva's maneuver. Otherwise, nasopharyngeal decongestant therapy may be helpful. If decongestant therapy fails, myringotomy and aspiration of middle ear fluid, followed by insertion of a polyethylene tube into the tympanic membrane, are necessary for immediate and prolonged equalization of pressure. The tube falls out spontaneously after 9 to 12 months.

Must use sparingly

Broad-spectrum antibiotics may be used to help prevent acute otitis media in high-risk patients. (In patients with recurring otitis media, antibiotics must be used sparingly and with discretion to prevent development of resistant strains of bacteria.)

Other treatment for acute otitis media includes:

I've got tubes, you don't have to shout. When they're done, they'll just fall out.... I got tubes, Babe.

• antibiotic therapy with ampicillin or amoxicillin, or cefaclor or co-trimoxazole for those who are allergic to penicillin derivatives
• acetaminophen or ibuprofen to help control pain and fever
• myringotomy for severe, painful bulging of the tympanic membrane.

When it goes on and on

For chronic otitis media, therapy includes:
• antibiotics for exacerbations of acute infection
• elimination of eustachian tube obstruction
• myringoplasty (tympanic membrane graft)
• tympanoplasty to reconstruct middle ear structures when thickening and scarring are present, and, possibly, mastoidectomy
• excision of cholesteatoma, if present.

What to do

After myringotomy:
• Maintain drainage flow. Don't place cotton or plugs deep in the ear canal. Instead, place sterile cotton loosely in the external ear to absorb drainage.
• To prevent infection, change the cotton whenever it gets damp and wash your hands before and after providing ear care.
• Watch for and report headache, fever, severe pain, or disorientation.

Tympano treatment

After tympanoplasty:
• Reinforce dressings, and observe for excessive bleeding from the ear canal. Administer an analgesic, if needed.
• After completing therapy for otitis media, evaluate the patient. Make sure the patient is free from pain and fever, his hearing is completely restored, he understands the importance of completing his antibiotic therapy, and he understands how to prevent recurrence. (See *Teaching the patient with otitis media.*)

Sinusitis

The prognosis is good for all types of sinusitis. The types include:
• acute, which usually results from the common cold and lingers in subacute form in only about 10% of patients
• chronic, which follows persistent bacterial infection
• allergic, which accompanies allergic rhinitis
• hyperplastic, which is a combination of purulent acute sinusitis and allergic sinusitis or rhinitis

Education edge

Teaching the patient with otitis media

• Teach the patient the causes, signs, and treatment of otitis media.
• Warn the patient against blowing his nose or getting his ears wet when bathing.
• Encourage the patient to complete the prescribed course of antibiotic treatment.
• Instruct the patient or caregiver about medications ordered, correct administration, dosage, and adverse effects.
• Suggest applying heat to the ear to relieve pain.
• Advise the patient with acute otitis media to watch for and immediately report pain and fever, which are signs of secondary infection.
• To promote eustachian tube patency, instruct the patient to perform Valsalva's maneuver several times daily.
• Urge prompt treatment of otitis media to prevent perforation of the tympanic membrane.
• Tell the patient to seek treatment at the earliest signs of an earache.

• viral, which follows an upper respiratory tract infection in which the virus penetrates the normal mucous membrane
• fungal, which is generally uncommon but is more common in immunosuppressed or debilitated patients.

What causes it

Sinusitis may result from:
• an upper respiratory tract infection, allergies, or rhinitis
• nasal polyps
• bacterial, viral, or fungal infection (possibly due to swimming in contaminated water or dental manipulation, for example).

Pathophysiology

Ordinarily, bacteria are swept from the sinuses through mucociliary clearance. When the ostia (openings to the sinuses) become obstructed by inflammation or mucus, however, these bacteria remain in the sinus cavity and multiply. The mucous membrane inside the cavity becomes swollen and inflamed, and the cavity fills with secretions.

What to look for

Signs and symptoms associated with sinusitis include:
• nasal congestion and pressure
• pain over the cheeks and upper teeth (in maxillary sinusitis)
• pain over the eyes (in ethmoid sinusitis)
• pain over the eyebrows (in frontal sinusitis)
• rarely, pain behind the eyes (in sphenoid sinusitis)
• edematous nasal mucosa and edema of the face and periorbital area
• fever (in acute sinusitis)
• nasal discharge (possibly purulent in acute and subacute sinusitis, continuous in chronic sinusitis, watery in the allergic sinusitis)
• nasal stuffiness, possible inflammation and pus on nasal examination.

What tests tell you

• Sinus X-rays reveal cloudiness in the affected sinus, air-fluid levels, or thickened mucosal lining.
• Antral puncture promotes drainage and removal of purulent material and may provide a specimen for culture and sensitivity identification of the infecting organism (rarely performed).

• Transillumination allows inspection of the sinus cavities by shining a light through them; however, purulent drainage prevents passage of light.

How it's treated

The primary treatment for acute sinusitis is antibiotic therapy. Other appropriate measures include:
• a vasoconstrictor, such as epinephrine or phenylephrine, to decrease nasal secretions
• an analgesic to help relieve pain
• steam inhalation to promote vasoconstriction and encourage drainage
• local application of heat to relieve pain and congestion
• an antibiotic or antifungal agent (for persistent infection).

The primary treatment for acute sinusitis is an antibiotic.

Only subacute

Antibiotic therapy is also the primary treatment for subacute sinusitis. A vasoconstrictor may reduce the amount of nasal secretions.

Allergic sinusitis? Treat rhinitis.

Treatment of allergic sinusitis involves treatment of allergic rhinitis, which includes:
• administration of an antihistamine
• identification of allergens by skin testing and desensitization by immunotherapy
• corticosteroids and epinephrine for severe allergic symptoms.

Anti's, irrigation, surgery

For chronic and hyperplastic sinusitis, an antihistamine, an antibiotic, and a steroid nasal spray may relieve pain and congestion. If irrigation fails to relieve symptoms, one or more sinuses may require surgery. Surgeries include:
• sinus tap and irrigation for acute sinusitis
• functional endoscopic sinus surgery
• external ethmoidectomy or sphenoethmoidectomy
• frontal sinusotomy for chronic sinusitis.

What to do

• Enforce bed rest with the head of the bed elevated.
• Encourage the patient to drink plenty of fluids to promote drainage.
• Use a humidifier and nasal saline sprays to decrease dryness.
• Monitor temperature to detect infection. Perform sinus irrigations as ordered.

• To relieve pain and promote drainage, apply warm compresses continuously or four times daily for 2-hour intervals.
• Watch for and report complications, such as vomiting, chills, fever, edema of the forehead or eyelids, blurred or double vision, and personality changes.
• Evaluate the patient. Make sure the patient is free from pain, congestion, headaches, and fever; maintains humidification and drainage of his sinuses; understands the importance of complying with antibiotic therapy; and is able to distinguish common smells. (See *Teaching the patient with sinusitis.*)

Quick quiz

1. During an otoscopic examination, the nurse should pull the superior posterior auricle of an adult patient's ear:

    A.   up and back.
    B.   up and forward.
    C.   down and back.
    D.   down and forward.

Answer: A. In the adult patient, the superior posterior auricle should be pulled up and back to straighten the ear canal.

2. To assess the frontal sinuses, the nurse should palpate:

    A.   the forehead.
    B.   below the cheekbones.
    C.   over the temporal areas.
    D.   over the preauricular areas.

Answer: A. The frontal sinuses are located in the forehead, the site of palpation for those structures.

3. After a tonsillectomy and adenoidectomy, do all of the following interventions except:

    A.   use a flashlight to check the throat.
    B.   watch for frequent swallowing.
    C.   allow the patient to use a straw and other utensils.
    D.   provide an ice collar for comfort.

Answer: C. Don't allow the patient to use straws and other utensils, in order to prevent dislodging clots.

Education edge

Teaching the patient with sinusitis

• Instruct the patient on how to apply compresses and take his antihistamine.
• Teach him about all prescribed medications, including dosage, frequency, and adverse effects.
• Tell him to finish the prescribed antibiotics, even if his symptoms disappear.
• Encourage the patient to keep all follow-up appointments with the doctor.

4. Pain elicited by palpating the patient's tragus or auricle indicates:

    A.   sinusitis.

    B.   pharyngitis.

    C.   otitis media.

    D.   otitis externa.

Answer: D. If palpating the tragus or auricle causes pain, the problem is otitis externa.

Scoring

☆☆☆ If you answered all four items correctly, yippee! Your sense of ENT disorders is top-notch.

☆☆ If you answered three items correctly, good for you! You're well on your way to shining a light on the ear, nose, and throat.

☆ If you answered fewer than three items correctly, keep your chin up! Sniff out the difficult areas, and try again!

Cardiovascular disorders

Just the facts

In this chapter you'll learn:

♦ anatomy and physiology of the heart

♦ history and physical assessment techniques that target cardiac function

♦ appropriate treatments to promote cardiac health

♦ common cardiovascular disorders.

A look at cardiovascular disorders

Although people are living longer than ever before, they're increasingly living with chronic conditions or the effects of acute ones. Of these conditions, cardiovascular disorders head the list. In North America, almost 60 million people suffer from some form of cardiovascular disorder, and many of them suffer from a combination of disorders. Year after year, the number of affected patients continues to rise.

Because of this upward trend, you'll be dealing with cardiovascular patients more often. To provide effective care for these patients, you need a clear understanding of cardiovascular anatomy and physiology, assessment techniques, diagnostic tests, and treatments as well as cardiovascular disorders.

The number of patients with cardiovascular disease continues to rise.

Anatomy and physiology

The cardiovascular system delivers oxygenated blood to tissues and removes waste products. The heart, controlled by the autonomic nervous system, pumps blood to all organs and tissues of the body. Arteries and veins (vascular network) carry blood throughout the body, keep the heart filled with blood, and maintain blood pressure. Let's look at each part of this critical system.

Heart

The heart is a hollow, muscular organ about the size of a closed fist. Located between the lungs in the mediastinum, it's about 5″ (12.5 cm) long and 3½″ (9 cm) in diameter at its widest point. It weighs between 8.8 and 10 oz (250 to 300 g).

Where's your heart?

The heart spans the area from the second to the fifth intercostal space. The right border of the heart lines up with the right border of the sternum. The left border lines up with the left midclavicular line. The exact position of the heart may vary slightly with each patient. Leading into and out of the heart are the great vessels:
- inferior vena cava
- superior vena cava
- aorta
- pulmonary artery
- four pulmonary veins.

Boy, aren't those some great vessels?! I sure think so.

Slip and slide

The heart is protected by a thin sac called the *pericardium*, which has an inner, or visceral, layer that forms the epicardium and an outer, or parietal, layer. The space between the two layers contains 10 to 30 ml of serous fluid, which prevents friction between the layers as the heart pumps.

Chamber made

The heart has four chambers (two atria and two ventricles) separated by a cardiac septum. The upper atria have thin walls and serve as reservoirs for blood. They also boost the amount of blood moving into the lower ventricles, which fill primarily by gravity. (See *Inside the heart.*)

Blood pathways

Blood moves to and from the heart through specific pathways.

Where there's no air

Deoxygenated venous blood returns to the right atrium through three vessels:

    superior vena cava—returning blood from the upper body

    inferior vena cava—returning blood from the lower body

    coronary sinus—returning blood from the heart muscle.

Inside the heart

The heart's internal structure consists of the pericardium, 3 layers of the heart wall, 4 chambers, 11 openings, and 4 valves.

Branches of right pulmonary artery

Superior vena cava

Right atrium

Right pulmonary veins

Tricuspid valve

Chordae tendineae

Right ventricle

Papillary muscle

Inferior vena cava

Descending aorta

Aortic arch

Pulmonary semilunar valve

Branches of left pulmonary artery

Pulmonary artery

Left atrium

Left pulmonary veins

Aortic semilunar valve

Mitral valve

Left ventricle

Myocardium

Interventricular septum

Heart wall

Endocardium

Myocardium

Serous pericardium (visceral layer)

Epicardium

Pericardial space

Serous pericardium (parietal layer)

Fibrous pericardium

Get some fresh air

Blood in the right atrium empties into the right ventricle and is then ejected through the pulmonic valve into the pulmonary artery when the ventricle contracts. The blood then travels to the lungs to be oxygenated.

Share the wealth

From the lungs, blood travels to the left atrium through the pulmonary veins. The left atrium empties the blood into the left ventricle, which then pumps the blood through the aortic valve into the aorta and throughout the body with each contraction. Because the left ventricle pumps blood against a much higher pressure than the right ventricle, its wall is three times thicker.

We work with the heart to oxygenate the blood that the heart sends to the rest of the body. Yeah, we're special that way.

Valves

Valves in the heart keep blood flowing in only one direction through the heart. Think of the valves as traffic cops at the entrances to one-way streets, preventing blood from traveling the wrong way despite great pressure to do so. Healthy valves open and close as a result of pressure changes within the four heart chambers.

Matching sets

There are two sets of valves:

    atrioventricular (between atria and ventricles)—tricuspid valve on the heart's right side and mitral valve on its left

    semilunar—pulmonic valve (between the right ventricle and pulmonary artery) and aortic valve (between the left ventricle and aorta).

On the cusp

Each valve has cusps (leaflets), which are anchored to the heart wall by cords of fibrous tissue (chordae tendineae). The cusps of the valves act to maintain tight closure. The tricuspid valve has three cusps. The mitral valve has two cusps. Each of the semilunar valves has three cusps.

Once I get the rhythm, around and around I go!

Cardiac cycle

Contractions of the heart occur in a rhythm—the cardiac cycle—and are regulated by impulses that normally begin at the sinoatrial (SA) node, the heart's pacemaker. The impulses are conducted from there throughout the heart. Impulses from the autonomic nervous system affect the SA node and alter its firing rate to meet the body's needs. The cardiac cycle consists of two phases: diastole and systole.

Diastole: Parts 1, 2, and 3

Diastole is the period when the heart relaxes and fills with blood and the heart muscle receives its own supply of blood from the coronary arteries. During diastole, the mitral and tricuspid valves are open, and the aortic and pulmonic valves are closed. There are three phases of diastole:

isovolumetric relaxation—when ventricular pressure drops below the pressure in the aorta and the pulmonary artery, allowing blood to back up toward the ventricles and causing the aortic and pulmonic valves to snap shut, leading to the second heart sound (S_2) and atrial filling (the beginning of the cardiac cycle)

ventricular filling (passive)—when 70% of the blood in the atria drains into the ventricles by gravity, which may cause vibrations heard as the third heart sound (S_3)

atrial contraction (active), also called *atrial kick*—when the remaining 30% of blood is pumped into the ventricles, which may cause the fourth heart sound (S_4).

The sound of systole

Systole is the period of ventricular contraction when the heart sends blood on its outward journey. There are two phases of systole:

isovolumetric contraction—when pressure within the ventricles rises (due to atrial kick) causing the mitral and tricuspid valves to snap closed, which makes the first heart sound (S_1)

ventricular ejection—when ventricular pressure rises above the pressure in the aorta and pulmonary artery, causing the aortic and pulmonic valves to open and blood to eject into the pulmonary artery and out to the lungs and into the aorta and out to the rest of the body.

It may seem like magic, but the three phases of diastole are simply about pressure and gravity.

Vascular system

The vascular system consists of a network of arteries, arterioles, capillaries, venules, and veins. This network is constantly filled with about 5 L of blood. The vascular system delivers oxygen, nutrients, and other substances to the body's cells and removes the waste products of cellular metabolism. (See *A close look at arteries and veins*.)

Arteries

Arteries carry blood away from the heart. Nearly all arteries carry oxygen-rich blood from the heart throughout the rest of the body. The only exception is the pulmonary artery, which carries oxygen-depleted blood from the right ventricle to the lungs.

Must be thick

Arteries are thick-walled because they transport blood under high pressure. Arterial walls contain a tough, elastic layer to help propel blood through the arterial system.

Pulse is pressure

Arterial pulses are pressure waves of blood generated by the pumping action of the heart. All vessels in the arterial system have pulsations, but the pulsations can be felt only where an artery lies near the skin. You can palpate for these peripheral pulses: temporal, carotid, brachial, radial, ulnar, femoral, popliteal, posterior tibial, and dorsalis pedis. The location of pulse points varies between individuals. In older adults, peripheral pulses may be diminished.

Without the vascular system, I'd be on my own trying to regulate the flow of blood. Talk about pressure!

Capillaries

The exchange of fluid, nutrients, and metabolic wastes between blood and cells occurs in the capillaries. The exchange can occur because capillaries are thin-walled and highly permeable. About 5% of the circulating blood volume at any given moment is contained within the capillaries. They're connected to arteries and veins through intermediary vessels called arterioles and venules, respectively.

Veins

Veins carry blood toward the heart. Nearly all veins carry oxygen-depleted blood, the sole exception being the pulmonary vein, which carries oxygenated blood from the lungs to the left atrium. Veins serve as a large reservoir for circulating blood.

Must be flexible

The wall of a vein is thinner and more pliable than the wall of an artery. That pliability allows the vein to accommodate variations in blood volume. Veins contain valves at periodic intervals to prevent blood from flowing backward.

A close look at the arteries and veins

This illustration shows major arteries and veins of the body.

Assessment

Baseline information regarding cardiovascular status obtained during assessment will help guide your intervention and follow-up care. Note, however, that if your patient is in a cardiac crisis you'll have to rethink your assessment priorities. The patient's condition and the clinical situation will dictate what steps to take.

If the patient is in a cardiac crisis, you'll have to rethink assessment priorities.

History

Begin the assessment with a thorough history. You'll find that patients with a cardiovascular problem typically cite specific complaints, including:
- chest, neck, arm, or jaw discomfort or pain
- difficulty breathing
- "fluttering" feeling in the chest
- cyanosis, pallor, or other skin changes (such as decreased hair distribution and a thin, shiny appearance to the skin)
- high or low blood pressure, weakness, fatigue, or dizziness.

Current health status

Ask the following questions to help the patient elaborate on his current illness:
- How long have you had this problem? When did it begin?
- Where's the pain located? Does the pain radiate to any area of your body? Rate the pain on a scale of 0 to 10.
- Do you recognize anything that precipitates, exacerbates, or relieves the pain?

Previous health status

Explore all of the patient's previous major illnesses, recurrent minor illnesses, accidents or injuries, surgical procedures, and allergies. Ask about any history of cardiac-related disorders, such as hypertension, rheumatic fever, scarlet fever, diabetes mellitus, hyperlipidemia, congenital heart defects, and syncope. Other questions to ask include:
- Have you ever had severe fatigue not caused by exertion?
- Do you consume alcohol, tobacco, and caffeine? How much do you consume?
- Are you taking any prescription, over-the-counter, or recreational drugs?
- Are you allergic to any drugs, foods, or other products? Can you describe the reaction you experienced?

Ask the patient about cardiac-related disorders, such as hypertension, rheumatic fever, scarlet fever... Ack! I'm feeling a little faint.

In addition, ask the female patient:
- Have you begun menopause?
- Do you use hormonal contraceptives or estrogen?
- Have you experienced any medical problems during pregnancy? Have you ever had pregnancy-induced hypertension?

Family history

Information about the patient's blood relatives may suggest a specific cardiac problem. Ask him if anyone in his family has ever had hypertension, myocardial infarction (MI), cardiomyopathy, diabetes mellitus, coronary artery disease (CAD), vascular disease, hyperlipidemia, or sudden death.

Lifestyle patterns

Always consider the patient's cultural and social background when planning care. For example, what's his religion? Does he actively practice his beliefs? Also note the patient's education level and occupation: Does he have a stable or erratic employment history? Does he live alone or with someone? Does he have any hobbies? How does he view his illness? Assess the patient's self-image as you gather this information.

Don't forget to ask about cultural and social background such as religion. Now, go in peace, my nurse. Tee hee!

Physical examination

The first step in the physical examination is to assess the factors that reflect cardiovascular function, including vital signs and physical appearance. After examining these factors, you may assess the patient's cardiovascular system using inspection, palpation, percussion, and auscultation.

Alter and explain

Combine parts of the assessment, as needed, to conserve time and the patient's energy. If the patient is experiencing cardiovascular difficulties, alter the order of your assessment as needed. For example, if he complains of chest pain and dyspnea, quickly check his vital signs and then auscultate the heart. If a female patient feels embarrassed about exposing her chest, explain each assessment step beforehand, use drapes appropriately, and expose only the area being assessed at the moment.

Vital signs

Assessing vital signs includes measurement of temperature, blood pressure, pulse rate, and respiratory rate.

Temperature

Temperature change can be caused by:
- cardiovascular inflammation or infection (higher than normal temperature)
- increased metabolism, which heightens cardiac workload (higher than normal temperature)
- poor perfusion and certain metabolic disorders such as hypothyroidism (lower than normal temperature).

Blood pressure

According to the American Heart Association (AHA), three successive readings of blood pressure above 140/90 mm Hg indicate hypertension. However, emotional stress caused by physical examination may elevate blood pressure. If the patient's blood pressure is high, allow him to relax for several minutes and then measure again to rule out stress.

When assessing a patient's blood pressure for the first time, take measurements in both arms. A difference of 10 mm Hg or more between arms may indicate thoracic outlet syndrome or other forms of arterial obstruction.

If the patient's blood pressure is high, allow him to relax and then measure again to rule out stress.

Heart rate

If you suspect cardiac disease, palpate a radial pulse for 1 full minute to detect any arrhythmias. Normally, an adult's pulse ranges from 60 to 100 beats/minute. Its rhythm should feel regular, except for a subtle slowing on expiration, caused by changes in intrathoracic pressure and vagal response. Note whether the pulse feels weak, normal, or bounding.

Respiration

Observe for eupnea—a regular, unlabored, and bilaterally equal breathing pattern. Tachypnea may indicate low cardiac output. Dyspnea, a possible indicator of heart failure, may not be evident at rest. However, the patient may pause after only a few words to take a breath. A Cheyne-Stokes respiratory pattern may accompany severe heart failure, although it's more commonly associated with coma. Shallow breathing may accompany acute pericarditis as the patient attempts to reduce the pain associated with deep respirations.

Physical appearance

Observe the patient's general appearance, noting:
- weight and muscle composition
- skin turgor, integrity, and color
- energy level

- appearance compared with age
- comfort level or apparent level of anxiety.

Apparent appendages?

Inspect the hair on the patient's arms and legs. Hair should be distributed symmetrically and should grow thicker on the anterior surface of the arms and legs. If not, it may indicate diminished arterial blood flow to the arms and legs.

Note whether the length of the arms and legs is proportionate to the length of the trunk. Long, thin arms and legs may indicate Marfan syndrome, a congenital disorder that causes cardiovascular problems, such as aortic dissection, aortic valve incompetence, and cardiomyopathy.

Inspect arm and leg hair for symmetry and thicker growth on the anterior surface. Variation may indicate diminished arterial blood flow.

I think I'm safe, what do you think?

Normal nails?

Fingernails normally appear pinkish with no markings. A bluish color in the nail beds indicates peripheral cyanosis. To estimate the rate of peripheral blood flow, assess the capillary refill in the fingernails or toenails by applying pressure to the nail for 5 seconds, then assessing the time it takes for color to return. In a patient with a good arterial supply, color should return in less than 3 seconds. Delayed capillary refill suggests reduced circulation to that area, a sign of low cardiac output that may lead to arterial insufficiency.

Inspection

Inspect the patient's chest and thorax. (See *Identifying cardiovascular landmarks*, page 238.) Expose the anterior chest and observe its general appearance. Normally, the lateral diameter is twice the size of the anteroposterior diameter. Note any deviations from typical chest shape.

Go for the jugular

When the patient is in a supine position, the jugular veins normally protrude; when the patient stands, the jugular veins normally lie flat. To check for jugular vein distention, place the patient in semi-Fowler's position with his head turned slightly away from the side being examined. Use tangential lighting (lighting from the side) to cast small shadows along the neck. This will allow you to see pulse wave movement better. If jugular veins appear distended, it indicates high right atrial pressure and an increase in fluid volume caused by right heart dysfunction.

Identifying cardiovascular landmarks

These views show where to find critical landmarks used in cardiovascular assessment.

Anterior thorax

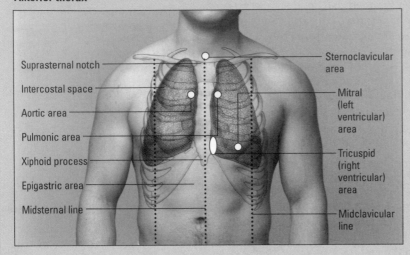

- Suprasternal notch
- Intercostal space
- Aortic area
- Pulmonic area
- Xiphoid process
- Epigastric area
- Midsternal line
- Sternoclavicular area
- Mitral (left ventricular) area
- Tricuspid (right ventricular) area
- Midclavicular line

Lateral thorax

- Anterior axillary line
- Midaxillary line
- Posterior axillary line

Precordium pulsations

Using tangential lighting, watch for chest wall movement, visible pulsations, and exaggerated lifts or heaves (strong outward thrusts over the chest during systole) in all areas of the precordium. Ask an obese patient or a patient with large breasts to sit during inspection to bring the heart closer to the anterior chest wall and make pulsations more noticeable.

Impulsive heart

Normally, you'll see pulsations at the point of maximal impulse of the apical impulse. The apical impulse (pulsation at the apex of the heart) normally appears in the fifth intercostal space at or just medial to the midclavicular line. This impulse reflects the location and size of the heart, especially of the left ventricle. In thin adults and in children, you may see a slight sternal movement and pulsations over the pulmonary arteries or the aorta as well as visible pulsations in the epigastric area.

Palpation

Palpate the peripheral pulses and precordium. Make sure the patient is positioned comfortably, draped appropriately, and kept

Call me impulsive, but I just love a good pulsation in my apex!

warm. Also, warm your hands and remember to use gentle to moderate pressure.

Palpating carotid pulses

Palpation of the radial pulse occurs during vital signs assessment. Palpation of the other major pulse points is necessary to assess blood flow to the tissues. Because the larger central arteries (the carotids) lie closer to the heart, they have slightly higher pressures than the peripheral arteries and, thus, are more easily palpated. Palpate only one carotid artery at a time; simultaneous palpation can slow the pulse or decrease blood pressure, causing the patient to faint.

I remember my arteries well. Those were some pulses. They'd just go on and on. One time... Oh, never mind, it's a vascular thing. You wouldn't understand...

What?! Suddenly I'm made of cardboard or something?

Other prominent pulses

After palpating the carotids, continue on to the brachial, radial, femoral, popliteal, dorsalis pedis, and posterior tibial pulses. (See *Assessing arterial pulses*, page 240.) These arteries are close to the body surface and lie over bones, making palpation easier. Press gently over these pulse sites; excess pressure can obliterate the pulsation, making the pulse appear absent. Look for the following:
• pulse rate — varies with age and other factors (usually 60 to 100 beats/minute in adults)
• pulse rhythm — regular
• symmetry — equally strong bilateral pulses
• contour — smooth, wavelike (upstroke and downstroke) pulse flow
• strength — easily palpated pulses (strong finger pressure required to obliterate pulse).

Making the grade

Pulses are graded on a scale:
• 4+ is bounding.
• 3+ is increased.
• 2+ is normal.
• 1+ is weak.
• 0 is absent.

Percussion

As a medical-surgical nurse, you won't routinely percuss the heart. If you note an abnormality in your overall assessment, check the patient's record for a chest X-ray, because it provides more accurate information and usually eliminates the need for percussion. Also, lung problems, which commonly accompany cardiovascular

Assessing arterial pulses

To assess arterial pulses, apply pressure with your index and middle fingers. The following illustrations show where to position your fingers when palpating for various pulses.

Carotid pulse
Lightly place your fingers just medial to the trachea and below the jaw angle. Never palpate both carotid arteries at the same time.

Brachial pulse
Position your fingers medial to the biceps tendon.

Radial pulse
Apply gentle pressure to the medial and ventral side of the wrist, just below the base of the thumb.

Femoral pulse
Press relatively hard at a point inferior to the inguinal ligament. For an obese patient, palpate in the crease of the groin, halfway between the pubic bone and the hip bone.

Popliteal pulse
Press firmly in the popliteal fossa at the back of the knee.

Posterior tibial pulse
Apply pressure behind and slightly below the malleolus of the ankle.

Dorsalis pedis pulse
Place your fingers on the medial dorsum of the foot while the patient points his toes down. The pulse is difficult to palpate here and may seem to be absent in healthy patients.

disorders, reduce the accuracy of percussion. However, percussion of the abdomen of a patient with right-sided heart failure may reveal dullness that extends several centimeters below the margin of the right ribs, indicating an enlarged liver.

Auscultation

The cardiovascular system requires more auscultation than any other body system.

Auscultation aficionado

Heart sounds are auscultated in the precordium. Identifying normal heart sounds, rates, and rhythms isn't routine practice for the medical-surgical nurse, but it's certainly a valuable skill to develop. Even so, expect some difficulty. Even with a stethoscope, the amount of tissue between the source of the sound and the outer

Dullness on percussion of the abdomen below the right ribs may indicate an enlarged liver. I'm thinking that's something none of us want.

Positioning the patient for auscultation

If heart sounds are faint or undetectable, try listening to them with the patient seated and leaning forward or lying on his left side, which brings the heart closer to the surface of the chest. These illustrations show how to position the patient for high- and low-pitched sounds.

Leaning forward
The forward-leaning position is best suited for hearing high-pitched sounds related to semilunar valve problems, such as aortic and pulmonic valve murmurs. To auscultate for these sounds, place the diaphragm of the stethoscope over the aortic and pulmonic areas in the right and left second intercostal spaces, as shown below.

Left lateral recumbent
The left lateral recumbent position is best suited for hearing low-pitched sounds, such as mitral valve murmurs and extra heart sounds. To hear these sounds, place the bell of the stethoscope over the apical area, as shown below.

chest wall can affect what you hear. Fat, muscle, and air tend to reduce sound transmission. When auscultating an obese patient or a patient with a muscular chest wall or hyperinflated lungs, sounds may seem distant. (See *Positioning the patient for auscultation*, page 241.)

See the sites

Identify cardiac auscultation sites. These include aortic, pulmonic, tricuspid, and mitral areas. Most normal heart sounds result from vibrations created by the opening and closing of the heart valves. When valves close, they suddenly terminate the motion of blood; when valves open, they accelerate the motion of blood. This sudden deceleration or acceleration produces heart sounds. Auscultation sites don't lie directly over the valves but over the pathways the blood takes as it flows through chambers and valves.

Sound it out

Listen to those lovely sounds. Lub-dub, lub-dub...

Listen for a few cycles to become accustomed to the rate and rhythm of the sounds. You'll differentiate heart sounds by their pitch (frequency), intensity (loudness), duration, quality (such as musical or harsh), location, and radiation. The timing of heart sounds in relation to the cardiac cycle is particularly important. Two sounds normally occur: S_1 and S_2. They have a relatively high pitch and are separated by a silent period. Normal heart sounds last only a fraction of a second, followed by slightly longer periods of silence. Listen for:
- S_1—the *lub* of *lub-dub*—beginning of systole when mitral and tricuspid valves close and blood is ejected into the circulation, which occurs within one-third of a second
- S_2—the *dub* of *lub-dub*—beginning of diastole when aortic and pulmonic valves close (louder in the aortic and pulmonary chest areas), coinciding with the pulse downstroke and followed by a silent period that normally exceeds the pause between S_1 and S_2.

Compare and contrast

At each auscultatory site, use the diaphragm to listen closely to S_1 and S_2 and compare them. Then auscultate again, using the bell of the stethoscope. If you hear any sounds during the diastolic or systolic period or any variations in S_1 and S_2, document the characteristics of the sound. Note the auscultatory site and the part of the cardiac cycle during which it occurred. If you have difficulty identifying normal heart sounds, palpate the patient's carotid artery with your stethoscope over the apex of the heart. The heart sound you hear at the time of the carotid pulse is S_1.

Abnormal findings

Auscultation may also reveal the third and fourth heart sounds as well as a summation gallop, murmur, click, snap, or rub.

Ridin' 3 white horses

Also known as S_3 or *ventricular gallop*, the third heart sound is a low-pitched noise heard best by placing the bell of the stethoscope at the apex of the heart. Its rhythm resembles a horse galloping, and its cadence resembles the word "Ken-tuc-ky" (*lub-dub-by*). Listen for S_3 with the patient in a supine or left-lateral decubitus position.

An S_3 usually occurs during early diastole to middiastole, at the end of the passive-filling phase of either ventricle. Listen for this sound immediately after S_2. It may signify that the ventricle isn't compliant enough to accept the filling volume without additional force. Noncompliance in the right ventricle can be heard in the tricuspid area, and in the mitral area if the left ventricle is noncompliant. A heave may be palpable when the sound occurs.

> The rhythm of ventricular gallop resembles a horse galloping to the sound of the word Kentucky. Giddyap!

Whoa, Nellie

An S_4 is an abnormal heart sound that occurs late in diastole, just before the pulse upstroke. It immediately precedes the S_1 of the next cycle and is associated with acceleration and deceleration of blood entering a chamber that resists additional filling. Known as *atrial gallop* or *presystolic gallop*, it occurs during atrial contraction.

The S_4 shares the same cadence as the word "Ten-nes-see" (*le-lub-dub*). Heard best with the bell of the stethoscope and with the patient in a supine position, S_4 may occur in the tricuspid or mitral area, depending on which ventricle is dysfunctional.

To sum up: A full stable

Occasionally, a patient may have both a third and a fourth heart sound. When this happens, S_3 and S_4 occur so closely together that they appear to be one sound, called *summation gallop*. Auscultation may reveal two separate abnormal heart sounds and two normal sounds. In this case, the patient usually has tachycardia and diastole is shortened.

Murmuring brook

Longer than a heart sound, a murmur occurs as a vibrating, blowing, or rumbling noise. Just as water in a stream "babbles" as it passes through a narrow point, turbulent blood flow produces a murmur. If you detect a murmur, identify its loudest location, pinpoint the time it occurs during the cardiac cycle, and describe its pitch, pattern, quality, and intensity. (See *Grading murmurs*.)

Clicking cusps

Clicks are high-pitched abnormal heart sounds that result from tensing of the chordae tendineae structures and mitral valve cusps. Initially, the mitral valve closes securely, but then a large cusp prolapses into the left atrium causing the sound. The click usually precedes a late systolic murmur caused by regurgitation of a little blood from the left ventricle into the left atrium. Clicks occur in 5% to 10% of young adults and affect more women than men.

To detect the high-pitched click of mitral valve prolapse, place the stethoscope diaphragm at the heart's apex and listen during midsystole to late systole. To enhance the sound, change the patient's position to sitting or standing, and listen along the lower left sternal border.

Sternal S_2 snaps

Place the stethoscope diaphragm medial to the apex along the lower left sternal border to detect a possible opening snap immediately after S_2. This sound results from a stenotic valve (a valve that's constricted or narrowed) attempting to open. The snap resembles the normal S_1 and S_2 in quality and its high pitch helps differentiate it from an S_3. Because the opening snap may accompany mitral or tricuspid stenosis, it usually precedes a middiastolic to late diastolic murmur (classic sign of stenosis).

Rub-a-lub-dub

To detect a pericardial friction rub, use the diaphragm of the stethoscope to auscultate in the third left intercostal space along the lower left sternal border. Listen for a harsh, scratchy, scraping, or squeaking sound that occurs throughout systole, diastole, or both. To enhance the sound, have the patient sit upright and lean forward or exhale. A rub usually indicates pericarditis.

Inaudible arteries

Auscultate the carotid, femoral, and popliteal arteries as well as the abdominal aorta. Over the carotid, femoral, and popliteal arteries, auscultation should reveal no sounds; over the abdominal aorta, it may detect bowel sounds but no vascular sounds.

That bruit is no hooey

During auscultation of the central and peripheral arteries, you may notice a bruit — a continuous sound caused by tur-

An opening snap after S_2 makes diagnosing stenosis a, well... a snap!

bulent blood flow. A bruit over the carotid artery usually indicates atherosclerosis; over the femoral or popliteal arteries, narrowed vessels; over the abdominal aorta, an aneurysm (sac formed at a weak point in the arterial wall) or a dissection (tear in layers of the arterial wall).

Diagnostic tests

Technological advances have improved the precision of diagnostic tests. Although cardiac marker studies and electrocardiograms (ECGs) are of great value, nuclear imaging tests can pinpoint the exact location and extent of cardiac damage within hours of an acute MI, allowing more effective treatment.

Cardiac marker studies

Analysis of cardiac markers (proteins) aids diagnosis of acute MI. After infarction, damaged cardiac tissue releases significant amounts of enzymes into the blood. Serial measurement of enzyme levels reveals the extent of damage and helps monitor healing progress. These cardiac enzymes include creatine kinase (CK), lactate dehydrogenase (LD), myoglobin, and troponin I and T.

CK

CK is present in heart muscle, skeletal muscle, and brain tissue. Its isoenzymes are combinations of the subunits M (muscle) and B (brain). CK-BB appears primarily in brain and nerve tissue; CK-MM, in skeletal muscles; and CK-MB, in the heart muscle. Elevated levels of CK-MB reliably indicate acute MI. Generally, CK-MB levels rise 4 to 8 hours after the onset of acute MI, peak after 20 hours, and may remain elevated for up to 72 hours.

Nursing considerations
• Explain to the patient that the test will help confirm or rule out MI.
• Inform him that blood specimens will be drawn at timed intervals.
• Muscle trauma caused by I.M. injections can raise CK levels.
• Handle the collection tube gently to prevent hemolysis and send the sample to the laboratory immediately.
• If a hematoma develops at the venipuncture site, apply warm soaks.

Grading murmurs

Use the system outlined below to describe the intensity of a murmur. When recording your findings, use Roman numerals as part of a fraction, always with VI as the denominator. For instance, a grade III murmur would be recorded as "grade III/VI."
• Grade I is a barely audible murmur.
• Grade II is audible but quiet and soft.
• Grade III is moderately loud, without a thrust or thrill.
• Grade IV is loud, with a thrill.
• Grade V is very loud, with a thrust or a thrill.
• Grade VI is loud enough to be heard before the stethoscope comes into contact with the chest.

LD

LD appears in almost all body tissues, but its five isoenzymes are organ-specific. The isoenzymes LD_1 and LD_2 appear primarily in the heart, red blood cells (RBCs), and kidneys; LD_3, primarily in the lungs; and LD_4 and LD_5, in the liver and the skeletal muscles. Usually, LD_1 and LD_2 levels rise 8 to 12 hours after acute MI, peak in 24 to 48 hours, and return to normal in 10 to 14 days if tissue necrosis doesn't persist. A flipped LD, in which LD_1 levels exceed LD_2 levels (the reversal of their normal pattern), reliably indicates acute MI. If measurement of CK doesn't take place within 24 hours of an acute MI, LD isoenzyme analysis becomes especially useful.

Nursing considerations

• Inform the patient that he need not restrict food or fluids before the test.
• Tell the patient with suspected MI that the test is likely to be repeated for the next few days to monitor changes.
• Muscle trauma caused by I.M. injections can raise LD levels.
• Handle the collection tube gently to prevent hemolysis and send the sample to the laboratory immediately.
• Prosthetic heart valves or recent surgery or pregnancy can cause elevated LD levels.
• If a hematoma develops at the venipuncture site, apply warm soaks to help ease discomfort.

LD is particularly useful if CK measurement isn't done in the first 24 hours after MI.

Myoglobin

Myoglobin is found in both the myocardium and skeletal muscle. Normally, small amounts of myoglobin are continually released into the bloodstream as a result of the turnover of muscle cells. It's then excreted by the kidneys. During acute MI, myoglobin levels rise as a larger quantity of myoglobin enters the bloodstream. Rising myoglobin levels may be the first marker of cardiac injury after acute MI. Levels may rise within 30 minutes to 4 hours, peak within 6 to 7 hours, and return to baseline by 24 hours. However, because skeletal muscle damage may cause myoglobin levels to rise, it isn't specific to myocardial injury. Myoglobin levels may be available within 30 minutes.

Rising myoglobin levels may be the first marker of cardiac injury after acute MI.

Nursing considerations

• I.M. injections, recent angina, cardioversion, acute alcohol intoxication, dermatomyositis, hypothermia, muscular dystrophy, polymyositis, severe burns, trauma, severe renal failure, and systemic lupus erythematosus (SLE) can cause elevated myoglobin levels.

• Handle the collection tube gently to prevent hemolysis and send the sample to the laboratory immediately.
• If a hematoma develops at the venipuncture site, apply warm soaks to help ease discomfort.

Troponin I and troponin T

Troponin is a protein found in skeletal and cardiac muscles. Troponin I and troponin T, two isotypes of troponin, are found in the myocardium. Troponin T may also be found in skeletal muscle. Troponin I, however, is found only in the myocardium — in fact, it's more specific to myocardial damage than CK, CK-MB isoenzymes, and myoglobin. Because troponin T levels can occur in certain muscle disorders or renal failure, it's less specific for myocardial injury than troponin I.

Rise time

 Troponin levels rise within 3 to 6 hours after myocardial damage. Troponin I peaks in 14 to 20 hours, with a return to baseline in 5 to 7 days, and troponin T peaks in 12 to 24 hours, with a return to baseline in 10 to 15 days. Because troponin levels stay elevated for a prolonged period of time, they can detect an infarction that occurred several days earlier. Rapid troponin T levels can be determined at the bedside in minutes, making them a useful tool for determining treatment in acute MI.

> Troponin takes its time. In fact, elevated levels last so long, they can help detect an infarction that occurred several days earlier.

Nursing considerations

• Inform the patient that he need not restrict food or fluids before the test.
• Tell him that multiple blood samples may be drawn.
• Sustained vigorous exercise, cardiotoxic drugs such as doxorubicin, renal disease, and certain surgical procedures can cause elevated troponin T levels.
• Handle the collection tube gently to prevent hemolysis and send the sample to the laboratory immediately.
• If a hematoma develops at the venipuncture site, apply warm soaks to help ease discomfort.

Graphic recording studies

Graphic recording studies to diagnose cardiac disorders include ECG, exercise ECG, and Holter monitoring.

What the ECG strip shows

On an electrocardiogram (ECG) strip, the horizontal axis correlates the length of each particular electrical event with its duration. Each small block on the horizontal axis represents 0.04 second. Five small blocks form the base of a large block, which in turn represents 0.2 second. The graphic display, or tracing, usually consists of the P wave, the QRS complex, and the T wave.

ECG

ECG, a valuable diagnostic test that's now a routine part of every cardiovascular evaluation, graphically records electrical current generated by the heart. (See *What the ECG strip shows*.) This test helps identify primary conduction abnormalities, arrhythmias, cardiac hypertrophy, pericarditis, electrolyte imbalance, and MI (site and extent).

Nursing considerations

• Tell the patient that an ECG only takes about 10 minutes and causes no discomfort.

- Explain that he must lie still, relax, breathe normally, and remain quiet.
- Evaluation of the recording will guide further treatment.
- Treat chest pain, if present (as ordered).

Exercise ECG

Exercise ECG is a noninvasive test that helps the doctor assess cardiovascular response to an increased workload. Commonly known as a stress test, it provides diagnostic information that can't be obtained from a resting ECG. This test may also assess response to treatment.

The test is stopped if the patient experiences chest pain, fatigue, or other signs and symptoms that reflect exercise intolerance. These may include severe dyspnea, claudication, weakness or dizziness, hypotension, pallor or vasoconstriction, disorientation, ataxia, ischemic ECG changes (with or without pain), rhythm disturbances or heart block, and ventricular conduction abnormalities.

Drugs do it, too

If the patient can't exercise, a stress test can be performed by I.V. injection of a coronary vasodilator, such as dipyridamole or adenosine. Other methods of stressing the heart include dobutamine administration and pacing (in the patient with a pacemaker). During the stress test, nuclear scanning or echocardiography may also be performed.

> A stress test can also be performed by I.V. injection of a coronary vasodilator.

Nursing considerations

- Inform the patient that he must not eat food, drink caffeinated beverages, or smoke cigarettes for 4 hours before the test.
- Explain that he should wear loose, lightweight clothing and snug-fitting but comfortable shoes and emphasize that he should immediately report any chest pain, leg discomfort, breathlessness, or fatigue.
- Check the doctor's orders to determine which cardiac drugs should be administered or withheld prior to the test. Beta-adrenergic blockers, for example, can limit the patient's ability to raise his heart rate.
- Inform the patient that he may receive an injection of thallium during the test so that the doctor can evaluate coronary blood flow. Reassure him that the injection involves negligible radiation exposure.
- Tell the patient that after the test, his blood pressure and ECG will be monitored for 10 to 15 minutes.
- Explain that he should wait at least 2 hours before showering, and then he should use warm water.

Holter monitoring

Also called ambulatory ECG, Holter monitoring allows recording of heart activity as the patient follows his normal routine. Like an exercise ECG, it can provide considerably more diagnostic information than a standard resting ECG. In addition, Holter monitoring can record intermittent arrhythmias.

This test usually lasts about 24 hours (about 100,000 cardiac cycles). The patient wears a small tape recorder connected to bipolar electrodes placed on his chest, and keeps a diary of his activities and associated symptoms.

Nursing considerations

• Urge the patient not to tamper with the monitor or disconnect lead wires or electrodes. Demonstrate how to check the recorder for proper function.
• Tell the patient that he can't bathe or shower while wearing the monitor. He also needs to avoid electrical appliances that can interfere with the monitor's recording.
• Emphasize to the patient the importance of keeping track of his activities, regardless of symptoms.
• Evaluation of the recordings will guide further treatment.

Holter monitoring records heart activity as the patient follows his normal routine.

Imaging studies

Imaging studies used to diagnose cardiovascular disorders include chest X-ray, echocardiography, magnetic resonance imaging (MRI), transesophageal echocardiography, and ultrafast computed tomography (CT) scan.

Chest X-ray

A chest X-ray may detect cardiac enlargement, pulmonary congestion, pleural effusion, calcium deposits in or on the heart, pacemaker placement, hemodynamic monitoring lines, and tracheal tube position.

Keep in mind that a chest X-ray alone can't rule out a cardiac problem. Also, clinical signs may reflect the patient's condition 24 to 48 hours before problems appear on an X-ray.

Nursing considerations

• Tell the patient that while this test takes only a few minutes, the doctor or technician will require extra time to evaluate the quality of the films.
• Inform him that he'll wear a gown without snaps but may keep his pants, socks, and shoes on. Instruct him to remove all jewelry from his neck and chest.

• Tell him that he'll need to take a deep breath and hold it as the technician takes the X-ray.
• Permit the patient to resume activities, as ordered.

Echocardiography

Echocardiography, a noninvasive imaging technique, records the reflection of ultra-high frequency sound waves directed at the patient's heart. It enables the doctor to visualize heart size and shape, myocardial wall thickness and motion, and cardiac valve structure and function. It also helps evaluate overall left ventricular function and detect some MI complications; mitral valve prolapse; mitral, tricuspid, or pulmonic valve insufficiency; cardiac tamponade; pericardial diseases; cardiac tumors; prosthetic valve function; subvalvular stenosis; ventricular aneurysms; cardiomyopathies; and congenital abnormalities.

Nursing considerations

• Reassure the patient that this 15- to 30-minute test doesn't cause pain or pose any risk.
• Mention that he may undergo other tests, such as ECG and phonocardiography, simultaneously. Tell him that two recordings will be made, one with him on his back, and one with him on his left side.
• Tell him he must sit still while recording is occurring because movement may distort results.
• Permit the patient to resume activities as ordered.

What's that noise? Do you hear that? I thought these walls were thick, but I guess not!

MRI

Also known as *nuclear magnetic resonance*, MRI yields high-resolution, tomographic, three-dimensional images of body structures. It takes advantage of certain body nuclei that are magnetically aligned and fall out of alignment after radio frequency transmission. The MRI scanner records the signals the nuclei emit as they realign in a process called *precession* and then translates the signals into detailed pictures of body structures. The resulting images show tissue characteristics without lung or bone interference.

MRI permits visualization of valve leaflets and structures, pericardial abnormalities and processes, ventricular hypertrophy, cardiac neoplasm, infarcted tissue, anatomic malformations, and structural deformities. Applications include monitoring the progression of ischemic heart disease and treatment effectiveness.

Nursing considerations

• Instruct the patient that he'll need to lie still during the test.
• Warn him that he'll hear a thumping noise.

Lose the jewels

• Have him remove all jewelry and other metallic objects before testing. A patient with an internal surgical clip, scalp vein needle, pacemaker, gold fillings, heart valve prosthesis, or other metal object in his body can't undergo an MRI.
• Permit the patient to resume activities, as ordered.

Transesophageal echocardiography

Transesophageal echocardiography directs high frequency sound waves at the heart through the esophagus or stomach. This test provides better resolution than echocardiography because the sound waves travel through less tissue. To perform this test, a flexible tube with a transducer at the tip is inserted endoscopically into the esophagus or stomach.

Nursing considerations

• Tell the patient that he must fast for 4 to 6 hours before the test.
• Reassure him that the test only lasts about 15 minutes and that short-acting I.V. sedation is commonly given to reduce anxiety and a topical anesthetic is sprayed in the back of the throat to prevent gagging.
• Inform him that ECG leads will be placed on his chest and his ECG will be continuously monitored.
• Explain that he'll be placed on his left side and will be asked to swallow while the lubricated catheter tip is advanced down his esophagus.
• Warn the patient that he won't be able to have anything to eat or drink after the procedure until his gag reflex has returned, typically in 2 hours.
• Observe the patient for signs of esophageal perforation, such as GI bleeding and complaints of pain.

Ultrafast CT scan

Ultrafast CT scan, also called *electron beam CT,* uses a scanner that takes images at fast speeds, resulting in high resolution pictures. This noninvasive test can identify microcalcifications in the coronary arteries, making it useful for detecting early CAD before symptoms occur, screening symptomatic people at risk for CAD, and evaluating chest pain. This test may also be used to diagnose pulmonary embolus, aortic dissection or aneurysm, congenital heart dis-

MRI is contraindicated in a patient with a metal object in his body, such as an internal surgical clip, a pacemaker, and gold fillings.

Until your gag reflex returns, you won't be able to eat or drink. Don't worry, though. It usually returns in about 2 hours.

ease, pericardial disease, and diseases of the great vessels (main vessels that supply organs).

Nursing considerations

• Explain to the patient that he 'll need to lie still as the images are obtained.
• Question him about allergies to contrast media in case a contrast medium is used during the test.
• If a contrast medium is used, encourage the patient to increase his fluid intake after the test.

Radionuclide imaging tests

Radionuclide imaging tests used to diagnose cardiovascular disorders include cardiac catheterization and coronary angiography, coronary flow and perfusion evaluation, digital subtraction angiography (DSA), multiple-gated acquisition (MUGA) scanning, technetium-99m (^{99m}Tc) pyrophosphate scanning, and thallium scanning.

Cardiac catheterization and coronary angiography

Cardiac catheterization and coronary angiography, two common invasive tests, use a catheter threaded through an artery (for a left-sided catheterization) or vein (for a right-sided catheterization) into the heart to determine the size and location of a coronary lesion, evaluate ventricular function, and measure heart pressures and oxygen saturation.

Cardiac catheterization and coronary angiography measure oxygen saturation, among other things.

Nursing considerations

• Make sure the patient understands why he's scheduled for catheterization.
• Check with the doctor before withholding any medication. Explain to the patient that he won't be able to have anything to eat or drink for 6 to 8 hours before the test.
• Explain that a mild I.V. or oral sedative may be given before or during the procedure and that a local anesthetic will be used at the insertion site.

A case of the head spins

• Warn him that he may feel light-headed, warm, or nauseated for a few moments after the dye injection. He may also receive nitroglycerin during the test to dilate coronary vessels and aid visualization.
• Tell the patient he must cough or breathe deeply as instructed during the test.

• Tell the patient he must lie on his back for several hours after the procedure. Instruct him to notify you if he has any chest pain.
• When the femoral approach is used, tell the patient to keep his leg straight for 12 hours or as ordered. Elevate the head of the bed no more than 30 degrees. When the brachial artery is used, tell the patient to keep his arm straight for at least 24 hours or as ordered. To immobilize the leg or arm, place a sandbag over it, as ordered.
• Several devices may be used to seal the arterial puncture site, including absorbable collagen protein plugs and a suture tool that's placed inside the puncture site so that the wound can be sutured from below the skin.
• For the 1st hour after catheterization, monitor the patient's vital signs every 15 minutes and inspect the dressing frequently for signs of bleeding.

Vital checks

• Check the patient's skin color, temperature, and pulses distal to the insertion site. An absent or weak pulse may signify an embolus or other problem requiring immediate attention. Notify the doctor of any changes in peripheral pulses.
• If the patient's vital signs change or if he has chest pain (possible indications of arrhythmias, angina, or MI), notify the doctor.
• After the 1st hour, assess the patient every 30 minutes for 1 hour, then every hour for 4 hours, then once every 4 hours.
• Monitor urine output, especially in cases of impaired renal function.

Measure pulses distal to the insertion site. An absent or weak pulse may signify an embolus or other problem.

Coronary flow and perfusion evaluation

Coronary flow and perfusion evaluation is used to assess blood flow through the coronary arteries, investigate myocardial anatomy and perfusion, and determine the extent of coronary lesions. A contrast medium injected into the coronary artery passes through the artery, entering cardiac tissue. A computer screen then displays a multicolored image, with each color representing blood flow during subsequent cardiac cycles. The completed picture, called a *contrast medium appearance picture*, shows how long it takes for the contrast medium to reach cardiac tissue.

Nursing considerations

Care for a patient undergoing a coronary flow and perfusion evaluation as you would for a patient undergoing cardiac catheterization.

DSA

DSA combines angiography with computer processing to produce high-resolution images of cardiovascular structures. The images are converted to digital signals with a number assigned to each color density from white to black. These images undergo a subtraction process that eliminates interference and extraneous structures, such as bone and soft tissue. DSA helps evaluate coronary arterial flow, myocardial perfusion, and left ventricular function and wall movement. It may also enable the doctor to visualize carotid and peripheral vessels.

Performed on an outpatient basis, DSA provides a clear view of arterial structures. Because the contrast medium is injected into a vein, DSA eliminates the risks associated with arterial puncture. Because the dilute, low-dose contrast medium doesn't depress cardiac and kidney function, the test is safer for patients with heart failure, diabetes, and renal impairment.

In DSA, images undergo a subtraction process to eliminate bone and soft tissue interference.

Nursing considerations

Care for a patient undergoing DSA as you would care for a patient undergoing cardiac catheterization.

MUGA scanning

MUGA scanning is cardiac blood pool imaging used to evaluate regional and global ventricular performance. During a MUGA scan, the camera records 14 to 64 points of a single cardiac cycle, yielding sequential images that can be studied like a motion picture film to evaluate regional wall motion and determine the ejection fraction and other indices of cardiac function.

Various variations

There are many variations of the MUGA scan. In the stress MUGA test, the same test is performed at rest and after exercise to detect changes in ejection fraction and cardiac output. In the nitroglycerin MUGA test, the scintillation camera records points in the cardiac cycle after the sublingual administration of nitroglycerin to assess the drug's effect on ventricular function.

I'm ready for my close-up, Mr. MUGA.

Nursing considerations

• An ECG is required to signal the computer and camera to take images for each cardiac cycle.
• If arrhythmias interfere with a reliable ECG, the test may need to be postponed.

^{99m}Tc pyrophosphate scanning

^{99m}Tc pyrophosphate scanning, also known as *hot spot imaging* or *PYP scanning*, helps diagnose acute myocardial injury by showing the location and size of newly damaged myocardial tissue. Especially useful for diagnosing transmural infarction, this test works best when performed 12 hours to 6 days after symptom onset. It also helps diagnose right ventricular infarctions; locate true posterior infarctions; assess trauma, ventricular aneurysm, and heart tumors; and detect myocardial damage from a recent electric shock such as defibrillation.

In this test, the patient receives an injection of ^{99m}Tc pyrophosphate, a radioactive material absorbed by injured cells. A scintillation camera scans the heart and displays damaged areas as "hot spots," or bright areas. A spot's size usually corresponds to the injury size.

I absorb ^{99m}Tc pyrophosphate more readily than healthy cells.

Nursing considerations

• Tell the patient that the doctor will inject ^{99m}Tc pyrophosphate into an arm vein about 3 hours before the start of this 45-minute test. Reassure him that the injection causes only transient discomfort and that it involves only negligible radiation exposure.
• Instruct the patient to remain still during the test.
• Permit the patient to resume activities as ordered.

Thallium scanning

Also known as *cold spot imaging*, thallium scanning evaluates myocardial blood flow and myocardial cell status. This test helps determine areas of ischemic myocardium and infarcted tissue. It can also help evaluate coronary artery and ventricular function as well as pericardial effusion. (See *Understanding thallium scanning*.) Thallium imaging can also detect a MI in its first few hours.

The test uses thallium-201, a radioactive isotope that emits gamma rays and closely resembles potassium. When injected I.V., the isotope enters healthy myocardial tissue rapidly but enters areas with poor blood flow and damaged cells slowly. A camera counts the gamma rays and displays an image. Areas with heavy isotope uptake appear light, while areas with poor uptake, known as "cold spots," look dark. Cold spots represent areas of reduced myocardial perfusion.

Nursing considerations

• Tell the patient to avoid heavy meals, cigarette smoking, and strenuous activity before the test.

- If your patient is scheduled for an exercise thallium scan, advise him to wear comfortable clothes or pajamas and snug-fitting shoes or slippers.
- Permit the patient to resume activities, as ordered.

Treatments

Ongoing technological advances in the treatment of cardiovascular disorders enable patients to live longer than ever before. These treatments include drug therapy, surgery, balloon catheter treatments, and emergency treatment for cardiac arrest.

Drug therapy

Drugs are critical to the treatment of many cardiovascular disorders. Drugs that may be used to treat cardiovascular disorders include:
- adrenergics
- antianginals
- antiarrhythmics
- antihypertensives
- antilipemics
- antiplatelet agents
- diuretics
- inotropic agents
- thrombolytics.

Surgery

Despite the drama of successful single- and multiple-organ transplants, improved immunosuppressants, and advanced ventricular assist devices (VADs), far more patients undergo conventional surgeries such as coronary artery bypass. However, for this and other cardiovascular surgeries, the patient initially recovers in the cardiac intensive care unit (ICU). The role of the medical-surgical nurse is to promote recovery and help smooth the transition from hospital to home using appropriate patient-teaching techniques.

Coronary artery bypass grafting

Coronary artery bypass grafting (CABG) circumvents an occluded coronary artery with an autogenous graft (usually a segment of the saphenous vein or internal mammary artery), thereby restoring blood flow to the myocardium. CABG techniques vary accord-

---

Understanding thallium scanning

In thallium scanning, areas with poor blood flow and ischemic cells fail to take up the isotope (thallium-201 or Cardiolite) and thus appear as cold spots on a scan. Thallium imaging should show normal distribution of the isotope throughout the left ventricle and no defects (cold spots).

To distinguish normal from infarcted myocardial tissue, the doctor may order an exercise thallium scan followed by a resting perfusion scan. A resting perfusion scan helps differentiate between an ischemic area and an infarcted or scarred area of the myocardium. Ischemic myocardium appears as a reversible defect (the cold spot disappears). Infarcted myocardium shows up as a nonreversible defect (the cold spot remains).

Bypassing coronary occlusions

In this example of coronary artery bypass grafting, the surgeon has used saphenous vein segments to bypass occlusions in three sections of the coronary artery.

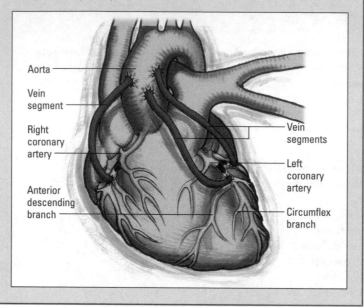

- Aorta
- Vein segment
- Right coronary artery
- Anterior descending branch
- Vein segments
- Left coronary artery
- Circumflex branch

ing to the patient's condition and the number of arteries needing bypass. The most common procedure, aortocoronary bypass, involves suturing one end of the autogenous graft to the ascending aorta and the other end to a coronary artery distal to the occlusion. (See *Bypassing coronary occlusions*.)

CABG caveat

More than 200,000 Americans (most of them male) undergo CABG each year, making it one of the most common cardiac surgeries. Prime candidates include patients with severe angina from atherosclerosis and others with CAD who have a high risk of MI. Successful CABG can relieve anginal pain, improve cardiac function and, possibly, enhance the patient's quality of life.

Even so, although the surgery relieves pain in about 90% of patients, its long-term effectiveness is unclear. Such problems as graft closure and development of atherosclerosis in other coronary arteries may make repeat surgery necessary. In addition, because CABG doesn't resolve the underlying disease associated with arterial blockage, CABG may not reduce the risk of MI recurrence. (See *TMR: New treatment for severe angina*.)

Because CABG doesn't resolve underlying disease, it may not reduce the risk of MI recurrence.

TMR: New treatment for severe angina

Transmyocardial revascularization (TMR) is a relatively new procedure. It can provide relief for severe angina when medical therapy fails or the patient isn't a candidate for angioplasty or bypass surgery.

How it's done

TMR is performed through an incision on the left side of the chest. The surgeon drills 20 to 40 1-mm channels approximately 1 cm apart into each wall of the left ventricle. These channels extend from the epicardium into the ventricle. As the heart pumps, blood is forced into them. Bleeding on the surface of the heart is stopped after a few minutes of pressure by the surgeon's finger.

Potential complications

Complications that may occur with TMR include arrhythmias; bleeding; damage to the great vessels, valves, and coronary arteries; and eye injury. The risk of arrhythmias is minimized by delivering the laser burst during the heart's refractory period.

Less invasive PTMR

Percutaneous TMR (PTMR) is a less invasive TMR procedure that can be performed under local anesthesia in a cardiac catheterization laboratory. Cannulas are inserted through the femoral artery and vein. While laser bursts are also used in this procedure to create channels in the myocardium, these bursts originate from a laser advanced into the left ventricle. The laser burst penetrates the endocardium through the myocardium but doesn't penetrate the epicardial layer of the ventricle. During this procedure, the patient is given heparin to reduce the risk of thrombus formation.

Advantages and complications

Advantages of PTMR include its minimal invasiveness; a reduced risk of infection and bleeding; no need for chest tubes, invasive monitoring, and intubation; only local anesthesia required; and less pain. Complications include arrhythmias, myocardial perforation, damage to nearby structures, bleeding, emboli, eye injury, and risks normally associated with cardiac catheterization.

Patient preparation

• Reinforce the doctor's explanation of the surgery for the patient. Also, explain the complex equipment and procedures used in the ICU or postanesthesia care unit (PACU).
• Restrict food and fluids after midnight and provide a sedative, if ordered.
• On the morning of surgery, also provide a sedative, as ordered, to help the patient relax.

Monitoring and aftercare

The patient requiring CABG will be monitored in the cardiac ICU before and after surgery. He'll be transferred to the medical-surgical unit for further postoperative care when his condition is stable. After transfer to the medical-surgical unit:

• Provide analgesia or encourage the use of patient-controlled analgesia (PCA), if appropriate.
• Monitor for postoperative complications, such as stroke, pulmonary embolism, pneumonia, and impaired renal perfusion.
• Gradually allow the patient to increase activities, as ordered.
• Monitor the incision site for signs of infection or drainage.
• Provide support to the patient and his family to help them cope with recovery and lifestyle changes.

Home care instructions

Instruct the patient to:
• watch for and immediately notify the doctor of any signs of infection (redness, swelling, or drainage from the leg or chest incisions; fever; or sore throat) or possible arterial reocclusion (angina, dizziness, dyspnea, rapid or irregular pulse, or prolonged recovery time from exercise)
• call the doctor in the case of weight gain greater than 3 lb (1.4 kg) in 1 week
• follow his prescribed diet, especially sodium and cholesterol restrictions
• maintain a balance between activity and rest by trying to sleep at least 8 hours each night, scheduling a short rest period each afternoon, and resting frequently when engaging in tiring physical activity
• follow exercise program or cardiac rehabilitation, if prescribed
• follow lifestyle modifications (no smoking, improved diet, and regular exercise) to reduce atherosclerotic progression
• contact a local chapter of the Mended Hearts Club and the AHA for information and support
• make sure he understands the dose, frequency of administration, and possible adverse effects of prescribed medications.

MIDCAB

Until recently, cardiac surgery required stopping the heart and using cardiopulmonary bypass to oxygenate and circulate blood. Now, minimally invasive direct coronary artery bypass (MIDCAB) can be performed on a pumping heart through a small thoracotomy incision. The patient may receive only right lung ventilation along with drugs such as beta-adrenergic blockers to slow the heart rate and reduce heart movement during surgery.

It's a good thing

Advantages of MIDCAB include shorter hospital stays, use of shorter-acting anesthetic agents, fewer postoperative complications, earlier extubation, reduced cost, smaller incisions, and earlier return to work. Patients eligible for MIDCAB include those with proximal left anterior descending lesions and some lesions of the right coronary and circumflex arteries.

Patient preparation
• Review the procedure with the patient and answer his questions. Tell the patient that he'll be extubated in the operating room or within 2 to 4 hours after surgery.
• Teach the patient to cough and breathe deeply through use of an incentive spirometer.
• Explain the use of pain medications after surgery as well as nonpharmacologic methods to control pain.
• Let the patient know that he should be able to walk with assistance the 1st postoperative day and be discharged within 48 hours.

Monitoring and aftercare
The patient undergoing MIDCAB may be monitored in a cardiac ICU or step-down unit after surgery. He'll be transferred to the medical-surgical unit for further postoperative care when his condition is stable. After transfer to the medical-surgical unit:
• Provide analgesia or encourage the use of PCA, if appropriate.
• Monitor for postoperative complications, such as stroke, pulmonary embolism, pneumonia, and impaired renal perfusion.
• Gradually allow the patient to increase activities, as ordered.
• Monitor the incision site for signs of infection or drainage. Depending on the procedure, the patient will have one to three small chest incisions.
• Provide support to the patient and his family to help them cope with recovery and lifestyle changes.

Depending on the procedure, the patient undergoing MIDCAB will have one to three small incisions.

Home care instructions
Instruct the patient to:
• continue with the progressive exercise started in the hospital
• perform coughing and deep-breathing exercises, splint the incision with a pillow to reduce pain while doing these exercises, and use the incentive spirometer to reduce pulmonary complications
• avoid lifting objects that weigh more than 10 lb (4.5 kg) for the next 4 to 6 weeks
• wait 2 to 4 weeks before resuming sexual activity
• check the incision site daily and immediately notify the doctor of any signs of infection (redness, foul-smelling drainage, or swelling) or possible graft occlusion (slow, rapid, or irregular pulse; angina; dizziness; or dyspnea)
• perform any necessary incisional care

• follow lifestyle modifications
• take medications, as prescribed, and report adverse effects to the doctor
• consider participation in a cardiac rehabilitation program.

Port access cardiac surgery

Port access cardiac surgery is another minimally invasive surgical technique that uses femorofemoral bypass through a small incision with the aid of videoscopes. This procedure requires a shorter hospital stay, promoting faster recovery. Also, because the heart can be turned, port access allows more bypass grafting to be performed.

Picture using ports

Port access surgery is performed using a small anterior thoracotomy and several small "port" chest incisions. The surgeon inserts a thorascope through the ports to view the heart. As with traditional cardiac surgery, cardiopulmonary bypass is conducted during port access. However, it's performed using the femoral artery and vein cannulation, reducing the risk of atrial fibrillation associated with atrial cannulation. In addition, rather than cross-clamping the aorta, increasing the risk of atherosclerotic emboli, port access surgery internally occludes the aorta with an inflated endo-aortic balloon, which prevents air and thrombotic emboli during bypass.

> Balloons prevent air and thrombotic emboli during bypass. Plus, they just make me happy.

Patient preparation
• Teach the patient to perform coughing and deep-breathing exercises and how to use an incentive spirometer.
• Tell the patient that he'll be assisted to a sitting position and allowed to ambulate as early as the 1st postoperative evening.

Monitoring and aftercare
The patient undergoing port access cardiac surgery will require nursing care similar to MIDCAB. After transfer to the medical-surgical unit:
• Provide analgesia or encourage the use of PCA, if appropriate.
• Monitor for postoperative complications, such as stroke, femoral artery dissection, and femoral artery or vein occlusion.
• Gradually allow the patient to increase activities, as ordered.
• Monitor the incision site for signs of infection, drainage, or bleeding.
• Provide support to the patient and his family to help them cope with recovery and lifestyle changes.

Home care instructions

Instruct the patient to:
• continue with the progressive exercise started in the hospital
• perform coughing and deep-breathing exercises, splint the incision with a pillow to reduce pain while doing these exercises, and use the incentive spirometer to reduce pulmonary complications
• avoid lifting objects that weigh more than 10 lb (4.5 kg) for the next 4 to 6 weeks
• wait 2 to 4 weeks before resuming sexual activity
• check the incision site daily and immediately notify the doctor of any signs and symptoms of infection (redness, foul-smelling drainage, or swelling) or possible graft occlusion (slow, rapid, or irregular pulse; angina; dizziness; or dyspnea)
• check for bleeding or hematoma at the femoral insertion sites
• follow lifestyle modifications
• take medications as prescribed and report adverse effects to the doctor
• comply with the laboratory schedule for monitoring International Normalized Ratio (INR) if the patient is receiving warfarin
• consider participation in a cardiac rehabilitation program.

Tell the patient to call the doctor if he has any symptoms of graft occlusion such as angina — ouch!

Vascular repair

Vascular repair may treat:
• vessels damaged by arteriosclerotic or thromboembolic disorders (such as aortic aneurysm or arterial occlusive disease), trauma, infections, or congenital defects
• vascular obstructions that severely compromise circulation
• vascular disease that doesn't respond to drug therapy or nonsurgical treatments such as balloon catheterization
• life-threatening dissecting or ruptured aortic aneurysms
• limb-threatening acute arterial occlusion.

Vascular repair includes aneurysm resection, grafting, embolectomy, vena caval filtering, endarterectomy, and vein stripping. The specific surgery used depends on the type, location, and extent of vascular occlusion or damage. (See *Understanding types of vascular repair*, page 264.)

In all vascular surgeries, there's a potential for vessel trauma, emboli, hemorrhage, infection, and other complications. Grafting carries added risks because the graft may occlude, narrow, dilate, or rupture.

Among other conditions, vascular repair treats vascular obstructions that compromise circulation.

Patient preparation

Vascular surgery may be performed as an emergency procedure or a scheduled event. Before surgery:

Understanding types of vascular repair

Vascular repair is performed to treat various conditions. Five common types of vascular repair are illustrated and described here.

Aortic aneurysm repair

Aortic aneurysm repair removes an aneurysmal segment of the aorta.

Procedure

The surgeon first makes an incision to expose the aneurysm site. If necessary, he places the patient on a cardiopulmonary bypass machine; then he clamps the aorta. The aneurysm is resected and the damaged portion of the aorta is repaired.

Vena caval filter insertion

Vena caval filter insertion traps emboli in the vena cava, preventing them from reaching the pulmonary vessels.

Umbrella

Direction of blood flow

Procedure

A vena caval filter or umbrella (shown at right) is inserted transvenously via a catheter. Once in place in the vena cava, the umbrella or filter traps emboli but allows venous blood flow.

Vein stripping

Vein stripping removes the saphenous vein and its branches to treat varicosities.

Stripper removing vein

Stripper in place

Procedure

The surgeon ligates the saphenous vein. He then threads the stripper into the vein, secures it, and pulls it back out, bringing the vein with it.

Embolectomy

Embolectomy removes an embolism from an artery.

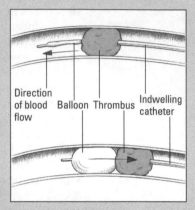

Direction of blood flow   Balloon   Thrombus   Indwelling catheter

Procedure

The surgeon inserts a balloon-tipped indwelling catheter into the artery and passes it through the thrombus (top). He then inflates the balloon and withdraws the catheter to remove the thrombus (bottom).

Bypass grafting

Bypass grafting bypasses an arterial obstruction resulting from arteriosclerosis.

Procedure

After exposing the affected artery, the surgeon anastomoses a synthetic or autogenous graft to divert blood flow around the occluded arterial segment. The autogenous graft may be a vein harvested from elsewhere in the patient's body. The illustration at right shows a femoropopliteal bypass.

• Reinforce all explanations regarding surgery and recovery.
• Perform and document a vascular assessment, focusing on the area that requires treatment.
• If the patient is awaiting surgery for aortic aneurysm repair, be on guard for signs and symptoms of acute dissection or rupture. Note especially sudden severe pain in the chest, abdomen, or lower back; severe weakness; diaphoresis; tachycardia; or a precipitous drop in blood pressure. If any of these conditions occur, call the doctor immediately; he may need to perform life-saving emergency surgery.

Be on the lookout for signs and symptoms of acute dissection or rupture, a condition requiring life-saving emergency treatment.

Monitoring and aftercare

After surgery, the patient will be cared for in the ICU. He'll be transferred to the medical-surgical unit for further postoperative care when his condition is stable. After transfer to the medical-surgical unit:
• Frequently assess peripheral pulses, using Doppler ultrasonography if palpation proves difficult.
• Assess extremities bilaterally for muscle strength and movement, color, temperature, and capillary refill time.
• Provide analgesia or encourage the use of PCA, if appropriate.
• Gradually allow the patient to increase activities, as ordered.
• Monitor the incision site for signs of infection or drainage.
• Monitor for complications, such as infection, bleeding, and vessel occlusion.
• Provide support to the patient and his family to help them cope with recovery and lifestyle changes.

Home care instructions

Instruct the patient to:
• check his pulse (or have a family member do it) in the affected extremity before rising from bed each morning and to notify the doctor if he can't palpate his pulse or he develops coldness, pallor, numbness, tingling, or pain in extremities
• continue with the progressive exercise started in the hospital
• perform coughing and deep-breathing exercises, splint the incision with a pillow to reduce pain while doing these exercises, and use the incentive spirometer to reduce pulmonary complications
• avoid lifting objects that weigh more than 10 lb (4.5 kg) for the next 4 to 6 weeks
• check the incision site daily and immediately notify the doctor of any signs and symptoms of infection
• take medications as prescribed and report adverse effects to the doctor
• comply with the laboratory schedule for monitoring INR if the patient is receiving warfarin.

Valve surgery

To prevent heart failure, a patient with valvular stenosis or insufficiency accompanied by severe, unmanageable symptoms may require valvuloplasty (valvular repair), commissurotomy (separation of the adherent, thickened leaflets of the mitral valve), or valve replacement (with a mechanical or prosthetic valve).

Because of the high pressure generated by the left ventricle during contraction, stenosis and insufficiency most commonly affect the mitral and aortic valves. Other indications for valve surgery depend on the patient's symptoms and on the affected valve:

• *aortic insufficiency* — valve replacement after symptoms (palpitations, dizziness, dyspnea on exertion, angina, and murmurs) have developed or the chest X-ray and ECG reveal left ventricular hypertrophy
• *aortic stenosis* — possibly asymptomatic with valve replacement (or balloon valvuloplasty) recommended if cardiac catheterization reveals significant stenosis
• *mitral stenosis* — valvuloplasty or commissurotomy indicated if the patient develops fatigue, dyspnea, hemoptysis, arrhythmias, pulmonary hypertension, or right ventricular hypertrophy
• *mitral insufficiency* — valvuloplasty or valve replacement when symptoms (dyspnea, fatigue, and palpitations) interfere with patient activities or in acute insufficiency (as in papillary muscle rupture).

Stenosis and insufficiency most commonly affect the mitral and aortic valves.

It gets complicated

Although valve surgery carries a low risk of mortality, it can cause serious complications. Hemorrhage, for instance, may result from unligated vessels, anticoagulant therapy, or coagulopathy resulting from cardiopulmonary bypass during surgery. Stroke may result from thrombus formation caused by turbulent blood flow through the prosthetic valve or from poor cerebral perfusion during cardiopulmonary bypass. In valve replacement, bacterial endocarditis can develop within days of implantation or months later. Valve dysfunction or failure may occur as the prosthetic device wears out.

Odds are against mortality as a result of valve surgery, but the stakes are higher when it comes to complications.

Patient preparation

• As necessary, reinforce and supplement the doctor's explanation of the procedure.
• Tell the patient that he'll awaken from surgery in an ICU or PACU. Mention that he'll be connected to a cardiac monitor and have I.V. lines, an arterial line and, possibly, a pulmonary artery or left atrial catheter in place.

• Explain that he'll breathe through an endotracheal tube connected to a mechanical ventilator and he'll have a chest tube in place.

Monitoring and aftercare

The patient undergoing valve surgery will be cared for in the cardiac ICU after surgery. He'll be transferred to the medical-surgical unit when his condition is stable. After transfer to the medical-surgical unit:
• Provide analgesia or encourage the use of PCA, if appropriate.
• Monitor for postoperative complications, such as stroke, pulmonary embolism, pneumonia, impaired renal perfusion, endocarditis, and hemolytic anemia.
• Gradually allow the patient to increase activities, as ordered.
• Monitor the incision site for signs of infection or drainage.
• Provide support to the patient and his family to help them cope with recovery and lifestyle changes.

Home care instructions

Instruct the patient to:
• immediately report chest pain, fever, or redness, swelling, or drainage at the incision site
• immediately notify the doctor if signs or symptoms of heart failure (weight gain, dyspnea, or edema) develop
• notify the doctor if signs or symptoms of postpericardiotomy syndrome (fever, muscle and joint pain, weakness, or chest discomfort) develop
• follow the prescribed medication regimen and report adverse effects
• follow his prescribed diet, especially sodium and fat restrictions
• maintain a balance between activity and rest
• follow exercise or rehabilitation program, if prescribed
• inform dentist and other doctors of his prosthetic valve before undergoing surgery or dental work and to take prophylactic antibiotics before such procedures.

Implantable cardioverter-defibrillator

The implantable cardioverter-defibrillator (ICD) has a programmable pulse generator and lead system that monitors the heart's activity, detects ventricular bradyarrhythmias and tachyarrhythmias, and responds with appropriate therapies. Its range of therapies includes antitachycardia and bradycardia pacing, cardioversion, and defibrillation. Some defibrillators also have the ability to pace the atrium and the ventricle.

Implantation of the ICD is similar to that of a permanent pacemaker. The cardiologist positions the lead (or leads) transvenous-

Emphasize the importance of following the prescribed diet, especially sodium and fat restrictions.

ly in the endocardium of the right ventricle (and the right atrium, if both chambers require pacing). The lead connects to a generator box, which is implanted in the right or left upper chest near the clavicle. (See *Location of an ICD.*)

Patient preparation
• Reinforce the cardiologist's instructions to the patient and his family, answering any questions they may have.
• Be sure to emphasize that the need for the device, the potential complications, and ICD terminology.
• Restrict food and fluid for 12 hours before the procedure.
• Provide a sedative on the morning of the procedure, as ordered, to help the patient relax.

Monitoring and aftercare
The patient undergoing ICD implantation will be monitored on a telemetry or medical-surgical unit.
• Monitor for arrhythmias and proper device functioning.
• Gradually allow the patient to increase activities, as ordered.
• Monitor the incision site for signs of infection or drainage.
• Provide support to the patient and his family to help them cope with recovery and lifestyle changes.
• Encourage family members to learn cardiopulmonary resuscitation (CPR).

Home care instructions
Instruct the patient to:
• avoid placing excessive pressure over the insertion site or moving or jerking the area until the postoperative visit
• check the incision site daily and immediately notify the doctor of any signs and symptoms of infection
• wear a medical identification band and carry information regarding his ICD at all times
• increase exercise and sexual activity as allowed by the doctor
• take medications as prescribed and report adverse effects to the doctor.

VAD

A temporary life-sustaining treatment for a failing heart, the VAD diverts systemic blood flow from a diseased ventricle into a pump, which then sends the blood into the aorta. Used most commonly to assist the left ventricle, this device may also assist the right ventricle or both. (See *VAD: Help for the failing heart.*)
  Candidates for a VAD include patients with:
• massive MI

Location of an ICD

To insert an implantable cardioverter-defibrillator (ICD), the cardiologist makes a small incision near the collarbone and accesses the subclavian vein. The lead wires are inserted through the subclavian vein, threaded into the heart, and placed in contact with the endocardium.

  The leads are connected to the pulse generator, which is placed under the skin in a specially prepared pocket in the right or left upper chest. (Placement is similar to that used for a pacemaker.) The cardiologist then closes the incision and programs the device.

VAD: Help for the failing heart

A ventricular assist device (VAD), commonly called a "bridge to transplant," is a mechanical pump that relieves the workload of the ventricle as the heart heals or until a donor heart is located. Many types of VAD systems are available. This illustration shows a VAD (from Baxter Novacor) implanted in the left abdominal wall connected to an external controller by a percutaneous lead. This patient also has a reserve power pack. The monitor is a backup power source that can run on electricity.

Typical types

The typical VAD is implanted in the upper abdominal wall. An inflow cannula drains blood from the left ventricle into a pump, which then pushes the blood into the aorta through the outflow cannula. There are two types of VADs:

• continuous flow pump, which fills continuously and returns blood to the aorta at a constant rate

• pulsatile pump, which may fill during systole and pump blood into the aorta during diastole, or pump irrespective of the patient's cardiac cycle.

Complications

VADs attempt to duplicate the seemingly simple task of the heart; pumping blood throughout the body. Designing a pump is fairly straightforward, but researchers still haven't solved the riddle of how blood swirls through the pulsing chambers of the heart without clotting. Despite the use of anticoagulants and special materials, the VAD usually causes thrombi formation, leading to pulmonary embolism, stroke, and other ominous complications. Thus, VADs aren't used until other measures have failed. Other possible complications from VAD use include:

• bleeding cardiac tamponade
• right-sided heart failure
• infection
• kidney and liver dysfunction
• hemolysis.

Implanted left ventricle assist device

Ascending aorta

Pulmonary artery

Left ventricle

Outflow cannula

Inflow cannula

Primary power pack

Pump unit

Percutaneous lead

Reserve power pack

External controller unit

• irreversible cardiomyopathy
• acute myocarditis
• inability to wean from cardiopulmonary bypass
• valvular disease
• bacterial endocarditis
• rejection of a heart transplant.

The device may also benefit patients awaiting a heart transplant, enabling them to live for months or years at home with a portable left VAD until a donor heart is located.

The downside

Unfortunately, the VAD carries a high risk of complications. For example, the device damages blood cells, creating the risk of thrombus formation and subsequent pulmonary embolism or stroke. As a result, if ventricular function hasn't improved in 96 hours, the doctor may consider a heart transplant.

> The VAD can damage us, increasing the risk of thrombus formation and pulmonary embolism or stroke. Yikes!

Patient preparation
• Explain to the patient that you must restrict his food and fluid intake before surgery.
• Tell the patient that his cardiac function will be continuously monitored using an ECG, a pulmonary artery catheter, and an arterial line.

Monitoring and aftercare
The patient having a VAD implanted will be monitored in the cardiac ICU. He'll be transferred to the medical-surgical unit when his condition is stable. After transfer to the medical-surgical unit:
• Provide analgesia or encourage the use of PCA, if appropriate.
• Monitor for postoperative complications, such as stroke, pulmonary embolism, pneumonia, and impaired renal perfusion.
• Gradually allow the patient to increase activities, as ordered.
• Monitor the incision site for signs of infection or drainage.
• Provide support to the patient and his family to help them cope with recovery and lifestyle changes.

> Monitor the VAD patient for complications, including impaired renal perfusion. Ack!

Home care instructions
Instruct the patient to:
• immediately report redness, swelling, or drainage at the incision site; chest pain; or fever
• immediately notify the doctor if signs or symptoms of heart failure (weight gain, dyspnea, or edema) develop
• follow the prescribed medication regimen and report adverse effects
• follow his prescribed diet, especially sodium and fat restrictions
• maintain a balance between activity and rest
• follow exercise or rehabilitation program (if prescribed)
• comply with the laboratory schedule for monitoring INR if the patient is receiving warfarin.

Balloon catheter treatments

Balloon catheter treatments for cardiovascular disorders include percutaneous balloon valvuloplasty and percutaneous transluminal coronary angioplasty (PTCA).

Percutaneous balloon valvuloplasty

Percutaneous balloon valvuloplasty, which can be performed in the cardiac catheterization laboratory, seeks to improve valvular function by enlarging the orifice of a stenotic heart valve caused by congenital defect, calcification, rheumatic fever, or aging. A small balloon valvuloplasty catheter is introduced through the skin at the femoral vein. While the treatment of choice for valvular heart disease remains surgery (valvuloplasty, valve replacement, or commissurotomy), percutaneous balloon valvuloplasty offers an alternative for individuals considered poor candidates for surgery.

Percutaneous balloon valvuloplasty is an alternative for patients who are considered poor candidates for surgery.

Balloon bungles

Unfortunately, elderly patients with aortic disease commonly experience restenosis 1 to 2 years after undergoing valvuloplasty. In addition, despite the decreased risks associated with more invasive procedures, balloon valvuloplasty can lead to complications, including:
• worsening valvular insufficiency by misshaping the valve so that it doesn't close completely
• pieces breaking off of the calcified valve, which may travel to the brain or lungs and cause embolism (rare)
• severely damaging delicate valve leaflets, requiring immediate surgery to replace the valve (rare)
• bleeding and hematoma at the arterial puncture site
• MI (rare), arrhythmias, myocardial ischemia, and circulatory defects distal to the catheter entry site.

Patient preparation

• Reinforce the doctor's explanation of the procedure, including its risks and alternatives.
• Restrict food and fluid intake for at least 6 hours before the procedure, or as ordered.

Monitoring and aftercare

The patient undergoing balloon valvuloplasty will be monitored in the cardiac ICU or PACU after the procedure. He'll be transferred to the medical-surgical unit when his condition is stable. After transfer to the medical-surgical unit:
• Monitor the effects of I.V. medications such as heparin.
• Assess the cannulation site for bleeding or infection.
• Monitor peripheral pulses distal to the insertion site and the color, temperature, and capillary refill time of the extremity. If pulses are difficult to palpate, use a Doppler stethoscope.
• Notify the doctor if pulses are absent.

If you're having difficulty finding a pulse using palpation, switch to a Doppler stethoscope.

Home care instructions

Instruct the patient to:
• resume normal activity
• notify the doctor if he experiences bleeding or increased bruising at the puncture site or recurrence of symptoms of valvular insufficiency, such as breathlessness or decreased exercise tolerance
• comply with regular follow-up visits.

PTCA

PTCA offers a nonsurgical alternative to coronary artery bypass surgery. The doctor uses a balloon-tipped catheter to dilate a coronary artery that has become narrowed because of atherosclerotic plaque. (See *Looking at angioplasty.*)

Performed in the cardiac catheterization laboratory under local anesthesia, PTCA doesn't involve a thoracotomy, so it's less costly and requires shorter hospitalization. Patients can usually walk the next day and return to work in 2 weeks.

Best working conditions

PTCA works best when lesions are readily accessible, noncalcified, less than 10 mm, concentric, discrete, and smoothly tapered. Patients with a history of less than 1 year of disabling angina make good candidates because their lesions tend to be softer and more compressible. Complications of PTCA are acute vessel closure and late restenosis. To prevent restenosis, such procedures as stenting, atherectomy, and laser angioplasty may be performed.

Patient preparation

• Tell the patient that a catheter will be inserted into an artery and a vein in the groin area and that he may feel pressure as the catheter moves along the vessel.
• Advise the patient that the entire procedure lasts from 1 to 4 hours and that he'll have to lie flat on a table during that time.
• Explain to the patient that he'll be awake during the procedure and may have to take deep breaths to allow visualization of the radiopaque balloon catheter and answer questions about how he's feeling during the procedure.
• Tell the patient to notify the cardiologist if he experiences any angina during the procedure.

Monitoring and aftercare

The patient undergoing PTCA may be monitored in the cardiac ICU or interventional care recovery area after the procedure. The patient will be transferred to the medical-surgical unit when stable. After transfer to the medical-surgical unit:

PTCA is especially effective in patients who have a history of less than 1 year of disabling angina.

Looking at angioplasty

Percutaneous transluminal coronary angioplasty can open an occluded coronary artery without opening the chest. This procedure is outlined in the steps below.

First, the doctor must thread the catheter into the artery. The illustration below shows the entrance of a guide catheter into the coronary artery.

When angiography shows the guide catheter positioned at the occlusion site, the doctor carefully inserts a smaller double-lumen balloon catheter through the guide catheter and directs the balloon through the occlusion.

The doctor then inflates the balloon, causing arterial stretching and plaque fracture. The balloon may need to be inflated or deflated several times until successful arterial dilation occurs.

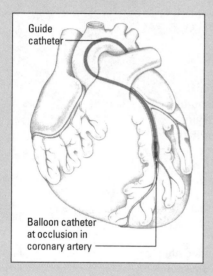

Guide catheter

Balloon catheter at occlusion in coronary artery

Plaque

Deflated balloon

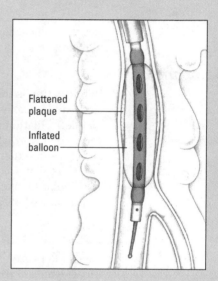

Flattened plaque

Inflated balloon

- Monitor the effects of I.V. medications such as heparin.
- Assess the cannulation site for bleeding or infection.
- Monitor peripheral pulses distal to the insertion site and the color, temperature, and capillary refill time of the extremity. If pulses are difficult to palpate, use a Doppler stethoscope.
- Notify the doctor if pulses are absent.

Home care instructions

If the patient doesn't experience complications from the procedure, he may go home in 6 to 12 hours. Instruct the patient to:
- call his doctor if he experiences any bleeding or bruising at the arterial puncture site
- return for a stress thallium imaging test and follow-up angiography, as recommended by his doctor

• report chest pain to the doctor because restenosis can occur after PTCA.

Emergency treatment for cardiac arrest

Emergency treatment for cardiac arrest may include defibrillation and pacemaker insertion.

Yowzer!
Alright, already,
I'm pacing, I'm
pacing!

Defibrillation

With defibrillation, a strong burst of electric current is delivered to the heart through defibrillator paddles applied to the patient's chest. This brief electric shock completely depolarizes the myocardium, allowing the heart's natural pacemaker to regain control of cardiac rhythm.

Best choice

Defibrillation is the treatment of choice for ventricular fibrillation and pulseless ventricular tachycardia. For every minute that defibrillation is delayed, the patient's chance of surviving ventricular fibrillation drops 7% to 10%. If ventricular fibrillation lasts for more than a few minutes, it causes irreparable brain damage. Note that, for patients with certain arrhythmias such as stable ventricular tachycardia, a technique similar to defibrillation called *synchronized cardioversion* may be necessary.

Pacemaker insertion

Pacemakers are battery-operated generators that emit timed electrical signals to trigger contraction of the heart muscle, thus controlling heart rate. Whether temporary or permanent, they're used when the heart's natural pacemaker fails to work properly.

From the temp pool

Temporary pacemakers are used to pace the heart during CPR or open-heart surgery, after cardiac surgery, and when sinus arrest, symptomatic sinus bradycardia, or complete heart block occurs. Temporary pacing may also correct tachyarrhythmias that fail to respond to drug therapy. In emergency situations, the patient may receive a temporary pacemaker if time or his condition doesn't permit or require implantation of a permanent pacemaker. The doctor may also use a temporary pacemaker to observe the effects of pacing on cardiac function so he can select an optimal rate before implanting a permanent pacemaker. The method of insertion depends on the device.

Pacemakers
are used when
the heart's
natural
pacemaker fails
to work properly.

Here to stay

Permanent pacemaker implantation is a common procedure; worldwide, about 110,000 people undergo it every year. Permanent pacemakers are inserted when the heart's natural pacemaker becomes irreversibly disrupted. Indications for a permanent pacemaker include:

- acquired atrioventricular (AV) block
- chronic bifascicular and trifascicular block
- AV block associated with acute MI
- sinus node dysfunction
- hypersensitive carotid sinus syndrome

Reviewing pacemaker codes

The North American Society of Pacing and Electrophysiology (NASPE) and the British Pacing and Electrophysiology Group (BPEG) developed a five-letter coding system called NASPE/BPEG Generic PaceMaker Code (NBG) to describe pacemaker type and function. Codes may consist of three to five letters. The fourth and fifth letters refer to newer pacemaker functions that aren't utilized in every pacemaker. Here's a summary of what each of the five letters of the code signifies:

heart chamber being paced—**A** (atrium), **V** (ventricle), **D** (dual, or both chambers), or **O** (none).

heart chamber that the pacemaker senses: **A, V, D,** or **O**.

how the pacemaker responds to the sensed event—**T** (triggered by the event), **I** (inhibited by the event), **D** (dual—triggered and inhibited by the event), or **O** (no response to sensing).

pacemaker's degree of programmability and rate responsiveness—**P** (simple programmable), **M** (multiprogrammable), **C** (communicating functions), **R** (rate responsiveness), or **O** (none).

how the pacemaker reacts to tachycardia—**P** (pacing), **S** (shock), **D** (dual—pacing and shock), or **O** (none).

Common pacing codes

The codes DDD and VVI are the most commonly used pacing codes. Below is a description of each, along with its advantages and disadvantages.

DDD

Paces: atrium and ventricle
Senses: atrium and ventricle
Response: inhibited and triggered
Summary: If the atrial rate falls below a preset lower limit, the atrium is paced. If the atrial rate is above this preset lower limit, the atrium isn't paced. However, the ventricle may be paced if the pacemaker doesn't sense a ventricular response within the present atrioventricular (AV) interval.
Advantages: Because both chambers may be paced, AV synchrony is preserved. Used for patients with an intact sinus node but AV block at or below the AV node. May have a rate responsive mode.
Disadvantages: Requires two leads.

VVI

Paces: ventricle
Senses: ventricle
Response: inhibited
Summary: This type of pacemaker paces only when the ventricular rate falls below a preset rate.
Advantages: Requires a single lead and is relatively simple to operate. May be used to treat chronic atrial fibrillation with a slow ventricular response. These patients don't require an atrial lead because a fibrillating atrium can't be paced. May have a rate responsive mode.
Disadvantages: Because only the ventricle is paced, it doesn't preserve AV synchrony.

• hypertrophic and dilated cardiomyopathy.

The many types of pacemakers are categorized according to capabilities. Choice of a pacemaker depends on the patient's age and condition, the doctor's preference and, increasingly, the cost of the device, which can be several thousand dollars. (See *Reviewing pacemaker codes*, page 275.)

Nursing diagnoses

When caring for patients with cardiovascular disorders, you'll find that several nursing diagnoses can be used frequently. These commonly used nursing diagnoses appear below, along with appropriate nursing interventions and rationales.

Activity intolerance

Related to an imbalance between oxygen supply and demand, *Activity intolerance* may be associated with such conditions as acute MI, valvular disorders, heart failure, peripheral vascular disorders, and other ailments.

Activity intolerance is related to an imbalance between oxygen supply and demand.

Expected outcomes
• Patient states a desire to increase his activity level.
• Patient identifies controllable factors that cause fatigue.
• Patient demonstrates skill in conserving energy while carrying out activities of daily living (ADLs) to tolerance level.

Nursing interventions and rationales
• Discuss with the patient the need for activity, which will improve physical and psychosocial well-being.
• Identify activities the patient considers desirable and meaningful to enhance their positive impact.
• Encourage the patient to help plan activity progression. Be sure to include activities he considers essential to help compliance.
• Instruct and help the patient to alternate periods of rest and activity to reduce the body's oxygen demand and prevent fatigue.
• Identify and minimize factors that diminish exercise tolerance to help increase activity level.
• Monitor physiologic responses to increased activity (including respirations, heart rate and rhythm, and blood pressure) to ensure they return to normal a few minutes after exercising.

Conserve and reserve

- Teach the patient how to conserve energy while performing ADLs—for example, sitting in a chair while dressing, wearing lightweight clothing that fastens with Velcro or a few large buttons, and wearing slip-on shoes. These measures reduce cellular metabolism and oxygen demand.
- Demonstrate exercises for increasing strength and endurance, which will improve breathing and gradually increase activity level.
- Support and encourage activity to the patient's level of tolerance to help develop his independence.
- Before discharge, formulate a plan with the patient and his caregivers that will enable the patient to continue functioning at maximum activity tolerance or to gradually increase the tolerance. For example, teach the patient and his caregivers how to monitor the patient's pulse during activities; recognize the need for oxygen, if prescribed; and use oxygen equipment properly. Participation in planning encourages patient satisfaction and compliance.

Decreased cardiac output

Related to reduced stroke volume, *Decreased cardiac output* may be associated with such conditions as angina, bacterial endocarditis, heart failure, MI, valvular heart disease, and other ailments.

Expected outcomes

- Patient maintains hemodynamic stability.
- Patient exhibits no arrhythmias.
- Patient maintains adequate cardiac output.

Nursing interventions and rationales

- Monitor and record level of consciousness (LOC), heart rate and rhythm, and blood pressure at least every 4 hours, or more often if necessary, to detect cerebral hypoxia possibly resulting from decreased cardiac output.
- Auscultate heart and breath sounds at least every 4 hours. Report abnormal sounds as soon as they develop. Extra heart sounds may indicate early cardiac decompensation. Adventitious breath sounds may indicate pulmonary congestion and decreased cardiac output.
- Measure and record intake and output. Reduced urine output without reduced fluid intake may indicate reduced renal perfusion, possibly from decreased cardiac output.
- Promptly treat life-threatening arrhythmias to avoid the risk of death.

> Monitor and record LOC, heart rate and rhythm, and blood pressure at least every 4 hours, or more often if necessary.

Biofeedback

Because stress increases the risk of developing hypertension, helping the patient reduce stress will improve his cardiovascular health. Biofeedback is an alternative therapy that teaches people how to exert conscious control over various autonomic functions with the help of electronic monitors. By observing on a monitor the fluctuations of a particular body function (such as breathing, heart rate, or blood pressure), the patient can learn how to bring them under control through mental adjustments. In time, he may be able to regulate conditions, such as high blood pressure, without medication or the use of monitors.

1-2-3, blue light

For example, using monitors initially, a patient with high blood pressure can be taught to recognize and ultimately regulate his body's response to stress. The patient is connected to a skin temperature monitor, which reflects the amount of blood flow beneath the skin. Changes in temperature caused by vasoconstriction or vasodilation signal lights on the monitor, indicating the stress response. A black light signals if the patient is tense, a blue light shows he's relaxed.

- Weigh the patient daily before breakfast to detect fluid retention.
- Inspect for pedal or sacral edema to detect venous stasis and decreased cardiac output.

Getting a facial

- Provide skin care every 4 hours to enhance skin perfusion and venous flow.
- Gradually increase the patient's activities within limits of prescribed heart rate to allow the heart to adjust to increased oxygen demand. Monitor pulse rate before and after activity to compare rates and gauge tolerance.
- Plan the patient's activities to avoid fatigue and increased myocardial workload.
- Maintain dietary restrictions as ordered to reduce complications and the risk of cardiac disease.
- Teach the patient stress-reduction techniques to reduce anxiety and provide a sense of control. (See *Biofeedback.*)
- Explain all procedures and tests to enhance understanding and reduce anxiety.

Teaching an old dog new tricks

- Teach the patient about chest pain and other reportable symptoms, prescribed diet, medications (name, dosage, frequency, therapeutic effects, and adverse effects), prescribed activity level, simple methods for lifting and bending, and stress-reduction techniques. These measures involve the patient and his family in care.

• Carry out the care plan, as ordered. Collaborative practice enhances overall care.
• Administer oxygen as ordered to increase supply to the myocardium.

> Collaborative practice enhances overall care.

Deficient knowledge

Related to heart disease, *Deficient knowledge* can apply to a particular disorder or the risk factors related to cardiovascular disease.

Expected outcomes

• Patient expresses an interest in learning new behaviors.
• Patient sets realistic learning goals.
• Patient practices new health-related behaviors during hospitalization (for example, selects appropriate diet, weighs himself daily, and monitors intake and output).

Nursing interventions and rationales

• Establish an environment of mutual trust and respect to enhance learning. Comfort with growing self-awareness, ability to share this awareness with others, receptiveness to new experiences, and consistency between actions and words form the basis of a trusting relationship.
• Help the patient develop goals for learning. Involving him in planning meaningful goals will encourage follow-through.
• Select teaching strategies (discussion, demonstration, role-playing, or visual materials) appropriate for the patient's individual learning style (specify) to enhance teaching effectiveness.
• Teach skills that the patient must use every day. Have him demonstrate each new skill to help him gain confidence.
• Have the patient incorporate learned skills into daily routine during hospitalization (specify skills) to allow him to practice new skills and receive feedback.
• Provide the patient with the names and telephone numbers of resource people or organizations to provide continuity of care and follow-up after discharge.

> Have the patient demonstrate each new skill to help him gain confidence.

Common cardiovascular disorders

Below are several common cardiovascular disorders, along with their causes, pathophysiology, signs and symptoms, diagnostic test findings, treatments, and nursing interventions.

Abdominal aortic aneurysm

Abdominal aortic aneurysm, an abnormal dilation in the arterial wall, most commonly occurs in the aorta between the renal arteries and iliac branches. More than 50% of all patients with untreated abdominal aneurysms die within 2 years of diagnosis, primarily from aneurysmal rupture. More than 85% die within 5 years.

My aorta's muscular layer is plenty strong. No easy target for an aneurysm here! No, siree!

What causes it

Aneurysms commonly result from atherosclerosis, which weakens the aortic wall and gradually distends the lumen. Other causes include:
• fungal infection (mycotic aneurysms) of the aortic arch and descending segments
• congenital disorders, such as coarctation of the aorta and Marfan syndrome
• trauma
• syphilis
• hypertension (in dissecting aneurysm).

Pathophysiology

Degenerative changes in the muscular layer of the aorta (tunica media) create a focal weakness, allowing the inner layer (tunica intima) and outer layer (tunica adventitia) to stretch outward. The resulting outward bulge is called an aneurysm. Blood pressure within the aorta progressively weakens the vessel walls and enlarges the aneurysm.

What to look for

• Asymptomatic pulsating mass in the periumbilical area
• Possible systolic bruit over the aorta on auscultation
• Possible abdominal tenderness on deep palpation
• Lumbar pain that radiates to the flank and groin (imminent rupture)
    If the aneurysm ruptures, look for:
• severe, persistent abdominal and back pain, mimicking renal or ureteral colic

- weakness
- sweating
- tachycardia
- hypotension.

What tests tell you

Several tests can confirm suspected abdominal aneurysm:
- Serial ultrasonography determines aneurysm size, shape, and location.
- Anteroposterior and lateral X-rays of the abdomen can detect aortic calcification, which outlines the mass, in at least 75% of patients.
- Aortography shows the condition of vessels proximal and distal to the aneurysm and the extent of the aneurysm but may underestimate aneurysm diameter because it visualizes only the flow channel and not the surrounding clot.

How it's treated

Usually, abdominal aneurysm requires resection of the aneurysm and replacement of the damaged aortic section with a Dacron graft. Large aneurysms or those that produce symptoms involve a significant risk of rupture and necessitate immediate repair. Patients with poor distal runoff may undergo external grafting.

If the aneurysm appears small and asymptomatic, the doctor may delay surgery, opting to first treat the patient's hypertension and reduce risk factors. Note, however, that small aneurysms may rupture. The patient must undergo regular physical examinations and ultrasound checks to detect enlargement, which may indicate imminent rupture.

Endovascular grafting, a relatively new procedure, may be used to repair an abdominal aortic aneurysm. In this minimally invasive procedure, a catheter with an attached graft is inserted through the femoral or iliac artery and advanced over a guide wire into the aorta, where it is positioned across the aneurysm. A balloon on the catheter expands, affixing the graft to the vessel wall.

Surgery may be delayed if the aneurysm is small, but regular exams and ultrasound checks are a must to detect enlargement.

What to do

- Be alert for signs of rupture, which may cause immediate death. Watch closely for any signs of acute blood loss, such as hypotension, increasing pulse and respiratory rate, cool and clammy skin, restlessness, and decreased sensorium.
- If rupture occurs, get the patient to surgery immediately.
- Evaluate the patient. Note whether the patient is free from pain and if he has adequate tissue perfusion with warm, dry skin; ade-

quate pulse and blood pressure; and absence of fatigue. (See *Teaching the patient with an abdominal aortic aneurysm*.)

Arterial occlusive disease

A common complication of atherosclerosis, arterial occlusive disease may affect the carotid, vertebral, innominate, subclavian, mesenteric, and celiac arteries. Arterial occlusions may be acute or chronic. Men suffer from arterial occlusive disease more commonly than women.

What causes it

Risk factors for arterial occlusive disease include smoking, aging, hypertension, hyperlipidemia, diabetes mellitus, and family history of vascular disorders, MI, or stroke. Causes include:
- emboli formation
- thrombosis
- trauma or fracture.

Pathophysiology

In arterial occlusive disease, obstruction or narrowing of the lumen of the aorta and its major branches causes an interruption of blood flow, usually to the legs and feet.

Location and timing

Prognosis depends on the location of the occlusion, the development of collateral circulation to counteract reduced blood flow and, in acute disease, the time elapsed between occlusion and its removal.

What to look for

Signs and symptoms depend on the severity and site of the arterial occlusion. Acute arterial occlusion may produce the five classic Ps:

 paralysis

 pain

 paresthesia

 pallor

 pulselessness.

Other signs and symptoms include:
• intermittent claudication
• severe burning pain in the toes (aggravated by elevating the extremity and sometimes relieved by keeping the extremity in a dependent position)
• ulcers, gangrene
• pallor on elevation, followed by redness with dependency
• delayed capillary filling, hair loss, or trophic nail changes
• diminished or absent pedal pulses.

What tests tell you

Pertinent supportive diagnostic tests include:
• arteriography, which demonstrates the type (thrombus or embolus), location, and degree of obstruction, and helps evaluate the collateral circulation, is particularly useful for diagnosing chronic forms of the disease and evaluating candidates for reconstructive surgery
• Doppler ultrasonography and plethysmography, which show reduced blood flow distal to the occlusion in acute disease
• ophthalmodynamometry, which helps determine degree of obstruction in the internal carotid artery by comparing ophthalmic artery pressure with brachial artery pressure on the affected side, with a difference greater than 20% suggesting insufficiency
• ankle-brachial indexes, which can determine the level of ischemia.

How it's treated

Treatment for arterial occlusive disease depends on the cause, location, and size of the obstruction. For patients with mild chronic disease, it usually consists of supportive measures, such as smoking cessation, hypertension control, and walking exercise.

Dextran and others

Drug therapy includes dextran and antiplatelet and hemorheologic drugs, such as aspirin, ticlopidine, pentoxifylline, and cilostazol. Thrombolytic therapy may be used to treat an arterial thrombosis. Patients with hyperlipidemia may be treated with antilipemic drugs.

Embolectomy, grafting, amputation — oh, my!

Appropriate surgical procedures may include embolectomy, thromboendarterectomy, patch grafting, bypass grafting, and lumbar sympathectomy. Amputation becomes necessary with failure of arterial reconstructive surgery or with the development of complications.

In mild disease, treatment consists of such supportive measures as — cough — smoking — cough — cessation. Thank goodness!

Lower the risk

Invasive endovascular techniques carry less risk than surgery and may include balloon angioplasty, atherectomy, and stenting. Other appropriate therapy includes heparin to prevent emboli (for embolic occlusion) and bowel resection after restoration of blood flow (for mesenteric artery occlusion).

What to do

• For information on nursing care of patients who undergo vascular surgery, see "Vascular repair," page 263.
• Following treatment, evaluate the patient. He should be able to increase exercise tolerance without developing pain and peripheral pulses should be normal. In addition, the patient should maintain good skin color and temperature in his extremities. (See *Teaching the patient with arterial occlusive disease.*)

CAD

CAD refers to any narrowing or obstruction of arterial lumina that interferes with cardiac perfusion. Deprived of sufficient blood, the myocardium can develop various ischemic diseases, including angina pectoris, MI, heart failure, sudden death, and cardiac arrhythmias.

CAD affects more Whites than Blacks, and more men than women. After menopause, however, the risk of CAD in women increases to equal that of men. CAD occurs more commonly in industrial countries than underdeveloped areas and affects affluent people more than poor people.

What causes it

Most commonly, atherosclerosis leads to CAD. Other possible causes include:
• arteritis
• coronary artery spasm
• certain infectious diseases
• congenital abnormalities.

Patients with certain risk factors appear to face a greater likelihood of developing CAD. These factors include:
• family history of heart disease
• obesity
• smoking
• high-fat, high-carbohydrate diet
• sedentary lifestyle
• menopause

Education edge

Teaching the patient with arterial occlusive disease

• Teach proper foot care or other appropriate measures, depending on the affected area.
• Instruct the patient about signs of recurrence (pain, pallor, numbness, paralysis, absence of pulse) that can result from a graft occlusion or occlusion at another site.
• Caution the patient against wearing constrictive clothing or crossing his legs while sitting.
• Advise the patient to stop smoking and refer him to a smoking-cessation program, if appropriate.
• Encourage the patient to closely follow his prescribed medication regimen.
• Advise the patient to avoid temperature extremes.
• Help the patient adjust to lifestyle constraints.

- stress
- diabetes
- hypertension
- hyperlipoproteinemia.

Pathophysiology

Fatty, fibrous plaques progressively occlude the coronary arteries, reducing the volume of blood that can flow through them, leading to myocardial ischemia.

A precarious balance

As atherosclerosis progresses, luminal narrowing is accompanied by vascular changes that impair the diseased vessel's ability to dilate. This causes a precarious balance between myocardial oxygen supply and demand, threatening the myocardium beyond the lesion. When oxygen demand exceeds what the diseased vessels can supply, localized myocardial ischemia results.

From aerobic to anaerobic

Transient ischemia causes reversible changes at the cellular and tissue levels, depressing myocardial function. Untreated, it can lead to tissue injury or necrosis. Oxygen deprivation forces the myocardium to shift from aerobic to anaerobic metabolism. As a result, lactic acid (the end product of anaerobic metabolism) accumulates and cellular pH decreases.

With each contraction, less blood

The combination of hypoxia, reduced energy availability, and acidosis rapidly impairs left ventricular function. The strength of contractions in the affected myocardial region is reduced as the fibers shorten inadequately with less force and velocity. In addition, the ischemic section's wall motion is abnormal. This generally results in less blood being ejected from the heart with each contraction. Restoring blood flow through the coronary arteries restores aerobic metabolism and contractility. Failure to do so results in MI.

What to look for

Angina, the classic symptom of CAD, occurs as a burning, squeezing, or crushing tightness in the substernal or precordial chest. It may radiate to the left arm, neck, jaw, or shoulder blade. Women, however, may experience atypical chest pain. (See *Atypical chest pain in women*.)

Atypical chest pain in women

Women with coronary artery disease commonly experience atypical chest pain, vague chest pain, or a lack of chest pain. However, they may also experience classic chest pain, which may occur without any relationship to activity or stress

While men tend to complain of crushing pain in the center of the chest, women are more likely to experience arm or shoulder pain; jaw, neck, or throat pain; toothache; back pain; or pain under the breastbone or in the stomach.

Other signs and symptoms women may experience include nausea or dizziness; shortness of breath; unexplained anxiety, weakness, or fatigue; and palpitations, cold sweat, or paleness.

Angina has four major forms:
• *stable* — pain that's predictable in frequency and duration and can be relieved with nitrates and rest
• *unstable* — increased pain that's easily induced
• *Prinzmetal's* or *variant* — from unpredictable coronary artery spasm
• *microvascular* — impairment of vasodilator reserve, which causes angina-like chest pain in a patient with normal coronary arteries).

Microvascular angina causes angina-like chest pain in a patient with normal coronary arteries. Owee!

Don't forget about these

Other signs and symptoms of CAD include:
• nausea
• vomiting
• weakness
• diaphoresis
• cool extremities.

What tests tell you

• ECG shows ischemia and, possibly, arrhythmias such as premature ventricular contractions. A pain-free patient may have a normal ECG. Arrhythmias may occur without infarction, secondary to ischemia.
• Exercise ECG may provoke chest pain and signs of myocardial ischemia in response to physical exertion.
• Coronary angiography reveals coronary artery stenosis or obstruction and collateral circulation and shows the condition of the arteries beyond the narrowing.
• Myocardial perfusion imaging with thallium-201 during treadmill exercise detects ischemic areas of the myocardium, visualized as "cold spots."
• Laboratory evaluation of cardiac markers may be performed to eliminate a diagnosis of MI. The patient may also undergo serum lipid studies to detect and classify hyperlipidemia.

Myocardial perfusion imaging during treadmill exercise detects ischemic areas of the myocardium.

Hey, shouldn't you be up here instead of me?

How it's treated

For patients with angina, the goal of CAD treatment is to reduce myocardial oxygen demand or increase oxygen supply. Nitrates reduce myocardial oxygen consumption. Beta-adrenergic blockers may be administered to reduce the workload and oxygen demands of the heart by reducing heart rate and peripheral resistance to blood flow. If angina is caused by coronary artery spasm, calcium channel blockers may be given. Antiplatelet drugs minimize platelet aggregation and the danger of coronary occlusion. Antilipemic drugs can reduce elevated serum cholesterol or triglyceride levels. Estrogen replacement therapy may be useful in some postmenopausal women to reduce the risk of CAD.

Obstructive lesions may necessitate coronary artery bypass surgery or PTCA. Other alternatives include laser angioplasty, minimally invasive surgery, rotational atherectomy, or stent placement.

What to do

During anginal episodes:
- Monitor blood pressure and heart rate.
- Take an ECG before administering nitroglycerin or other nitrates.
- Record duration of pain, amount of medication required to relieve it, and accompanying symptoms. Keep nitroglycerin available for immediate use.
- Evaluate the patient. Note if the patient experiences pain or shortness of breath at rest or with usual activity. Assess whether he can tolerate activity. (See *Teaching the patient with coronary artery disease.*)

Dilated cardiomyopathy

Dilated cardiomyopathy occurs when myocardial muscle fibers become extensively damaged. This disorder interferes with myocardial metabolism and grossly dilates every heart chamber, giving the heart a globular shape. Dilated cardiomyopathy leads to intractable heart failure, arrhythmias, and emboli. Usually not diagnosed until its advanced stages, this disorder carries a poor prognosis.

What causes it

The primary cause of dilated cardiomyopathy is unknown. Although the relationship remains unclear, it occasionally occurs secondary to:
- viral or bacterial infections
- hypertension
- peripartum syndrome (related to toxemia)
- ischemic heart disease or valvular disease
- drug hypersensitivity or chemotherapy
- cardiotoxic effects of drugs or alcohol.

Education edge

Teaching the patient with coronary artery disease

- Explain all procedures and tests, answer questions appropriately and provide support.
- Instruct the patient to immediately seek medical attention if he feels symptoms of angina.
- Help the patient determine which activities precipitate episodes of pain. Help him identify and select more effective coping mechanisms to deal with stress.
- Stress the need to follow the prescribed drug regimen.
- Encourage the patient to maintain the prescribed diet.
- Encourage regular moderate exercise. Refer the patient to a local cardiac rehabilitation center, if appropriate.
- If the patient smokes, refer him to a smoking-cessation program.
- Refer the patient to the American Heart Association for more information and support.

Pathophysiology

Dilated cardiomyopathy is characterized by a grossly dilated, hypodynamic ventricle that contracts poorly and, to a lesser degree, myocardial hypertrophy. All four chambers become dilated as a result of increased volumes and pressures. Thrombi commonly develop within these chambers due to blood pooling and stasis, which may lead to embolization.

If hypertrophy coexists, the heart ejects blood less efficiently. A large volume remains in the left ventricle after systole, causing heart failure.

What to look for

The patient may develop:
- shortness of breath (orthopnea, exertional dyspnea, or paroxysmal nocturnal dyspnea)
- fatigue
- irritating dry cough at night
- edema
- liver engorgement
- jugular vein distention
- peripheral cyanosis
- sinus tachycardia
- atrial fibrillation
- diffuse apical impulses
- pansystolic murmur (mitral and tricuspid insufficiency secondary to cardiomegaly and weak papillary muscles)
- S_3 and S_4 gallop rhythms.

What tests tell you

- ECG and angiography rule out ischemic heart disease. ECG may also show biventricular hypertrophy, sinus tachycardia, atrial enlargement and, in 20% of patients, atrial fibrillation.
- Chest X-ray demonstrates cardiomegaly (usually affecting all heart chambers), pulmonary congestion, or pleural effusion.
- MUGA scanning and echocardiography show decreased left ventricular function and decreased wall motion.

How it's treated

Treatment seeks to correct the underlying causes and to improve the heart's pumping ability. Angiotensin-converting enzyme (ACE) inhibitors reduce afterload through vasodilation, thereby reducing heart failure. Diuretics are commonly given with an ACE inhibitor to reduce fluid retention.

Chest X-ray demonstrates cardiomegaly, pulmonary congestion, or pleural effusion.

When the ACE doesn't fly right

For those without improvement of symptoms on an ACE inhibitor and diuretic, digoxin may improve myocardial contractility. Hydralazine and isosorbide dinitrate, in combination, produce vasodilation. Antiarrhythmics, cardioversion, and pacemakers may be used to control arrhythmias. Although controversial, anticoagulants may be prescribed to reduce the risk of emboli. Treatment may also include oxygen, a sodium-restricted diet, and bed rest.

Surgery sometimes

Surgical interventions in carefully selected patients may include revascularization, such as CABG, if ischemia is the cause of dilated cardiomyopathy. Valvular repair or replacement may help if dilated cardiomyopathy is due to valve dysfunction. Cardiomyoplasty, in which the latissimus dorsi muscle is wrapped around the ventricles to assist the ventricles to pump more efficiently, may also be considered when medical treatment fails. A cardiomyostimulator delivering bursts of electrical impulses during systole can help the myocardium contract. Heart transplantation may also be considered for patients who fail to respond to other treatments.

Shake the habit

Lifestyle modifications such as smoking cessation; low-fat, low-sodium diet; physical activity; and abstinence from alcohol are also important.

What to do

- Monitor for signs of progressive heart failure (decreased arterial pulses and increased jugular vein distention) and compromised renal perfusion (oliguria, increased blood urea nitrogen [BUN] and serum creatinine levels, and electrolyte imbalances)
- Weigh the patient daily.
- Check blood pressure and heart rate frequently.
- Monitor the patient receiving diuretics for signs of resolving congestion (decreased crackles and dyspnea) or too vigorous diuresis. Check serum potassium level for hypokalemia, especially if therapy includes digoxin.
- Offer support and encourage the patient to express his feelings.
- Evaluate the patient. Look for adequate tissue perfusion, as evidenced by good color; warm, dry skin; and clear lungs. The patient should maintain his weight and level of activity. Blood pressure should be adequate and dizziness and edema absent. (See *Teaching the patient with dilated cardiomyopathy*.)

Education edge

Teaching the patient with dilated cardiomyopathy

- Before discharge, teach the patient about his illness and its treatment.
- Emphasize the need to restrict sodium intake and watch for weight gain.
- Explain the need to take digoxin as prescribed and watch for such adverse effects as anorexia, nausea, vomiting, and yellow vision.
- Because the patient faces an increased risk of sudden cardiac arrest, encourage family members to learn cardiopulmonary resuscitation.

Endocarditis

Endocarditis, infection of the endocardium, heart valves, or cardiac prosthesis, results from bacterial or fungal invasion.

Untreated endocarditis usually proves fatal, but with proper treatment, 70% of patients recover. Prognosis becomes much worse when endocarditis causes severe valvular damage (leading to insufficiency and heart failure) or when it involves a prosthetic valve.

What causes it

Most cases of endocarditis occur in patients who abuse I.V. drugs or those with:
- prosthetic heart valves
- mitral valve prolapse
- rheumatic heart disease.

Other predisposing conditions include congenital abnormalities (coarctation of aorta and tetralogy of Fallot), subaortic and valvular aortic stenosis, ventricular septal defects, pulmonary stenosis, Marfan syndrome, degenerative heart disease, and syphilis. Causative organisms may include group A nonhemolytic streptococci, *Pneumococcus*, *Staphylococcus*, *Enterococcus* and, rarely, *Gonococcus*.

Pathophysiology

Infection causes fibrin and platelets to aggregate on the valve tissue and engulf circulating bacteria or fungi. They form friable verrucous (wartlike) vegetative growths on the heart valves, endocardial lining of a heart chamber, or endothelium of a blood vessel. Such vegetations may cover the valve surfaces, causing ulceration and necrosis; they may also extend to the cordae tendineae. Ultimately, they may embolize to the spleen, kidneys, central nervous system, and lungs. (See *Effects of endocarditis.*)

What to look for

Early clinical features are usually nonspecific and include:
- weakness
- fatigue
- weight loss
- anorexia
- arthralgia
- night sweats
- intermittent fever (may recur for weeks)

A closer look

Effects of endocarditis

This illustration shows vegetative growths on the endocardium produced by fibrin and platelet deposits on infection sites.

Vegetative growths

• loud, regurgitant murmur, which is typical of the underlying rheumatic or congenital heart disease
• murmur that changes or appears suddenly, accompanied by fever.

Lots of spots

Other indications of endocarditis include:
• petechiae on the skin (especially common on the upper anterior trunk); the buccal, pharyngeal, or conjunctival mucosa; and the nails (splinter hemorrhages)
• Osler's nodes
• Roth's spots
• Janeway lesions (rare).

Endo with embo

In subacute endocarditis, embolization from vegetating lesions or diseased valve tissue may produce:
• splenic infarction—pain in the left upper quadrant that radiates to the left shoulder, and abdominal rigidity
• renal infarction—hematuria, pyuria, flank pain, and decreased urine output
• cerebral infarction—hemiparesis, aphasia, and other neurologic deficits
• pulmonary infarction, most commonly in right-sided endocarditis (common among I.V. drug abusers and after cardiac surgery)—cough, pleuritic pain, pleural friction rub, dyspnea, and hemoptysis
• peripheral vascular occlusion—numbness and tingling in an arm, leg, finger, or toe or impending peripheral gangrene.

What tests tell you

• Three or more blood cultures, with samples drawn at least 1 hour apart during a 24-hour period, identify the causative organism in up to 90% of patients. The remaining 10% may have negative blood cultures, possibly suggesting fungal infection.
• Echocardiography, including transesophageal echocardiography, may identify vegetations and valvular damage.
• ECG readings may show atrial fibrillation and other arrhythmias that accompany valvular disease.
• Laboratory abnormalities include elevated white blood cell (WBC) count; abnormal histocytes (macrophages); elevated erythrocyte sedimentation rate (ESR); normocytic, normochromic anemia (in subacute bacterial endocarditis); and rheumatoid factor (occurs in about one-half of all patients).

> Spots can be an indication of endocarditis. Yikes — not you, Spot!

How it's treated

Treatment seeks to eradicate the infecting organism. It should start promptly and continue over several weeks. The doctor bases antibiotic selection on sensitivity studies of the infecting organism — or the probable organism, if blood cultures are negative. I.V. antibiotic therapy usually lasts 4 to 6 weeks and may be followed by oral antibiotics.

Supportive treatment includes bed rest, antipyretics for fever and aches, and sufficient fluid intake. Severe valvular damage, especially aortic insufficiency, or infection of a cardiac prosthesis may require corrective surgery if refractory heart failure develops.

What to do

- Obtain a patient history of allergies.
- Administer antibiotics on time to maintain consistent blood levels. Check dilutions for compatibility with other patient medications, and use a compatible solution (for example, add methicillin to a buffered solution).
- Evaluate the patient. The patient has recovered from endocarditis if he maintains a normal temperature, clear lungs, stable vital signs, adequate tissue perfusion, and is able to tolerate activity for a reasonable period and to maintain normal weight. (See *Teaching the patient with endocarditis.*)

Femoral and popliteal aneurysms

Progressive atherosclerotic changes in the medial layer of the femoral and popliteal arteries may lead to aneurysm. Aneurysmal formations may be fusiform (spindle-shaped) or saccular (pouch-like). Fusiform aneurysms are three times more common than saccular aneurysms.

Femoral and popliteal aneurysms may occur as single or multiple segmental lesions, in many cases affecting both legs, and may accompany aneurysms in the abdominal aorta or iliac arteries. This condition occurs most commonly in men over age 50. Elective surgery before complications arise greatly improves prognosis.

What causes it

- Atherosclerosis
- Congenital weakness in the arterial wall (rare)
- Blunt or penetrating trauma
- Bacterial infection

Education edge

Teaching the patient with endocarditis

- Teach the patient about the anti-infective medication that he'll continue to take. Stress the importance of taking the medication and restricitng activity for as long as recommended.
- Tell the patient to watch for and report signs of embolization and to watch closely for fever, anorexia, and other signs of relapse that could occur about 2 weeks after treatment stops.
- Discuss the importance of completing the full course of antibiotics, even if he's feeling better. Make sure susceptible patients understand the need for prophylactic antibiotics before, during, and after dental work, childbirth, and genitourinary, GI, or gynecologic procedures.

• Peripheral vascular reconstructive surgery (which causes "suture line" aneurysms, whereby a blood clot forms a second lumen; also called false aneurysms).

Pathophysiology

An aneurysm is a localized outpouching or dilation of a weakened arterial wall. This weakness can result from either atherosclerotic plaque formation that erodes the vessel wall or the loss of elastin and collagen in the vessel wall.

I wish it were this easy to get rid of atherosclerotic plaque!

What to look for

If large enough to compress the medial popliteal nerve and vein, popliteal aneurysms may cause:
• pain in the popliteal space
• edema
• vein distention
• possibly symptoms of severe ischemia (in the leg or foot).
  Signs of a femoral aneurysm include:
• pulsating mass above or below the inguinal ligament found on bilateral palpation
• firm, nonpulsating mass, which identifies thrombosis.

What tests tell you

If palpation doesn't provide a positive identification, these tests may help with diagnosis:
• Arteriography may help identify femoral and popliteal aneurysms. It may also detect associated aneurysms, especially those in the abdominal aorta and the iliac arteries.
• Ultrasound can help identify aneurysms and may help to determine the size of the popliteal or femoral artery.

How it's treated

Femoral and popliteal aneurysms require surgical bypass and reconstruction of the artery, usually with an autogenous saphenous vein graft replacement. Arterial occlusion that causes severe ischemia and gangrene may require leg amputation.

Femoral and popliteal aneurysms require surgical bypass and reconstruction of the artery.

What to do

• Administer prophylactic antibiotics, antihypertensives, or anticoagulants, as ordered.
• Prepare the patient for surgery. (For information on nursing care of patients who undergo vascular surgery, see "Vascular repair," page 263.)

• Evaluate the patient. Note whether the patient shows good color and temperature of extremities and if he has ceased to experience pain. Pulses should be present in his extremities. (See *Teaching the patient with a femoral or popliteal aneurysm.*)

Heart failure

When the myocardium can't pump effectively enough to meet the body's metabolic needs, heart failure occurs. Pump failure usually occurs in a damaged left ventricle, but may also happen in the right ventricle. Usually, left-sided heart failure develops first. Heart failure is classified as:
• acute or chronic
• left-sided or right-sided (see *Understanding left- and right-sided heart failure*)
• systolic or diastolic. (See *Classifying heart failure*, page 298.)

Quality time

Symptoms of heart failure may restrict a person's ability to perform ADLs and severely affect quality of life. Advances in diagnostic and therapeutic techniques have greatly improved outcomes for these patients. However, prognosis still depends on the underlying cause and its response to treatment.

What causes it

Cardiovascular disorders that lead to heart failure include:
• atherosclerotic heart disease
• MI
• hypertension
• rheumatic heart disease
• congenital heart disease
• ischemic heart disease
• cardiomyopathy
• valvular diseases
• arrhythmias.
  Noncardiovascular causes of heart failure include:
• pregnancy and childbirth
• increased environmental temperature or humidity
• severe physical or mental stress
• thyrotoxicosis
• acute blood loss
• pulmonary embolism
• severe infection
• chronic obstructive pulmonary disease.

Education edge

Teaching the patient with a femoral or popliteal aneurysm

• Explain what an aneurysm is and how it occurs. Provide emotional support and address concerns.
• Provide preoperative and postoperative teaching. Be sure to explain how to care for the incision after surgery and how to recognize complications.
• Teach the patient how to assess daily for a pulse in the affected extremity.
• Tell the patient to immediately report recurrence of symptoms.
• Explain to the patient with popliteal artery resection that swelling may persist. Make sure antiembolism stockings fit properly, and teach the patient how to apply them. Warn against wearing constrictive clothes.
• If the patient is receiving anticoagulant therapy, suggest measures to prevent accidental bleeding.

A closer look

Understanding left- and right-sided heart failure

These illustrations show how myocardial damage leads to heart failure.

Left-sided heart failure

Increased workload and end-diastolic volume enlarge the left ventricle (see illustration below). Because of lack of oxygen, the ventricle enlarges with stretched tissue rather than functional tissue. The patient may experience increased heart rate, pale and cool skin, tingling in the extremities, decreased cardiac output, and arrhythmias.

Diminished left ventricular function allows blood to pool in the ventricle and the atrium and eventually back up into the pulmonary veins and capillaries, as shown below. At this stage, the patient may experience dyspnea on exertion, confusion, dizziness, orthostatic hypotension, decreased peripheral pulses and pulse pressure, cyanosis, and an S_3 gallop.

As the pulmonary circulation becomes engorged, rising capillary pressure pushes sodium (Na) and water (H_2O) into the interstitial space (as shown below), causing pulmonary edema. You'll note coughing, subclavian retractions, crackles, tachypnea, elevated pulmonary artery pressure, diminished pulmonary compliance, and increased partial pressure of carbon dioxide.

When the patient lies down, fluid in the extremities moves into the systemic circulation. Because the left ventricle can't handle the increased venous return, fluid pools in the pulmonary circulation, worsening pulmonary edema. You may note decreased breath sounds, dullness on percussion, crackles, and orthopnea.

The right ventricle may now become stressed because it's pumping against greater pulmonary vascular resistance and left ventricular pressure (see illustration below). When this occurs, the patient's symptoms worsen.

Right-sided heart failure

The stressed right ventricle enlarges with the formation of stretched tissue (see illustration below). Increasing conduction time and deviation of the heart from its normal axis can cause arrhythmias. If the patient doesn't already have left-sided heart failure, he may experience increased heart rate, cool skin, cyanosis, decreased cardiac output, palpitations, and dyspnea.

(continued)

Understanding left- and right-sided heart failure *(continued)*

 Blood pools in the right ventricle and right atrium. The backed-up blood causes pressure and congestion in the vena cava and systemic circulation (see illustration below). The patient will have elevated central venous pressure, jugular vein distention, and hepatojugular reflux.

 Backed-up blood also distends the visceral veins, especially the hepatic vein. As the liver and spleen become engorged (see illustration below), their function is impaired. The patient may develop anorexia, nausea, abdominal pain, palpable liver and spleen, weakness, and dyspnea secondary to abdominal distention.

 Rising capillary pressure forces excess fluid from the capillaries into the interstitial space (see illustration below). This causes tissue edema, especially in the lower extremities and abdomen. The patient may experience weight gain, pitting edema, and nocturia.

Pathophysiology

The patient's underlying condition determines whether heart failure is acute or insidious. Heart failure is commonly associated with systolic or diastolic overloading and myocardial weakness. As stress on the heart muscle reaches a critical level, the muscle's contractility is reduced and cardiac output declines. Venous input to the ventricle remains the same, however.

The body's responses to decreased cardiac output include:
• reflex increase in sympathetic activity
• release of renin from the juxtaglomerular cells of the kidney
• anaerobic metabolism by affected cells
• increased extraction of oxygen by the peripheral cells.

Adept at adaptation

When blood in the ventricles increases, the heart compensates, or adapts. Compensation may occur for long periods before signs and symptoms develop. Adaptations may be:
• *short-term.* As the end-diastolic fiber length increases, the ventricular muscle responds by dilating and increasing the force of contractions. (This is called the Frank-Starling curve.)
• *long-term.* Ventricular hypertrophy increases the heart muscle's ability to contract and push its volume of blood into the circulation.

You'd think an increase in sympathetic activity would mean more pity for me — but it doesn't. Ooooh!

What to look for

Clinical signs of left-sided heart failure include:
- dyspnea, initially upon exertion
- paroxysmal nocturnal dyspnea
- Cheyne-Stokes respirations
- cough
- orthopnea
- tachycardia
- fatigue
- muscle weakness
- edema and weight gain
- irritability
- restlessness
- shortened attention span
- ventricular gallop (heard over the apex)
- bibasilar crackles.
  The patient with right-sided heart failure may develop:
- edema, initially dependent
- jugular vein distention
- hepatomegaly.

What tests tell you

- Blood tests may show elevated BUN and creatinine levels, elevated serum norepinephrine levels, and elevated transaminase and bilirubin levels if hepatic function is impaired.
- Elevated blood levels of brain natriuretic peptide may correctly identify heart failure in as many as 83% of patients.
- ECG reflects heart strain or ventricular enlargement (ischemia). It may also reveal atrial enlargement, tachycardia, and extrasystoles, suggesting heart failure.
- Chest X-ray shows increased pulmonary vascular markings, interstitial edema, or pleural effusion and cardiomegaly.
- MUGA scan shows a decreased ejection fraction in left-sided heart failure.
- Cardiac catheterization may show ventricular dilation, coronary artery occlusion, and valvular disorders (such as aortic stenosis) in both left- and right-sided heart failure.
- Echocardiography may show ventricular hypertrophy, decreased contractility, and valvular disorders in both left- and right-sided heart failure. Serial echocardiograms may help assess the patient's response to therapy.
- Cardiopulmonary exercise testing to evaluate the patient's ventricular performance during exercise may show decreased oxygen uptake.

Increased levels of natriuretic peptide in me may correctly identify heart failure in as many as 83% of patients. Wow, I'm good!

Classifying heart failure

Heart failure is classified according to its pathophysiology. It may be left- or right-sided, systolic or diastolic, and acute or chronic.

Right-sided or left-sided

Right-sided heart failure is the result of ineffective right ventricular contraction. It may be caused by an acute right ventricular infarction or pulmonary embolus. However, the most common cause is profound backward flow due to left-sided heart failure.

Left-sided heart failure is the result of ineffective left ventricular contraction. It may lead to pulmonary congestion or pulmonary edema and decreased cardiac output. Left ventricular myocardial infarction, hypertension, and aortic and mitral valve stenosis or regurgitation are common causes. As the decreased pumping ability of the left ventricle persists, fluid accumulates, backing up into the left atrium and then into the lungs. If this worsens, pulmonary edema and right-sided heart failure may also result.

Systolic or diastolic

In systolic heart failure, the left ventricle can't pump enough blood out to the systemic circulation during systole and the ejection fraction falls. Consequently, blood backs up into the pulmonary circulation, pressure rises in the pulmonary venous system, and cardiac output falls.

In diastolic heart failure, the left ventricle can't relax and fill properly during diastole and the stroke volume falls. Therefore, larger ventricular volumes are needed to maintain cardiac output.

Acute or chronic

Acute refers to the timing of the onset of symptoms and whether compensatory mechanisms kick in. Typically, fluid status is normal or low, and sodium and water retention don't occur.

In chronic heart failure, signs and symptoms have been present for some time, compensatory mechanisms have taken effect, and fluid volume overload persists. Drugs, diet changes, and activity restrictions usually control symptoms.

How it's treated

Treatment for heart failure can be determined by using the New York Heart Association classification system and the American College of Cardiology/American Heart Association (ACC/AHA) guidelines. (See *Classifying signs and symptoms to determine treatment.*)

Measures include diuretics that reduce preload by decreasing total blood volume and circulatory congestion. ACE inhibitors dilate blood vessels and decrease systemic vascular resistance, thereby reducing the workload of the heart. Vasodilators may be given to the patient who can't tolerate ACE inhibitors. Vasodilators increase cardiac output by reducing impedance to ventricular outflow, thereby decreasing afterload.

Strengthening medicine

Digoxin may help strengthen myocardial contractility. Beta-adrenergic blockers may prevent cardiac remodeling (left ventricular dilation and hypertrophy). Nesiritide, a human B-type natriuretic peptide, may be administered to augment diuresis and to decrease afterload. Positive inotropic agents, such as I.V. dopamine or dobutamine, are reserved for those with end-stage heart failure or those awaiting heart transplantion.

Classifying signs and symptoms to determine treatment

Two sets of guidelines are available to help direct treatment of the patient with heart failure. The New York Heart Association (NYHA) classification is based on functional capacity. The American College of Cardiology/American Heart Association (ACC/AHA) guidelines are based on objective assessment. These guidelines are compared side-by-side below.

NYHA classification	ACC/AHA guidelines	Recommendations
	Stage A. Patient at high risk for developing heart failure (HF) but without structural heart disease or signs and symptoms of HF	• Treatment of hypertension, lipid disorders, and diabetes • Encouraging patient to stop smoking and to exercise regularly • Discouraging use of alcohol and illicit drugs • Angiotensin-converting enzyme (ACE) inhibitor if indicated
Class I. Ordinary physical activity doesn't cause undue fatigue, palpitations, dyspnea, or angina.	*Stage B.* Structural heart disease, but without signs and symptoms of HF	• All stage A therapies • ACE inhibitor (unless contraindicated) • Beta-adrenergic blocker (unless contraindicated)
Class II. Slight limitation of physical activity but asymptomatic at rest. Ordinary physical activity causes fatigue, palpitations, dyspnea, or anginal pain. *Class III.* Marked limitation of physical activity, but typically asymptomatic at rest. Less than ordinary physical activity causes fatigue, palpitations, dyspnea, or angina.	*Stage C.* Structural heart disease with prior or current signs and symptoms of HF	• All stage A and B therapies • Sodium-restricted diet • Diuretics • Digoxin • Avoiding or withdrawing antiarrhythmic agents, most calcium channel blockers, and nonsteroidal anti-inflammatory drugs • Drug therapy, including aldosterone antagonists, angiotensin receptor blockers, hydralazine, and nitrates
Class IV. Unable to perform any physical activity without discomfort; symptoms may be present at rest. Discomfort increases with physical activity.	*Stage D.* End-stage disease requiring specialized treatment strategies, such as mechanical circulatory support, continuous inotropic infusion, or heart transplant	• All therapies for stages A, B, and C • Mechanical assist device, such as biventricular pacemaker or left ventricular assist device • Continuous inotropic therapy • Hospice care

Used with permission from Davis, S.L. "How The Heart Failure Picture Has Changed," *Nursing2002* (32)11:36-44, November 2002.

Stop and go

The patient must alternate periods of rest with periods of activity and follow a sodium-restricted diet with smaller, more frequent meals. He may have to wear antiembolism stockings to prevent venostasis and possible thromboembolism formation. The doctor may also order oxygen therapy.

Surgery isn't a sure thing

Although controversial, surgery may be performed if the patient's heart failure doesn't improve after therapy and lifestyle modifications. If the patient with valve dysfunction has recurrent acute heart failure, he may undergo surgical valve replacement. CABG, PTCA, or stenting may be performed in a patient with heart failure caused by ischemia.

Remodeling show

The Dor procedure, also called *partial left ventriculectomy* or *ventricular remodeling*, involves the removal of nonviable heart muscle to reduce the size of the hypertrophied ventricle, thereby allowing the heart to pump more efficiently. Patients with severe heart failure may benefit from a mechanical VAD or cardiac transplantation. An internal cardioverter-defibrillator may be implanted to treat life-threatening arrhythmias. A biventricular pacemaker may be placed to control ventricular dyssynchrony.

What to do

• Frequently monitor BUN, serum creatinine, potassium, sodium, chloride, and magnesium levels.
• Reinforce the importance of adhering to the prescribed diet. If fluid restrictions have been ordered, arrange a mutually acceptable schedule for allowable fluids.
• Weigh the patient daily to assess for fluid overload.
• To prevent deep vein thrombosis from vascular congestion, assist the patient with range-of-motion (ROM) exercises. Enforce bed rest, and apply antiembolism stockings. Watch for calf pain and tenderness. Organize activities to provide periods of rest.
• Evaluate the patient. Successful recovery should reveal clear lungs, normal heart sounds, adequate blood pressure, and absence of dyspnea or edema. The patient should be able to perform ADLs and maintain his normal weight. (See *Teaching the patient with heart failure*.)

Hypertension

Hypertension refers to an intermittent or sustained elevation in diastolic or systolic blood pressure. Essential (idiopathic) hypertension is the most common form. Secondary hypertension results from a number of disorders. Malignant hypertension is a severe, fulminant form of hypertension common to both types.

Hypertension represents a major cause of stroke, cardiac disease, and renal failure. Detecting and treating it before complications develop greatly improves the patient's prognosis. Severely elevated blood pressure may become fatal.

Education edge

Teaching the patient with heart failure

• Teach the patient about lifestyle changes. Advise him to avoid foods high in sodium to help curb fluid overload. Explain that the potassium he loses through diuretic therapy must be replaced by a prescribed potassium supplement and eating high-potassium foods. Stress the need for regular checkups and the benefits of balancing activity and rest.
• Stress the importance of taking cardiac glycosides exactly as prescribed. Tell him to watch for and report signs of toxicity.
• Tell him to notify the doctor if his pulse is unusually irregular or less than 60 beats/minute; if he experiences symptoms including dizziness, blurred vision, shortness of breath, paroxysmal nocturnal dyspnea, swollen ankles, or decreased urine output; or if he gains 3 to 5 lb (1.5 to 2.5 kg) in 1 week.

What causes it

Scientists haven't been able to identify a single cause for essential hypertension. The disorder probably reflects an interaction of multiple homeostatic forces, including changes in renal regulation of sodium and extracellular fluids, in aldosterone secretion and metabolism, and in norepinephrine secretion and metabolism.

Secondary hypertension may be caused by renal vascular disease, pheochromocytoma, primary hyperaldosteronism, Cushing's syndrome, or dysfunction of the thyroid, pituitary, or parathyroid glands. It may also result from coarctation of the aorta, pregnancy, and neurologic disorders.

Certain risk factors appear to increase the likelihood of hypertension. These include:
- family history of hypertension
- race (more common in blacks)
- gender
- diabetes mellitus
- stress
- obesity
- high dietary intake of saturated fats or sodium
- tobacco use
- hormonal contraceptive use
- sedentary lifestyle
- aging.

Family history of hypertension places a person at increased risk for the disease.

Pathophysiology

Essential hypertension usually begins insidiously as a benign disease, slowly progressing to a malignant state. If left untreated, even mild cases can cause major complications and death.

Why? Why? Why?

Several theories help to explain the development of hypertension. It's thought to arise from:
- changes in the arteriolar bed causing increased resistance.
- abnormally increased tone in the sensory nervous system that originates in the vasomotor system centers, causing increased peripheral vascular resistance.
- increased blood volume resulting from renal or hormonal dysfunction.
- increased arteriolar thickening caused by genetic factors, leading to increased peripheral vascular resistance.
- abnormal renin release resulting in the formation of angiotensin II, which constricts the arterioles and increases blood volume. (See *Blood vessel damage*, page 302.)

A closer look

Blood vessel damage

Sustained hypertension damages blood vessels. Vascular injury begins with alternating areas of dilation and constriction in the arterioles. The illustrations below show how damage occurs.

 Increased intra-arterial pressure damages the endothelium.

Angiotensin induces endothelial wall contraction, allowing plasma to leak through interendothelial spaces.

Plasma constituents deposited in the vessel wall cause medial necrosis.

Damage from increased blood pressure

Angiotensin

Platelet

Fibrinogen

Medial necrosis

Protein with fibrin deposits

Secondary isn't small

The pathophysiology of secondary hypertension is related to the underlying disease. For example, consider these points:

• The most common cause of secondary hypertension is chronic renal disease. Insult to the kidney from chronic glomerulonephritis or renal artery stenosis interferes with sodium excretion, the renin-angiotensin-aldosterone system, or renal perfusion. This causes blood pressure to rise.

• In Cushing's syndrome, increased cortisol levels raise blood pressure by increasing renal sodium retention, angiotensin II levels, and vascular response to norepinephrine.

• In primary aldosteronism, increased intravascular volume, altered sodium concentrations in vessel walls, or very high aldosterone levels cause vasoconstriction (increased resistance).

• Pheochromocytoma is a secreting tumor of chromaffin cells, usually of the adrenal medulla. It causes hypertension due to increased secretion of epinephrine and norepinephrine. Epinephrine functions mainly to increase cardiac contractility and rate. Norepinephrine functions mainly to increase peripheral vascular resistance.

The most common cause of secondary hypertension is chronic renal disease. We're all in this together.

What to look for

Signs and symptoms may include:
• blood pressure measurements of more than 140/90 mm Hg on two or more readings taken at two or more visits after an initial screening
• throbbing occipital headaches upon waking
• drowsiness
• confusion
• vision problems
• nausea.

Expect a patient with secondary hypertension to have clinical manifestations of the primary disease. Other clinical effects don't appear until complications develop as a result of vascular changes in target organs. These effects include:
• left ventricular hypertrophy
• angina
• MI
• heart failure
• stroke
• transient ischemic attack
• nephropathy
• peripheral arterial disease
• retinopathy.

What tests tell you

Along with patient history, the following tests may show predisposing factors and help identify an underlying cause:
• *urinalysis*. Protein, RBCs, and WBCs may indicate glomerulonephritis.
• *blood glucose*. Elevated blood glucose levels may indicate diabetes.
• *complete blood count*. Anemia may cause a high output state resulting in hypertension. Polycythemia I increases the risk of hypertension and stroke.
• *lipid profile*. Elevated total cholesterol and low-density lipoprotein levels increase the risk of atherosclerosis.
• *excretory urography*. Renal atrophy indicates chronic renal disease; one kidney more than ⅝″ (1.5 cm) shorter than the other suggests unilateral renal disease.

Elevated blood glucose levels may indicate diabetes, a condition that predisposes the patient to hypertension.

304

• *serum potassium level*. Levels less than 3.5 mEq/L may indicate adrenal dysfunction (primary hyperaldosteronism).
• *BUN and creatinine levels*. BUN level normal or elevated to more than 20 mg/dl and creatinine level normal or elevated to more than 1.5 mg/dl suggest renal disease.

Other tests help detect cardiovascular damage and other complications. ECG may show left ventricular hypertrophy or ischemia. Echocardiography may show left ventricular hypertrophy. Chest X-ray may show cardiomegaly.

How it's treated

Treatment of secondary hypertension includes correcting the underlying cause and controlling hypertensive effects. Although essential hypertension has no cure, lifestyle modifications along with drug therapy can control it. Lifestyle modifications, initiated on all patients, may include changes in diet, adoption of relaxation techniques, regular exercise, smoking cessation, limited intake of alcohol, and restriction of sodium and saturated fat intake.

The need for drug therapy is determined by blood pressure and the presence of target organ damage or risk factors. Drug therapy for uncomplicated hypertension usually begins with a thiazide diuretic, an ACE inhibitor, or a beta-adrenergic blocker. Other antihypertensive drugs include angiotensin II receptor blockers, alpha-receptor blockers, direct arteriole dilators, and calcium channel blockers.

What to do

• If a patient enters the hospital with hypertension, find out if he was taking prescribed medication. If not, help the patient to identify reasons for noncompliance. If the patient can't afford the medication, refer him to an appropriate social service agency. If he suffered severe adverse effects, he may need different medication.
• Routinely screen all patients for hypertension, especially those at high risk.
• Evaluate the patient. After successful treatment for hypertension, the patient will demonstrate blood pressure under 140/ 90 mm Hg at rest, ability to tolerate activity, absence of enlargement of left ventricle (as revealed by ECG or chest X-ray). (See *Teaching the patient with hypertension*.)

Hypertrophic cardiomyopathy

Hypertrophic cardiomyopathy is a primary disease of the cardiac muscle characterized by disproportionate, asymmetrical thicken-

Education edge

Teaching the patient with hypertension

• Teach the patient to use a self-monitoring blood pressure cuff and to record readings at the same time of the day at least twice weekly to review with his primary health care provider.
• Warn the patient that uncontrolled hypertension may cause a stroke or myocardial infarction.
• To encourage compliance with antihypertensive therapy, suggest that the patient establish a daily routine for taking medication. Tell him to report drug adverse effects and to keep a record of the effectiveness of drugs. Advise him to avoid high-sodium antacids and over-the-counter cold and sinus medications, which contain harmful vasoconstrictors.
• Help the patient examine and modify his lifestyle and encourage necessary diet changes.
• If the patient smokes, encourage quitting and refer him to a smoking-cessation program.

ing of the interventricular septum, particularly in the anterior-superior part. It affects both diastolic and systolic function. As the septum hypertrophies, blood flow through the aortic valve becomes obstructed. Mitral insufficiency develops as the papillary muscles become affected. The course of illness varies; some patients demonstrate progressive deterioration. Others remain stable for several years. Sudden cardiac death may also occur.

What causes it

Almost all patients inherit hypertrophic cardiomyopathy as a non–sex-linked autosomal dominant trait.

Pathophysiology

In hypertrophic cardiomyopathy, hypertrophy of the left ventricle and interventricular septum obstruct left ventricular outflow. The heart compensates for the decreased cardiac output (due to obstructed outflow) by increasing the rate and force of contractions. The hypertrophied ventricle becomes stiff and unable to relax and fill during diastole. As left ventricular volume diminishes and filling pressure rises, pulmonary venous pressure also rises, leading to venous congestion and dyspnea.

Hypertrophic cardiomyopathy is almost always a genetically inherited disorder.

What to look for

Clinical features include:
- angina pectoris
- arrhythmias
- dyspnea
- syncope
- heart failure
- systolic ejection murmur (of medium pitch, heard along the left sternal border and at the apex)
- pulsus biferiens
- irregular pulse (with atrial fibrillation).

What tests tell you

- Echocardiography shows increased thickness of the interventricular septum and abnormal motion of the anterior mitral leaflet during systole.
- Cardiac catheterization reveals elevated left ventricular end-diastolic pressure and possibly mitral insufficiency.
- ECG usually demonstrates left ventricular hypertrophy, ST-segment and T-wave abnormalities, deep waves (from hypertro-

phy, not infarction), left anterior hemiblock, ventricular arrhythmias and, possibly, atrial fibrillation.
• Phonocardiography confirms an early systolic murmur.

How it's treated

Treatment seeks to relax the ventricle and to relieve outflow tract obstruction. Propranolol, a beta-adrenergic blocker, slows heart rate and increases ventricular filling by relaxing the obstructing muscle, thereby reducing angina, syncope, dyspnea, and arrhythmias. However, propranolol may aggravate symptoms of cardiac decompensation. Calcium channel blockers may be prescribed to relax the heart muscle and improve ventricular filling. Antiarrhythmic drugs may be prescribed to treat arrhythmias. Atrial fibrillation necessitates cardioversion to treat the arrhythmia and, because of the high risk of systemic embolism, anticoagulant therapy until fibrillation subsides.

Surgery: Second choice

If drug therapy fails, the patient may undergo surgery. Ventricular myotomy (resection of the hypertrophied septum) alone or combined with mitral valve replacement may ease outflow tract obstruction and relieve symptoms. This is an experimental procedure and can cause complications, such as complete heart block and ventricular septal defect. Dual-chamber pacing can prevent progression of hypertrophy and obstruction. Implantable defibrillators may be used in patients with ventricular arrhythmias.

What to do

• Administer medication, as ordered. Warn the patient not to stop taking propranolol abruptly because doing so may cause rebound effects, resulting in MI or sudden death. Before dental work or surgery, administer prophylaxis for subacute bacterial endocarditis.
• Provide psychological support. Refer the patient for psychosocial counseling to help him and his family accept his restricted lifestyle and cope with his poor prognosis. Urge parents of a school-age child to arrange for continuation of studies in the hospital.
• Evaluate the patient. If treatment proves successful, the patient will show adequate tissue perfusion, clear lungs, and absence of edema and syncopal episodes. He'll be able to maintain his weight and tolerate activity. Blood pressure will remain adequate. (See *Teaching the patient with hypertrophic cardiomyopathy.*)

Education edge

Teaching the patient with hypertrophic cardiomyopathy

• Instruct the patient to take his medication as ordered.
• Warn the patient against strenuous physical activity such as running. Syncope or sudden death may follow well-tolerated exercise. Advise him to avoid Valsalva's maneuver or sudden position changes; both may worsen obstruction.
• Inform the patient that before dental work or surgery he needs antibiotic prophylaxis to prevent bacterial endocarditis.
• Because the patient is at risk for sudden cardiac arrest, urge his family to learn cardiopulmonary resuscitation.

MI

MI is an occlusion of a coronary artery that leads to oxygen deprivation, myocardial ischemia, and eventual necrosis. (See *Understanding MI*, pages 308 and 309.)

The extent of functional impairment and the patient's prognosis depend on the size and location of the infarct, the condition of the uninvolved myocardium, the potential for collateral circulation, and the effectiveness of compensatory mechanisms. In the United States, MI is the leading cause of death in adults.

> In the United States, MI is the leading cause of death.

What causes it

MI can arise from any condition in which the myocardial oxygen supply can't keep pace with demand, including:
- CAD
- coronary artery emboli
- thrombus
- coronary artery spasm
- severe hematologic and coagulation
- myocardial contusion
- congenital coronary artery anomalies.

Certain risk factors increase a patient's vulnerability to MI. These factors include family history of MI, gender (men are more susceptible), hypertension, smoking, elevated serum triglyceride, cholesterol, and low-density lipoprotein (LDL) levels, diabetes mellitus, obesity, sedentary lifestyle, aging, stress, and menopause.

Pathophysiology

MI results from prolonged ischemia to the myocardium with irreversible cell damage and muscle death. Functionally, MI causes:
- reduced contractility with abnormal wall motion
- altered left ventricular compliance
- reduced stroke volume
- reduced ejection fraction
- elevated left ventricular end-diastolic pressure.

What to look for

The patient experiences severe, persistent chest pain that's unrelieved by rest or nitroglycerin. He may describe the pain as crushing or squeezing. Usually substernal, pain may radiate to the left arm, jaw, neck, or shoulder blades. Other signs and symptoms include a feeling of impending doom, fatigue, nausea and vomiting, shortness of breath, cool extremities, perspiration, anxiety, hypotension or hypertension, palpable precordial pulse and, possibly, muffled heart sounds.

A closer look

Understanding MI

In myocardial infarction (MI), blood supply to the myocardium is interrupted. Here's what happens.

Injury to the endothelial lining of the coronary arteries causes platelets, white blood cells, fibrin, and lipids to gather at the injured site, as shown below. Foam cells, or resident macrophages, gather beneath the damaged lining and absorb oxidized cholesterol, forming a fatty streak that narrows the arterial lumen.

As the arterial lumen narrows gradually, collateral circulation develops, which helps to maintain myocardial perfusion distal to the obstructed vessel lumen. The illustration below shows collateral circulation.

When myocardial demand for oxygen is more than the collateral circulation can supply, myocardial metabolism shifts from aerobic to anaerobic, producing lactic acid, which stimulates nerve endings, as shown below.

Lacking oxygen, the myocardial cells die. This decreases contractility, stroke volume, and blood pressure.

Hypotension stimulates baroreceptors, which in turn stimulate the adrenal glands to release epinephrine and norepinephrine. This cycle is shown below. These catecholamines increase heart rate and cause peripheral vasoconstriction, further increasing myocardial oxygen demand.

Damaged cell membranes in the infarcted area allow intracellular contents into the vascular circulation, as shown below. Ventricular arrhythmias then develop with elevated serum levels of potassium, creatine kinase (CK), CK-MB, aspartate aminotransferase, and lactate dehydrogenase.

Understanding MI (continued)

 All myocardial cells are capable of spontaneous depolarization and repolarization, so the electrical conduction system may be affected by infarct, injury, or ischemia. The illustration below shows an injury site.

 Extensive damage to the left ventricle may impair its ability to pump, allowing blood to back up into the left atrium and, eventually, into the pulmonary veins and capillaries, as shown in the illustration below. Crackles may be heard in the lungs on auscultation. Pulmonary artery wedge pressure is increased.

 As back pressure rises, fluid crosses the alveolar-capillary membrane, impeding diffusion of oxygen (O_2) and carbon dioxide (CO_2). Arterial blood gas measurements may show decreased partial pressure of arterial oxygen and arterial pH and increased partial pressure of arterial carbon dioxide.

What tests tell you

- Serial 12-lead ECG may show no abnormalities or may prove inconclusive during the first few hours after MI. When present, characteristic abnormalities show serial ST-T changes in subendocardial MI, and Q waves representing transmural MI.
- ST-segment monitoring tracks the heart's response to MI. Continuous monitoring can immediately detect ischemic episodes. ST-segment monitoring can identify patients at high risk for reocclusion after PTCA or MI and permits prompt intervention if reocclusion occurs. After MI, ST-segment monitoring may reduce or eliminate the need for angiography in patients receiving thrombolytic drugs by gauging the efficacy of the drugs.
- Serial serum cardiac marker measurements show elevated CK, especially the CK-MB isoenzyme (the cardiac muscle fraction of CK), troponin I and T, and myoglobin.
- Echocardiography shows ventricular wall dyskinesia (with transmural MI).

How it's treated

Primary treatment for MI seeks to relieve pain, stabilize heart rhythm, revascularize the coronary artery, preserve myocardial tissue, and reduce cardiac workload. These treatments include

Serial 12-lead ECG may be inconclusive or show no abnormalities during the first few hours after MI.

thrombolytic therapy and PTCA. To preserve myocardial tissue, thrombolytic therapy should be started within 3 hours of the onset of symptoms (unless contraindications exist). This therapy involves administration of streptokinase, alteplase, anistreplase, or reteplase. PTCA is another option for opening blocked or narrowed arteries. If PTCA is performed soon after the onset of symptoms, the thrombolytic agent can be administered directly into the coronary artery.

Other options

Other treatments include:
• delivering oxygen to increase oxygenation of the blood
• administering nitroglycerin sublingually to relieve chest pain, unless systolic blood pressure is less than 90 mm Hg or heart rate is less than 50 or greater than 100 beats/minute
• administering morphine for analgesia (because pain stimulates the sympathetic nervous system, leading to an increase in heart rate and vasoconstriction)
• administering aspirin to inhibit platelet aggregation
• administering I.V. heparin for patients who have received tissue plasminogen activator to increase the chances of patency in the affected coronary artery (only limited evidence that I.V. or subcutaneous (S.C.) heparin is beneficial in patients with acute MI treated with a nonspecific thrombolytic drug, such as streptokinase and anistreplase)

Pain stimulates the sympathetic nervous system, which gets me going. Thank goodness for analgesics!

Cutting down the workload

• limiting physical activity for the first 12 hours to reduce cardiac workload, thereby limiting the area of necrosis
• administering atropine, procainamide, lidocaine, transcutaneous pacing patches (or transvenous pacemaker), defibrillation, or epinephrine if arrhythmias are present
• administering I.V. nitroglycerin for 24 to 48 hours in patients without hypotension, bradycardia, or excessive tachycardia to reduce afterload and preload and relieve chest pain
• administering glycoprotein IIb/IIIa inhibitors to patients with continued unstable angina, acute chest pain, or following invasive cardiac procedures, to reduce platelet aggregation
• providing an early I.V. beta-adrenergic blocker to patients with an evolving acute MI, followed by oral therapy (if no contraindications exist) to reduce heart rate and myocardial contractile force in order to reduce myocardial oxygen requirements

Remodeling the heart

• administering an ACE inhibitor to those with an evolving MI with ST-segment elevation or left bundle-branch block but without

hypotension or other contraindications, to reduce afterload and preload and prevent remodeling
• performing laser angioplasty, atherectomy, stent placement, or transmyocardial revascularization
• administering lipid-lowering drugs to patients with elevated LDL and cholesterol levels.

What to do

When caring for post-MI patients, direct your efforts toward detecting complications, preventing further myocardial damage, and promoting comfort, rest, and emotional well-being. Many patients with MI receive treatment in the ICU, under constant observation for complications. Expect to perform these nursing measures:
• Monitor and record ECG readings, blood pressure, temperature, and heart and breath sounds.
• Assess pain and administer analgesics, as ordered. Always record the severity and duration of pain. Avoid giving I.M. injections because absorption from the muscle is unpredictable. Also, muscle damage increases CK, myoglobin, and LD levels, making diagnosis of MI more difficult.
• Check the patient's blood pressure after giving nitroglycerin, especially the first dose.
• Frequently monitor ECG to detect rate changes or arrhythmias.
• During episodes of chest pain, obtain ECG, blood pressure, and pulmonary artery catheter measurements to determine changes.
• Watch for signs and symptoms of fluid retention (crackles, cough, tachypnea, and edema), which may indicate impending heart failure. Carefully monitor daily weight, intake and output, respirations, serum enzyme levels, and blood pressure. Auscultate for adventitious breath sounds periodically (patients on bed rest commonly have atelectatic crackles), and for S_3 or S_4 gallops.

Promoting comfort, rest, and emotional well-being is an important objective in nursing care for MI patients.

Do not disturb

• Organize patient care and activities to maximize his periods of uninterrupted rest.
• Ask the dietary department to provide a clear liquid diet until nausea subsides. A low-cholesterol, low-sodium diet may be ordered.
• Provide a stool softener to prevent straining, which causes vagal stimulation and may slow heart rate. Allow the patient to use a bedside commode, and provide as much privacy as possible.
• Assist with ROM exercises and ambulation, as allowed. If the patient is completely immobilized by a severe MI, turn him often.

Education edge

Teaching the patient with MI

• Explain procedures and answer questions.
• Carefully prepare the patient with a myocardial infarction (MI) for discharge. To promote compliance with the prescribed medication regimen and other treatment measures, thoroughly explain dosages and therapy. Warn about drug adverse effects, and advise the patient to watch for and report signs of toxicity. If the patient has a Holter monitor in place, explain its purpose and use.
• Counsel the patient about lifestyle changes. Review dietary restrictions. If the patient must follow a low-sodium or low-fat and low-cholesterol diet, provide a list of undesirable foods. Ask the dietitian to speak to the patient and his family.
• Advise the patient to resume sexual activity progressively, usually after 2 to 4 weeks.

• Stress the need to stop smoking. Refer him to a smoking-cessation program.
• Advise the patient to control hypertension, strive for ideal body weight and, if necessary, manage blood glucose levels.
• Help the patient learn about support groups and community resources. Refer him to the American Heart Association for further information and support.
• Recommend his participation in a cardiac rehabilitation program for exercise, education, symptom management, and support with risk modification.
• Instruct the patient to report chest pain. Postinfarction syndrome may develop, producing chest pain that must be differentiated from recurrent MI, pulmonary infarct, or heart failure.

Antiembolism stockings help prevent venostasis and thrombophlebitis in patients on prolonged bed rest.
• Provide emotional support, and help reduce stress and anxiety; administer tranquilizers, as needed. Involve his family as much as possible in his care.
• Evaluate the patient. When assessing treatment outcome, look for clear breath sounds; normal heart sounds and blood pressure; absence of arrhythmias, chest pain, shortness of breath, fatigue, and edema; and evidence of ability to tolerate exercise. In addition, cardiac output should be adequate, as shown by a normal LOC; warm, dry skin; and an absence of dizziness. (See *Teaching the patient with MI.*)

Involve the patient's family as much as possible in his care.

Myocarditis

Myocarditis, a focal or diffuse inflammation of the cardiac muscle (myocardium), may be acute or chronic and can strike at any age. In many cases, myocarditis fails to produce specific cardiovascular symptoms or ECG abnormalities. The patient will commonly experience spontaneous recovery without residual defects. Occasionally, myocarditis is complicated by heart failure and, rarely, leads to cardiomyopathy.

What causes it

Potential causes of myocarditis include:
• viral infections (most common cause in the United States), such as coxsackievirus A and B strains and, possibly, poliomyelitis, influenza, rubeola, rubella, adenoviruses, and echoviruses
• bacterial infections, such as diphtheria, tuberculosis, typhoid fever, tetanus, and staphylococcal, pneumococcal, and gonococcal infections
• hypersensitivity reactions, such as acute rheumatic fever and postcardiotomy syndrome
• radiation therapy to the chest in treating lung or breast cancer
• chronic alcoholism
• parasitic infections, such as toxoplasmosis and, especially, South American trypanosomiasis (Chagas' disease) in infants and immunosuppressed adults
• helminthic infections such as trichinosis.

Pathophysiology

Damage to the myocardium occurs when an infectious organism triggers an autoimmune, cellular, or humoral reaction; a noninfectious cause can lead to toxic inflammation. In either case, the resulting inflammation may lead to hypertrophy, fibrosis, and inflammatory changes of the myocardium and conduction system. The heart muscle weakens and contractility is reduced. The heart muscle becomes flabby and dilated and pinpoint hemorrhages may develop.

What to look for

Signs and symptoms of myocarditis may include:
• fatigue
• dyspnea
• palpitations
• fever
• mild, continuous pressure or soreness in the chest
• signs and symptoms of heart failure (with advanced disease).

What tests tell you

• Laboratory tests may reveal elevated cardiac enzymes, such as CK and CK-MB, an increased WBC count and ESR, and elevated

My muscle isn't flabby. Who are you calling flabby?!

antibody titers (such as antistreptolysin-O titer in rheumatic fever).
• ECG changes provide the most reliable diagnostic aid. Typically, the ECG shows diffuse ST-segment and T-wave abnormalities such as occurs with pericarditis, conduction defects (prolonged PR interval), and other supraventricular ectopic arrhythmias.
• Stool and throat cultures may identify bacteria.
• Endomyocardial biopsy provides a definitive diagnosis.

How it's treated

Treatment includes antibiotics for bacterial infection, modified bed rest to decrease heart workload, and careful management of complications. Thromboembolism requires anticoagulant therapy. Inotropic drugs, such as amrinone, dobutamine, or dopamine, may be necessary. Nitroprusside and nitroglycerin may be administered for afterload reduction. Treatment with immunosuppressive drugs is controversial but may be helpful after the acute inflammation has passed. Patients with low cardiac output may benefit from intra-aortic balloon pulsation and left VADs. Heart transplantation is performed as a last resort.

What to do

• Assess cardiovascular status frequently, watching for signs of heart failure, such as dyspnea, hypotension, and tachycardia.
• Assist the patient with bathing, as necessary. Provide a bedside commode because this stresses the heart less than using a bedpan.
• Evaluate the patient. After successful treatment, the patient's cardiac output should be adequate as evidenced by normal blood pressure, warm and dry skin, normal LOC, and absence of dizziness. He should be able to tolerate a normal level of activity. His temperature should be normal, and he shouldn't be dyspneic. (See *Teaching the patient with myocarditis*.)

Education edge

Teaching the patient with myocarditis

• Teach the patient about anitinfective drugs. Stress the importance of taking the prescribed drug as ordered.
• Reassure the patient that activity limitations are temporary. Offer diversional activities that are physically undemanding.
• Stress the importance of bed rest. During recovery, recommend that the patient resume normal activities slowly and avoid competitive sports.

Pericarditis

Pericarditis is an acute or chronic inflammation that affects the pericardium, the fibroserous sac that envelops, supports, and protects the heart. Acute pericarditis can be fibrinous or effusive, with purulent serous or hemorrhagic exudate. Chronic constrictive pericarditis characteristically leads to dense fibrous pericardial thickening. Because pericarditis commonly coexists with other conditions, diagnosis of acute pericarditis depends on typical clinical features and the elimination of other possible causes.

Prognosis depends on the underlying cause. Most patients recover from acute pericarditis, unless constriction occurs.

What causes it

Pericarditis may result from:
- bacterial, fungal, or viral infection (infectious pericarditis)
- neoplasms (primary or metastatic from lungs, breasts, or other organs)
- high-dose radiation to the chest
- uremia
- hypersensitivity or autoimmune diseases, such as rheumatic fever (the most common cause of pericarditis in children), SLE, and rheumatoid arthritis
- postcardiac injury, such as MI (which later causes an autoimmune reaction [Dressler's syndrome] in the pericardium), trauma, and surgery that leaves the pericardium intact but causes blood to leak into the pericardial cavity
- drugs, such as hydralazine and procainamide
- idiopathic factors (most common in acute pericarditis)
- less commonly, aortic aneurysm with pericardial leakage, and myxedema with cholesterol deposits in the pericardium.

Pathophysiology

As the pericardium becomes inflamed, it may become thickened and fibrotic. If it doesn't heal completely after an acute episode, it may calcify over a long period and form a firm scar around the heart. This scarring interferes with diastolic filling of the ventricles.

What to look for

Signs and symptoms of pericarditis include:
- sharp, sudden pain that usually starts over the sternum and radiates to the neck, shoulders, back, and arms. Unlike the pain of MI, pericardial pain is usually pleuritic, increasing with deep inspiration and decreasing when the patient sits up and leans forward.
- pericardial friction rub. A classic sign, this grating sound occurs as the heart moves. You will usually hear the friction rub best during forced expiration while the patient leans forward or is on his hands and knees in bed. Occasionally, friction rub is heard only briefly or not at all.
- signs similar to those of chronic right-sided heart failure, such as fluid retention, ascites, and hepatomegaly (with chronic constrictive pericarditis).

Rheumatic fever is the most common cause of pericarditis in children.

What tests tell you

• Laboratory results don't establish a diagnosis. They indicate the presence of inflammation and may identify its cause. They may include normal or elevated WBC count (especially in infectious pericarditis), an elevated ESR, and slightly elevated cardiac enzymes (with associated myocarditis).
• A culture of pericardial fluid obtained by open surgical drainage or cardiocentesis sometimes identifies a causative organism in bacterial or fungal pericarditis.
• Echocardiography may establish the diagnosis of pericardial effusion by revealing an echo-free space between the ventricular wall and the pericardium.
• Chest X-ray may show an enlarged cardiac silhouette (with large effusion).

Get the rhythm

ECG changes in acute pericarditis may include:
• elevation of ST segments in the standard limb leads and most precordial leads without the significant changes in QRS morphology that occur with MI
• atrial ectopic rhythms such as atrial fibrillation
• diminished QRS voltage (in pericardial effusion).

How it's treated

Treatment for pericarditis seeks to relieve symptoms and manage underlying systemic disease. In acute idiopathic pericarditis, post-MI pericarditis, and postthoracotomy pericarditis, treatment consists of bed rest as long as fever and pain persist, and nonsteroidal anti-inflammatory drugs, such as aspirin and indomethacin, to relieve pain and reduce inflammation. If these drugs fail to relieve symptoms, expect to administer corticosteroids.

Infection on the left

Infectious pericarditis that results from disease of the left pleural space, mediastinal abscesses, or septicemia requires antibiotics, surgical drainage, or both. If cardiac tamponade develops, the doctor may perform emergency pericardiocentesis. Signs of cardiac tamponade include pulsus paradoxus, jugular vein distention, dyspnea, and shock.

Here it comes again

Recurrent pericarditis may necessitate partial pericardectomy, which creates a "window" that allows fluid to drain into the pleural space. In constrictive pericarditis, total pericardectomy to permit adequate filling and contraction of the heart may be necessary.

Lab results don't establish a diagnosis of pericarditis but can indicate inflammation and may help identify a cause.

Education edge

Teaching the patient with pericarditis

• Explain tests and treatments to the patient.
• Instruct him to resume his daily activities slowly and to schedule rest periods into his daily routine.
• Show him how to position himself to relieve pain.

Treatment must also include management of rheumatic fever, uremia, tuberculosis, and other underlying disorders.

What to do

• Encourage complete bed rest.
• Assess pain in relation to respiration and body position to distinguish pericardial pain from myocardial ischemic pain.
• Place the patient in an upright position to relieve dyspnea and chest pain.
• Provide analgesics and oxygen, as ordered.
• Reassure the patient with acute pericarditis that his condition is temporary and treatable.
• Monitor for signs of cardiac compression or cardiac tamponade, which are possible complications of pericardial effusion. Signs include decreased blood pressure, increased central venous pressure, jugular vein distention, and pulsus paradoxus. Because cardiac tamponade requires immediate treatment, keep a pericardiocentesis set at bedside whenever pericardial effusion is suspected.
• Evaluate the patient. Evidence of successful treatment includes normal temperature, absence of pain and shortness of breath, adequate blood pressure, and warm, dry skin. (See *Teaching the patient with pericarditis.*)

Treatment for pericarditis includes management of underlying disorders such as tuberculosis.

Raynaud's disease

Raynaud's disease is one of several primary arteriospastic diseases characterized by episodic vasospasm in the small peripheral arteries and arterioles. It occurs bilaterally and usually affects the hands or, less commonly, the feet. Upon exposure to cold or stress, the patient experiences skin color changes. He may develop minimal cutaneous gangrene or no gangrene at all. Arterial pulses are normal. This benign condition requires no specific treatment and doesn't lead to any serious sequelae.

What causes it

The cause of Raynaud's disease is unknown. However, Raynaud's phenomenon is a condition commonly associated with several connective tissue disorders, such as systemic sclerosis, SLE, and polymyositis, and has a progressive course, leading to ischemia, gangrene, and amputation. Distinction between the two disorders is difficult; some patients who experience mild symptoms of Raynaud's disease for several years may later develop overt connective tissue disease — especially systemic sclerosis.

Pathophysiology

Raynaud's disease is a syndrome of episodic constriction of the arterioles and arteries of the extremities, resulting in pallor and cyanosis of the fingers and toes. Several mechanisms may account for the reduced digital blood flow, including:
• intrinsic vascular wall hyperactivity to cold
• increased vasomotor tone due to sympathetic stimulation
• antigen-antibody immune response (most likely because abnormal immunologic test results accompany Raynaud's phenomenon).

Although they may share some symptoms, don't assume they're the same...

...One disorder is much more serious than the other.

What to look for

After exposure to cold or stress, the patient will typically experience:
• blanching of the skin on the fingertips, which then becomes cyanotic before changing to red and from cold to normal temperature
• numbness and tingling of fingers
• sclerodactyly (in long-standing disease)
• ulcerations (in long-standing disease)
• chronic paronychia (in long-standing disease).

What tests tell you

Diagnosis requires that clinical symptoms last at least 2 years. The patient may undergo tests to rule out secondary disease processes, such as chronic arterial occlusive or connective tissue disease. Antinuclear antibody (ANA) titer may identify autoimmune disease as an underlying cause of Raynaud's phenomenon. More specific tests must be performed if ANA titer is positive. Doppler ultrasonography may show reduced blood flow if symptoms are due to arterial occlusive disease. Arteriography can rule out arterial occlusive disease.

How it's treated

Initially, the patient must avoid cold, safeguard against mechanical or chemical injury, and quit smoking. Drug therapy is usually reserved for patients with unusually severe symptoms.

Calcium channel blockers, such as nifedipine, diltiazem, and nicardipine, may be prescribed to produce vasodilation and prevent vaso-spasm. Adrenergic blockers, such as phenoxybenzamine or reserpine, may improve blood flow to fingers or toes. If conservative measures fail to prevent ischemic ulcers, the patient may undergo sympathectomy.

What to do

• For a patient with a less advanced form of illness, provide reassurance that symptoms are benign. As the disorder progresses, try to allay the patient's fears regarding disfigurement.
• Evaluate the patient. The patient who responds well to treatment will have warm hands and feet. The skin of his hands and feet will retain its normal color. (See *Teaching the patient with Raynaud's disease.*)

Restrictive cardiomyopathy

Characterized by restricted ventricular filling and failure to contract completely during systole, restrictive cardiomyopathy is a rare disorder of the myocardial musculature that results in low cardiac output, and eventually endocardial fibrosis and thickening. If severe, it's irreversible.

What causes it

The cause of primary restrictive cardiomyopathy remains unknown. In amyloidosis, infiltration of amyloid into the intracellular spaces in the myocardium, endocardium, and subendocardium may lead to restrictive cardiomyopathy syndrome.

Pathophysiology

In restrictive cardiomyopathy, left ventricular hypertrophy and endocardial fibrosis limit myocardial contraction and emptying during systole as well as ventricular relaxation and filling during diastole. As a result, cardiac output falls.

What to look for

Restrictive cardiomyopathy produces:
• fatigue
• dyspnea
• orthopnea
• chest pain
• generalized edema
• liver engorgement
• peripheral cyanosis
• pallor
• S_3 or S_4 gallop rhythms.

Education edge

Teaching the patient with Raynaud's disease

• Warn against exposure to the cold. Tell the patient to wear mittens or gloves in cold weather or when handling cold items.
• Advise the patient to avoid stressful situations and to stop smoking. Refer him to a smoking-cessation program, if needed.
• Encourage the patient to avoid decongestants and caffeine to reduce vasoconstriction.
• Instruct the patient to inspect his skin frequently and to seek immediate care for signs of skin breakdown or infection.
• Teach the patient about prescribed drugs, their use, and their adverse effects.

What tests tell you

- ECG may show low-voltage complexes, hypertrophy, or AV conduction defects. Arterial pulsation reveals blunt carotid upstroke with small volume.
- Chest X-ray shows massive cardiomegaly, affecting all four chambers of the heart (in advanced stages).
- Echocardiography rules out constrictive pericarditis as the cause of restricted filling by detecting increased left ventricular muscle mass and differences in end-diastolic pressures between the ventricles.
- Cardiac catheterization demonstrates increased left ventricular end-diastolic pressure and also rules out constrictive pericarditis as the cause of restricted filling.
- Endomyocardial biopsy may reveal amyloidosis.

How it's treated

Although no therapy currently exists for restricted ventricular filling, digoxin, diuretics, and a sodium-restricted diet can ease symptoms. Anticoagulant therapy may prevent thrombophlebitis in the patient on prolonged bed rest.

What to do

In the acute phase:
- Monitor heart rate and rhythm, blood pressure, and urine output.
- Be supportive and understanding, and encourage the patient to express his fears.
- Provide appropriate diversionary activities for the patient restricted to prolonged bed rest.
- If the patient needs additional help in coping with his restricted lifestyle, refer him for psychosocial counseling.
- Evaluate the patient. When assessing his response to therapy, look for adequate tissue perfusion, demonstrated by good color; warm, dry skin; and clear lungs. The patient should maintain his weight and level of activity. Blood pressure should be adequate and dizziness and edema absent. (See *Teaching the patient with restrictive cardiomyopathy*.)

Education edge

Teaching the patient with restrictive cardiomyopathy

- Teach the patient to watch for and report signs of digoxin toxicity (anorexia, nausea, vomiting, yellow vision).
- Advise the patient to record his weight daily and report weight gain of 2 lb (0.9 kg) in 1 day or 5 lb (2.3 kg) in 1 week.
- If the patient must restrict sodium intake, tell him to avoid canned foods, pickles, smoked meats, and excessive use of table salt.

Thrombophlebitis

An acute condition characterized by inflammation and thrombus formation, thrombophlebitis may occur in deep (intermuscular or intramuscular) or superficial (subcutaneous) veins. Deep vein thrombophlebitis affects small veins, such as the soleal venous sinuses, or large veins, such as the vena cava and the femoral, iliac, and subclavian veins. Usually progressive, this disorder may lead to pulmonary embolism, a potentially fatal condition. Superficial thrombophlebitis is usually self-limiting and rarely leads to pulmonary embolism.

What causes it

While deep vein thrombophlebitis may be idiopathic, it usually results from endothelial damage, accelerated blood clotting, or reduced blood flow. Superficial thrombophlebitis may follow:

- trauma
- infection
- I.V. drug abuse
- chemical irritation caused by extensive I.V. use.

Extensive I.V. use may cause superficial thrombophlebitis.

Risk on the rise

Certain risk factors appear to increase the risk of developing deep vein or superficial thrombophlebitis. These include:

- prolonged bed rest
- trauma
- childbirth
- use of hormonal contraceptives.

Pathophysiology

Alteration in the epithelial lining causes platelet aggregation and fibrin entrapment of RBCs, WBCs, and additional platelets. The thrombus initiates a chemical inflammatory process in the vessel epithelium that leads to fibrosis, which may occlude the vessel lumen or embolize.

What to look for

Clinical features vary with the site and length of the affected vein. Deep vein thrombophlebitis may produce:

- severe pain
- fever
- chills
- malaise
- swelling and cyanosis of the affected arm or leg
- affected area possibly warm to the touch
- positive Homans' sign (pain on dorsiflexion of the foot). (False-positives are common.)

Superficial swell

Superficial thrombophlebitis may produce the following signs and symptoms along the length of the affected vein:

- heat
- pain
- swelling
- redness
- tenderness
- induration
- lymphadenitis (with extensive vein involvement).

What tests tell you

- Doppler ultrasonography identifies reduced blood flow to a specific area and any obstruction to venous flow, particularly in iliofemoral deep vein thrombophlebitis.
- Plethysmography shows decreased circulation distal to the affected area.
- Phlebography (also called venography), which usually confirms diagnosis, shows filling defects and diverted blood flow.

How it's treated

Treatment aims to control thrombus development, prevent complications, relieve pain, and prevent recurrence of the disorder. Symptomatic measures include bed rest, with elevation of the affected arm or leg; warm, moist soaks to the affected area; and analgesics, as ordered. After an acute episode of deep vein thrombophlebitis subsides, the patient may begin to walk while wearing antiembolism stockings (applied before getting out of bed).

Drugs and surgery

Treatment for thrombophlebitis may also include anticoagulants (initially, unfractionated or low-molecular-weight heparin; later, warfarin) to prolong clotting time. Before any surgical procedure, discontinue the full anticoagulant dose as ordered to reduce the risk of hemorrhage. After some types of surgery, especially major abdominal or pelvic operations, prophylactic doses of anticoagulants may reduce the risk of deep vein thrombophlebitis and pulmonary embolism.

Big and not so cute

For lysis of acute, extensive deep vein thrombosis, treatment may include thrombolytics (such as streptokinase). In rare cases, deep vein thrombophlebitis may cause complete venous occlusion, which necessitates venous interruption through simple ligation to vein plication, or clipping. Embolectomy may also be performed.

Superficial treatment

Therapy for severe superficial thrombophlebitis may include an anti-inflammatory drug, such as indomethacin, along with antiem-

Thrombophlebitis causes filling defects and diverted blood flow detected with phlebography...

...which usually confirms the diagnosis.

bolism stockings, warm soaks, and elevation of the patient's leg. A patient with a high risk for thrombophlebitis and pulmonary embolus combined with contraindications to anticoagulant therapy or with a high risk for bleeding complications might undergo insertion of a vena caval umbrella or filter.

What to do

Include the following steps for the patient with thrombophlebitis:
• To prevent thrombophlebitis in high-risk patients, perform ROM exercises while the patient is on bed rest. Use an intermittent external compression device during lengthy surgical or diagnostic procedures. Apply antiembolism stockings postoperatively, and encourage early ambulation.
• Remain alert for signs of pulmonary emboli, such as crackles, dyspnea, hemoptysis, sudden changes in mental status, restlessness, and hypotension.
• Closely monitor anticoagulant therapy to prevent serious complications such as internal hemorrhage. Watch for signs of bleeding, such as dark, tarry stools; coffee-ground vomitus; and ecchymoses. Encourage the patient to use an electric razor and to avoid medications that contain aspirin.

Make Veno go

To prevent venostasis in patients with thrombophlebitis, take the following steps:
• Enforce bed rest, as ordered, and elevate the patient's affected arm or leg. If you plan to use pillows for elevating the leg, place them to support the entire length of the affected extremity and to prevent possible compression of the popliteal space.
• Apply warm soaks to improve circulation to the affected area and to relieve pain and inflammation. Give analgesics to relieve pain, as ordered.
• Measure and record the circumference of the affected arm or leg daily. Compare this with the circumference of the other arm or leg. To ensure accuracy and consistency of serial measurements, mark the skin over the area and measure at the same spot daily.
• Administer heparin I.V. or S.C. as ordered. If necessary, use an infusion monitor or pump to control the flow rate of I.V. infusions.
• Evaluate the patient. After successful therapy, the patient shouldn't feel pain in the affected area or have a fever. Skin temperature and pulses in the affected arm or leg should be normal. (See *Teaching the patient with thrombophlebitis.*)

Education edge

Teaching the patient with thrombophlebitis

• To prepare the patient with thrombophlebitis for discharge, emphasize the importance of follow-up blood studies to monitor anticoagulant therapy. If the doctor has ordered postdischarge heparin therapy, teach the patient or a family member how to give subcutaneous injections. If he requires further assistance, arrange for a visiting nurse.
• Tell the patient to avoid prolonged sitting or standing to help prevent recurrence.
• Teach him how to apply and use antiembolism stockings properly.
• Tell the patient to immediately report signs of blocked blood flow such as cold, blue toes.

Quick quiz

1. The test that's most specific for myocardial damage is:
A. CK.
B. CK-MB.
C. troponin I.
D. myoglobin.

Answer: C. Troponin is a protein found in skeletal and cardiac muscles. However, troponin I is found only in the myocardium; it's more specific to myocardial damage than the other choices.

2. Modifiable risk factors associated with CAD include:
A. age, weight, cholesterol level.
B. smoking, diet, blood pressure.
C. family history, weight, blood pressure.
D. blood glucose level, activity level, family history.

Answer: B. Smoking, diet, and blood pressure are modifiable risk factors. Age and family history aren't modifiable.

3. A primary goal in the treatment of MI is to:
A. prevent blood loss.
B. decrease blood pressure.
C. relieve pain.
D. administer I.V. fluids.

Answer: C. The primary goals in the treatment of MI are to relieve pain, stabilize heart rhythm, revascularize the coronary artery, preserve myocardial tissue, and reduce cardiac workload.

4. One sign of arterial occlusive disease is:
A. bounding pulse.
B. abdominal pain.
C. high blood pressure.
D. intermittent claudication.

Answer: D. Intermittent claudication is a sign of arterial occlusive disease.

Scoring

☆☆☆ If you answered all four items correctly, yahoo! You got to the heart of cardiovascular disorders.

☆☆ If you answered three items correctly, terrific! You are pumping cardiovascular information very efficiently.

☆ If you answered fewer than three items correctly, don't get tachycardic! Review the chapter, take deep breaths, and try again.

Respiratory disorders

Just the facts

In this chapter, you'll learn:

♦ anatomy and physiology of the respiratory system

♦ important questions and discussion topics for the health history

♦ how to inspect, palpate, percuss, and auscultate respiratory structures

♦ relevant nursing diagnoses with nursing interventions and rationales

♦ nursing care for common respiratory disorders.

The respiratory system functions primarily to maintain the exchange of oxygen and carbon dioxide in the lungs and tissues and to regulate acid-base balance. Any change in this system affects every other body system. Conversely, changes in other body systems may reduce the lungs' ability to provide oxygen and eliminate carbon dioxide.

Anatomy and physiology

The respiratory system consists of the airways, lungs, bony thorax, and respiratory muscles and functions in conjunction with the central nervous system (CNS). (See *A close look at the respiratory system*, page 326.) These structures work together to deliver oxygen to the bloodstream and remove excess carbon dioxide from the body.

The respiratory system delivers oxygen to the bloodstream and removes excess carbon dioxide from the body — and I help!

A close look at the respiratory system

The major structures of the upper and lower airways are illustrated below. The alveolus, or acinus, is shown in the insert.

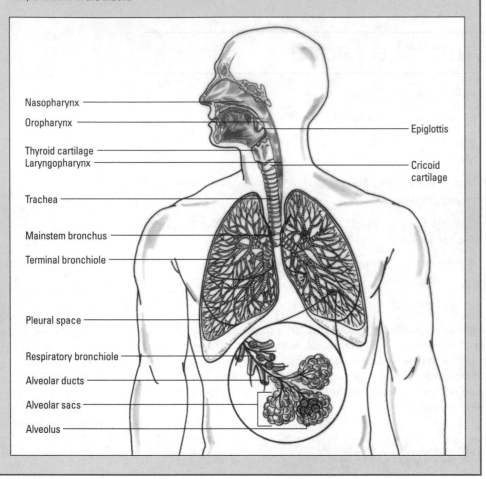

Nasopharynx
Oropharynx
Thyroid cartilage
Laryngopharynx
Trachea
Mainstem bronchus
Terminal bronchiole
Pleural space
Respiratory bronchiole
Alveolar ducts
Alveolar sacs
Alveolus

Epiglottis
Cricoid cartilage

Airways

The airways are divided into the upper and lower airways. The upper airways include the nasopharynx (nose), oropharynx (mouth), laryngopharynx, and larynx. Their purpose is to warm, filter, and humidify inhaled air. They also help make sound and send air to the lower airways.

The flap that protects

The epiglottis is a flap of tissue that closes over the top of the larynx when the patient swallows. The epiglottis protects the patient from aspirating food or fluid into the lower airways.

Lovely larynx

The larynx is located at the top of the trachea and houses the vocal cords. It's the transition point between the upper and lower airways.

Lowdown on the lower airways

The lower airways begin with the trachea, which then divides into the right and left mainstem bronchial tubes. The mainstem bronchi divide into the lobar bronchi, which are lined with mucus-producing ciliated epithelium, one of the lungs' major defense systems.

The lobar bronchi then divide into secondary bronchi, tertiary bronchi, terminal bronchioles, respiratory bronchioles, alveolar ducts and, finally, into the alveoli, the gas-exchange units of the lungs. The lungs in a typical adult contain about 300 million alveoli.

Lungs

Each lung is wrapped in a lining called the visceral pleura. The right lung is larger and has three lobes: upper, middle, and lower. The left lung is smaller and has only an upper and a lower lobe.

Smooth sliding

The lungs share space in the thoracic cavity with the heart, great vessels, trachea, esophagus, and bronchi. All areas of the thoracic cavity that come in contact with the lungs are lined with parietal pleura.

A small amount of fluid fills the area between the two layers of the pleura. This pleural fluid allows the layers of the pleura to slide smoothly over one another as the chest expands and contracts. The parietal pleura also contains nerve endings that transmit pain signals when inflammation occurs.

Pleural fluid allows layers of the pleura to slide smoothly over one another as the chest expands and contracts. Yippee!

Thorax

The bony thorax includes the clavicles, sternum, scapula, 12 sets of ribs, and 12 thoracic vertebrae. You can use specific parts of the

Respiratory assessment landmarks

The illustrations below show common landmarks used in respiratory assessment.

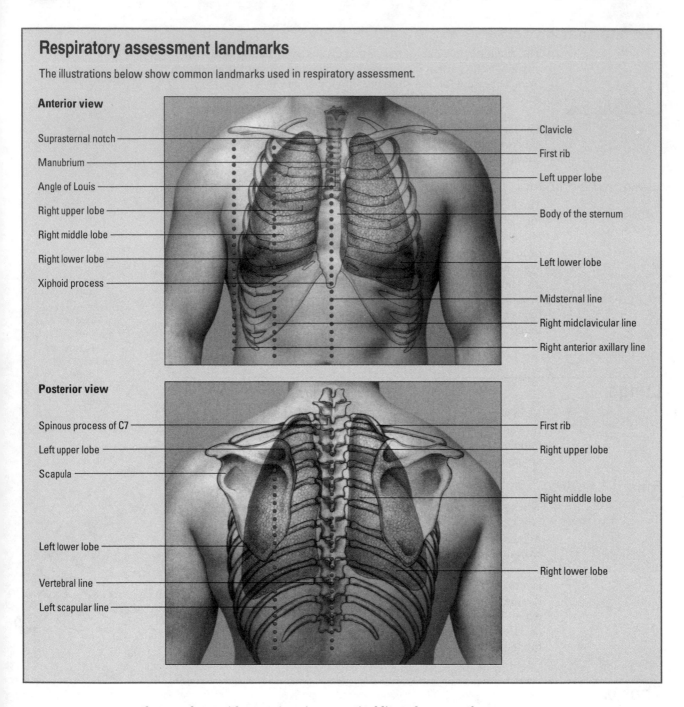

Anterior view

- Suprasternal notch
- Manubrium
- Angle of Louis
- Right upper lobe
- Right middle lobe
- Right lower lobe
- Xiphoid process

- Clavicle
- First rib
- Left upper lobe
- Body of the sternum
- Left lower lobe
- Midsternal line
- Right midclavicular line
- Right anterior axillary line

Posterior view

- Spinous process of C7
- Left upper lobe
- Scapula
- Left lower lobe
- Vertebral line
- Left scapular line

- First rib
- Right upper lobe
- Right middle lobe
- Right lower lobe

thorax, along with some imaginary vertical lines drawn on the chest, to help describe the locations of your findings. (See *Respiratory assessment landmarks*.)

A close look at breathing

These illustrations show how mechanical forces, such as the movement of the diaphragm and intercostal muscles, produce a breath. A plus sign (+) indicates positive pressure, and a minus sign (−) indicates negative pressure.

At rest
- Inspiratory muscles relax.
- Atmospheric pressure is maintained in the tracheobronchial tree.
- No air movement occurs.

Inhalation
- Inspiratory muscles contract.
- The diaphragm descends.
- Negative alveolar pressure is maintained.
- Air moves into the lungs.

Exhalation
- Inspiratory muscles relax, causing the lungs to recoil to their resting size and position.
- The diaphragm ascends.
- Positive alveolar pressure is maintained.
- Air moves out of the lungs.

Ribs are made of bone and cartilage and allow the chest to expand and contract during each breath. All ribs attach to the vertebrae. The first seven ribs also attach directly to the sternum. The 8th and 9th ribs attach to the 7th rib. The 11th and 12th ribs are called floating ribs because they don't attach to anything in the front.

Respiratory muscles

The diaphragm and the external intercostal muscles are the primary muscles used in breathing. They contract when the patient inhales and relax when the patient exhales. The respiratory center in the medulla initiates each breath by sending messages to the primary respiratory muscles over the phrenic nerve. Impulses from the phrenic nerve adjust the rate and depth of breathing, depending on the carbon dioxide and pH levels in the cerebrospinal fluid (CSF). (See *A close look at breathing*.)

The medulla initiates each breath by sending messages to primary respiratory muscles.

Yeah, hey, thanks for that!

My pleasure!

Accessory to breathing

Accessory inspiratory muscles also assist in breathing. They include the trapezius, sternocleidomastoid, and scalenes, which work together to elevate the scapula, clavicle, sternum, and upper ribs. That elevation expands the front-to-back diameter of the chest when use of the diaphragm and intercostal muscles isn't effective. In addition, if the patient has an airway obstruction, he may use the abdominal muscles and internal intercostal muscles to exhale.

Pulmonary circulation

Oxygen-depleted blood enters the lungs from the pulmonary artery off the right ventricle, then flows through the main pulmonary vessels into the pleural cavities and the main bronchi, where it continues to flow through progressively smaller vessels until it reaches the single-celled endothelial capillaries serving the alveoli. Here, oxygen and carbon dioxide diffusion takes place.

Movin' and diffusin'

In diffusion, molecules of oxygen and carbon dioxide move in opposite directions between the alveoli and the capillaries. Partial pressure — the pressure exerted by one gas in a mixture of gases — dictates the direction of movement, which is always from an area of greater concentration to one of lesser concentration. During diffusion, oxygen moves across the alveolar and capillary membranes into the bloodstream, where it's taken up by the hemoglobin (Hb) in the red blood cells (RBCs). This oxygen movement displaces the carbon dioxide in those RBCs, which then moves back through the alveoli.

Heh, ho! heh, ho! C-O-2 has got to go!

Take a deep breath and join the oxygen movement

Where do we go from here?

After passing through the pulmonary capillaries, the oxygenated blood flows through progressively larger vessels, enters the main pulmonary vein, and flows into the left atrium for distribution throughout the body. (See *Understanding pulmonary circulation.*)

Acid-base balance

The lungs help maintain acid-base balance in the body by maintaining external respiration (gas exchange in the lungs) and internal respiration (gas exchange in the tissues). Oxygen collected in the lungs is transported to the tissues by the circulatory system,

Understanding pulmonary circulation

The right and left pulmonary arteries carry deoxygenated blood from the right side of the heart to the lungs. These arteries divide into distal branches, called arterioles, which eventually terminate as a concentrated capillary network in the alveoli and alveolar sacs, where gas exchange occurs. The end branches of the pulmonary veins, called venules, collect the oxygenated blood from the capillaries and transport it to larger vessels, which lead to the pulmonary veins. The pulmonary veins enter the left side of the heart and deliver the oxygenated blood for distribution throughout the body.

During the gas exchange process, oxygen and carbon dioxide continuously diffuse across a very thin pulmonary membrane. To understand the direction of movement, remember that gases travel from areas of greater to lesser concentration. Carbon dioxide diffuses from the venous end of the capillary into the alveolus, and oxygen diffuses from the alveolus into the capillary.

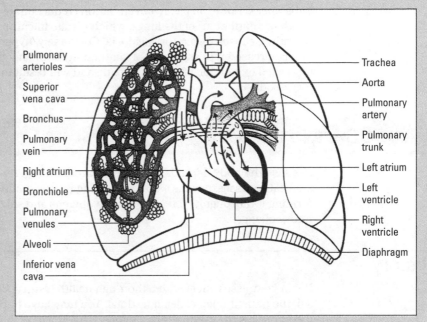

Pulmonary arterioles
Superior vena cava
Bronchus
Pulmonary vein
Right atrium
Bronchiole
Pulmonary venules
Alveoli
Inferior vena cava
Trachea
Aorta
Pulmonary artery
Pulmonary trunk
Left atrium
Left ventricle
Right ventricle
Diaphragm

which exchanges it for the carbon dioxide produced by cellular metabolism. Because carbon dioxide is 20 times more soluble than oxygen, it dissolves in the blood, where most of it forms bicarbonate (base) and smaller amounts form carbonic acid (acid).

In control

The lungs control bicarbonate levels by converting bicarbonate to carbon dioxide and water for excretion. In response to signals from the medulla, the lungs can change the rate and depth of ventilation. Such changes maintain acid-base balance by adjusting the amount of carbon dioxide that's lost. For example, in metabolic alkalosis, which results from excess bicarbonate retention, the rate and depth of ventilation decrease so that carbon dioxide is retained. This increases carbonic acid levels. In metabolic acidosis (a condition resulting from excess acid retention or excess bicarbonate loss), the lungs increase the rate and depth of ventilation to exhale excess carbon dioxide, thereby reducing carbonic acid levels.

When things go wrong

Inadequately functioning lungs, however, can produce acid-base imbalances. For example, hypoventilation (reduced rate and depth of ventilation) of the lungs, which results in carbon dioxide retention, causes respiratory acidosis. Conversely, hyperventilation (increased rate and depth of ventilation) of the lungs leads to increased exhalation of carbon dioxide and will result in respiratory alkalosis.

If I'm not at the top of my game, acid-base imbalances result. And they can lead to a world of trouble!

Assessment

Because the body depends on the respiratory system for survival, respiratory assessment is a critical nursing responsibility. By performing it thoroughly, you can evaluate obvious and subtle respiratory changes.

History

Begin your assessment with a thorough health history. Be sure to ask the patient open-ended questions. You may have to conduct the interview in several short sessions, depending on the severity of your patient's condition.

Current health status

Ask your patient to tell you about his reason for seeking care. Because many respiratory disorders are chronic, be sure to ask him how the latest episode compared with the previous episode, and what relief measures were helpful or unhelpful. A patient with a respiratory disorder may complain of shortness of breath, cough, sputum production, wheezing, and chest pain.

Short and severe

Gain a history of the patient's shortness of breath by determining its severity. (See *Grading dyspnea.*) Ask the patient:
• What do you do to relieve the shortness of breath?
• How well does it work?

Less rest, more pillows

A patient with orthopnea (shortness of breath when lying down) tends to sleep with his upper body elevated. Ask this patient how many pillows he uses. The answer describes the severity of orthopnea. For instance, a

Orthopnea is described using the number of pillows the patient uses to ease his shortness of breath when lying down.

patient who uses three pillows can be said to have "three-pillow orthopnea."

Off the cough

Ask the patient with a cough these questions:
- Is the cough productive?
- If the cough is chronic, has it changed recently? If so, how?
- What makes the cough better?
- What makes it worse?

Sputum size

When a patient produces sputum, ask him to estimate the amount produced in teaspoons or some other common measurement. Also ask him these questions:
- At what time of day do you cough most often?
- What's the color and consistency of the sputum?
- If sputum is a chronic problem, has it changed recently? If so, how?

Tell me about the wheeze, please

If a patient wheezes, ask these questions:
- At what time of day does wheezing occur?
- What makes you wheeze?
- Do you wheeze loudly enough for others to hear it?
- What helps stop your wheezing?

Chest pain particulars

Chest pain that occurs from a respiratory problem is usually the result of pleural inflammation, inflammation of the costochondral junctions, soreness of chest muscles because of coughing, or indigestion. Less common causes of pain include rib or vertebral fractures caused by coughing or by osteoporosis. If the patient has chest pain, ask him these questions:
- Where is the pain exactly?
- What does it feel like? Is it sharp, stabbing, burning, or aching?
- Does it move to another area?
- How long does it last?
- What causes it to occur?
- What makes it better?

Previous health status

Focus your questions on identifying previous respiratory problems, such as asthma or emphysema. A history of these conditions provides instant clues to the patient's current condition. Then ask about childhood illnesses. Infantile eczema, atopic dermatitis, or allergic rhinitis, for example, may precipitate current respiratory problems such as asthma.

Grading dyspnea

To assess dyspnea as objectively as possible, ask your patient to briefly describe how various activities affect his breathing. Then document his response using the grading system below.

Grade 0: Not troubled by breathlessness except with strenuous exercise

Grade 1: Troubled by shortness of breath when hurrying on a level path or walking up a slight hill

Grade 2: Walks more slowly on a level path because of breathlessness than people of the same age, or has to stop to breathe when walking on a level path at his own pace

Grade 3: Stops to breathe after walking about 100 yards (91.4 m) on a level path

Grade 4: Too breathless to leave the house or breathless when dressing or undressing

Family history

Ask the patient if anyone in his family has had cancer, diabetes, sickle cell anemia, heart disease, or a chronic illness, such as asthma or emphysema. Be sure to determine whether the patient lives with anyone who has an infectious disease, such as influenza or tuberculosis (TB).

Lifestyle patterns

The patient's history should also include information about lifestyle, community, and other environmental factors that might affect his respiratory status or how he deals with respiratory problems. Most importantly, ask the patient if he smokes; if he does, ask when he started and how many cigarettes he smokes per day.

Also ask about interpersonal relationships, mental status, stress management, and coping style. Keep in mind that a patient's sex habits or drug use may be connected with acquired immunodeficiency syndrome-related respiratory disorders.

Physical examination

In most cases, you'll proceed with the physical examination after you have taken the patient's history. However, you won't have the chance to obtain a history if the patient develops an ominous sign such as acute respiratory distress. (See *Emergency respiratory assessment.*)

A physical examination of the respiratory system follows four steps: inspection, palpation, percussion, and auscultation. Before you begin, introduce yourself, if necessary, and explain what you'll be doing. Then make sure the room is well lit and warm.

When performing a physical examination of the chest, make sure the room is well lit and warm.

Back, then front

Examine the back of the chest first, using inspection, palpation, percussion, and auscultation. Always compare one side with the other. Then examine the front of the chest using the same sequence. The patient can lie back when you examine the front of the chest if that's more comfortable for him.

Inspection

First, inspect the chest. Help the patient into an upright position. The patient should be undressed from the waist up or clothed in an examination gown that allows easy access to his chest.

What do I do?

Emergency respiratory assessment

When your patient is in acute respiratory distress, immediately assess his airway, breathing, and circulation (ABCs). If they're compromised, call for help and start cardiopulmonary resuscitation as necessary. If his airway is patent and he's breathing and has a pulse, proceed with the following rapid assessment.

Crisis questions

Quickly check for these signs of impending crisis:
- Is the patient having trouble breathing?
- Is he using accessory muscles to breathe? If chest excursion is less than the normal 1⅛" to 2⅜" (3 to 6 cm), he'll use accessory muscles when he breathes. Look for shoulder elevation, intercostal muscle retraction, and the use of scalene and sternocleidomastoid muscles.
- Has his level of consciousness diminished?
- Is he confused, anxious, or agitated?
- Does he change his body position to ease breathing?
- Does his skin look pale or cyanotic?
- Is he diaphoretic?

Setting priorities

When your patient is in respiratory distress, establish priorities for your nursing assessment. Don't assume the obvious. Note positive and negative factors, starting with the most critical (the ABCs) and progressing to less critical factors.

Although you won't have time to go through each step of the nursing process, make sure you gather enough data to clarify the problem. Remember, a single sign or symptom has many possible meanings. Rely on a group of findings for problem solving and appropriate intervention.

Beauty in symmetry

Note masses or scars that indicate trauma or surgery. Look for chest wall symmetry. Both sides of the chest should be equal at rest and expand equally as the patient inhales. The diameter of the chest from front to back should be about half the width of the chest.

A new angle

Also, look at the angle between the ribs and the sternum at the point immediately above the xiphoid process. This angle — the costal angle — should be less than 90 degrees in an adult. The angle will be larger if the chest wall is chronically expanded because of an enlargement of the intercostal muscles, as can happen with chronic obstructive pulmonary disease (COPD).

Breathing rate and pattern

To find the patient's respiratory rate, count his respirations for a full minute — longer if you note abnormalities. Don't tell him what you're doing, or he might alter his natural breathing pattern.

> Count respirations for more than a minute if you notice abnormalities.

Adults normally breathe at a rate of 12 to 20 breaths/minute. The respiratory pattern should be even, coordinated, and regular, with occasional sighs. The inspiratory-expiratory ratio is about 1:2.

Muscles in motion

When the patient inhales, his diaphragm should descend and the intercostal muscles should contract. This dual motion causes the abdomen to push out and the lower ribs to expand laterally.

When the patient exhales, his abdomen and ribs return to their resting position. The upper chest shouldn't move much. Accessory muscles may hypertrophy with frequent use. Frequent use of accessory muscles may be normal in some athletes, but for other patients it indicates a respiratory problem, particularly when the patient purses his lips and flares his nostrils when breathing.

Inspecting related structures

Inspection of the skin, tongue, mouth, fingers, and nail beds may also provide information about respiratory status.

Skin color and nail beds

Skin color varies considerably among patients, but in all cases, a patient with a bluish tint to his skin and mucous membranes is considered cyanotic. Cyanosis, which occurs when oxygenation to the tissues is poor, is a late sign of hypoxemia.

The most reliable place to check for cyanosis is the tongue and mucous membranes of the mouth. A chilled patient may have cyanotic nail beds, nose, or ears, indicating low blood flow to those areas but not necessarily to major organs.

Clubbing clues

When you check the fingers, look for clubbing, a possible sign of long-term hypoxia. A fingernail normally enters the skin at an angle of less than 180 degrees. When clubbing occurs, the angle is greater than or equal to 180 degrees.

Palpation

Palpation of the chest provides important information about the respiratory system and the processes involved in breathing. Here's what to look for when palpating the chest.

> The most reliable place to check for cyanosis is the tongue and mucous membranes of the mouth.

No extra air

The chest wall should feel smooth, warm, and dry. Crepitus indicates subcutaneous air in the chest, an abnormal condition. Crepitus feels like puffed-rice cereal crackling under the skin and indicates that air is leaking from the airways or lungs.

If a patient has a chest tube, you may find a small amount of subcutaneous air around the insertion site. If the patient has no chest tube or the area of crepitus is getting larger, alert the doctor immediately.

No pain

Gentle palpation shouldn't cause the patient pain. If the patient complains of chest pain, check for painful areas on the chest wall. Painful costochondral joints are typically located at the midclavicular line or next to the sternum. Rib or vertebral fractures will be quite painful over the fracture, though pain may radiate around the chest as well. Pain may also be caused by sore muscles as a result of protracted coughing or a collapsed lung.

Vibratin' fremitus

Palpate for tactile fremitus, palpable vibrations caused by the transmission of air through the bronchopulmonary system. Fremitus is decreased over areas where pleural fluid collects, at times when the patient speaks softly, and within pneumothorax, atelectasis, and emphysema. Fremitus is increased normally over the large bronchial tubes and abnormally over areas in which alveoli are filled with fluid or exudate, as happens in pneumonia. (See *Checking for tactile fremitus*, page 338.)

Measure up

To evaluate the patient's chest wall symmetry and expansion, place your hands on the front of the chest wall, with your thumbs touching each other at the second intercostal space. As the patient inhales deeply, watch your thumbs. They should separate simultaneously and equally, to a distance several centimeters away from the sternum. Repeat the measurement at the fifth intercostal space. The same measurement may be made on the back of the chest near the tenth rib.

To evaluate chest wall symmetry and expansion, watch your thumbs!

Percussion

Percuss the chest to find the boundaries of the lungs; determine whether the lungs are filled with air, fluid, or solid material; and evaluate the distance the diaphragm travels between the patient's inhalation and exhalation. (See *Percussing the chest*, page 339.)

Checking for tactile fremitus

When you check the back of the thorax for tactile fremitus, ask the patient to fold his arms across his chest. This movement shifts the scapulae out of the way.

What to do

Check for tactile fremitus by lightly placing your open palms on both sides of the patient's back, as shown, without touching his back with your fingers. Ask the patient to repeat the phrase "ninety-nine" loudly enough to produce palpable vibrations. Then palpate the front of the chest using the same hand positions.

What the results mean

Vibrations that feel more intense on one side than the other indicate tissue consolidation on that side. Less intense vibrations may indicate emphysema, pneumothorax, or pleural effusion. Faint or no vibrations in the upper posterior thorax may indicate bronchial obstruction or a fluid-filled space.

Different sites, different sounds

Percussion allows you to assess structures as deep as 3″ (7.6 cm). You'll hear different percussion sounds in different areas of the chest. (See *Percussion sounds*, page 340.)

You also may hear different sounds after certain treatments. For instance, if your patient has atelectasis and you percuss his chest before chest physiotherapy, you'll hear a high-pitched, dull, soft sound. After physiotherapy, you should hear a low-pitched, hollow sound.

Ringing with resonance

You'll hear resonant sounds over normal lung tissue, which you should find over most of the chest. In the left front chest, from the third or fourth intercostal space at the sternum to the third or fourth intercostal space at the midclavicular line, you should hear a dull sound. Percussion is dull here because that's the space occupied by the heart. Resonance resumes at the sixth intercostal space.

Movement of the diaphragm

Percussion also allows you to assess how much the diaphragm moves during inspiration and expiration. The normal diaphragm

Normally, my percussion isn't dull — except over the heart, of course!

Percussing the chest

To percuss the chest, hyperextend the middle finger of your left hand if you're right-handed or the middle finger of your right hand if you're left-handed. Place your hand firmly on the patient's chest. Use the tip of the middle finger of your dominant hand—your right hand if you're right-handed, left hand if you're left-handed—to tap on the middle finger of your other hand just below the distal joint (as shown).

The movement should come from the wrist of your dominant hand, not your elbow or upper arm. Keep the fingernail you use for tapping short so you won't hurt yourself. Follow the standard percussion sequence over the front and back chest walls.

descends 1⅛″ to 2″ (3 to 5 cm) when the patient inhales. The diaphragm doesn't move as far in patients with emphysema, respiratory depression, diaphragm paralysis, atelectasis, obesity, or ascites. (See *Measuring diaphragm movement*, page 341.)

Auscultation

Auscultation helps you determine the condition of the alveoli and surrounding pleura. As air moves through the bronchial tubes, it creates sound waves that travel to the chest wall. The sounds produced by breathing change as air moves from larger airways to smaller airways. Sounds also change if they pass through fluid, mucus, or narrowed airways.

Preparing to auscultate

Auscultation sites are the same as percussion sites. Listen to a full inspiration and a full expiration at each site, using the diaphragm of the stethoscope. Ask the patient to breathe through his mouth; nose breathing alters the pitch of breath sounds. If the patient has abundant chest hair, mat it down with a damp washcloth so the hair doesn't make sounds like crackles.

Auscultation sites are the same as percussion sites. Easy peasey!

Percussion sounds

Use the chart below to become more comfortable with percussion and interpret percussion sounds quickly. Learn the different percussion sounds by practicing on yourself, your patients, and any other person willing to help.

Sound	Description	Clinical significance
Flat	Short, soft, high-pitched, extremely dull, found over the thigh	Consolidation, as in atelectasis and extensive pleural effusion
Dull	Medium in intensity and pitch, moderate length, thudlike, found over the liver	Solid area as in pleural effusion
Resonant	Long, loud, low-pitched, hollow	Normal lung tissue
Hyperresonant	Very loud, lower-pitched, found over the stomach	Hyperinflated lung, as in emphysema or pneumothorax
Tympanic	Loud, high-pitched, moderate length, musical, drumlike, found over a puffed-out cheek	Air collection, as in a gastric air bubble or air in the intestines

Be firm

To auscultate for breath sounds, press the stethoscope firmly against the skin. Remember that if you listen through clothing or dry chest hair, you may hear unusual, deceptive sounds.

Normal breath sounds

You'll hear four types of breath sounds over normal lungs. The type of sound you hear depends on where you listen:
• Tracheal breath sounds, heard over the trachea, are harsh, discontinuous sounds. They occur when a patient inhales or exhales.
• Bronchial breath sounds, usually heard next to the trachea, are loud, high-pitched, and discontinuous. They're loudest when the patient exhales.
• Bronchovesicular sounds, heard when the patient inhales or exhales, are medium-pitched and continuous. They're best heard over the upper third of the sternum and between the scapula.
• Vesicular sounds, heard over the rest of the lungs, are soft and low-pitched. They're prolonged during inhalation and shortened during exhalation.

Interpreting what you hear

Classify each sound according to its intensity, location, pitch, duration, and characteristic. Note whether the sound occurs when the patient inhales, exhales, or both. If you hear a sound in an area

Measuring diaphragm movement

You can measure how much the diaphragm moves by asking the patient to exhale. Percuss the back on one side to locate the upper edge of the diaphragm, the point at which normal lung resonance changes to dullness. Use a pen to mark the spot indicating the diaphragm at full expiration on that side of the back.

Then ask the patient to inhale as deeply as possible. Percuss the back when the patient has breathed in fully until you locate the diaphragm. Use the pen to mark this spot as well. Repeat on the opposite side of the back.

Measure

Use a rule or tape measure to determine the distance between the marks. The distance, normally 1⅛″ to 2″ (3 to 5 cm), should be equal on the right and left sides.

other than where you would expect to hear it, consider the sound abnormal.

For instance, bronchial or bronchovesicular breath sounds found in an area where vesicular breath sounds would normally be heard indicates that the alveoli and small bronchioles in that area might be filled with fluid or exudate, as occurs in pneumonia and atelectasis. You won't hear vesicular sounds in those areas because no air is moving through the small airways.

The next step

A patient with abnormal findings during a respiratory assessment may be further evaluated using such diagnostic tests as arterial blood gas (ABG) analysis or pulmonary function tests.

If you hear a sound in an area where you wouldn't expect to hear it, consider it abnormal.

Vocal fremitus

Vocal fremitus is the sound produced by chest vibrations as the patient speaks. Abnormal transmission of voice sounds may occur over consolidated areas. The most common abnormal voice sounds are:

• *bronchophony.* Ask the patient to say "ninety-nine" or "blue moon." Over normal lung tissue, the words sound muffled. Over consolidated areas, the words sound unusually loud.

• *egophony.* Ask the patient to say "E." Over normal lung tissue, the sound is muffled. Over consolidated lung tissue, it will sound like the letter a.

• *whispered pectoriloquy.* Ask the patient to whisper "1, 2, 3." Over normal lung tissue, the numbers will be almost indistinguishable. Over consolidated lung tissue, the numbers will be loud and clear.

Diagnostic tests

If the history and physical examination reveal evidence of respiratory dysfunction, diagnostic tests will help identify and evaluate the dysfunction. These tests include blood and sputum studies and endoscopic and imaging tests as well as other diagnostic tests, such as pulse oximetry, thoracentesis, and pulmonary function tests.

Blood and sputum studies

Blood and sputum studies include ABG analysis and sputum analysis.

ABG analysis

ABG analysis is one of the first tests ordered to assess respiratory status because it helps evaluate gas exchange in the lungs by measuring:

• *pH.* An indication of hydrogen ion (H^+) concentration in the blood, pH shows the blood's acidity or alkalinity.

• *partial pressure of arterial carbon dioxide* ($Paco_2$). Known as the respiratory parameter, $Paco_2$ reflects the adequacy of the lungs' ventilation and carbon dioxide elimination.

• *partial pressure of arterial oxygen* (Pao_2). Pao_2 reflects the body's ability to pick up oxygen from the lungs.

• *bicarbonate* (HCO_3^-) *level.* Known as the metabolic parameter, HCO_3^- reflects the kidneys' ability to retain and excrete HCO_3^-.

ABG analysis is one of the first tests used to assess respiratory status because it evaluates gas exchange in the lungs.

Teamwork

The respiratory and metabolic systems work together to keep the body's acid-base balance within normal limits. If respiratory acidosis develops, for example, the kidneys attempt to compensate by conserving HCO_3^-. Therefore, if respiratory acidosis is present, expect to see the HCO_3^- value rise above normal. Similarly, if metabolic acidosis develops, the lungs try to compensate by increasing the respiratory rate and depth to eliminate carbon dioxide. Therefore, expect to see the $Paco_2$ level fall below normal. (See *Understanding acid-base disorders*, page 344.)

Nursing considerations

• Blood for an ABG analysis should be drawn from an arterial line if the patient has one. If a percutaneous puncture must be done, the site must be chosen carefully. The brachial, radial, and femoral arteries can be used.
• After the sample is obtained, apply pressure to the puncture site for 5 minutes and tape a gauze pad firmly in place. (Don't apply tape around the arm; it could restrict circulation.) Regularly monitor the site for bleeding and check the arm for signs of complications (such as swelling, discoloration, pain, numbness, and tingling).
• Make sure it's noted on the slip whether the patient is breathing room air or oxygen. If oxygen, document the number of liters. If the patient is receiving mechanical ventilation, the fraction of inspired oxygen should be documented.
• Keep in mind that certain conditions may interfere with test results—for example, failing to properly heparinize the syringe before drawing a blood sample or exposing the sample to air. Venous blood in the sample may lower Pao_2 levels and elevate $Paco_2$ levels.

Don't forget to heparinize me to avoid interfering with ABG test results.

Sputum analysis

Analysis of a sputum specimen (the material expectorated from a patient's lungs and bronchi during deep coughing) helps diagnose respiratory disease, determine the cause of respiratory infection (including viral and bacterial causes), identify abnormal lung cells, and manage lung disease.

A sputum specimen is stained and examined under a microscope and, depending on the patient's condition, sometimes cultured. Culture and sensitivity testing identifies a specific microorganism and its antibiotic sensitivities. A negative culture may suggest a viral infection.

Understanding acid-base disorders

Disorder and ABG findings	Possible causes	Signs and symptoms
Respiratory acidosis (excess carbon dioxide retention) pH <7.35 HCO_3^- >26 mEq/L (if compensating) $Paco_2$ >45 mm Hg	• Central nervous system depression due to drugs, injury, or disease • Asphyxia • Hypoventilation due to pulmonary, cardiac, musculoskeletal, or neuromuscular disease	Diaphoresis, headache, tachycardia, confusion, restlessness, apprehension, flushed face
Respiratory alkalosis (excess carbon dioxide excretion) pH >7.45 HCO_3^- <22 mEq/L (if compensating) $Paco_2$ <35 mm Hg	• Hyperventilation due to anxiety, pain, or improper ventilator settings • Respiratory stimulation due to drugs, disease, hypoxia, fever, or high room temperature • Gram-negative bacteremia	Rapid, deep respirations; paresthesia; light-headedness; twitching; anxiety; fear
Metabolic acidosis (HCO_3^- loss, acid retention) pH <7.35 HCO_3^- <22 mEq/L $Paco_2$ <35 mm Hg (if compensating)	• HCO_3^- depletion due to diarrhea • Excessive production of organic acids due to hepatic disease, endocrine disorders, shock, or drug intoxication • Inadequate excretion of acids due to renal disease	Rapid, deep breathing; fruity breath; fatigue; headache; lethargy; drowsiness; nausea; vomiting; coma (if severe); abdominal pain
Metabolic alkalosis (HCO_3^- retention, acid loss) pH >7.45 HCO_3^- >26 mEq/L $Paco_2$ >45 mm Hg (if compensating)	• Loss of hydrochloric acid due to prolonged vomiting or gastric suctioning • Loss of potassium due to increased renal excretion (as in diuretic therapy) or steroids • Excessive alkali ingestion	Slow, shallow breathing; hypertonic muscles; restlessness; twitching; confusion; irritability; apathy; tetany; seizures; coma (if severe)

Nursing considerations
• Encourage the patient to increase his fluid intake the night before sputum collection to aid expectoration.
• When ready to expectorate, instruct the patient to take three deep breaths and force a deep cough.
• To prevent foreign particles from contaminating the specimen, instruct the patient not to eat, brush his teeth, or use a mouthwash before expectorating. He may rinse his mouth with water.
• Before sending the specimen to the laboratory, make sure it's sputum, not saliva. Saliva has a thinner consistency and more bubbles (froth) than sputum.

Endoscopic and imaging tests

Endoscopic and imaging tests include bronchoscopy, chest X-ray, magnetic resonance imaging (MRI), pulmonary angiography, thoracic computed tomography (CT) scan, and ventilation-perfusion ($\dot{V}/\dot{Q}$) scan.

Bronchoscopy

Bronchoscopy is direct inspection of the trachea and bronchi through a flexible fiber-optic or rigid bronchoscope. It allows the doctor to determine the location and extent of pathologic processes, assess resectability of a tumor, diagnose bleeding sites, collect tissue or sputum specimens, and remove foreign bodies, mucus plugs, or excessive secretions.

Bronchoscopy inspects the trachea and me through a bronchoscope. How do I look? Am I fabulous or what?!

Nursing considerations

• Tell the patient that he'll receive a sedative, such as diazepam (Valium), midazolam (Versed), or meperidine (Demerol).
• Explain that the doctor will introduce the bronchoscope tube through the patient's nose or mouth into the airway. Then he'll flush small amounts of anesthetic through the tube to suppress coughing and gagging.
• Explain to the patient that he'll be asked to lie on his side or sit with his head elevated at least 30 degrees until his gag reflex returns. Food, fluid, and oral drugs will be withheld as well until this time. Hoarseness or a sore throat is temporary, and when his gag reflex returns, he can have throat lozenges or a gargle.
• Report bloody mucus, dyspnea, wheezing, or chest pain to the doctor immediately. A chest X-ray will be taken after the procedure and the patient may receive an aerosolized bronchodilator treatment.
• Watch for subcutaneous crepitus around the patient's face and neck, which may indicate tracheal or bronchial perforation.
• Monitor the patient for breathing problems from laryngeal edema or laryngospasm; call the doctor immediately if you note labored breathing.
• Observe the patient for signs of hypoxia, pneumothorax, bronchospasm, or bleeding.
• Keep resuscitative equipment and a tracheostomy tray available during the procedure and for 24 hours afterward.

Chest X-ray

Because normal pulmonary tissue is radiolucent, foreign bodies, infiltrates, fluids, tumors, and other abnormalities appear as densities (white areas) on a chest X-ray. It's most useful when compared with the patient's previous films, which allows the radiologist to detect changes.

By itself, a chest X-ray film may not provide information for a definitive diagnosis. For example, it may not reveal mild to moderate obstructive pulmonary disease. Even so, it can show the location and size of lesions and identify structural abnormalities that influence ventilation and diffusion. Examples of abnormalities visible on X-ray include pneumothorax, fibrosis, atelectasis, and infiltrates.

A chest X-ray alone may not confirm a diagnosis, but it can show structural abnormalities and lesion location and size.

Nursing considerations

• Tell the patient that he must wear a gown without snaps and must remove all jewelry from his neck and chest, but need not remove his pants, socks, and shoes.

• If the test is performed in the radiology department, tell the patient that he'll stand or sit in front of a machine. If it's performed at the bedside, someone will help him to a sitting position and a cold, hard film plate will be placed behind his back. He'll be asked to take a deep breath and to hold it for a few seconds while the X-ray is taken. He should remain still for those few seconds.

• Reassure the patient that the amount of radiation exposure is minimal. Facility personnel will leave the area when the technician takes the X-ray because they're potentially exposed to radiation many times each day.

• Explain that female patients of childbearing age will wear a lead apron. Males will be given a protective shield for the testes.

MRI

MRI is a noninvasive test that employs a powerful magnet, radio waves, and a computer to help diagnose respiratory disorders. It provides high-resolution, cross-sectional images of lung structures and traces blood flow. MRI's greatest advantage is its ability to "see through" bone and to delineate fluid-filled soft tissue in great detail, without using ionizing radiation or contrast media.

Nursing considerations

• Tell the patient that he must remove all jewelry and take everything out of his pockets. No metal can be in the test room. The powerful magnet may demagnetize the magnetic strip on a credit card or stop a watch from ticking. If he has any metal inside his body, such as a pacemaker, orthopedic pins or disks, and bullets or shrapnel fragments, he must notify his doctor.

(Text continues on page 347.)

Heart failure

Normal cardiac circulation

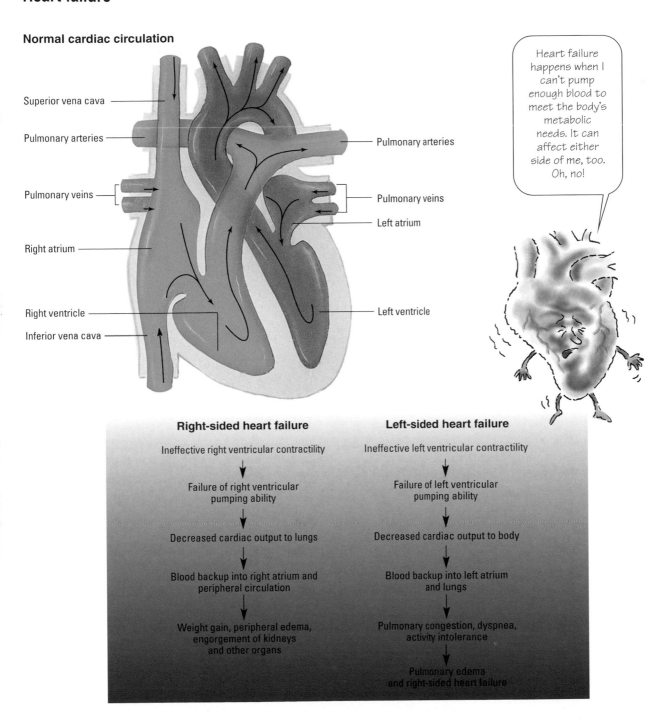

Superior vena cava

Pulmonary arteries

Pulmonary veins

Right atrium

Right ventricle

Inferior vena cava

Pulmonary arteries

Pulmonary veins

Left atrium

Left ventricle

Heart failure happens when I can't pump enough blood to meet the body's metabolic needs. It can affect either side of me, too. Oh, no!

Right-sided heart failure

Ineffective right ventricular contractility

↓

Failure of right ventricular pumping ability

↓

Decreased cardiac output to lungs

↓

Blood backup into right atrium and peripheral circulation

↓

Weight gain, peripheral edema, engorgement of kidneys and other organs

Left-sided heart failure

Ineffective left ventricular contractility

↓

Failure of left ventricular pumping ability

↓

Decreased cardiac output to body

↓

Blood backup into left atrium and lungs

↓

Pulmonary congestion, dyspnea, activity intolerance

↓

Pulmonary edema and right-sided heart failure

Myocardial infarction

All infarcts have a central area of necrosis surrounded by an area of potentially viable hypoxic injury. This viable area can be salvaged if circulation is restored. If not, it may progress to necrosis. The zone of injury, in turn, is surrounded by viable ischemic tissue.

Tissue destruction in myocardial infarction

Superior vena cava

Arch of aorta

Pulmonary trunk

Right atrium

Left atrium

Right coronary artery

Circumflex branch of left coronary artery

Left anterior descending artery

Papillary muscle

Damaged muscle from myocardial infarction

Zones of myocardial infarction

Reversible ischemia

Severe ischemia (recovery possible with revascularization)

Necrosis

Reduced blood flow through one or more of my coronary arteries leads to myocardial ischemia and necrosis. And that can lead to...YIKES!... myocardial infarction!

Pulmonary edema

Normal alveoli

Smooth muscle

Pulmonary artery

Alveolar duct

Alveolar sac

Alveolar pores

Bronchiole

Pulmonary vein

Alveoli

Capillary beds covering all alveoli

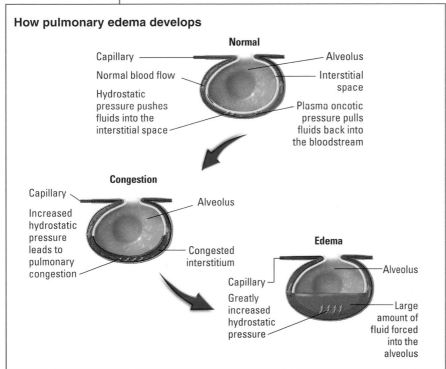

How pulmonary edema develops

Normal

Capillary

Normal blood flow

Hydrostatic pressure pushes fluids into the interstitial space

Alveolus

Interstitial space

Plasma oncotic pressure pulls fluids back into the bloodstream

Congestion

Capillary

Increased hydrostatic pressure leads to pulmonary congestion

Alveolus

Congested interstitium

Edema

Capillary

Greatly increased hydrostatic pressure

Alveolus

Large amount of fluid forced into the alveolus

A common complication of cardiac disorders, pulmonary edema may be chronic or develop quickly and become fatal.

Alzheimer's disease

Abnormal cellular structures in Alzheimer's disease

How and why neurons die in Alzheimer's disease is largely unknown. However, several characteristic abnormal cellular structures, which scientists believe cause cell malfunction or cell death, are found in the brain of every patient with Alzheimer's disease. These structures include excessive granulovacuoles, neurofibrillary tangles, and amyloid plaques.

Granulovacuolar degeneration

Granulovacuolar degeneration is found inside the neurons of the hippocampus. An abnormally high number of fluid-filled spaces, called *vacuoles*, enlarge the cell's body, possibly causing the cell to malfunction or die.

Neurofibrillary tangles

Neurofibrillary tangles are bundles of filaments inside the neuron that abnormally twist around one another. Numerous neurofibrillary tangles are found in areas of the brain associated with memory and learning (hippocampus), fear and aggression (amygdala), and thinking (cerebral cortex). Scientists believe the neurofibrillary tangles play a role in the memory loss and personality changes that the patient with Alzheimer's disease suffers.

Amyloid plaques

Amyloid plaques (senile plaques) are found outside neurons in the extracellular space of the cerebral cortex and hippocampus. They contain a core of beta amyloid protein that's surrounded by abnormal nerve endings, or neurites. Amyloid plaques also occur in the walls of cerebral blood vessels, causing the condition called *amyloid angiopathy*.

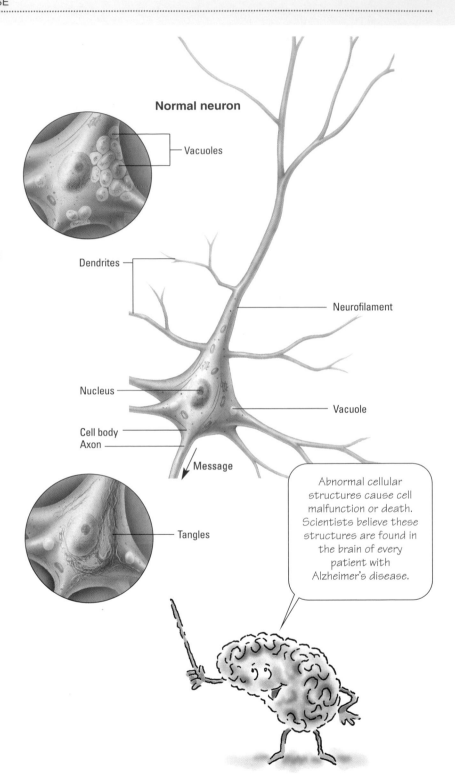

Normal neuron

Vacuoles

Dendrites

Neurofilament

Nucleus

Vacuole

Cell body
Axon

Message

Tangles

Abnormal cellular structures cause cell malfunction or death. Scientists believe these structures are found in the brain of every patient with Alzheimer's disease.

• Explain to the patient that he'll be asked to lie on a table that slides into an 8′ (2.4-m) tunnel inside the magnet.
• Tell him to breathe normally but not talk or move during the test to avoid distorting the results; the test usually takes 15 to 30 minutes but may take up to 45 minutes.
• Warn the patient that the machinery will be noisy with sounds ranging from an constant ping to a loud bang. He may feel claustrophobic or bored. Suggest that he try to relax and concentrate on breathing or a favorite subject or image.

> Tell the patient he'll lie on a table that slides into an 8′ tunnel. Urge him to relax by focusing on breathing or a favorite subject.

Pulmonary angiography

Pulmonary angiography, also called pulmonary arteriography, allows radiographic examination of the pulmonary circulation. After injecting a radioactive contrast dye through a catheter inserted into the pulmonary artery or one of its branches, a series of X-rays is taken to detect blood flow abnormalities, possibly caused by emboli or pulmonary infarction. This test provides more reliable results than a $\dot{V}/\dot{Q}$ scan but carries higher risks, including cardiac arrhythmias.

Nursing considerations

• Tell the patient who will perform the test and where and when it will be done. Explain that the test takes about 1 hour and allows confirmation of pulmonary emboli.
• Tell the patient he must fast for 6 hours before the test or as ordered. He may continue his prescribed drug regimen unless the doctor orders otherwise.
• Explain that he'll be given a sedative, such as diazepam, as ordered. Diphenhydramine (Benadryl) may also be given to reduce the risk of a reaction to the dye.
• Explain the procedure to the patient. The doctor will make a percutaneous needle puncture in an antecubital, femoral, jugular, or subclavian vein. The patient may feel pressure at the site. The doctor will then insert and advance a catheter.
• After catheter insertion, check the pressure dressing for bleeding and assess for arterial occlusion by checking the patient's temperature, sensation, color, and peripheral pulse distal to the insertion site.
• After the test, monitor the patient for hypersensitivity to the contrast medium or to the local anesthetic. Keep emergency equipment nearby and watch for dyspnea.

Thoracic CT scan

A thoracic CT scan provides cross-sectional views of the chest by passing an X-ray beam from a computerized scanner through the body at different angles and depths. The CT scan provides a three-dimensional image of the lung, allowing the doctor to assess abnormalities in the configuration of the trachea or major bronchi and evaluate masses or lesions, such as tumors and abscesses, and abnormal lung shadows. A contrast agent is sometimes used to highlight blood vessels and to allow greater visual discrimination.

Nursing considerations

• Tell the patient that, if a contrast dye will be used, he should fast for 4 hours before the test.
• Explain that he'll lie on a large, noisy, tunnel-shaped machine. When the dye is injected into his arm vein, he may experience transient nausea, flushing, warmth, and a salty taste.
• Tell him that the equipment may make him feel claustrophobic. He shouldn't move during the test but try to relax and breathe normally. Movement may invalidate the results and require repeat testing.
• Reassure the patient that radiation exposure during the test is minimal.

A thoracic CT scan allows assessment of the trachea and bronchi for abnormalities, masses, lesions, and — gulp — abnormal shadows.

Ventilation-perfusion scan

Although less reliable than pulmonary angiography, a $\dot{V}/\dot{Q}$ scan carries fewer risks. This test indicates lung perfusion and ventilation. It's used to evaluate $\dot{V}/\dot{Q}$ mismatch, to detect pulmonary emboli, and to evaluate pulmonary function, particularly in preoperative patients with marginal lung reserves.

Nursing considerations

• Tell the patient that a $\dot{V}/\dot{Q}$ scan requires injection of a radioactive contrast dye. Explain that he'll lie in a supine position on a table as a radioactive protein substance is injected into an arm vein.
• While he remains supine, a large camera will take pictures, continuing as he lies on his side, lies prone, and sits up. When he's prone, more dye will be injected.
• Reassure the patient that the amount of radioactivity in the dye is minimal. However, he may experience some discomfort from the venipuncture and from lying on a cold, hard table. He may also feel claustrophobic when surrounded by the camera equipment.

Other diagnostic tests

Other diagnostic tests include pulse oximetry, thoracentesis, and pulmonary function tests (PFTs).

Pulse oximetry

Pulse oximetry is a continuous noninvasive study of arterial blood oxygen saturation using a clip or probe attached to a sensor site (usually an earlobe or a fingertip). The percentage expressed is the ratio of oxygen to Hb. (See *Pulse oximetry levels*.)

Nursing considerations

• Place the probe or clip over the finger or other intended sensor site so that the light beams and sensors are opposite each other.
• Protect the transducer from exposure to strong light. Check the transducer site frequently to make sure the device is in place and examine the skin for abrasion and circulatory impairment.
• Rotate the transducer at least every 4 hours to avoid skin irritation.
• If oximetry has been performed properly, the oxygen saturation readings are usually within 2% of ABG values when saturations range between 84% and 98%.

Thoracentesis

Thoracentesis, also known as pleural fluid aspiration, is used to obtain a sample of pleural fluid for analysis, relieve lung compression and, occasionally, obtain a lung tissue biopsy specimen.

Nursing considerations

• Tell the patient that his vital signs will be taken and then the area around the needle insertion site will be shaved.
• The doctor will clean the needle insertion site with a cold antiseptic solution, then inject a local anesthetic. He may feel a burning sensation as the doctor injects the anesthetic.
• Explain to him that after his skin is numb, the doctor will insert the needle. He'll feel pressure during needle insertion and withdrawal. He'll need to remain still during the test to avoid the risk of lung injury. He should try to relax and breathe normally during the test and shouldn't cough, breathe deeply, or move.
• Emphasize that he should tell the doctor if he experiences dyspnea, palpitations, wheezing, dizziness, weakness, or diaphoresis, as these symptoms may indicate respiratory distress. After withdrawing the needle, the doctor will apply slight pressure to the site and then an adhesive bandage.
• Tell the patient to report fluid or blood leakage from the needle insertion site as well as signs and symptoms of respiratory distress.

Pulse oximetry levels

Pulse oximetry may be intermittent or continuous and is used to monitor arterial oxygen saturation. Normal oxygen saturation levels are 95% to 100% for adults and 94% to 100% for full-term neonates. Lower levels may indicate hypoxemia and warrant intervention.

Interfering factors

Certain factors can interfere with accuracy. For example, an elevated bilirubin level may falsely lower oxygen saturation readings, whereas elevated carboxyhemoglobin or methemoglobin levels can falsely elevate oxygen saturation readings. Certain intravascular substances, such as lipid emulsions and dyes, can also affect readings. Other interfering factors include excessive light (such as from phototherapy or direct sunlight), excessive patient movement, excessive ear pigment, severe peripheral vascular disease, hypothermia, hypotension, and vasoconstriction.

PFTs

PFTs are of two types: volume and capacity. These tests aid diagnosis in patients with suspected respiratory dysfunction. The doctor orders these tests to:

- evaluate ventilatory function through spirometric measurements
- determine the cause of dyspnea
- assess the effectiveness of medications, such as bronchodilators and steroids
- determine whether a respiratory abnormality stems from an obstructive or restrictive disease process
- evaluate the extent of dysfunction.

How do we do it? Volume, volume, volume!

Volume, volume, volume

Of the five pulmonary volume tests, tidal volume and expiratory reserve volume are measurements obtained through direct spirography. Minute volume, inspiratory reserve volume, and residual volume are calculated from the results of other pulmonary function tests.

Calculating capacity

Of the pulmonary capacity tests, functional residual capacity, total lung capacity, and maximal midexpiratory flow must be calculated. Vital capacity and inspiratory capacity may be measured directly or calculated indirectly. Direct spirographic measurements include forced vital capacity, forced expiratory volume, and maximal voluntary ventilation. The amount of carbon monoxide exhaled permits calculation of the diffusing capacity for carbon monoxide. (See *Interpreting pulmonary function test results.*)

Nursing considerations

- For some tests, the patient will sit upright and wear a noseclip. For others, he may sit in a small airtight box called a body plethysmograph and not need a noseclip. In this case, warn him that he may experience claustrophobia. Reassure him that he won't suffocate and that he'll be able to communicate with the technician through the window in the box.
- Explain that he may receive an aerosolized bronchodilator. Administration of the bronchodilator may be repeated in order to evaluate the drug's effectiveness.
- Emphasize that the test will proceed quickly if the patient follows directions, tries hard, and keeps a tight seal around the mouthpiece or tube to ensure accurate results.
- Instruct the patient to loosen tight clothing so he can breathe freely. Tell him he must not smoke or eat a large meal for 4 hours before the test.

Tell the patient to refrain from smoking or eating a large meal for 4 hours before a pulmonary function test.

Interpreting pulmonary function test results

You may need to interpret pulmonary test results in your assessment of a patient's respiratory status. Use the chart below as a guide to common pulmonary function tests.

Restrictive and obstructive

The chart mentions restrictive and obstructive defects. A restrictive defect is one in which a person can't inhale a normal amount of air. It may occur with chest-wall deformities, neuromuscular diseases, or acute respiratory tract infections.

An obstructive defect is one in which something obstructs the flow of air into or out of the lungs. It may occur with such disorders as asthma, chronic bronchitis, emphysema, and cystic fibrosis.

Test	Implications
Tidal volume (V_T): amount of air inhaled or exhaled during normal breathing	Decreased V_T may indicate restrictive disease and indicates the need for further tests, such as full pulmonary function studies and chest X-rays.
Minute volume (MV): amount of air breathed per minute	Normal MV can occur in emphysema. Decreased MV may indicate other diseases such as pulmonary edema.
Inspiratory reserve volume (IRV): amount of air inhaled after normal inspiration	Abnormal IRV alone doesn't indicate respiratory dysfunction. IRV decreases during normal exercise.
Expiratory reserve volume (ERV): amount of air that can be exhaled after normal expiration	ERV varies, even in healthy people.
Vital capacity (VC): amount of air that can be exhaled after maximum inspiration	Normal or increased VC with decreased flow rates may indicate reduction in functional pulmonary tissue. Decreased VC with normal or increased flow rates may indicate respiratory effort, decreased thoracic expansion, or limited movement of the diaphragm.
Inspiratory capacity (IC): amount of air that can be inhaled after normal expiration	Decreased IC indicates restrictive disease.
Forced vital capacity (FVC): amount of air that can be exhaled after maximum inspiration	Decreased FVC indicates flow resistance in the respiratory system from obstructive disorders, such as chronic bronchitis, emphysema, and asthma.
Forced expiratory volume (FEV): volume of air exhaled in the first (FEV_1), second (FEV_2), or third (FEV_3) FVC maneuver	Decreased FEV_1 and increased FEV_2 and FEV_3 may indicate obstructive disease. Decreased or normal FEV_1 may indicate restrictive disease.

• Keep in mind that anxiety can affect test accuracy. Also remember that medications, such as analgesics and bronchodilators, may produce misleading results. You may be asked to withhold bronchodilators and other respiratory treatments before the test. If the patient receives a bronchodilator during the test, don't give another dose for 4 hours.

Treatments

Respiratory disorders interfere with airway clearance, breathing patterns, and gas exchange. If not corrected, they can adversely affect many other body systems and can be life-threatening. Treatments for respiratory disorders include drug therapy, surgery, inhalation therapy, and chest physiotherapy.

Drug therapy

Drugs are used for airway management in such disorders as bronchial asthma and chronic bronchitis, and may include:
• xanthines (theophylline and derivatives) and adrenergics to dilate bronchial passages and reduce airway resistance, making it easier for the patient to breathe and allowing sufficient ventilation
• corticosteroids to reduce inflammation and make the airways more responsive to bronchodilators
• antihistamines, antitussives, and expectorants to help suppress coughing and mobilize secretions
• antimicrobials to reduce or eliminate infective organisms.

Surgery

If drugs or other therapeutic approaches fail to maintain airway patency and protect healthy tissues from disease, surgical intervention may be necessary. Respiratory surgeries include tracheotomy, chest tube insertion, and thoracotomy. Lung resection, lung reduction, pneumonectomy, or lung transplant surgery may also be indicated.

Tracheotomy

A tracheotomy provides an airway for an intubated patient who needs prolonged mechanical ventilation and helps remove lower tracheobronchial secretions in a patient who can't clear them. It's also performed in emergencies when endotracheal (ET) intubation isn't possible, to prevent an unconscious or paralyzed patient from aspirating food or secretions, and to bypass upper airway obstruction due to trauma, burns, epiglottiditis, or a tumor.

A tracheotomy helps remove lower tracheobronchial secretions in a patient who can't clear them. Phew!

Comparing tracheostomy tubes

Tracheostomy tubes are made of plastic or metal and come in uncuffed, cuffed, or fenestrated varieties. Tube selection depends on the patient's condition and the doctor's preference. Make sure you're familiar with the advantages and disadvantages of these commonly used tracheostomy tubes.

Uncuffed
(plastic or metal)

Plastic cuffed
(low pressure and high volume)

Fenestrated

Advantages
- Free flow of air around tube and through larynx
- Reduced risk of tracheal damage
- Mechanical ventilation possible in patient with neuromuscular disease

Disadvantages
- Increased risk of aspiration in adults due to lack of cuff
- Adapter possibly needed for ventilation

Advantages
- Disposable
- Cuff bonded to tube (won't detach accidentally inside trachea)
- Low cuff pressure that's evenly distributed against tracheal wall (no need to deflate periodically to lower pressure)
- Reduced risk of tracheal damage

Disadvantages
- Possibly more expensive than other tubes

Advantages
- Speech possible through upper airway when external opening is capped and cuff is deflated
- Breathing by mechanical ventilation possible with inner cannula in place and cuff inflated
- Easy removal of inner cannula for cleaning

Disadvantages
- Possible occlusion of fenestration
- Possible dislodgment of inner cannula
- Cap removal necessary before inflating cuff

After the doctor creates the surgical opening, he inserts a tracheostomy tube to permit access to the airway. He may select from several tube styles, depending on the patient's condition. (See *Comparing tracheostomy tubes.*)

Patient preparation

- For an emergency tracheotomy, briefly explain the procedure to the patient as time permits and quickly obtain supplies or a tracheotomy tray.

- For a scheduled tracheotomy, explain the procedure and the need for general anesthesia to the patient and his family. If possible, mention whether the tracheostomy will be temporary or permanent.
- Set up a communication system with the patient (letter board or flash cards), and practice it with him to ensure he'll be able to communicate comfortably while his speech is limited.
- Introduce a patient requiring a long-term or permanent tracheostomy to someone who has experienced the procedure and has adjusted well to tracheostomy care.
- Ensure that samples for ABG analysis and other diagnostic tests have been collected and that the patient or a responsible family member has signed a consent form.

Monitoring and aftercare

- Auscultate breath sounds every 2 hours after the procedure. Note crackles, rhonchi, or diminished breath sounds.
- Turn the patient every 2 hours to avoid pooling tracheal secretions. As ordered, provide chest physiotherapy to help mobilize secretions, and note their quantity, consistency, color, and odor.

Humidity lost

- Replace humidity lost in bypassing the nose, mouth, and upper airway mucosa to reduce the drying effects of oxygen on mucous membranes. Humidification will also help to thin secretions. Oxygen administered through a T-piece or tracheostomy mask should be connected to a nebulizer or heated cascade humidifier.
- Monitor ABG results and compare them with baseline values to check adequacy of oxygenation and carbon dioxide removal. Also monitor the patient's oximetry values as ordered.
- Suction the tracheostomy using sterile technique to remove excess secretions when necessary. Avoid suctioning a patient for longer than 10 seconds at a time and discontinue the procedure if the patient develops respiratory distress.
- Make sure the tracheostomy ties are secure but not too tight. To prevent accidental tube dislodgment or expulsion, avoid changing the ties until the stoma track is stable. Report any tube pulsation to the doctor; this may indicate the tube is close to the innominate artery, which predisposes the patient to hemorrhage.

Keeping it clean

- Change the tracheostomy dressing when soiled or once per shift, using aseptic technique, and check the color, odor, amount, and type of drainage. Also check for swelling, crepitus, erythema, and bleeding at the site and report excessive bleeding or unusual

Avoid suctioning the patient for longer than 10 seconds at a time and stop if the patient develops respiratory distress.

drainage immediately. Wear goggles, gloves, and mask when changing tracheostomy tubes.
• Keep a sterile tracheostomy tube (with obturator) at the patient's bedside and be prepared to replace an expelled or contaminated tube. Also keep available a sterile tracheostomy tube (with obturator) that's one size smaller than the tube currently being used. The smaller tube may be necessary if the trachea begins to close after tube expulsion, making insertion of the same size tube difficult.

Home care instructions

• Tell the patient or his family to notify the doctor of breathing problems, chest or stoma pain, or a change in the amount or color of his secretions.
• Ensure that the patient or family can care for the stoma and tracheostomy tube effectively.
• Tell the patient to place a foam filter over his stoma in winter to warm the inspired air and to wear a bib over the filter.
• Teach the patient to bend at the waist during coughing to help expel secretions. Tell him to keep a tissue handy to catch expelled secretions.

Tell the patient or his family to notify his doctor of breathing problems, chest or stoma pain, or changes in the color or amount of secretions.

Chest tube insertion

A chest tube may be required to help treat pneumothorax, hemothorax, empyema, pleural effusion, or chylothorax. Inserted into the pleural space, the tube allows blood, fluid, pus, or air to drain and allows the lung to reinflate. In pneumothorax, the tube restores negative pressure to the pleural space through an underwater-seal drainage system. The water in the system prevents air from being sucked back into the pleural space during inspiration. If a leak occurs through the bronchi and can't be sealed, suction applied to the underwater-seal system removes air from the pleural space faster than it can collect.

Patient preparation

• If time permits, the doctor will obtain a signed consent form after explaining the procedure. Reassure the patient that chest tube insertion will help him breathe more easily.
• Obtain baseline vital signs and administer a sedative as ordered.

Using the underwater seal

• Collect necessary equipment, including a thoracotomy tray and an underwater-seal drainage system. Prepare lidocaine (Xylocaine) for local anesthesia as directed. The doctor will clean the insertion site with povidone-iodine solution. Set up the underwater-seal drainage system according to the manufacturer's instructions and

Closed chest drainage system

One-piece, disposable plastic drainage systems, such as the Pleur-evac, contain three chambers. The drainage chamber is on the right and has three calibrated columns that display the amount of drainage collected. When the first column fills, drainage carries over into the second and, when that fills, into the third. The water-seal chamber is located in the center. The suction-control chamber on the left is filled with water to achieve various suction levels. Rubber diaphragms are provided at the rear of the device to change the water level or remove samples of drainage. A positive-pressure relief valve at the top of the water-seal chamber vents excess pressure into the atmosphere, preventing pressure buildup.

place it at bedside, below the patient's chest level. Stabilize the unit to avoid knocking it over. (See *Closed chest drainage system.*)

Monitoring and aftercare

• When the patient's chest tube is stabilized, instruct him to take several deep breaths to inflate his lungs fully and help push pleural air out through the tube.
• Obtain vital signs immediately after tube insertion and every 15 minutes thereafter, according to facility policy (usually for 1 hour).
• Routinely assess chest tube function. Describe and record the amount of drainage on the intake and output sheet.
• After most of the air has been removed, the drainage system should bubble only during forced expiration unless the patient has a bronchopleural fistula. Constant bubbling in the system may indicate that a connection is loose or that the tube has advanced slightly out of the patient's chest. Promptly correct any loose connections to prevent complications.

Describe and record the amount of chest tube drainage on the intake and output sheet.

What do I do?

Combating tension pneumothorax

Tension pneumothorax, the entrapment of air within the pleural space, can be fatal without prompt treatment.

What causes it?

An obstructed or dislodged chest tube is a common cause of tension pneumothorax. Other causes include blunt chest trauma or high-pressure mechanical ventilation. In such cases, increased positive pressure within the patient's chest cavity compresses the affected lung and the mediastinum, shifting them toward the opposite lung. This impairs venous return and cardiac output and may cause the lung to collapse.

Telltale signs

Suspect tension pneumothorax if the patient develops dyspnea, chest pain, an irritating cough, vertigo, syncope, or anxiety after a blunt chest trauma or if the patient has a chest tube in place. Is his skin cold, pale, and clammy? Are his respiratory and pulse rates unusually rapid? Does the patient have equal bilateral chest expansion?

If you note these signs and symptoms, palpate the patient's neck, face, and chest wall for subcutaneous emphysema and palpate his trachea for deviation from midline. Auscultate the lungs for decreased or absent breath sounds on one side. Then percuss them for hyperresonance. If you suspect tension pneumotorax, notify the doctor at once and help identify the cause.

• Change the dressing daily (or as per facility policy) to clean the site and remove drainage.
• If the chest tube becomes dislodged, cover the opening immediately with petroleum gauze and apply pressure to prevent negative inspiratory pressure from sucking air into the chest. Call the doctor and have an assistant collect equipment for tube reinsertion while you keep the opening closed. Reassure the patient and monitor him closely for signs of tension pneumothorax. (See *Combating tension pneumothorax*.)
• The doctor will remove the patient's chest tube after the lung is fully reexpanded. As soon as the tube is removed, apply an airtight, sterile petroleum dressing.

Home care instructions

Typically, a patient is discharged with a chest tube only if it's used to drain a loculated empyema, which doesn't require an underwater-seal drainage system. Teach this patient how to care for his tube, perform wound care and dressing changes, and dispose of soiled dressings.

Teach the patient with a recently removed chest tube how to clean the wound site and change dressings. Tell him to report any signs of infection.

Thoracotomy

A thoracotomy is the surgical removal of all or part of a lung; it aims to spare healthy lung tissue from disease. Lung excision may involve a pneumonectomy, lobectomy, segmental resection, or wedge resection.

Whole shebang

A pneumonectomy is the excision of an entire lung; it's usually performed to treat bronchogenic carcinoma but may also be used to treat TB, bronchiectasis, or a lung abscess. It's used only when a less radical approach can't remove all diseased tissue. Chest cavity pressures stabilize after a pneumonectomy and, over time, fluid enters the cavity where lung tissue was removed, preventing significant mediastinal shift.

One lobe out of five ain't bad

A lobectomy is the removal of one of the five lung lobes; it's used to treat bronchogenic carcinoma, TB, a lung abscess, emphysematous blebs or bullae, benign tumors, and localized fungal infections. After this surgery, the remaining lobes expand to fill the entire pleural cavity.

Segments and wedges

A segmental resection is the removal of one or more lung segments; it preserves more functional tissue than lobectomy and is commonly used to treat bronchiectasis. A wedge resection is the removal of a small portion of the lung without regard to segments; it preserves the most functional tissue of all the surgeries but can treat only a small, well-circumscribed lesion. Remaining lung tissue must be reexpanded after both types of resection.

Patient preparation

• Explain the anticipated surgery to the patient and inform him that he'll receive a general anesthetic.
• Inform the patient that postoperatively he may have chest tubes in place and may receive oxygen.
• Teach him deep-breathing techniques and explain that he'll perform these after surgery to facilitate lung reexpansion. Also teach him to use an incentive spirometer; record the volumes he achieves to provide a baseline.

Monitoring and aftercare

• After a pneumonectomy, the patient should lie only on the operative side or on his back until stabilized. This

Thoracotomy surgically removes all or part of a lung. Pneumonectomy is the excision of the entire lung. Oh, dear!

Let me show you how to use this incentive spirometer. I'll record the volumes you achieve now so we have a baseline for later.

prevents fluid from draining into the unaffected lung if the sutured bronchus opens.
• Make sure the chest tube is functioning, if present, and observe for signs of tension pneumothorax.
• Provide analgesics as ordered.
• Have the patient begin coughing and deep-breathing exercises as soon as his condition is stable. Auscultate his lungs, place him in semi-Fowler's position, and have him splint his incision to facilitate coughing and deep breathing.
• Perform passive range-of-motion (ROM) exercises the evening of surgery and two or three times daily thereafter. Progress to active ROM exercises.

Home care instructions

• Tell the patient to continue his coughing and deep-breathing exercises to prevent complications. Advise him to report changes in sputum characteristics to his doctor.
• Instruct the patient to continue performing ROM exercises to maintain mobility of his shoulder and chest wall.
• Tell the patient to avoid contact with people who have an upper respiratory tract infection and to refrain from smoking.
• Provide instructions for wound care and dressing changes as necessary.

Inhalation therapy

Inhalation therapy employs carefully controlled ventilation techniques to help the patient maintain optimal ventilation in the event of respiratory failure. Techniques include mechanical ventilation, continuous positive airway pressure (CPAP), and oxygen therapy.

Mechanical ventilation

Mechanical ventilation corrects profoundly impaired ventilation, evidenced by hypercapnia and symptoms of respiratory distress (such as nostril flaring, intercostal retractions, decreased blood pressure, and diaphoresis). Typically requiring an ET or tracheostomy tube, it delivers up to 100% room air under positive pressure or oxygen-enriched air in concentrations up to 100%.

Positive, negative, and high

Major types of mechanical ventilation systems include positive-pressure, negative-pressure, and high-frequency ventilation (HFV). Positive-pressure systems, the most commonly used, can be volume-cycled or pressure-cycled. During a cycled breath, inspiration ceases when a preset pressure or volume is met. Negative-

Mechanical ventilation corrects profoundly impaired ventilation.

pressure systems provide ventilation for patients who can't generate adequate inspiratory pressures. HFV systems provide high ventilation rates with low peak airway pressures, synchronized to the patient's own inspiratory efforts.

In control

Mechanical ventilators can be programmed to assist, control, or assist-control. In assist mode, the patient initiates inspiration and receives a preset tidal volume from the machine, which augments his ventilatory effort while letting him determine his own rate. In control mode, a ventilator delivers a set tidal volume at a prescribed rate, using predetermined inspiratory and expiratory times. This mode can fully regulate ventilation in a patient with paralysis or respiratory arrest. In assist-control mode, the patient initiates breathing and a backup control delivers a preset number of breaths at a set volume.

Synchronicity

In synchronized intermittent mandatory ventilation (SIMV), the ventilator delivers a set number of specific-volume breaths. The patient may breathe spontaneously between the SIMV breaths at volumes that differ from those on the machine, however. Commonly used as a weaning tool, SIMV may also be used for ventilation and helps to condition respiratory muscles.

> SIMV helps condition respiratory muscles.

Patient preparation
• Describe to the patient what mechanical ventilation system will be used, including its benefits and what he may experience.
• Set up a communication system with the patient (such as a letter board) and reassure him that a nurse will always be nearby. Keep in mind that an apprehensive patient may fight the machine, defeating its purpose.
• Place the patient in semi-Fowler's position, if possible, to promote lung expansion. Obtain baseline vital signs and ABG readings.

Monitoring and aftercare
If the patient doesn't have an ET or tracheostomy tube in place, he may start on a noninvasive form of mechanical ventilation to avoid intubation or tracheotomy. If more conservative measures fail, the patient may be intubated to establish an artificial airway. A bite block is commonly used with an oral ET tube to prevent the patient from biting the tube. Arrange for a chest X-ray after intubation to evaluate tube placement. Make sure he has a communication device and a call bell within reach.

Check ABG levels as ordered. Overventilation may cause respiratory alkalosis from decreased carbon dioxide levels. Inadequate alveolar ventilation or atelectasis from an inappropriate tidal volume may cause respiratory acidosis.

Perform the following steps every 1 to 2 hours and as needed:
• Check all connections between the ventilator and the patient. Make sure critical alarms are turned on, such as the low-pressure alarm that indicates a disconnection in the system and is set at not less than 3 cm H_2O and the high-pressure alarm that prevents excessive airway pressures. The high-pressure alarm should be set 20 to 30 cm H_2O greater than the patient's peak airway pressure. Volume alarms should also be used if available. Ensure that the patient can reach his call bell.

Check ABG levels as ordered to detect respiratory alkalosis or acidosis.

Choosing a cycle

• Verify that ventilator settings are correct and that the ventilator is operating at those settings; compare the patient's respiratory rate with the setting and, for a volume-cycled machine, watch that the spirometer reaches the correct volume. For a pressure-cycled machine, use a respirometer to check exhaled tidal volume.
• Check the humidifier and refill it if necessary. Check the corrugated tubing for condensation; drain collected water into a container and discard. Don't drain condensation, which may be contaminated with bacteria, into the humidifier and be careful not to drain condensation into the patient's airway.
• If ordered, give the patient several deep breaths (usually two or three) each hour by setting the sigh mechanism on the ventilator or by using a handheld resuscitation bag.
• Check oxygen concentration every 8 hours and ABG values whenever ventilator settings are changed. Assess respiratory status at least every 2 hours in the acute patient and every 4 hours in the stable chronic patient to detect the need for suctioning and to evaluate the response to treatment. Suction the patient as necessary, noting the amount, color, odor, and consistency of secretions. Auscultate for decreased breath sounds on the left side — an indication of tube slippage into the right mainstem bronchus.

Also perform the following:
• Monitor the patient's fluid intake and output and his electrolyte balance. Weigh him as ordered.
• Using aseptic technique, change the humidifier, nebulizer, and ventilator tubing according to facility protocol.
• Reposition the patient frequently, and perform chest physiotherapy as necessary.

To detect tube slippage in a patient receiving mechanical ventilation, auscultate for decreased breath sounds on the left side of the chest.

No more heartburn

• Provide emotional support to reduce stress, and give antacids and other medications, as ordered, to reduce gastric acid production and to help prevent GI complications.

• Monitor for decreased bowel sounds and abdominal distention, which may indicate paralytic ileus.

• Check nasogastric (NG) aspirate and stools for blood; stress ulcers are a common complication of mechanical ventilation.

• If the patient is receiving high-pressure ventilation, assess for signs of a pneumothorax (absent or diminished breath sounds on the affected side, acute chest pain and, possibly, tracheal deviation or subcutaneous or mediastinal emphysema).

• If he's receiving a high oxygen concentration, watch for signs of toxicity (substernal chest pain, increased coughing, tachypnea, decreased lung compliance and vital capacity, and decreased $Paco_2$ without a change in oxygen concentration).

• If the patient resists mechanical ventilation and ineffective ventilation results, give him a sedative, an antianxiety agent, or a neuromuscular blocking agent, as ordered, and observe him closely.

> If the patient resists mechanical ventilation, give him a sedative, antianxiety agent, or a neuromuscular blocking agent, as ordered.

Home care instructions

If the patient requires a ventilator at home, teach him and a family member:

• how to check the device and its settings for accuracy and the nebulizer and oxygen equipment for proper functioning at least once per day

• to refill his humidifier as necessary

• that his ABG levels will be measured periodically to evaluate his therapy

• how to count his pulse rate and to report changes in rate or rhythm as well as chest pain, fever, dyspnea, or swollen extremities

• to bring his ventilator with him if he needs to be treated for an acute problem because it may be possible to stabilize him without hospitalization but, if hospitalization is required, that he may not be able to use his own ventilator

• to call his doctor or respiratory therapist if he has questions or problems.

Continuous positive airway pressure

As its name suggests, CPAP ventilation maintains positive pressure in the airways throughout the patient's respiratory cycle. Originally delivered only with a ventilator, CPAP may now be de-

Using nasal CPAP

The illustration below shows the continuous positive airway pressure apparatus used to apply positive pressure to the airway to prevent obstruction during inspiration in patients with sleep apnea.

Inlet valve

Positive end-expiratory pressure valve

Oxygen tubing

Inflation valve

livered to intubated or nonintubated patients through an artificial airway, a mask, or nasal prongs by means of a ventilator or a separate high-flow generating system. (See *Using nasal CPAP*.)

Goes with the flows

CPAP is available as a continuous-flow system and a demand system. In the continuous-flow system, an air-oxygen blend flows through a humidifier and a reservoir bag into a T-piece. In the demand system, a valve opens in response to the patient's inspiratory flow.

Other talents

In addition to treating respiratory distress syndrome, CPAP has been used successfully in pulmonary edema, pulmonary emboli, bronchiolitis, fat emboli, pneumonitis, viral pneumonia, and postoperative atelectasis. In mild to moderate cases of these disorders, CPAP provides an alternative to intubation and mechanical ventilation. It increases the functional residual capacity by distending collapsed alveoli, which improves PaO_2 and decreases intrapulmonary shunting and oxygen consumption. It also reduces the work of breathing. CPAP can also be used to wean a patient from mechanical ventilation.

CPAP has successfully treated respiratory distress syndrome, pulmonary edema and emboli, bronchiolitis, and the list goes on. CPAP is my hero!

Through the nose

Nasal CPAP has proved successful as a long-term treatment for obstructive sleep apnea. In this type of CPAP, high-flow compressed air is directed into a mask that covers only the patient's nose. The pressure supplied through the mask serves as a back-pressure splint, preventing the unstable upper airway from collapsing during inspiration.

Not so positive

CPAP may cause gastric distress if the patient swallows air during the treatment (most common when CPAP is delivered without intubation). The patient may feel claustrophobic. Because mask CPAP can also cause nausea and vomiting, it shouldn't be used in patients who are unresponsive or at risk for vomiting and aspiration. Rarely, CPAP causes barotrauma or lowers cardiac output.

Patient preparation

• If the patient is intubated or has a tracheostomy, you can accomplish CPAP with a mechanical ventilator by adjusting the settings. Assess vital signs and breath sounds during CPAP.
• If CPAP is to be delivered through a mask, a respiratory therapist usually sets up the system and fits the mask. The mask should be transparent and lightweight, with a soft, pliable seal. A tight seal isn't required as long as pressure can be maintained. Obtain ABG results and bedside pulmonary function studies to establish a baseline.

Monitoring and aftercare

• Check for decreased cardiac output, which may result from increased intrathoracic pressure associated with CPAP.
• Watch closely for changes in respiratory rate and pattern. Uncoordinated breathing patterns may indicate severe respiratory muscle fatigue that can't be helped by CPAP. Report this to the doctor; the patient may need mechanical ventilation.
• Check the CPAP system for pressure fluctuations.
• Keep in mind that high airway pressures increase the risk of pneumothorax, so monitor for chest pain and decreased breath sounds.
• Use oximetry, if possible, to monitor oxygen saturation, especially when you remove the CPAP mask to provide routine care.
• If the patient is stable, remove his mask briefly every 2 to 4 hours to provide mouth and skin care along with fluids. Don't apply oils or lotions under the mask — they may react with the mask seal material. Increase the length of time the mask is off as the patient's ability to maintain oxygenation without CPAP improves.

Watch closely for uncoordinated breathing patterns that may indicate severe respiratory muscle fatigue that can't be helped by CPAP.

• Check closely for air leaks around the mask near the eyes (an area difficult to seal); escaping air can dry the eyes, causing conjunctivitis or other problems.
• If the patient is using a nasal CPAP device for sleep apnea, observe for decreased snoring and mouth breathing while he sleeps. If these symptoms don't subside, notify the doctor; either the system is leaking or the pressure is inadequate.

Home care instructions

CPAP for sleep apnea is the only treatment requiring instructions for home care.
• Have the patient demonstrate his ability to maintain the prescribed pressures without excess leakage in the system. Teach him how to clean the mask and change the air filter.
• Explain to the patient that he must use nasal CPAP every night, even when feeling better after initial treatments; apneic episodes will recur if CPAP isn't used as directed. He should call his doctor if symptoms recur despite consistent use.
• If the patient is obese, explain that CPAP treatments might be decreased or eliminated with weight loss.

Oxygen therapy

In oxygen therapy, oxygen is delivered by mask, nasal prongs, nasal catheter, or transtracheal catheter to prevent or reverse hypoxemia and reduce the work of breathing. Possible causes of hypoxemia include emphysema, pneumonia, Guillain-Barré syndrome, heart failure, and myocardial infarction (MI).

Fully equipped

Oxygen therapy prevents or reverses hypoxemia and reduces the work of breathing. Thank you!

The equipment depends on the patient's condition and the required fraction of inspired oxygen (FIO_2). High-flow systems, such as a Venturi mask and ventilators, deliver a precisely controlled air-oxygen mixture. Low-flow systems, such as nasal prongs, a nasal catheter, a simple mask, a partial rebreather mask, and a nonrebreather mask, allow variation in the oxygen percentage delivered, based on the patient's respiratory pattern.

Compare and contrast

Nasal prongs deliver oxygen at flow rates from 0.5 to 6 L/minute. Inexpensive and easy to use, the prongs permit talking, eating, and suctioning—interfering less with the patient's activities than other devices. Even so, the prongs may cause nasal drying and can't deliver high oxygen concentrations. In contrast, a nasal catheter can deliver low-flow oxygen at somewhat higher concentrations, but it isn't commonly used because of discomfort and drying of the mucous membranes. Masks deliver up to 100% oxygen concentrations but can't be used to deliver controlled oxygen concentrations. In addition, they may fit poorly causing discomfort and must be removed to eat. Transtracheal oxygen catheters, used for patients requiring chronic oxygen therapy, permit highly efficient oxygen delivery and increased mobility with portable oxygen systems and avoid the adverse effects of nasal delivery systems. Even so, they may become a source of infection and require close monitoring and follow-up after insertion as well as daily maintenance care.

Patient preparation
• Instruct the patient, his roommates, and visitors not to use improperly grounded radios, televisions, electric razors, or other equipment. Place an OXYGEN PRECAUTIONS sign on the outside of the patient's door.
• Perform a cardiopulmonary assessment, and check that baseline ABG or oximetry values have been obtained.
• Check the patency of the patient's nostrils (he may need a mask if they're blocked). Consult the doctor if a change in administration route is necessary.
• Assemble the equipment, check the connections, and turn on the oxygen source. Make sure the humidifier bubbles and oxygen flows through the prongs, catheter, or mask.
• Set the flow rate as ordered. If necessary, have the respiratory care practitioner check the flowmeter for accuracy.

Make sure that baseline ABG or oximetry values have been obtained.

Procedure
• When applying a nasal cannula, direct the curved prongs inward, following the nostrils' natural curvature. Hook the tubing behind the patient's ears and under his chin. Set the flow rate as ordered.
• If you're inserting a nasal catheter, determine the length to insert by stretching one end of the catheter from the tip of the patient's nose to his earlobe. Mark this spot. Then lubricate the catheter with sterile water or water-soluble lubricant and gently insert the catheter through the nostril into the nasopharynx to the premeasured length. Use a flashlight and a tongue blade to check that the catheter is positioned correctly: It should be directly behind the uvula but not beyond it (misdirected airflow may cause gastric distention). If the catheter causes the patient to gag or choke, withdraw it slightly. Secure the catheter by taping it at the nose and cheek and set the flow rate as ordered.

• When applying a mask, make sure the flow rate is at least 5 L/minute. Lower flow rates won't flush carbon dioxide from the mask. Place the mask over the patient's nose, mouth, and chin and press the flexible metal strip so it fits the bridge of the patient's nose. Use gauze padding to ensure comfort and proper fit.

• The partial rebreather mask has an attached reservoir bag that conserves the first portion of the patient's exhalation and fills with 100% oxygen before the next breath. The mask delivers oxygen concentrations ranging from 40% at a flow rate of 8 L/minute to 60% at a flow rate of 15 L/minute and depends on the patient's breathing pattern and rate. The nonrebreather mask also has a reservoir bag and can deliver oxygen concentrations ranging from 60% at a flow rate of 8 L/minute to 90% at a flow rate of 15 L/minute. Set flow rates for these masks as ordered but keep in mind that the reservoir bag should deflate only slightly during inspiration. If it deflates markedly or completely, increase the flow rate until only slight deflation occurs.

If the reservoir bag deflates markedly or completely, increase the flow rate until only slight deflation occurs.

Blocked ports

• The Venturi mask, another alternative, delivers the most precise oxygen concentrations (to within 1% of the setting). When using this mask, make sure its air entrainment ports don't become blocked or the patient's FIO_2 level could rise dangerously. Venturi masks are available with adapters that allow various oxygen concentrations ranging from 24% to 60%. Be sure to adjust oxygen flow to the rate indicated on the adapter.

• If a transtracheal oxygen catheter will be used to deliver oxygen, the doctor will give the patient a local anesthetic before inserting this device into the patient's trachea.

Monitoring and aftercare

• Periodically perform a cardiopulmonary assessment on the patient receiving any form of oxygen therapy.

• If the patient is on bed rest, change his position frequently to ensure adequate ventilation and circulation.

Don't neglect the skin

• Provide good skin care to prevent irritation and breakdown caused by the tubing, prongs, or mask.

• Be sure to humidify oxygen flow exceeding 3 L/minute to help prevent drying of mucous membranes. However, humidity isn't added with Venturi masks, because water can block the Venturi jets.

• Assess for signs of hypoxia, including decreased level of consciousness (LOC), tachycardia, arrhythmias, diaphoresis, restlessness, altered blood pressure or respiratory rate, clammy skin, and cyanosis. If these occur, notify the doctor, obtain a pulse oximetry reading, and check the oxygen delivery equipment to see if it's malfunctioning. Be especially alert for changes in respiratory status when you change or discontinue oxygen therapy.

• If your patient is using a nonrebreather mask, periodically check the valves to see if they're functioning properly. If the valves stick closed, the patient is reinhaling carbon dioxide and not receiving adequate oxygen. Replace the mask if necessary.

• If the patient receives high oxygen concentrations (exceeding 50%) for more than 24 hours, ask about symptoms of oxygen toxicity, such as burning, substernal chest pain, dyspnea, and dry cough. Atelectasis and pulmonary edema may also occur. Encourage coughing and deep breathing to help prevent atelectasis. Monitor ABG levels frequently and reduce oxygen concentrations as soon as ABG results indicate this is feasible.

• Use a low flow rate if your patient has chronic pulmonary disease. However, don't use a simple face mask because low flow rates won't flush carbon dioxide from the mask, and the patient will rebreathe carbon dioxide. Watch for alterations in LOC, heart rate, and respiratory rate, which may signal carbon dioxide narcosis or worsening hypoxemia.

If the valves of the nonrebreather mask stick, I get more carbon dioxide instead of the oxygen I need.

Home care instructions

If the patient needs oxygen at home, the doctor will order the flow rate, the number of hours per day to be used, and the conditions of use. Several types of delivery systems are available, including a tank, concentrator, and liquid oxygen system. Choose the system based on the patient's needs and the system's availability and cost. Make sure the patient can use the prescribed system safely and effectively. He'll need regular follow-up care to evaluate his response to therapy.

Chest physiotherapy

Chest physiotherapy is usually performed with other treatments, such as suctioning, incentive spirometry, and administration of such medications as small-volume nebulizer aerosol treatments and expectorants. (See *Types of chest physiotherapy.*) Recent studies indicate that percussional vibration isn't an effective treatment for most diseases; exceptions include cystic fibrosis and bronchiectasis. Improved breath sounds, increased Pao_2, sputum production, and improved airflow suggest successful treatment.

Patient preparation

• Administer pain medication before the treatment as ordered, and teach the patient to splint his incision.

Performing chest physiotherapy

Chest physiotherapy may be performed using postural drainage, percussion, or vibration. Outlined below is the procedure for each method.

Postural drainage
• Position the patient as ordered. (The doctor usually determines a position sequence after auscultation and chest X-ray review.) Be sure to position the patient so drainage is always oriented toward larger, more central airways.
• If the patient has a localized condition, such as pneumonia in a specific lobe, expect to start with that area first to avoid infecting uninvolved areas. If the patient has a diffuse disorder, such as bronchiectasis, expect to start with the lower lobes and work toward the upper ones.

Percussion
• Place your cupped hands against the patient's chest wall and rapidly flex and extend your wrists, generating a rhythmic, popping sound (a hollow sound helps verify correct performance of the technique).
• Percuss each segment for a minimum of 3 minutes. The vibrations you generate pass through the chest wall and help loosen secretions from the airways.

• Perform percussion throughout inspiration and expiration and encourage the patient to take slow, deep breaths.
• Don't percuss over the spine, sternum, liver, kidneys, or the female patient's breasts because you may cause trauma, especially in elderly patients.
• Percussion is painless when done properly, and the impact is diminished by a cushion of air formed in the cupped palm. This technique requires practice.

Vibration
• Ask the patient to inhale deeply and then exhale slowly through pursed lips.
• During exhalation, firmly press your fingers and the palms of your hands against the chest wall. Tense the muscles of your arms and shoulders in an isometric contraction to send fine vibrations through the chest wall.
• Repeat vibration for five exhalations over each chest segment.
• When the patient says "ah" on exhalation, you should hear a tremble in his voice.

Types of chest physiotherapy

Especially important for the bedridden patient, chest physiotherapy improves secretion clearance and ventilation and helps prevent or treat atelectasis and pneumonia. Procedures include:
• postural drainage, which uses gravity to promote drainage of secretions from the lungs and bronchi into the trachea
• percussion, which involves cupping the hands and fingers together and clapping them alternately over the patient's lung fields to loosen secretions (also achieved with the gentler technique of vibration)
• vibration, which can be used with percussion or as an alternative to it in a patient who's frail, in pain, or recovering from thoracic surgery or trauma
• deep-breathing exercises, which help loosen secretions and promote more effective coughing
• coughing, which helps clear the lungs, bronchi, and trachea of secretions and prevents aspiration.

• Auscultate the lungs to determine baseline status, and check the doctor's order to determine which lung areas require treatment.
• Obtain pillows and a tilt board if necessary.
• Don't schedule therapy immediately after a meal; wait 2 to 3 hours to reduce the risk of nausea and vomiting.
• Make sure the patient is adequately hydrated to facilitate removal of secretions.
• If ordered, administer bronchodilator and mist therapies before the treatment.
• Provide tissues, an emesis basin, and a cup for sputum.
• Set up suction equipment if the patient doesn't have an adequate cough to clear secretions.
• If he needs oxygen therapy or is borderline hypoxemic without it, provide adequate flow rates of oxygen during therapy. (See *Performing chest physiotherapy*.)

Monitoring and aftercare

• Evaluate the patient's tolerance for therapy and make adjustments as needed. Watch for fatigue and remember that the patient's ability to cough and breathe deeply diminishes as he tires.
• Assess for difficulty expectorating secretions. Use suction if the patient has an ineffective cough or a diminished gag reflex.
• Provide oral hygiene after therapy; secretions may taste foul or have an unpleasant odor.
• Be aware that postural drainage positions can cause nausea, dizziness, dyspnea, and hypoxemia.

Home care instructions

• The patient with chronic bronchitis, bronchiectasis, or cystic fibrosis may need chest physiotherapy at home.
• Teach him and his family the appropriate techniques and positions.
• Arrange for the patient to get a mechanical percussion and vibration device if necessary.

Be aware that postural drainage positions can cause nausea, dizziness, dyspnea, and hypoxemia.

Nursing diagnoses

After completing your assessment, you're ready to analyze the findings and select nursing diagnoses. Below you'll find nursing diagnoses commonly used in patients with respiratory problems. For each diagnosis, you'll also find nursing interventions along with rationales.

Ineffective breathing pattern

Related to decreased energy or increased fatigue, *Ineffective breathing pattern* is commonly associated with such conditions as COPD and pulmonary embolus.

Expected outcomes

• Patient reports feeling comfortable when breathing.
• Patient achieves maximum lung expansion with adequate ventilation.
• Patient's respiratory rate remains within 5 breaths/minute of baseline.

Nursing interventions and rationales

• Auscultate breath sounds at least every 4 hours to detect decreased or adventitious breath sounds.
• Assess adequacy of ventilation to detect early signs of respiratory compromise.
• Teach breathing techniques to help the patient improve ventilation.
• Teach relaxation techniques to help reduce the patient's anxiety and enhance his feeling of self-control.
• Administer bronchodilators to help relieve bronchospasm and wheezing.
• Administer oxygen as ordered to help relieve hypoxemia and respiratory distress.

Ineffective airway clearance

Related to the presence of tracheobronchial secretions or obstruction, *Ineffective airway clearance* commonly accompanies such conditions as asthma, COPD, interstitial lung disease, cystic fibrosis, and pneumonia.

Ineffective airway clearance is related to the presence of tracheobronchial secretions or obstruction.

Expected outcomes

• Patient coughs effectively.
• Patient's airway remains patent.
• Adventitious breath sounds are absent.

Nursing interventions and rationales

• Teach coughing techniques to promote chest expansion and ventilation, enhance clearance of secretions from airways, and involve the patient in his own care.
• Perform postural drainage, percussion, and vibration to facilitate secretion movement.
• Encourage fluids to ensure adequate hydration and liquefy secretions.
• Give expectorants and mucolytics as ordered to enhance airway clearance.
• Provide an artificial airway as needed to maintain airway patency.

Impaired gas exchange

Related to altered oxygen supply or oxygen-carrying capacity of the blood, *Impaired gas exchange* can be associated with acute respiratory failure (ARF), COPD, pneumonia, pulmonary embolism, and other respiratory problems.

Expected outcomes

- Patient's respiratory rate remains within 5 breaths/minute of baseline.
- Patient has normal breath sounds.
- Patient's ABG levels return to baseline.

Nursing interventions and rationales

- Give antibiotics, as ordered, and monitor their effectiveness in treating infection and improving alveolar expansion.
- Teach deep breathing and incentive spirometry to enhance lung expansion and ventilation.
- Monitor ABG values and notify the doctor immediately if Pao_2 drops or $Paco_2$ rises. If needed, start mechanical ventilation to improve ventilation.
- Provide CPAP or positive end-expiratory pressure (PEEP) as needed to improve the driving pressure of oxygen across the alveolocapillary membrane, enhance arterial blood oxygenation, and increase lung compliance.

Monitor ABG values and notify the doctor immediately if Pao_2 drops or $Paco_2$ rises.

Common respiratory disorders

Below are several common respiratory disorders, along with their causes, pathophysiology, signs and symptoms, diagnostic test findings, treatments, and nursing interventions.

Acute respiratory distress syndrome

A form of pulmonary edema that leads to ARF, acute respiratory distress syndrome (ARDS) results from increased permeability of the alveolocapillary membrane. Although severe ARDS may be fatal, recovering patients may have little or no permanent lung damage.

What causes it

ARDS may result from:
- aspiration of gastric contents
- sepsis (primarily gram-negative)
- trauma (such as lung contusion, head injury, and long-bone fracture with fat emboli)

It says here that patients who recover from ARDS will have little or no permanent lung damage. Well, that's just spiffy!

Med-Surg Nursing made Incredibly E-Z

- oxygen toxicity
- viral, bacterial, or fungal pneumonia
- microemboli (fat or air emboli or disseminated intravascular coagulation)
- drug overdose (such as barbiturates, glutethimide, and narcotics)
- blood transfusion
- smoke or chemical inhalation (such as nitrous oxide, chlorine, ammonia, and organophosphate)
- hydrocarbon or paraquat ingestion
- pancreatitis, uremia, or miliary TB (rare)
- near drowning.

Pathophysiology

In ARDS, fluid accumulates in the lung interstitium, alveolar spaces, and small airways, causing the lung to stiffen. This impairs ventilation and reduces oxygenation of pulmonary capillary blood. (See *What happens in ARDS*, page 375.)

What to look for

Assess your patient for the following signs and symptoms:
- rapid, shallow breathing; dyspnea; hypoxemia
- tachycardia
- intercostal and suprasternal retractions, crackles, and rhonchi
- restlessness, apprehension, mental sluggishness, motor dysfunction.

What tests tell you

- ABG values on room air show decreased PaO_2 (less than 60 mm Hg) and $PaCO_2$ (less than 35 mm Hg). As ARDS becomes more severe, ABG values show respiratory acidosis, with $PaCO_2$ values elevated above 45 mm Hg. Metabolic acidosis is also present, with HCO_3^- values below 22 mEq/L. The patient's PaO_2 decreases despite oxygen therapy.
- Pulmonary artery catheterization helps identify the cause of pulmonary edema by evaluating pulmonary artery wedge pressure; allows collection of pulmonary artery blood, which shows decreased oxygen saturation a sign of tissue hypoxia; measures pulmonary artery pressure; and measures cardiac output by thermodilution techniques.
- Serial chest X-rays initially show bilateral infiltrates. In later stages, the X-rays have a ground-glass appearance and, as hypoxemia becomes irreversible, "whiteouts" are seen in both lung fields.

• Other tests may be done to detect infections, drug ingestion, or pancreatitis.

How it's treated

Treatment aims to correct the underlying cause of ARDS to prevent its progression toward potentially fatal complications. Supportive medical care includes humidified oxygen through a tight-fitting mask, allowing the use of CPAP. When hypoxemia doesn't respond to these measures, patients require ventilatory support with intubation, volume ventilation, and PEEP. Other supportive measures include fluid restriction, diuretics, and correction of electrolyte and acid-base abnormalities.

Anxiety control

Patients who receive mechanical ventilation commonly require sedatives and narcotics or neuromuscular blocking agents, such as vecuronium and pancuronium, to minimize anxiety. Decreasing anxiety enhances ventilation by reducing oxygen consumption and carbon dioxide production. If given early, a short course of high-dose steroids may be beneficial to patients with ARDS that results from fat emboli or chemical injury to the lungs. Treatment with sodium bicarbonate may be necessary to reverse severe metabolic acidosis. Fluids and vasopressors are administered to maintain the patient's blood pressure. Nonviral infections require antimicrobial drugs.

What to do

ARDS requires careful monitoring and supportive care. To prepare your patient for transfer to an ICU, do the following:
• Frequently assess the patient's respiratory status. Be alert for retractions on inspiration. Note the rate, rhythm, and depth of respirations and watch for dyspnea and the use of accessory muscles of respiration. On auscultation, listen for adventitious or diminished breath sounds. Check for pink, frothy sputum, which may indicate pulmonary edema.
• Observe and document the hypoxemic patient's neurologic status. Assess his LOC and observe for mental sluggishness.
• Maintain a patent airway by suctioning the patient as needed.
• Closely monitor heart rate and rhythm and blood pressure.
• Reposition the patient often and observe for hypotension, increased secretions, or elevated body temperature—all signs of deterioration.
• Evaluate the patient. After successful treatment, he should have normal ABG values, a normal respiratory rate, depth, and pattern, and clear breath sounds. (See *Teaching the patient with ARDS*.)

Education edge

Teaching the patient with ARDS

• Provide emotional support. Advise the patient with acute respiratory distress syndrome (ARDS) that recovery will take some time with a gradual return to strength.
• If the patient requires mechanical ventilation, provide him with an alternate means of communication.

A closer look

What happens in ARDS

The illustrations below show the development of acute respiratory distress syndrome (ARDS).

Injury reduces normal blood flow to the lungs, allowing platelets to aggregate. These platelets release substances, such as serotonin (S), bradykinin (B), and histamine (H), that inflame and damage the alveolar membrane and later increase capillary permeability.

As capillary permeability increases, proteins and more fluid leak out, causing pulmonary edema.

The patient breathes faster, but sufficient oxygen (O_2) can't cross the alveolar capillary membrane. Carbon dioxide (CO_2), however, crosses more easily and is lost with every exhalation. Both O_2 and CO_2 levels in the blood decrease.

Histamines (H) and other inflammatory substances increase capillary permeability. Fluids shift into the interstitial space.

Fluid in the alveoli and decreased blood flow damage surfactant in the alveoli. This reduces the alveolar cells' ability to produce more surfactant. Without surfactant, alveoli collapse, impairing gas exchange.

Pulmonary edema worsens. Meanwhile, inflammation leads to fibrosis, which further impedes gas exchange. The resulting hypoxemia leads to respiratory acidosis.

Acute respiratory failure

ARF occurs when the lungs no longer meet the body's metabolic needs. In patients with essentially normal lung tissue, ARF usually means $Paco_2$ above 50 mm Hg and Pao_2 below 50 mm Hg. These limits, however, don't apply to patients with COPD, who commonly have a consistently high $Paco_2$ and low Pao_2. In patients with COPD, only acute deterioration in ABG values, with corresponding clinical deterioration, indicates ARF.

What causes it

ARF may develop from any condition that increases the work of breathing and decreases the respiratory drive. Respiratory tract infections, such as bronchitis and pneumonia, are the most common precipitating factors but bronchospasm or accumulated secretions due to cough suppression can also lead to ARF. Other causes of ARF include:
• CNS depression—head trauma or injudicious use of sedatives, narcotics, tranquilizers, or oxygen
• cardiovascular disorders—MI, heart failure, or pulmonary emboli
• airway irritants—smoke or fumes
• endocrine and metabolic disorders—myxedema or metabolic alkalosis
• thoracic abnormalities—chest trauma, pneumothorax, or thoracic or abdominal surgery.

Pathophysiology

Respiratory failure results from impaired gas exchange, when the lungs don't oxygenate the blood adequately and fail to prevent carbon dioxide retention. Any condition associated with hypoventilation (a reduction in the volume of air moving into and out of the lung), $\dot{V}/\dot{Q}$ mismatch (too little ventilation with normal blood flow or too little blood flow with normal ventilation), or intrapulmonary shunting (right-to-left shunting in which blood passes from the heart's right side to its left without being oxygenated) can cause ARF if left untreated.

What to look for

Patients with ARF experience hypoxemia and acidemia affecting all body organs, especially the central nervous, respiratory, and cardiovascular systems. Although specific symptoms vary with the underlying cause, you should always assess for:
• altered respirations (increased, decreased, or normal rate; shallow, deep, or alternating shallow and deep respirations; possible

How about that! Respiratory tract infections are the most common precipitating factor in ARF.

cyanosis; crackles, rhonchi, wheezes, or diminished breath sounds on chest auscultation)
• altered mentation (restlessness, confusion, loss of concentration, irritability, tremulousness, diminished tendon reflexes, or papilledema)
• cardiac arrhythmias (from myocardial hypoxia)
• tachycardia (occurs early in response to low Pao_2)
• pulmonary hypertension (increased pressures on the right side of the heart, elevated neck veins, enlarged liver, and peripheral edema).

What tests tell you

Progressive deterioration in ABG levels and pH, when compared with the patient's baseline values, strongly suggests ARF. (In patients with essentially normal lung tissue, a pH value below 7.35 usually indicates ARF. However, COPD patients display an even greater deviation in pH values, along with deviations in $Paco_2$ and Pao_2.) Other findings include:
• HCO_3^- level—increased in metabolic alkalosis or from metabolic compensation for chronic respiratory acidosis
• hematocrit and Hb levels—abnormally low possibly from blood loss, indicating decreased oxygen-carrying capacity
• serum electrolyte levels—hypokalemia possibly from compensatory hyperventilation (an attempt to correct alkalosis) and hypochloremia, which is common in metabolic alkalosis
• white blood cell (WBC) count—elevated if ARF results from bacterial infection (pathogens identified using Gram stain and sputum culture)
• chest X-ray—pulmonary abnormalities, such as emphysema, atelectasis, lesions, pneumothorax, infiltrates, and effusions
• electrocardiogram (ECG)—arrhythmias, which commonly suggest cor pulmonale and myocardial hypoxia.

How it's treated

In COPD patients, ARF is an emergency requiring cautious oxygen therapy (using nasal prongs or a Venturi mask) to raise the patient's Pao_2. If significant respiratory acidosis persists, mechanical ventilation through an ET or a tracheostomy tube may be necessary. HFV may be used if the patient doesn't respond to conventional mechanical ventilation. Prone positioning may also prove beneficial. Treatment routinely includes antibiotics for infection, bronchodilators and, possibly, steroids.

Progressive deterioration in ABG levels and pH strongly suggests ARF.

What to do

ARF requires close attention to airway patency and oxygen supply. Follow these steps:

• To reverse hypoxemia, administer oxygen at appropriate concentrations to maintain PaO_2 at a minimum of 50 mm Hg. Patients with COPD usually require only small amounts of supplemental oxygen. Watch for a positive response, such as improvement in ABG results and the patient's breathing and color.

• Maintain a patent airway. If the patient is intubated and lethargic, turn him every 1 to 2 hours. Use postural drainage and chest physiotherapy to help clear secretions.

• In an intubated patient, suction the airways as required, after hyperoxygenation. Observe for changes in quantity, consistency, and color of sputum. To prevent aspiration and reduce the risk of ventilator-associated pneumonia, always suction the oropharynx and the area above the cuff of the ET tube before deflating the cuff. Provide humidity to liquefy secretions.

• Observe the patient closely for respiratory arrest. Auscultate for breath sounds. Monitor ABG levels and report any changes immediately.

Balancing fluids

• Monitor serum electrolyte levels and correct imbalances; monitor fluid balance by recording fluid intake and output and daily weight.

• Check the cardiac monitor for arrhythmias.

• If the patient requires mechanical ventilation and is unstable he'll probably be transferred to an intensive care unit (ICU). Arrange for his safe transfer.

• If the patient isn't on mechanical ventilation and is retaining carbon dioxide, encourage him to cough and breathe deeply with pursed lips. If the patient is alert, teach and encourage him to use an incentive spirometer.

• Evaluate the patient. Make sure that ABG values are normal, with a PaO_2 greater than 50 mm Hg, and that the patient can make a normal respiratory effort. (See *Teaching the patient with ARF.*)

Education edge

Teaching the patient with ARF

• If the patient isn't on mechanical ventilation and is retaining carbon dioxide, encourage him to cough and breathe deeply with pursed lips.

• If the patient is alert, teach and encourage him to use an incentive spirometer.

Atelectasis

Atelectasis (collapsed or airless condition of all or part of the lung) may be chronic or acute and commonly occurs to some degree in patients undergoing abdominal or thoracic surgery. The prognosis depends on prompt removal of airway obstruction, relief of hypoxia, and reexpansion of the collapsed lobules or lung.

What causes it

Atelectasis may result from:
• bronchial occlusion by mucus plugs (a common problem in heavy smokers or people with COPD, bronchiectasis, or cystic fibrosis)
• occlusion by foreign bodies
• bronchogenic carcinoma
• inflammatory lung disease
• oxygen toxicity
• pulmonary edema
• any condition that inhibits full lung expansion or makes deep breathing painful, such as abdominal surgical incisions, rib fractures, tight dressings, and obesity
• prolonged immobility
• mechanical ventilation using constant small tidal volumes without intermittent deep breaths
• CNS depression (as in drug overdose), which eliminates periodic sighing.

Atelectasis may be caused by bronchial occlusion, a common problem in heavy smokers. So, ixnay on the okingsmay!

Pathophysiology

In atelectasis, incomplete expansion of lobules (clusters of alveoli) or lung segments leads to partial or complete lung collapse. Because parts of the lung are unavailable for gas exchange, unoxygenated blood passes through these areas unchanged, resulting in hypoxemia.

What to look for

Your assessment findings will vary with the cause and degree of hypoxia and may include:
• dyspnea (possibly mild and subsiding without treatment if atelectasis involves only a small area of the lung or severe if massive collapse occurs)
• cyanosis, decreased breath sounds
• anxiety, diaphoresis
• dull sound on percussion if a large portion of the lung is collapsed
• hypoxemia, tachycardia
• substernal or intercostal retraction
• compensatory hyperinflation of unaffected areas of the lung
• mediastinal shift to the affected side.

What tests tell you

• Chest X-ray shows characteristic horizontal lines in the lower lung zones. Dense shadows accompany segmental or lobar collapse and are commonly associated with hyperinflation of neigh-

boring lung zones during widespread atelectasis. However, extensive areas of "micro-atelectasis" may exist without showing abnormalities on the patient's chest X-ray.
• When the cause of atelectasis is unknown, bronchoscopy may be performed to rule out an obstructing neoplasm or a foreign body.

How it's treated

Atelectasis is treated with incentive spirometry, chest percussion, postural drainage, and frequent coughing and deep-breathing exercises. If these measures fail, bronchoscopy may help remove secretions. Humidity and bronchodilators can improve mucociliary clearance and dilate airways and are sometimes used with a nebulizer. Atelectasis secondary to an obstructing neoplasm may require surgery or radiation therapy.

What to do

Your goal is to keep the patient's airways clear and relieve hypoxia. To achieve this, follow these guidelines:
• To prevent atelectasis, encourage the patient to cough, turn, and breathe deeply every 1 to 2 hours as ordered. Teach the patient to splint his incision when coughing. Gently reposition a postoperative patient often and help him walk as soon as possible. Administer adequate analgesics to control pain.
• During mechanical ventilation, tidal volume should be maintained at 10 to 15 ml/kg of the patient's body weight to ensure adequate lung expansion. Use the sigh mechanism on the ventilator, if appropriate, to intermittently increase tidal volume at the rate of three to four sighs per hour.
• Humidify inspired air and encourage adequate fluid intake to mobilize secretions. Loosen and clear secretions with postural drainage and chest percussion.
• Assess breath sounds and ventilatory status frequently and report any changes.
• Evaluate the patient. Secretions should be clear and the patient should show no signs of hypoxia. (See *Teaching the patient with atelectasis.*)

Bronchiectasis

An irreversible condition marked by chronic abnormal dilation of bronchi and destruction of bronchial walls, bronchiectasis can occur throughout the tracheobronchial tree or can be confined to one segment or lobe. However, it's usually bilateral, involving the basilar segments of the lower lobes. It affects people of both sexes and all ages.

What causes it

Bronchiectasis may be caused by such conditions as:
• mucoviscidosis (cystic fibrosis of the pancreas)
• immunologic disorders such as agammaglobulinemia
• recurrent, inadequately treated bacterial respiratory tract infections such as TB
• measles, pneumonia, pertussis, or influenza
• obstruction by a foreign body, tumor, or stenosis associated with recurrent infection
• inhalation of corrosive gas or repeated aspiration of gastric juices into the lungs.

Pathophysiology

Bronchiectasis results from repeated damage of bronchial walls and abnormal mucociliary clearance that causes breakdown of supportive tissue adjacent to the airways. This disease has three forms: cylindrical (fusiform), varicose, and saccular (cystic). (See *Forms of bronchiectasis*, page 382.)

What to look for

Initially, bronchiectasis may not produce symptoms. Assess your patient for a chronic cough that produces copious, foul-smelling, mucopurulent secretions, possibly totaling several cupfuls daily (classic symptom). Other characteristic findings include:
• coarse crackles during inspiration over involved lobes or segments
• occasional wheezes
• dyspnea
• weight loss, malaise
• clubbing
• recurrent fever, chills, and other signs of infection.

What tests tell you

In addition to aiding diagnosis, the following tests also help determine the physiologic severity of the disease and the effects of therapy and help evaluate the patient for surgery:
• Bronchography is the most reliable diagnostic test and reveals the location and extent of disease.
• Chest X-rays show peribronchial thickening, areas of atelectasis, and scattered cystic changes.
• Bronchoscopy helps identify the source of secretions or the site of bleeding in hemoptysis.
• Sputum culture and Gram stain identify predominant organisms.

Watch for chronic cough that produces up to several cupfuls of foul-smelling, mucopurulent secretions. Suddenly, I'm no longer thirsty.

Forms of bronchiectasis

The different forms of bronchiectasis may occur separately or simultaneously. In cylindrical bronchiectasis, the bronchi expand unevenly, with little change in diameter, and end suddenly in a squared-off fashion. In varicose bronchiectasis, abnormal, irregular dilation and narrowing of the bronchi give the appearance of varicose veins. In saccular bronchiectasis, many large dilations end in sacs. These sacs balloon into pus-filled cavities as they approach the periphery and are then called saccules.

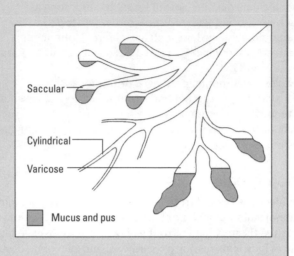

Saccular

Cylindrical

Varicose

Mucus and pus

• Complete blood count and WBC differential identify anemia and leukocytosis.
• PFTs detect decreased vital capacity and decreased expiratory flow.
• ABG analysis shows hypoxemia.

How it's treated

Treatment for bronchiectasis includes:
• antibiotics given by mouth or I.V. for 7 to 10 days or until sputum production decreases
• bronchodilators, with postural drainage and chest percussion, to help remove secretions if the patient has bronchospasm and thick, tenacious sputum
• bronchoscopy used occasionally to aid removal of secretions
• oxygen therapy for hypoxemia
• lobectomy or segmental resection for severe hemoptysis.

What to do

• Provide a warm, quiet, comfortable environment and urge the patient to rest as much as possible.
• Administer antibiotics as ordered.
• Perform chest physiotherapy several times per day (early morning and bedtime are best); include postural drainage and chest percussion for involved lobes. Have the patient maintain each position for 10 minutes; then perform percussion and tell him to cough.

Treatment includes antibiotics and bronchoscopy. Also, encourage plenty of fluids to aid expectoration.

• Encourage balanced, high-protein meals to promote good health and tissue healing and plenty of fluids to aid expectoration.
• Provide frequent mouth care to remove foul-smelling sputum.
• Evaluate the patient. His secretions should be thin and clear or white. (See *Teaching the patient with bronchiectasis*.)

Chronic obstructive pulmonary disease

COPD is an umbrella term that could refer to emphysema, chronic bronchitis, asthma and, more commonly, any combination of these conditions (usually bronchitis and emphysema). The most common chronic lung disease, COPD affects an estimated 30 million Americans, and its incidence is rising. It now ranks third among the major causes of death in the United States. The disorder affects more men than women, probably because until recently men were more likely to smoke heavily. However, the rate of COPD among women is increasing. Early COPD may not produce symptoms and may cause only minimal disability in many patients, but it tends to worsen with time.

What causes it

COPD may be caused by:
• cigarette smoking
• recurrent or chronic respiratory tract infection
• allergies
• familial and hereditary factors such as alpha$_1$-antitrypsin deficiency.

Pathophysiology

Smoking, one of the major causes of COPD, impairs ciliary action and macrophage function and causes inflammation in the airways, increased mucus production, destruction of alveolar septa, and peribronchiolar fibrosis. Early inflammatory changes may reverse if the patient stops smoking before lung disease becomes extensive.

The mucus plugs and narrowed airways cause air trapping, as in chronic bronchitis and emphysema. Hyperinflation of the alveoli occurs on expiration. On inspiration, airways enlarge, allowing air to pass beyond the obstruction; on expiration, airways narrow and gas flow is prevented. Air trapping (also called ball valving) occurs commonly in asthma and chronic bronchitis.

Education edge

Teaching the patient with bronchiectasis

• Explain all diagnostic tests.
• Show family members how to perform postural drainage and percussion. Also, teach the patient coughing and deep-breathing techniques to promote good ventilation and the removal of secretions.
• Advise the patient to stop smoking, which stimulates secretions and irritates the airways. Refer the patient to a local self-help group.
• Teach the patient to properly dispose of secretions.
• Tell the patient to avoid air pollutants and people with upper respiratory tract infections. Instruct him to take medications (especially antibiotics) exactly as ordered.
• To help prevent this disease, vigorously treat bacterial pneumonia and stress the need for immunization to prevent childhood diseases.

What to look for

The typical COPD patient is asymptomatic until middle age, when the following signs and symptoms may occur:
• reduced ability to exercise or do strenuous work
• productive cough
• dyspnea with minimal exertion.

What tests tell you

For specific diagnostic tests used to determine COPD, see *Types of COPD*, pages 386 to 389.

How it's treated

Treatment for COPD aims to relieve symptoms and prevent complications. Most patients receive beta-agonist bronchodilators (albuterol or salmeterol), anticholinergic bronchodilators (ipratropium), and corticosteroids (beclomethasone or triamcinolone). These drugs are usually given by metered dose inhaler.

What to do

• Administer antibiotics, as ordered, to treat respiratory tract infections.
• Administer low concentrations of oxygen as ordered.
• Check ABG levels regularly to determine oxygen need and to avoid carbon dioxide narcosis.
• Evaluate the patient. The patient's chest X-rays, respiratory rate and rhythm, ABG values, and pH should be normal. PaO_2 should be greater than 60 mm Hg. Body weight and urine output should also be normal. (See *Teaching the patient with COPD*.)

Pleural effusion

Pleural effusion is an excess of fluid in the pleural space. Normally this space contains a small amount of extracellular fluid that lubricates the pleural surfaces. Increased production or inadequate removal of this fluid results in transudative or exudative pleural effusion. Empyema is the accumulation of pus and necrotic tissue in the pleural space.

What causes it

Transudative pleural effusion can stem from:
• heart failure
• hepatic disease with ascites

Education edge

Teaching the patient with COPD

• Urge the patient to stop smoking and to avoid other respiratory irritants. Suggest that an air conditioner with an air filter may prove helpful.
• Explain that bronchodilators alleviate bronchospasm and enhance mucociliary clearance of secretions. Familiarize the patient with prescribed bronchodilators. Teach or reinforce the correct method of using an inhaler.
• To strengthen the muscles of respiration, teach the patient to take slow, deep breaths and exhale through pursed lips.
• Teach the patient how to cough effectively to help mobilize secretions. If secretions are thick, urge the patient to drink 12 to 15 glasses of fluid per day.
• If the patient is to continue oxygen therapy at home, teach him how to use the equipment correctly.

- peritoneal dialysis
- hypoalbuminemia
- disorders resulting in overexpanded intravascular volume.
  Exudative pleural effusion can stem from:
- TB
- subphrenic abscess
- esophageal rupture
- pancreatitis
- bacterial or fungal pneumonitis or empyema
- cancer
- pulmonary embolism with or without infarction
- collagen disorders (such as lupus erythematosus and rheumatoid arthritis)
- myxedema
- chest trauma.

Pathophysiology

In transudative pleural effusion, excessive hydrostatic pressure or decreased osmotic pressure allows excessive fluid to pass across intact capillaries, resulting in an ultrafiltrate of plasma containing low concentrations of protein. In exudative pleural effusion, capillaries exhibit increased permeability, with or without changes in hydrostatic and colloid osmotic pressures, allowing protein-rich fluid to leak into the pleural space. Empyema is usually associated with infection in the pleural space.

What to look for

Assess your patient for the following signs and symptoms:
- dyspnea, dry cough
- pleural friction rub
- possible pleuritic pain that worsens with coughing or deep breathing
- dullness on percussion
- tachycardia, tachypnea
- decreased chest motion and breath sounds.

What tests tell you

Examination of pleural fluid obtained by thoracentesis reveals the following:
- In transudative effusions, specific gravity is usually less than 1.015 and protein less than 3 g/dl.
- In exudative effusions, specific gravity is greater than 1.02, and the ratio of protein in pleural fluid to serum is equal to or greater than 0.5. Pleural fluid lactate dehydrogenase (LD) is equal to or

Assess your patient for decreased breath sounds, a sign of pleural effusion.

(Text continues on page 388.)

Types of COPD

The chart below lists the types of chronic obstructive pulmonary disease (COPD) along with their causes, pathophysiology, clinical features, confirming diagnostic measures, and management.

Disease	Causes and pathophysiology	Clinical features
Emphysema • Abnormal, irreversible enlargement of air spaces distal to terminal bronchioles due to destruction of alveolar walls, resulting in decreased elastic recoil properties of lungs • Most common cause of death from respiratory disease in the United States	• Cigarette smoking and congenital deficiency of alpha$_1$-antitrypsin • Recurrent inflammation associated with release of proteolytic enzymes from cells in lungs that causes bronchiolar and alveolar wall damage and, ultimately, destruction; decreased elastic recoil and airway collapse on expiration due to loss of lung supporting structure; decreased surface area for gas exchange due to alveolar wall destruction	• Insidious onset, with dyspnea the predominant symptom • *Other signs and symptoms of long-term disease:* anorexia, weight loss, malaise, barrel chest, use of accessory muscles of respiration, prolonged expiratory period with grunting, pursed-lip breathing, and tachypnea • *Complications:* recurrent respiratory tract infections, cor pulmonale, respiratory failure
Chronic bronchitis • Excessive mucus production with productive cough for at least 3 months per year for 2 successive years • Development of significant airway obstruction in only a minority of patients with the clinical syndrome of chronic bronchitis	• Severity of disease related to amount and duration of smoking; symptoms exacerbated by respiratory infection • Hypertrophy and hyperplasia of bronchial mucous glands, increased goblet cells, damage to cilia, squamous metaplasia of columnar epithelium, and chronic leukocytic and lymphocytic infiltration of bronchial walls; resistance in small airways and severe ventilation-perfusion imbalance due to widespread inflammation, distortion, narrowing of airways, and mucus within the airways	• Insidious onset, with productive cough and exertional dyspnea predominant symptoms • *Other signs and symptoms:* colds associated with increased sputum production and worsening dyspnea, which take progressively longer to resolve; copious sputum (gray, white, or yellow); weight gain due to edema; cyanosis; tachypnea; wheezing; prolonged expiratory time; use of accessory muscles of respiration
Asthma • Increased bronchial reactivity to various stimuli, which produces episodic bronchospasm and airway obstruction in conjunction with airway inflammation	• Possibly caused by allergy (family tendency and seasonal occurrence); release of mast cell vasoactive and bronchospastic mediators in response to allergic reaction • Attack possibly caused by upper airway infection, exercise, anxiety or, rarely, coughing or laughing; commonly accompanied by nocturnal flare-ups	• History of intermittent attacks of dyspnea and wheezing • Mild wheezing progressing to severe dyspnea, audible wheezing, chest tightness (a feeling of not being able to breathe), and cough producing thick mucus

Confirming diagnostic measures	Management
• *Physical examination:* hyperresonance on percussion, decreased breath sounds, expiratory prolongation, and quiet heart sounds • *Chest X-ray:* in advanced disease, flattened diaphragm, reduced vascular markings at lung periphery, hyperinflation of lungs, vertical heart, enlarged anteroposterior chest diameter, large retrosternal air space • *Pulmonary function tests:* increased residual volume, total lung capacity, and compliance; decreased vital capacity, diffusing capacity, and expiratory volumes • *Arterial blood gas* (ABG) *analysis:* reduced partial pressure of arterial oxygen (PaO_2) with normal partial pressure of arterial carbon dioxide ($PaCO_2$) until late in disease • *Electrocardiogram* (ECG): tall, symmetrical P waves in leads II, III, and aV_F vertical QRS axis; signs of right ventricular hypertrophy late in disease • *Red blood cell* (RBC) *count:* increased hemoglobin late in disease when persistent severe hypoxia is present	• Oxygen at low-flow settings to treat hypoxia • Avoidance of smoking and air pollutants • Breathing techniques to control dyspnea • Treatment only slightly helpful for emphysema component of COPD • Lung volume reduction surgery for selected patients
• *Physical examination:* rhonchi and wheezes on auscultation, prolonged expiration, jugular vein distention, and pedal edema • *Chest X-ray:* possibly hyperinflation and increased bronchovascular markings • *Pulmonary function tests:* increased residual volume, decreased vital capacity and forced expiratory volumes, normal static compliance and diffusing capacity • *ABG analysis:* decreased PaO_2, normal or increased $PaCO_2$ • *ECG:* may show atrial arrhythmias; peaked P waves in leads II, III, and aV_F; and, occasionally, right ventricular hypertrophy	• Antibiotics for infections • Avoidance of smoking and air pollutants • Bronchodilators to relieve bronchospasm and facilitate mucociliary clearance • Adequate fluid intake and chest physiotherapy to mobilize secretions • Ultrasonic or mechanical nebulizer treatments to loosen secretions and aid in mobilization • Occasionally, corticosteroids • Diuretics for edema • Oxygen for hypoxemia
• *Physical examination:* usually normal between attacks; rhonchi and wheezing throughout lung fields on expiration and, at times inspiration, revealed during auscultation; absent or diminished breath sounds during severe obstruction; grossly audible loud bilateral wheezing; hyperinflated chest • *Chest X-ray:* hyperinflated lungs with air trapping during attack; normal during remission • *Sputum:* presence of Curschmann's spirals (casts of airways), Charcot-Leyden crystals, and eosinophils	• Aerosol containing beta-adrenergic agents, such as metaproterenol or albuterol; also oral beta-adrenergic agents (terbutaline) and oral methylxanthines (theophylline); inhaled, oral, or I.V. corticosteroids required by most patients • *Emergency treatment:* oxygen therapy, corticosteroids, and bronchodilators, such as subcutaneous epinephrine, I.V. theophylline, and inhaled agents (such as metaproterenol, albuterol, and ipratropium)

(continued)

Types of COPD *(continued)*

Disease	Causes and pathophysiology	Clinical features
Asthma *(continued)* • Asthma with onset in adulthood: typically without distinct allergies; asthma with onset in childhood: commonly associated with definite allergens; status asthmaticus: an acute asthma attack with severe bronchospasm that fails to clear with bronchodilator therapy • Asymptomatic status achieved in adulthood for more than one-half of asthmatic children; persistent disease with occasional severe attacks in more than one-half of asthmatics with onset after age 15	• Paroxysmal airway obstruction associated with nasal polyps possible in response to aspirin or indomethacin ingestion • Airway obstruction from spasm of bronchial smooth muscle, which narrows airways; inflammatory edema of the bronchial wall and inspissation of tenacious mucoid secretions are also significant, particularly in status asthmaticus.	• *Other signs:* prolonged expiration, intercostal and supraclavicular retraction on inspiration, use of accessory muscles of respiration, flaring nostrils, tachypnea, tachycardia, perspiration, flushing; commonly, symptoms of eczema and allergic rhinitis (hay fever) • Without prompt treatment, status asthmaticus progressing to respiratory failure

greater than 200 IU, and the ratio of LD in pleural fluid to LD in serum is equal to or greater than 0.6.
• If a pleural effusion results from esophageal rupture or pancreatitis, amylase levels in aspirated fluid are usually higher than serum levels.
• In empyema, cell analysis shows leukocytosis.
• Aspirated fluid may also be tested for lupus erythematosus cells, antinuclear antibodies, and neoplastic cells. It may be analyzed for color and consistency; acid-fast bacillus, fungal, and bacterial cultures; and triglycerides (in chylothorax).
• Chest X-ray shows radiopaque fluid in dependent regions.
• Pleural biopsy may be particularly useful for confirming TB or cancer.

How it's treated

Depending on the amount of fluid present, symptomatic effusion requires either thoracentesis to remove fluid or careful monitoring of the patient's own fluid reabsorption. Hemothorax requires drainage to prevent fibrothorax formation. Associated hypoxia requires supplemental oxygen.

Confirming diagnostic measures	Management
• *Pulmonary function tests:* during attacks, decreased forced expiratory volumes that improve significantly after inhaled bronchodilator; increased residual volume and, occasionally, total lung capacity; possibly normal between attacks • *ABG analysis:* decreased Pao_2; $Paco_2$ possibly decreased, normal, or (in severe attack) increased • *ECG:* sinus tachycardia during an attack; signs of cor pulmonale (right axis deviation, peaked P wave) in severe attack that resolve after the attack • *Skin tests:* identification of possible allergens	• Monitoring for deteriorating respiratory status and documenting sputum characteristics; adequate fluid intake and oxygen as ordered • *Prevention:* patient's avoidance of possible triggers as well as use of inhaled corticosteroids, antihistamines, decongestants, cromolyn powder by inhalation, and oral or aerosol bronchodilators, as ordered; teaching about the influence of stress and anxiety on asthma as well as its frequent association with exercise (particularly running), cold air, and nighttime flare-ups • Assisting the patient in identifying triggers and teaching about how to use a metered dose inhaler and a peak flow meter

What to do

• Administer oxygen as ordered.
• Provide meticulous chest tube care and use aseptic technique for changing dressings around the tube insertion site in empyema. Record the amount, color, and consistency of tube drainage.
• If the patient has open drainage through a rib resection or an intercostal tube, use hand and dressing precautions. Because weeks of such drainage are usually necessary to obliterate the space, make visiting nurse referrals for patients who will be discharged with the tube in place.
• If pleural effusion was a complication of pneumonia or influenza, advise prompt medical attention for chest colds.
• Evaluate the patient. He should have minimal chest discomfort, be afebrile, and have a normal respiratory pattern. (See *Teaching the patient with pleural effusion.*)

Pneumonia

Pneumonia is an acute infection of the lung parenchyma that commonly impairs gas exchange. The prognosis is usually good for people who have normal lungs and adequate host defenses before the onset of pneumonia; however, bacterial pneumonia is the fifth

Education edge

Teaching the patient with pleural effusion

• Explain thoracentesis to the patient.
• Reassure him during the procedure and observe for complications during and after the procedure.
• Encourage the patient to do deep-breathing exercises to promote lung expansion and use an incentive spirometer to promote deep breathing.

leading cause of death in debilitated patients. The disorder occurs in primary and secondary forms.

What causes it

Pneumonia is caused by an infecting pathogen (bacterial or viral) or by a chemical or other irritant (such as aspirated material). Certain predisposing factors increase the risk of pneumonia. For bacterial and viral pneumonia, these include:
- chronic illness and debilitation
- cancer (particularly lung cancer)
- abdominal and thoracic surgery
- atelectasis, aspiration
- colds or other viral respiratory infections
- chronic respiratory disease, such as COPD, asthma, bronchiectasis, and cystic fibrosis
- smoking, alcoholism
- malnutrition
- sickle cell disease
- tracheostomy
- exposure to noxious gases
- immunosuppressive therapy.

    Aspiration pneumonia is more likely to occur in elderly or debilitated patients, those receiving NG tube feedings, and those with an impaired gag reflex, poor oral hygiene, or a decreased LOC.

Pathophysiology

In general, the lower respiratory tract can be exposed to pathogens by inhalation, aspiration, vascular dissemination, or direct contact with contaminated equipment such as suction catheters. After pathogens are inside, they begin to colonize and infection develops.

Stasis report

In bacterial pneumonia, which can occur in any part of the lungs, an infection initially triggers alveolar inflammation and edema. This produces an area of low ventilation with normal perfusion. Capillaries become engorged with blood, causing stasis. As the alveolar capillary membrane breaks down, alveoli fill with blood and exudate, resulting in atelectasis (lung collapse). In severe bacterial infections, the lungs look heavy and liverlike — similar to ARDS.

Exposure to noxious gases can increase the risk of pneumonia.

Virus attack!

In viral pneumonia, the virus first attacks bronchiolar epithelial cells. This causes interstitial inflammation and desquamation. The virus also invades bronchial mucous glands and goblet cells. It then spreads to the alveoli, which fill with blood and fluid.

Subtracting surfactant

In aspiration pneumonia, inhalation of gastric juices or hydrocarbons triggers inflammatory changes and inactivates surfactant over a large area. Decreased surfactant leads to alveolar collapse. Acidic gastric juices may damage the airways and alveoli. Particles containing aspirated gastric juices may obstruct the airways and reduce airflow, leading to secondary bacterial pneumonia.

What to look for

The five cardinal signs and symptoms of early bacterial pneumonia are:

 coughing

 sputum production

 pleuritic chest pain

 shaking chills

 fever.

Other signs vary widely, ranging from diffuse, fine crackles to signs of localized or extensive consolidation and pleural effusion.

There are five cardinal signs and symptoms of bacterial pneumonia.

What tests tell you

• Chest X-rays showing infiltrates and a sputum smear demonstrating acute inflammatory cells support the diagnosis.
• Positive blood cultures in patients with pulmonary infiltrates strongly suggest pneumonia produced by the organisms isolated from the blood cultures.
• Occasionally, a transtracheal aspirate of tracheobronchial secretions or bronchoscopy with brushings may be done to obtain material for smear and culture.
• Early *Pneumocystis carinii* pneumonia (PCP) can be detected only by a $\dot{V}/\dot{Q}$ scan.

How it's treated

Antimicrobial therapy varies with the infecting agent. Therapy should be reevaluated early in the course of treatment. Supportive measures include:
- humidified oxygen therapy for hypoxemia
- mechanical ventilation for respiratory failure
- a high-calorie diet and adequate fluid intake
- bed rest
- an analgesic to relieve pleuritic chest pain.

What to do

These interventions aim to increase patient comfort, avoid complications, and speed recovery:
- Maintain a patent airway and adequate oxygenation. Measure ABG levels, especially in hypoxic patients. Administer supplemental oxygen as ordered. Patients with underlying COPD should be given oxygen cautiously.
- Administer antibiotics as ordered and pain medication as needed. Fever and dehydration may require I.V. fluids and electrolyte replacement.
- Maintain adequate nutrition to offset extra calories burned during infection. Ask the dietary department to provide a high-calorie, high-protein diet consisting of soft, easy-to-eat foods. Encourage the patient to eat. Monitor fluid intake and output.
- To control the spread of infection, dispose of secretions properly. Tell the patient to sneeze and cough into a disposable tissue; tape a waxed bag to the side of the bed for used tissues.
- To prevent aspiration during NG tube feedings, elevate the patient's head, check the position of the tube, and administer feedings slowly. Don't give large volumes at one time because this could cause vomiting. If the patient has a tracheostomy or an ET tube, inflate the tube cuff. Keep his head elevated for at least 30 minutes after feeding.
- Be aware that antimicrobial agents used to treat cytomegalovirus, PCP, and respiratory syncytial virus pneumonia may be hazardous to fetal development. Pregnant health care workers or those attempting conception should minimize exposure to these agents (such as acyclovir, ribavirin, and pentamidine).
- Evaluate the patient. His chest X-rays should be normal and his ABG levels should show PaO_2 of 50 to 60 mm Hg. (See *Teaching the patient with pneumonia*.)

Education edge

Teaching the patient with pneumonia

- Teach the patient how to cough and perform deep-breathing exercises to clear secretions.
- Urge all postoperative and bedridden patients to perform deep-breathing exercises frequently. Position patients properly to promote full ventilation and drainage of secretions.
- Encourage annual influenza and pneumococcal vaccination for high-risk patients, such as those with COPD chronic heart disease, or sickle cell disease.
- To prevent pneumonia, advise the patient to avoid using antibiotics indiscriminately during minor viral infections because this may result in upper airway colonization with antibiotic-resistant bacteria. If the patient then develops pneumonia, the infecting organisms may require treatment with more toxic antibiotics.

Pneumothorax

In pneumothorax, air or gas accumulates between the parietal and visceral pleurae, causing the lungs to collapse. The amount of air or gas trapped determines the degree of lung collapse. In some cases, venous return to the heart is impeded, causing a life-threatening condition called tension pneumothorax.

Spontaneous or traumatic?

Pneumothorax is classified as either traumatic or spontaneous. Traumatic pneumothorax may be further classified as open (sucking chest wound) or closed (blunt or penetrating trauma). Note that an open (penetrating) wound may cause closed pneumothorax if communication between the atmosphere and the pleural space seals itself off. Spontaneous pneumothorax, which is also considered closed, can be further classified as primary (idiopathic) or secondary (related to a specific disease).

Sometimes being spontaneous isn't a good thing!

What causes it

Spontaneous pneumothorax can result from:
• ruptured congenital blebs
• ruptured emphysematous bullae
• tubercular or malignant lesions that erode into the pleural space
• interstitial lung disease, such as eosinophilic granuloma.
    Traumatic pneumothorax can result from:
• insertion of a central venous pressure line
• thoracic surgery
• thoracentesis or closed pleural biopsy
• penetrating chest injury
• transbronchial biopsy.
    Tension pneumothorax can develop from either spontaneous or traumatic pneumothorax. (See *Understanding tension pneumothorax*, page 394.)

Pathophysiology

The pathophysiology of pneumothorax varies according to classification.

A change in atmosphere

Open pneumothorax results when atmospheric air (positive pressure) flows directly into the pleural cavity (negative pressure). As the air pressure in the pleural cavity becomes positive, the lung collapses on the affected side. Lung collapse leads to decreased total lung capacity. The patient then develops $\dot{V}/\dot{Q}$ imbalance leading to hypoxia.

Understanding tension pneumothorax

In tension pneumothorax, air accumulates intrapleurally and can't escape. Intrapleural pressure rises, collapsing the ipsilateral lung.

On inspiration, the mediastinum shifts toward the unaffected lung, impairing ventilation.

On expiration, the mediastinal shift distorts the vena cava and reduces venous return.

A leak within the lung

Closed pneumothorax occurs when air enters the pleural space from within the lung, causing increased pleural pressure and preventing lung expansion during inspiration. It may be called traumatic pneumothorax when blunt chest trauma causes lung tissue to rupture, resulting in air leakage.

Rupture!

Spontaneous pneumothorax is a type of closed pneumothorax. The usual cause is rupture of a subpleural bleb (a small cystic space) at the surface of the lung. This rupture causes air leakage into the pleural spaces; then the lung collapses, causing decreased total lung capacity, vital capacity, and lung compliance — leading, in turn, to hypoxia.

What to look for

Spontaneous pneumothorax may not produce symptoms in mild cases, but profound respiratory distress occurs in moderate to severe cases. Weak and rapid pulse, pallor, jugular vein distention, and anxiety indicate tension pneumothorax. In most cases, look for these symptoms:
• sudden, sharp, pleuritic pain

- asymmetrical chest wall movement
- shortness of breath
- cyanosis
- decreased or absent breath sounds over the collapsed lung
- hyperresonance on the affected side
- crackling beneath the skin on palpation (subcutaneous emphysema).

What tests tell you

- Chest X-rays show air in the pleural space and may reveal mediastinal shift.
- If pneumothorax is significant, ABG findings include pH less than 7.35, PaO_2 less than 80 mm Hg, and $PaCO_2$ above 45 mm Hg.

To identify and treat pneumothorax, chest X-rays detect air in the pleural space and may reveal mediastinal shift.

How it's treated

Treatment is conservative for spontaneous pneumothorax in cases where no signs of increased pleural pressure appear, lung collapse is less than 30%, and the patient shows no signs of dyspnea or other indications of physiologic compromise. Such treatment consists of:
- bed rest or activity as tolerated by the patient
- careful monitoring of blood pressure, pulse rate, and respirations
- oxygen administration
- in some cases, needle aspiration of air with a large-bore needle attached to a syringe.

Also, keep in mind these treatment pointers:
- When more than 30% of the lung has collapsed, reexpansion of the lung is performed by placing a thoracotomy tube in the second or third intercostal space at the midclavicular line. This procedure is done to allow air to rise to the top of the intrapleural space. The tube is connected to an underwater seal with suction at low pressures.
- Recurring spontaneous pneumothorax requires thoracotomy and pleurectomy. These procedures prevent recurrence by causing the lung to adhere to the parietal pleura.
- Traumatic or tension pneumothorax requires chest tube drainage.
- Traumatic pneumothorax may also require surgical repair.

In the patient with pneumothorax, carefully monitor vital signs at least every hour.

What to do

- Watch for pallor, gasping respirations, and sudden chest pain.
- Carefully monitor vital signs at least every hour for indications of shock, increasing respiratory distress, or mediastinal shift. Lis-

ten for breath sounds over both lungs. Falling blood pressure with rising pulse and respiratory rates may indicate tension pneumothorax, which can be fatal if not promptly treated.

• Make the patient as comfortable as possible — a patient with pneumothorax is usually most comfortable sitting upright.

• Urge the patient to control coughing and gasping during thoracotomy.

Take a deep breath

• After the chest tube is in place, encourage him to cough and breathe deeply at least once per hour to facilitate lung expansion.

• In the patient undergoing chest tube drainage, watch for continuing air leakage (bubbling) in the water-seal chamber. This indicates the lung defect has failed to close and may require surgery. Also observe for increasing subcutaneous emphysema by checking around the neck or at the tube insertion site for crackling beneath the skin. If the patient is on a ventilator, be alert for any difficulty in breathing in time with the ventilator as you monitor its gauges for pressure increases.

• Change dressings around the chest tube insertion site as needed and as per your facility's policy. Be careful not to reposition or dislodge the tube. If the tube dislodges, immediately place a petroleum gauze dressing over the opening to prevent rapid lung collapse.

• Observe the chest tube site for leakage and note the amount and color of drainage. Walk the patient as ordered (usually on the 1st postoperative day) to facilitate deep inspiration and lung expansion.

• Reassure the patient by explaining what occurs with pneumothorax, its causes, and all accompanying diagnostic tests and procedures.

• Evaluate the patient. Chest X-rays, respiratory rate and depth, and vital signs should be normal. (See *Teaching the patient with pneumothorax*.)

Education edge

Teaching the patient with pneumothorax

• Encourage the patient to perform hourly deep-breathing exercises when awake.

• Discuss the potential for recurrent spontaneous pneumothorax, and review its signs and symptoms. Emphasize the need for immediate medical intervention if these occur.

Pulmonary embolism and infarction

Pulmonary embolism is an obstruction of the pulmonary arterial bed by a dislodged thrombus or foreign substance. Pulmonary infarction, or lung tissue death from a pulmonary embolus, is sometimes mild and may not produce symptoms. However, when a massive embolism occurs involving more than 50% obstruction of pulmonary arterial circulation, it can be rapidly fatal.

What causes it

Pulmonary embolism usually results from dislodged thrombi that originate in the leg veins. Other less common sources of thrombi

An embolism involving an obstruction of more than 50% of the pulmonary arterial circulation can be rapidly fatal.

are the pelvic veins, renal veins, hepatic vein, right side of the heart, and arms.

Pathophysiology

Trauma, clot dissolution, sudden muscle spasm, intravascular pressure changes, or a change in peripheral blood flow can cause the thrombus to loosen or fragmentize. Then the thrombus — now called an embolus — floats to the heart's right side and enters the lung through the pulmonary artery. There, the embolus may dissolve, continue to fragmentize, or grow.

Collapse, atelectasis, death

If the embolus occludes the pulmonary artery, alveoli collapse and atelectasis develops. If the embolus enlarges, it may clog most or all of the pulmonary vessels and cause death.

Rare but serious

Rarely, the emboli contain air, fat, amniotic fluid, tumor cells, or talc from drugs intended for oral administration that are injected I.V. by addicts. Pulmonary embolism may lead to pulmonary infarction, especially in patients with chronic heart or pulmonary disease.

What to look for

Total occlusion of the main pulmonary artery is rapidly fatal; smaller or fragmented emboli produce symptoms that vary with the size, number, and location of the emboli. Dyspnea is usually the first symptom of pulmonary embolism and may be accompanied by anginal or pleuritic chest pain. Other clinical features include tachycardia, productive cough (sputum may be blood-tinged), and low-grade fever.

Other signs

Less common signs include massive hemoptysis, splinting of the chest, and leg edema. A large embolus may produce cyanosis, syncope, and distended neck veins. Signs of shock (such as weak, rapid pulse and hypotension) and signs of hypoxia (such as restlessness) may also occur. Cardiac auscultation occasionally reveals a right ventricular S_3 audible at the lower sternum and increased intensity of a pulmonary component of S_2. Crackles and a pleural friction rub may be heard at the infarction site.

What tests tell you

The following test results can help confirm pulmonary embolism or infarction:

• Chest X-ray shows a characteristic wedge-shaped infiltrate suggestive of pulmonary embolism. X-ray studies may rule out other pulmonary diseases and reveal areas of atelectasis, an elevated diaphragm, pleural effusion, and a prominent pulmonary artery.
• Lung scan shows perfusion defects in areas beyond occluded vessels; a normal lung scan rules out pulmonary embolism.
• Pulmonary angiography is the most definitive test but poses some risk to the patient (such as allergic reaction to the dye, infection at the catheter site, and kidney failure related to difficulty excreting dye). Its use depends on the uncertainty of the diagnosis and the need to avoid unnecessary anticoagulant therapy (treatment of pulmonary embolism) in high-risk patients.
• ECG is inconclusive but helps distinguish pulmonary embolism from MI. In extensive embolism, the ECG may show right axis deviation; right bundle-branch block; tall, peaked P waves; depressed ST segments and T-wave inversions (indicating right heart strain); and supraventricular tachyarrhythmias.
• ABG measurements showing decreased PaO_2 and $PaCO_2$ are characteristic but don't always occur.

In pulmonary embolism, chest X-rays show a characteristic wedge-shaped infiltrate.

How it's treated

Treatment aims to maintain adequate cardiovascular and pulmonary function as the obstruction resolves and to prevent recurrence. Because most emboli resolve within 10 days, treatment consists of oxygen therapy as needed and anticoagulation with heparin to inhibit new thrombus formation.

Massive means more

Patients with massive pulmonary embolism and shock may require thrombolytic therapy with tissue plasminogen activator or streptokinase to enhance fibrinolysis of the pulmonary emboli and remaining thrombi. Hypotension related to pulmonary emboli may be treated with vasopressors.

Seek the septic source

Treatment for septic emboli requires antibiotic therapy as well as evaluation of the source of infection, particularly in cases of endocarditis. Anticoagulants aren't used to treat septic emboli.

To treat septic emboli, you must evaluate the source of the infection.

Surgery saved for last

Surgery to interrupt the inferior vena cava is reserved for patients for whom anticoagulants are contraindicated (for example, because of age, recent surgery, or blood dyscrasia) or who have recurrent emboli during anticoagulant therapy. It should only be performed when pulmonary embolism is confirmed by angiography.

Surgery consists of vena caval ligation, plication, or insertion of an umbrella filter for blood returning to the heart and lungs. A combination of low-dose heparin and dihydroergotamine (Migranal) may be administered to prevent postoperative venous thromboembolism.

What to do

- Give oxygen by nasal cannula or mask.
- Check ABG levels if fresh emboli develop or dyspnea worsens.
- Be prepared to provide equipment for ET intubation and assisted ventilation if breathing is severely compromised. If necessary, prepare to transfer the patient to an ICU per facility policy.
- Administer heparin as ordered through I.V. push or continuous drip.
- Monitor coagulation studies daily and after changes in heparin dosage. Maintain adequate hydration to avoid the risk of hypercoagulability.
- After the patient is stable, encourage him to move about often and assist with isometric and ROM exercises. Check temperature and color of feet to detect venostasis. Never vigorously massage the patient's legs. Walk the patient as soon as possible after surgery to prevent venostasis.
- Report frequent pleuritic chest pain so that analgesics can be prescribed.
- Evaluate the patient. His vital signs should be within normal limits, and he should show no signs of bleeding after anticoagulant therapy. (See *Teaching the patient with pulmonary embolism and infarction*.)

Tuberculosis

TB is an acute or chronic infection characterized by pulmonary infiltrates and formation of granulomas with caseation, fibrosis, and cavitation. The American Lung Association estimates that active TB afflicts nearly 7 out of every 100,000 people. The prognosis is excellent with correct treatment.

What causes it

Mycobacterium tuberculosis is the major cause of TB. Other strains of mycobacteria may also be involved. Several factors increase the risk of infection, including:

- gastrectomy
- uncontrolled diabetes mellitus
- Hodgkin's disease

Education edge

Teaching the patient with pulmonary embolism and infarction

- Teach the patient how to use an incentive spirometer to assist in deep breathing.
- Warn him not to cross his legs; this promotes thrombus formation.
- Encourage family participation in care. Most patients need treatment with an oral anticoagulant (such as warfarin) for 4 to 6 months after a pulmonary embolism.
- Advise the patient to watch for signs of bleeding from anticoagulants, to take the prescribed medication exactly as ordered, and to avoid taking any additional medication (even for headaches or colds) or changing medication dosages without consulting his doctor.
- Stress the importance of follow-up laboratory tests to monitor anticoagulant therapy.

• leukemia
• treatment with corticosteroid therapy or immunosuppressant therapy
• silicosis
• human immunodeficiency virus infection.

The first step in TB infection is inhalation of my infected droplets. Heh, heh, heh!

Pathophysiology

TB spreads by inhalation of droplet nuclei when infected persons cough or sneeze. Here's what happens:
• *Transmission* — An infected person coughs or sneezes, spreading infected droplets. When someone without immunity inhales these droplets, the bacilli are deposited in the lungs.
• *Immune response* — The immune system responds by sending leukocytes, and inflammation results. After a few days, leukocytes are replaced by macrophages. Bacilli are then ingested by the macrophages and carried off by the lymphatics to the lymph nodes.
• *Tubercle formation* — Macrophages that ingest the bacilli fuse to form epithelioid cell tubercles (tiny nodules surrounded by lymphocytes). Within the lesion, caseous necrosis develops and scar tissue encapsulates the tubercle. The organism may be killed in the process.
• *Dissemination* — If the tubercles and inflamed nodes rupture, the infection contaminates the surrounding tissue and may spread through the blood and lymphatic circulation to distant sites. This process is called hematogenous dissemination.

What to look for

In primary infection, the disease usually doesn't produce symptoms. However, it may produce nonspecific symptoms such as:
• fatigue
• weakness
• anorexia
• weight loss
• night sweats
• low-grade fever.

In reinfection, the patient may experience cough, productive mucopurulent sputum, and chest pain.

What tests tell you

• Chest X-rays show nodular lesions, patchy infiltrates (many in upper lobes), cavity formation, scar tissue, and calcium deposits. However, they may not distinguish active from inactive TB.

• Tuberculin skin tests detect exposure to TB but don't distinguish the disease from uncomplicated infection. Patients from non–North American countries may test positive for TB by skin test due to the positive antibody titer produced by the bacille Calmette-Guérin live vaccine they received as children.
• Stains and cultures of sputum, CSF, urine, drainage from abscess, or pleural fluid show heat-sensitive, nonmotile, aerobic, acid-fast bacilli and confirm the diagnosis.

How it's treated

Antitubercular therapy with daily oral doses of isoniazid, rifampin, and pyrazinamide (and sometimes with ethambutol or streptomycin) for at least 6 months usually cures TB. After 2 to 4 weeks, the disease is typically no longer infectious, and the patient can resume his normal lifestyle while continuing to take medication. The patient with atypical mycobacterial disease or drug-resistant TB may require second-line drugs, such as capreomycin, streptomycin, para-aminosalicylic acid, cycloserine, amikacin, and quinolones.

What to do

• Isolate the infectious patient in a negative-pressure room until he's no longer contagious.
• Be alert for adverse effects of medications. Pyridoxine (vitamin B_6) is sometimes recommended to prevent peripheral neuropathy caused by large doses of isoniazid. If the patient receives ethambutol, watch for optic neuritis; if it develops, discontinue the drug. Observe for hepatitis and purpura in patients receiving rifampin.
• Evaluate the patient. His sputum culture should be negative and secretions should be thin and clear. (See *Teaching the patient with tuberculosis.*)

Quick quiz

1. Which of the following breath sounds are medium-pitched, continuous, occur over the upper third of the sternum in the interscapular area, and are equally audible during inspiration and expiration?
    A.   Vesicular
    B.   Bronchial
    C.   Bronchovesicular
    D.   Tracheal

Answer: C. Bronchovesicular breath sounds demonstrate these characteristics.

2.   Your patient's ABG analysis shows a pH less than 7.35, HCO_3^- greater than 26 mEq/L and a $Paco_2$ greater than 45 mm Hg. He's diaphoretic, has tachycardia, and is restless. Which of the following conditions does he probably have?
  A.   Respiratory alkalosis
  B.   Respiratory acidosis
  C.   Metabolic alkalosis
  D.   Metabolic acidosis

Answer: B. The patient with respiratory acidosis can display all of these signs and symptoms and can also have headache, confusion, apprehension, and a flushed face.

3.   When suctioning a patient you should do which of the following?
  A.   Apply suction intermittently as you insert the catheter.
  B.   Suction the patient for longer than 10 seconds at a time.
  C.   Oxygenate the patient's lungs before and after suctioning.
  D.   Apply suction continuously as you insert the catheter.

Answer: C. Oxygenate the patient before and after to reduce the risk of hypoxemia. In addition, you should avoid suctioning for longer than 10 seconds and apply suction intermittently as you withdraw the catheter.

4.   TB is transmitted through:
  A.   inhalation of infected droplets.
  B.   contact with blood.
  C.   the fecal-oral route.
  D.   skin to skin contact.

Answer: A. TB spreads by inhalation of droplet nuclei when an infected person coughs or sneezes.

Scoring

☆☆☆   If you answered all four items correctly, way to go! You can breathe easy about your knowledge of respiratory disorders.

☆☆   If you answered three items correctly, great! Your understanding of respiratory disorders is circulating well!

☆   If you answered fewer than three items correctly, no worries! Take a deep breath, oxygenate those tissues, and review the chapter!

Gastrointestinal disorders

Just the facts

In this chapter, you'll learn:

♦ the anatomy and physiology of the GI system

♦ important questions and discussion topics for the health history

♦ how to assess the GI system and interpret abnormal findings

♦ nursing responsibilities for common diagnostic tests

♦ relevant nursing diagnoses with nursing interventions and rationales

♦ nursing care for common GI disorders.

As the site of the body's digestive processes, the GI system has the critical task of supplying essential nutrients to fuel the brain, heart, and lungs. GI function also profoundly affects the quality of life through its impact on overall health.

Anatomy and physiology

The GI system's major functions include ingestion and digestion of food and elimination of waste products. When these processes are interrupted, the patient can experience problems ranging from loss of appetite to acid-base imbalances.

The GI system consists of two major divisions: the GI tract and the accessory organs. (See *GI system structures*, page 404.)

The GI system consists of the GI tract and the accessory organs.

GI system structures

This illustration shows the GI system's major anatomic structures. Knowing these structures will help you conduct an accurate physical assessment.

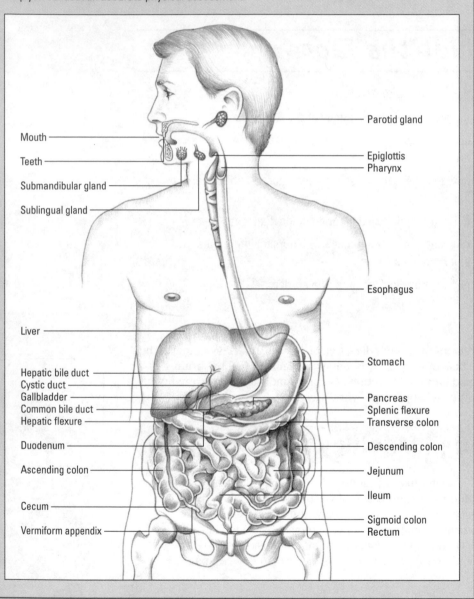

Mouth

Teeth

Submandibular gland

Sublingual gland

Liver

Hepatic bile duct

Cystic duct

Gallbladder

Common bile duct

Hepatic flexure

Duodenum

Ascending colon

Cecum

Vermiform appendix

Parotid gland

Epiglottis

Pharynx

Esophagus

Stomach

Pancreas

Splenic flexure

Transverse colon

Descending colon

Jejunum

Ileum

Sigmoid colon

Rectum

GI tract

The GI tract is a hollow tube that begins at the mouth and ends at the anus. About 258 (7.5 m) long, it consists of smooth muscle alternating with blood vessels and nerve tissue. Specialized circular and longitudinal fibers contract, causing peristalsis, which aids in propelling food through the GI tract. The GI tract includes the pharynx, esophagus, stomach, small intestine, and large intestine.

Start at the mouth

Digestive processes begin in the mouth with chewing, salivating, and swallowing. The tongue provides the sense of taste. Saliva is produced by three pairs of glands: the parotid, submandibular, and sublingual.

Proceed to the pharynx

The pharynx, or throat, allows the passage of food from the mouth to the esophagus. The pharynx assists in the swallowing process and secretes mucus that aids in digestion. The epiglottis—a thin, leaf-shaped structure made of fibrocartilage—is directly behind the root of the tongue. When food is swallowed, the epiglottis closes over the larynx, and the soft palate lifts to block the nasal cavity. These actions keep food and fluid from being aspirated into the airway.

Down the esophagus

The esophagus is a muscular, hollow tube about 10″ (25.5 cm) long that moves food from the pharynx to the stomach. When food is swallowed, the upper esophageal sphincter relaxes, and the food moves into the esophagus. Peristalsis then propels the food toward the stomach. The gastroesophageal sphincter at the lower end of the esophagus normally remains closed to prevent reflux of gastric contents. The sphincter opens during swallowing, belching, and vomiting.

Stay awhile in the stomach

The stomach, a reservoir for food, is a dilated, saclike structure that lies obliquely in the left upper quadrant below the esophagus and diaphragm, to the right of the spleen, and partly under the liver. The stomach contains two important sphincters: the cardiac sphincter, which protects the entrance to the stomach, and the pyloric sphincter, which guards the exit.

The stomach has three major functions. It:

stores food

mixes food with gastric juices (hydrochloric acid)

No matter what you choose, your sense of taste is provided by your tongue.

passes chyme—a watery mixture of partly digested food and digestive juices—into the small intestine for further digestion and absorption.

An average meal can remain in the stomach for 3 to 4 hours. Accordion-like folds in the stomach lining called *rugae* allow the stomach to expand when large amounts of food and fluid are ingested.

Slip through the small intestine

The small intestine is about 20′ (6 m) long and is named for its diameter, not its length. It has three sections: the duodenum, the jejunum, and the ileum. As food passes into the small intestine, the end products of digestion are absorbed through its thin mucous membrane lining into the bloodstream.

Carbohydrates, fats, and proteins are broken down in the small intestine. Enzymes from the pancreas, bile from the liver, and hormones from glands of the small intestine all aid digestion. These secretions mix with the food as it moves through the intestines by peristalsis.

Finally, the large intestine

The large intestine, or colon, is about 5′ (1.5 m) long and is responsible for:
- absorbing excess water and electrolytes
- storing food residue
- eliminating waste products in the form of feces.

The large intestine includes the cecum; the ascending, transverse, descending, and sigmoid colons; the rectum; and the anus—in that order. The appendix, a fingerlike projection, is attached to the cecum. Bacteria in the colon produce gas or flatus.

I can hold on to an average meal for 3 to 4 hours. Thanks to my rugae, I can expand for those larger-than-average meals, too!

Accessory organs

Accessory GI organs include the liver, pancreas, gallbladder, and bile ducts. The abdominal aorta and the gastric and splenic veins also aid the GI system.

Look at the liver

The liver is located in the right upper quadrant under the diaphragm. It has two major lobes, divided by the falciform ligament. The liver is the heaviest organ in the body, weighing about 3 lb (1.5 kg) in an adult.

The liver's functions include:

- metabolizing carbohydrates, fats, and proteins
- detoxifying blood
- converting ammonia to urea for excretion
- synthesizing plasma proteins, nonessential amino acids, vitamin A, and essential nutrients, such as iron and vitamins D, K, and B_{12}.

The liver also secretes bile, a greenish fluid that helps digest fats and absorb fatty acids, cholesterol, and other lipids. Bile also gives stool its color.

I'm a metabolizing, detoxifying, synthesizing wonder!

Gape at the gallbladder

The gallbladder is a small, pear-shaped organ about 4″ (10 cm) long that lies halfway under the right lobe of the liver. Its main function is to store bile from the liver until the bile is emptied into the duodenum. This process occurs when the small intestine initiates chemical impulses that cause the gallbladder to contract.

Probe the pancreas

The pancreas, which measures 6″ to 8″ (15 to 20.5 cm) in length, lies horizontally in the abdomen behind the stomach. It consists of a head, tail, and body. The body of the pancreas is located in the right upper quadrant, and the tail is in the left upper quadrant, attached to the duodenum. The tail of the pancreas touches the spleen. The pancreas releases insulin and glycogen into the bloodstream and produces pancreatic enzymes that are released into the duodenum for digestion.

Behold the bile ducts

The bile ducts provide a passageway for bile to travel from the liver to the intestines. Two hepatic ducts drain the liver, and the cystic duct drains the gallbladder. These ducts converge into the common bile duct, which then empties into the duodenum.

Visualize the vascular structures

The abdominal aorta supplies blood to the GI tract. It enters the abdomen, separates into the common iliac arteries, and then branches into many arteries extending the length of the GI tract.

The gastric and splenic veins drain absorbed nutrients into the portal vein of the liver. After entering the liver, the venous blood circulates and then exits the liver through the hepatic vein, emptying into the inferior vena cava.

Assessment

GI disorders can have many baffling signs and symptoms. To help sort out significant symptoms, you'll need to take a thorough patient history. Then you'll probe further by conducting a thorough physical examination, using inspection, auscultation, palpation, and percussion.

History

To help track the development of relevant signs and symptoms over time, you'll need to develop a detailed patient history.

Never underestimate the value of a thorough health history. It can directly impact your ability to provide care.

Current health status

Ask the patient if he's taking any medications. Several drugs — including aspirin, sulfonamides, nonsteroidal anti-inflammatory drugs (NSAIDs), and some antihypertensives — can cause nausea, vomiting, diarrhea, constipation, and other GI signs and symptoms.

Be sure to ask about laxative use; habitual use may cause constipation. Also ask the patient if he's allergic to medications or foods. Such allergies commonly cause GI symptoms.

In addition, ask the patient about changes in appetite, difficulty eating or chewing, and changes in bowel habits. Has he noticed a change in the color, amount, and appearance of his stool? Has he ever seen blood in his stool?

Previous health status

To determine if your patient's problem is new or recurring, ask about past GI illnesses, such as an ulcer, gallbladder disease, inflammatory bowel disease, or GI bleeding. Also ask if he has had abdominal surgery or trauma.

Family history

Because some GI disorders are hereditary, ask the patient whether anyone in his family has had a GI disorder. Disorders with a familial link include:
- ulcerative colitis
- colon cancer
- stomach ulcers
- diabetes
- alcoholism
- Crohn's disease.

Lifestyle patterns

Inquire about your patient's occupation, home life, financial situation, stress level, and recent life changes. Be sure to ask about al-

cohol, caffeine, and tobacco use as well as food consumption, exercise habits, and oral hygiene. Also ask about sleep patterns:
• How many hours of sleep does he feel he needs?
• How many does he get?

> Sleep deprivation can have a negative effect on health, so be sure to ask your patient about his sleep habits.

Physical examination

Physical assessment of the GI system includes evaluation of the mouth, abdomen, liver, and rectum. To perform an abdominal assessment, use this sequence: inspection, auscultation, percussion, and palpation. Palpating or percussing the abdomen before you auscultate it can change the character of the patient's bowel sounds and lead to an inaccurate assessment.

Mouth

Use inspection and palpation to assess the mouth.

Open wide

First, inspect the patient's mouth and jaw for asymmetry and swelling. Check his bite, noting malocclusion from an overbite or underbite. Inspect the inner and outer lips, teeth, and gums with a penlight. Note bleeding, gum ulcerations, and missing, displaced, or broken teeth. Palpate the gums for tenderness and the inner lips and cheeks for lesions.

Assess the tongue, checking for coating, tremors, swelling, and ulcerations. Note unusual breath odors. Finally, examine the pharynx, looking for uvular deviation, tonsillar abnormalities, lesions, plaques, and exudate.

Abdomen

Use inspection, auscultation, percussion, and palpation to examine the abdomen. Assess painful areas last to help prevent the patient from experiencing increased discomfort and tension.

Inspection

Begin inspecting the abdomen by mentally dividing it into four quadrants and then imagining the organs in each quadrant. (See *Abdominal quadrants*, page 410.)

It's all in the terms

You can more accurately pinpoint your physical findings by knowing these three terms:

Abdominal quadrants

To perform a systematic GI assessment, try to visualize abdominal structures by dividing the abdomen into four quadrants, as shown here.

Right upper quadrant
• Right lobe of liver
• Gallbladder
• Pylorus
• Duodenum
• Head of the pancreas
• Hepatic flexure of the colon
• Portions of the ascending and transverse colon

Left upper quadrant
• Left lobe of liver
• Stomach
• Body of the pancreas
• Splenic flexure of the colon
• Portions of the transverse and descending colon

Right lower quadrant
• Cecum and appendix
• Portion of the ascending colon

Left lower quadrant
• Sigmoid colon
• Portion of the descending colon

 epigastric — above the umbilicus and between the costal margins

 umbilical — around the navel

 suprapubic — above the symphysis pubis.

Checking for a bulge

Observe the abdomen for symmetry, checking for bumps, bulges, or masses. Also note the patient's abdominal shape and contour.

Assess the umbilicus, which should be located midline in the abdomen and inverted. If his umbilicus protrudes, the patient may have an umbilical hernia.

Knowing the language can aid in your assessment. N'est-ce pas?

Scouring the skin

The skin of the abdomen should be smooth and uniform in color. Note stretch marks, or *striae*, and dilated veins. Record the length of any surgical scars on the abdomen.

Riding the peristaltic wave

Note abdominal movements and pulsations. Usually, waves of peristalsis can't be seen; if they're visible, they look like slight, wavelike motions. Visible rippling waves may indicate bowel obstruction and should be reported immediately. In thin patients, pulsation of the aorta is visible in the epigastric area. Marked pulsations may occur with hypertension, aortic aneurysm, and other conditions causing widening pulse pressure.

Auscultation

Lightly place the stethoscope diaphragm in the right lower quadrant, slightly below and to the right of the umbilicus. Auscultate in a clockwise fashion in each of the four quadrants, spending at least 2 minutes in each area. Note the character and quality of bowel sounds in each quadrant. In some cases, you may need to auscultate for 5 minutes before you hear sounds. Be sure to allow enough time for listening in each quadrant before you decide that bowel sounds are absent.

Before auscultating the abdomen of a patient with a gastric or an abdominal tube connected to suction, such as a nasogastric (NG) tube, briefly clamp the tube or turn off the suction. Suction noises can obscure or mimic actual bowel sounds.

Pardon my borborygmus

Normal bowel sounds are high-pitched, gurgling noises caused by air mixing with fluid during peristalsis. The noises vary in frequency, pitch, and intensity and occur irregularly from 5 to 34 times per minute. They're loudest before mealtimes. Borborygmus, or stomach growling, is the loud, gurgling, splashing bowel sound heard over the large intestine as gas passes through it.

Bowel sounds are classified as normal, hypoactive, or hyperactive.

Voice of the vessels

Auscultate for vascular sounds with the bell of the stethoscope. (See *Vascular sounds*.) Using firm pressure, listen over the aorta and renal, iliac, and femoral arteries for bruits, venous hums, and friction rubs.

Vascular sounds

Use the bell of your stethoscope to auscultate for vascular sounds at the sites shown in this illustration.

Right renal artery   Aorta   Left renal artery

Right femoral artery   Left femoral artery

Right iliac artery   Left iliac artery

Percussion

Direct or indirect percussion is used to detect the size and location of abdominal organs and to detect air or fluid in the abdomen, stomach, or bowel. In direct percussion, strike your hand or finger directly against the patient's abdomen. In indirect percussion, use the middle finger of your dominant hand or a percussion hammer to strike a finger resting on the patient's abdomen. Begin percussion in the right lower quadrant and proceed clockwise, covering all four quadrants.

Sometimes, skip it

Don't percuss the abdomen of a patient with an abdominal aortic aneurysm or a transplanted abdominal organ. Doing so can precipitate a rupture or organ rejection.

Hollow or dull?

Normally, you'll hear two sounds during percussion of the abdomen: tympany and dullness. When you percuss over hollow organs, such as an empty stomach or bowel, you hear a clear, hollow sound like a drum beating. This sound, tympany, predominates because air is normally present in the stomach and bowel. The degree of tympany depends on the amount of air and gastric dilation.

When you percuss over solid organs — such as the liver, kidney, or feces-filled intestines — the sound changes to dullness. Note where percussed sounds change from tympany to dullness.

How large is the liver?

Percussion of the liver can help you estimate its size. (See *Percussing and measuring the liver*.) Hepatomegaly is commonly associated with hepatitis and other liver diseases. Liver borders may be obscured and difficult to assess.

Splenic dullard

The spleen is located at about the level of the 10th rib, in the left midaxillary line. Percussion may produce a small area of dullness, generally 7″ (17.8 cm) or less in adults. However, the spleen usually can't be percussed because tympany from the colon masks the dullness of the spleen.

To assess a patient for splenic enlargement, ask him to breathe deeply. Then percuss along the 9th to 11th intercostal spaces on the left, listening for a change from tympany to dullness. Measure the area of dullness.

Palpation

Palpate all four quadrants, leaving painful and tender areas for last.

Percussing and measuring the liver

To percuss and measure the liver, follow these steps:

• Identify the upper border of liver dullness. Start in the right midclavicular line in an area of lung resonance, and percuss downward toward the liver. Use a pen to mark the spot where the sound changes to dullness.

• Start in the right midclavicular line at a level below the umbilicus, and lightly percuss upward toward the liver. Mark the spot where the sound changes from tympany to dullness.

• Use a ruler to measure the vertical span between the two marked spots, as shown. In an adult, a normal liver span ranges from 2½″ to 4¾″ (6.5 to 12 cm).

Light touch

Light palpation helps identify muscle resistance and tenderness as well as the location of some superficial organs. To palpate, put the fingers of one hand close together, depress the skin about ½″ (1.25 cm) with your fingertips, and make gentle, rotating movements. Avoid short, quick jabs.

The abdomen should be soft and nontender. As you palpate the four quadrants, note organs, masses, and areas of tenderness or increased resistance.

In deep

To perform deep palpation, push the abdomen down about 2″ to 3″ (5 to 7.5 cm). In an obese patient, put one hand on top of the other and push. Palpate the entire abdomen in a clockwise direction, checking for tenderness, pulsations, organ enlargement, and masses.

If the patient's abdomen is rigid, don't palpate it. He could have peritoneal inflammation, and palpation could cause pain or could rupture an inflamed organ. (See *Emergency signals*, page 414.)

Lively liver, special spleen

Palpate the patient's liver to check for enlargement and tenderness. (See *Palpating the liver*, page 415.) Unless the spleen is enlarged, it isn't palpable. To attempt to palpate the spleen, stand on the patient's right side. Use your left hand to support his posterior

If the patient's abdomen is rigid, don't palpate it, or you could rupture an inflamed organ.

What do I do?

Emergency signals

When assessing a patient with a GI problem, stay alert for the signs and symptoms described here because they may signal an emergency. If you note any of these signs or symptoms, notify the doctor and assess the patient for deterioration such as signs of shock. Intervene, as necessary, by providing oxygen therapy and I.V. fluids, as ordered. Place the patient on a cardiac monitor if appropriate. Provide emotional support.

Abdominal pain
• Progressive, severe, or colicky pain for more than 6 hours without improvement
• Acute pain associated with hypertension
• Acute pain in an elderly patient (Such a patient may have minimal tenderness, even with a ruptured abdominal organ or appendicitis.)
• Severe pain with guarding and a history of recent abdominal surgery
• Pain accompanied by X-ray evidence of free intraperitoneal air (gas) or mediastinal gas
• Disproportionately severe pain under benign conditions (soft abdomen with normal physical findings)

Vomitus and stools
• Vomitus containing fresh blood
• Prolonged vomiting or heaving, with or without obstipation (intractable constipation)
• Bloody or black, tarry stools

Abdominal tenderness
• Abdominal tenderness and rigidity, even when the patient is distracted
• Rebound tenderness

Other signs
• Fever
• Tachycardia
• Hypotension
• Dehydration

left lower rib cage, and ask him to take a deep breath. Then, with your right hand on his abdomen, press up and in toward the spleen. If you do feel the spleen, stop palpating immediately because compression can cause rupture.

Rectum and anus

If the patient is age 40 or older, perform a rectal examination as part of your GI assessment. Be sure to explain the procedure to him.

Inspect the outside

First, inspect the perianal area. Put on gloves and spread the buttocks to expose the anus and surrounding tissue, checking for fissures, lesions, scars, inflammation, discharge, rectal prolapse, and external hemorrhoids. Ask the patient to strain as if he's having a bowel movement; this may reveal internal hemorrhoids, polyps, or

Palpating the liver

These illustrations show the correct hand positions for two ways of palpating the liver.

Simple palpation

• Place the patient in the supine position. Standing at his right side, place your left hand under his back at the approximate location of the liver.

• Place your right hand slightly below the mark you made at the liver's upper border during percussion and measurement. Point the fingers of your right hand toward the patient's head just under the right costal margin.

• As the patient inhales deeply, gently press in and up on the abdomen until the liver brushes under your right hand. The edge should be smooth, firm, and somewhat round. Note any tenderness.

Hooking

• Hooking is an alternate way of palpating the liver. To hook the liver, stand next to the patient's right shoulder, facing his feet. Place your hands side-by-side, and hook your fingertips over the right costal margin, below the lower mark of dullness.

• Ask the patient to take a deep breath as you push your fingertips in and up. If the liver is palpable, you may feel its edge as it slides down in the abdomen as he breathes in.

fissures. The skin in the perianal area is normally somewhat darker than that of the surrounding area.

Palpate the inside

Next, palpate the rectum. Apply a water-soluble lubricant to your gloved index finger. Tell the patient to relax, and warn him that he'll feel some pressure. Then insert your finger into the rectum, toward the umbilicus. To palpate as much of the rectal wall as possible, rotate your finger clockwise and then counterclockwise. The rectal walls should feel soft and smooth, without masses, fecal impaction, or tenderness.

Inspect and test

Remove your finger from the rectum, and inspect the glove for stool, blood, and mucus. Test fecal matter adhering to the glove for occult blood using a guaiac test.

Diagnostic tests

Many tests provide information that will help direct your care of the patient with a GI problem. Even if you don't participate in testing, you'll need to know why the doctor ordered each test, what the results mean, and what responsibilities you'll need to carry out before, during, and after the test.

It's essential to know the reasons for a test, the meaning of results, and your responsibilities before and after.

Endoscopy

Using a fiber-optic endoscope, the doctor can directly view hollow visceral linings to diagnose inflammatory, ulcerative, and infectious diseases; benign and malignant neoplasms; and other esophageal, gastric, and intestinal mucosal lesions. Endoscopy can also be used for therapeutic interventions or to obtain biopsy specimens.

Lower GI endoscopy

Lower GI endoscopy, also called *colonoscopy* or *proctosigmoidoscopy*, aids diagnosis of inflammatory and ulcerative bowel disease, pinpoints lower GI bleeding, and detects lower GI abnormalities, such as tumors, polyps, hemorrhoids, and abscesses.

Nursing considerations

Explain these measures to the patient:
• He must maintain a clear liquid diet for up to 48 hours before the test and, as ordered, fast the morning of the test.
• He should continue any oral drug regimen as ordered (except for anticoagulants, aspirin, and NSAIDs).
• Dietary restrictions and bowel preparation are essential to clear the lower GI tract for a better view.
• In general, sigmoidoscopes are performed without sedation, and colonoscopies are performed using I.V. sedation.
• The doctor will insert a flexible tube into the patient's rectum.
• The patient may feel some lower abdominal discomfort and the urge to move his bowels as the tube is advanced. To control the urge to defecate and ease the discomfort, instruct him to breathe deeply and slowly through his mouth.

- Explain that air may be introduced into the bowel through the tube. If he feels the urge to expel some air, tell him not to try to control it.
- He may hear and feel a suction machine removing any liquid that may obscure the doctor's view, but it won't cause any discomfort.
- He can eat after recovering from the sedative, usually about 1 hour after the test.
- If air was introduced into the bowel, he may pass large amounts of flatus.
- He should report any blood in his stool.

Upper GI endoscopy

Upper GI endoscopy, also called *esophagogastroduodenoscopy*, identifies abnormalities of the esophagus, stomach, and small intestine, such as esophagitis, inflammatory bowel disease, Mallory-Weiss syndrome, lesions, tumors, gastritis, and polyps. During endoscopy, biopsies may be taken to detect the presence of *Helicobacter pylori* or to rule out gastric carcinoma.

Nursing considerations
Explain these measures to the patient:
- He must restrict food and fluids for at least 6 hours before the test.
- If the test is an emergency procedure, inform the patient that he'll have his stomach contents suctioned to permit better visualization.
- The test is performed using I.V. sedation for patient comfort.
- Before insertion of the tube, the patient's throat will be sprayed with a local anesthetic. The spray tastes unpleasant and will make his mouth feel swollen and numb, causing difficulty in swallowing.
- He'll have a mouthguard to protect his teeth from the tube.
- Before the test, tell the patient to remove dentures and bridges.
- As the tube is inserted and advanced, he can expect pressure in the abdomen and some fullness or bloating as air is introduced to inflate the stomach for a better view.
- The patient can resume eating when his gag reflex returns — usually in about 1 hour.

H. pylori is my name and infecting the alimentary canal is my game.

Laboratory tests

Common laboratory tests used to diagnose GI disorders include studies of stool, urine, and esophageal, gastric, and peritoneal contents as well as percutaneous liver biopsy.

Acid perfusion test

The lower esophageal sphincter (LES) normally prevents gastric reflux. However, if this sphincter is incompetent, the recurrent backflow of acidic juices (and of bile salts, if the pyloric sphincter is also incompetent) into the esophagus inflames the esophageal mucosa. This inflammation (esophagitis) manifests in burning epigastric or retrosternal pain that radiates to the back or arms. To distinguish such pain from that caused by angina pectoris or other disorders, normal saline and acidic solutions are perfused separately into the esophagus through an NG tube.

Ambulatory pH monitoring offers continuous measurement of esophageal pH up to 24 hours.

Ambling pH

Ambulatory pH monitoring has largely replaced the acid perfusion test because it offers continuous measurement of esophageal pH for up to 24 hours. It's especially useful in monitoring nocturnal symptoms. The test is done by placing an NG tube that records pH continuously over a set period. The patient may perform regular activities with the monitor in place. The patient should record symptoms of reflux and dyspepsia while being monitored to help correlate activity with pH.

Nursing considerations

Explain to the patient that he should refrain from antacids for 24 hours, food for 12 hours, and fluids and smoking for 8 hours before the test, as ordered.

After the test, if the patient continues to experience pain or burning, administer an antacid, as ordered. If he complains of a sore throat, provide soothing lozenges or obtain an order for an ice collar.

Fecal studies

Normal stool appears brown and formed but soft. Narrow, ribbon-like stool signals spastic or irritable bowel, or partial bowel or rectal obstruction. Diet and medication can cause constipation. Diarrhea may indicate spastic bowel or viral infection. Soft stool mixed with blood and mucus can signal bacterial infection; mixed with blood and pus, colitis.

Yellow or green stool suggests severe, prolonged diarrhea; black stool suggests GI bleeding or intake of iron supplements or raw-to-rare meat. Tan or white stool shows hepatic-duct or gallbladder-duct blockage, hepatitis, or cancer. Red stool may signal colon or rectal bleeding, but some drugs and foods can also cause this coloration.

Some drugs can cause constipation and red stools, signs that might otherwise be serious.

Fecal and urine tests

This table lists fecal and urine tests along with their normal values and purpose as well as the implications of abnormal results.

Test and normal values	Purpose	Implications of abnormal results
Bilirubin None	Detects bile pigments in urine	• Presence: biliary obstruction
Clostridium difficile *toxin assay* Negative	Detects pseudomembranous enterocolitis	• Indicates presence of *C. difficile* • False-negative result possible
Fecal lipid Less than 7 g/24 hours	Tests 72-hour stool collection for increased fat content if malabsorption is suspected	• Elevated: possible malabsorption caused by insufficient pancreatic enzyme excretion
Fecal occult blood test 2 to 2.5 ml/day	Measures occult (concealed) blood in stool samples	• Positive: GI bleeding or colorectal cancer, anal outlet bleeding
Fecal urobilinogen Males: 0.3 to 2.1 Ehrlich units/2 hours Females: 0.1 to 1.1 Ehrlich units/2 hours	Detects impaired liver function	• Elevated: impaired liver function • Lowered: total biliary obstruction
Stool culture No pathogens	Bacteriologic examination of stool sample detects pathogens causing GI disease	• Presence of pathogens: bacterial, viral, or fungal GI infection
Stool examination for ova and parasites No parasites or ova in stool	Confirms or rules out intestinal parasitic infestation and disease	• Presence of parasites or ova: parasitic infestation and possible infection

Most stool contains 10% to 20% fat. However, higher fat content can turn stool pasty or greasy — a possible sign of intestinal malabsorption or pancreatic disease. (See *Fecal and urine tests.*)

Nursing considerations

When collecting a stool specimen:
• Collect the stool specimen in a clean, dry container.
• Don't use stool that has been in contact with toilet-bowl water or urine.
• Send the specimen to the laboratory immediately for accurate results.
• Serial stool specimens are usually collected once per day with the first morning stool.
• Instruct the patient being tested for fecal occult blood to avoid eating red meat, poultry, fish, turnips, or horseradish or taking

iron preparations, ascorbic acid, or anti-inflammatory agents for 48 to 72 hours before the specimens are collected.
• Use commercial Hemoccult slides as a simple method of testing for blood in stool. Follow the package directions.

Percutaneous liver biopsy

A percutaneous liver biopsy involves the needle aspiration of a core of liver tissue for histologic analysis. It's done under local or general anesthesia. This biopsy can detect hepatic disorders and cancer after ultrasonography, computed tomography (CT) scans, and radionuclide studies have failed. Because many patients with hepatic disorders have clotting defects, a clotting profile (prothrombin time [PT], partial thromboplastin time [PTT]) along with type and crossmatching should precede liver biopsy.

In a liver biopsy, a Menghini needle attached to a 5-ml syringe containing normal saline solution is introduced through the chest wall and intercostal space. Negative pressure is created in the syringe. The needle is then pushed rapidly into the liver and pulled out of the body entirely to obtain a tissue specimen.

Percutaneous liver biopsy can detect hepatic disorders and cancer. Gulp.

Nursing considerations

Explain these measures to the patient:
• The patient should avoid food and fluids for at least 4 hours before the test.
• The patient will be awake during the test and, although the test is uncomfortable, medication is available to help him relax.
• The doctor will drape and clean an area on his abdomen. Then he'll administer a local anesthetic, which may sting and cause brief discomfort.
• The patient will be instructed how and when to hold his breath and to lie still as the doctor inserts the biopsy needle into the liver.
• The needle may cause a sensation of pressure and some discomfort in his right upper back, but will remain in his liver for only a few seconds.
• The patient must remain in bed on his right side for 2 hours and maintain bed rest for 24 hours.
• The patient may experience discomfort for several hours and may take ibuprofen but no aspirin.
• The patient may resume his normal diet.

After percutaneous liver biopsy, the patient may resume his normal diet.

When it's all over

After the procedure:
• Watch for bleeding and symptoms of bile peritonitis—tenderness and rigidity around the biopsy site.

• Be alert for symptoms of a pneumothorax, such as rising respiratory rate, depressed breath sounds, dyspnea, persistent shoulder pain, and pleuritic chest pain. Report these complications promptly.
• Apply a gauze dressing to the puncture site. Check the dressing frequently, whenever you check vital signs. Reinforce or apply a pressure dressing if needed.
• Maintain the patient in a right side-lying position for several hours because the pressure will enhance coagulation at the site.
• Monitor urine output for at least 24 hours and watch for hematuria, which may indicate bladder trauma.

Peritoneal fluid analysis

The peritoneal fluid analysis series includes examination of gross appearance, erythrocyte and leukocyte counts, cytologic studies, microbiological studies for bacteria and fungi, and determinations of protein, glucose, amylase, ammonia, and alkaline phosphatase levels. A sample of peritoneal fluid is obtained by paracentesis, which involves inserting a trocar and cannula through the abdominal wall with the patient under a local anesthetic. If the sample of fluid is being removed for therapeutic purposes, the cannula can be connected to a drainage system.

Nursing considerations

Follow these measures for the patient undergoing peritoneal fluid analysis:
• Before the procedure, have the patient empty his bladder.
• Observe the patient for dizziness, pallor, perspiration, and increased anxiety.
• Check the site for peritoneal fluid leakage.
• Watch for signs of hemorrhage, shock, and increasing pain and abdominal tenderness. These signs may indicate a perforated intestine or, depending on the site of the paracentesis, puncture of the inferior epigastric artery, hematoma of the anterior cecal wall, or rupture of the iliac vein or bladder.

You don't need a crystal ball to know that increasing pain and abdominal tenderness after paracentesis could be serious.

Urine tests

Urinalysis provides valuable information about hepatic and biliary function. Urinary bilirubin and urobilinogen tests are commonly used to evaluate liver function.

Billy, Billy Rubin

Bilirubin results from the breakdown of the heme fraction of hemoglobin. In the liver, free bilirubin conjugates with glucuronic acid, which allows bilirubin to be filtered by the glomeruli (unconjugated bilirubin isn't filtered). Bilirubin is normally excreted in bile as its principal pigment, but it occurs abnormally in urine. Conjugated bilirubin is present in urine when serum levels rise, as in biliary tract obstruction or hepatocellular damage, and is accompanied by jaundice.

You're no Billy Nogen!

Formed in the intestine by bacterial action on conjugated bilirubin, urobilinogen is primarily excreted in stool, producing its characteristic brown color. A small amount is reabsorbed by the portal system and is mainly reexcreted in bile, although the kidneys do excrete some. As a result, elevated urine urobilinogen levels may be an early indication of hepatic damage. In biliary obstruction, urine urobilinogen levels decline.

Nursing considerations

Follow these measures when collecting a urine sample:
• Collect a freshly voided random urine specimen in the container provided.
• Bilirubin may be analyzed at the patient's bedside using dip strips. Wait 20 seconds before interpreting the color change on the dip strip. Bilirubin must be tested within 30 minutes (before it disintegrates). If it's to be tested in the laboratory, send it immediately and record the collection time on the patient's chart.
• For urobilinogen, obtain a random specimen and send it to the laboratory immediately; it must be tested within 30 minutes, before the sample deteriorates.

> Nuclear imaging and ultrasonography enhance visual evaluation of disease processes.

Nuclear imaging and ultrasonography

Nuclear imaging methods, which include liver-spleen scanning and magnetic resonance imaging (MRI), analyze concentrations of injected or ingested radiopaque substances to enhance visual evaluation of possible disease processes. Nuclear imaging methods are used to study the liver, spleen, and other abdominal organs.

Ultrasonography is used to create images of internal organs, such as the gallbladder and liver. Gas-filled structures, such as the intestines, can't be seen with this technique.

Liver-spleen scan

In a liver-spleen scan, a scanner or gamma camera records the distribution of radioactivity within the liver and spleen after I.V. injection of a radioactive colloid. Most of this colloid is taken up by

Kupffer's cells in the liver, while smaller amounts lodge in the spleen and bone marrow. By registering the extent of this absorption, the imaging device detects such abnormalities as tumors, cysts, and abscesses. Because the test demonstrates disease nonspecifically (as an area that fails to take up the colloid, or a *cold spot*), test results usually require confirmation by ultrasonography, CT scan, gallium scan, or biopsy.

Nursing considerations

Explain these measures to the patient:
- This test examines the liver and spleen through pictures taken with a special scanner or camera.
- He'll receive an injection of a radioactive substance (technetium-99m) through an I.V. line in his hand or arm to allow better visualization of the liver and spleen.
- The patient should immediately report any adverse reactions, such as flushing, fever, light-headedness, or difficulty breathing.
- The injection contains only trace amounts of radioactivity, and he won't be radioactive after the test.
- If the test uses a rectilinear scanner, he'll hear a soft, irregular clicking noise as the scanner moves across his abdomen.
- If the test uses a gamma camera, the patient will feel the camera lightly touch his abdomen. He should lie still, relax, and breathe normally. He may be asked to hold his breath briefly to ensure good-quality pictures.

Because a liver-spleen scan doesn't specify disease, results usually require confirmation by another test such as a biopsy.

Magnetic resonance imaging

MRI is used in imaging the liver and abdominal organs. The image is generated by energizing protons into a strong magnetic field. Radio waves emitted as protons return to former equilibrium state and are recorded. No ionizing radiation is transmitted during the scan. Disadvantages are the closed, tubelike space that's required for the scan. Newer MRI centers offer a less confining "open-MRI" scan. The test can't be performed on patients with metal or implanted devices. MRI is useful in evaluating liver disease to help characterize tumors, masses, or cysts found on previous studies.

Nursing considerations

Explain these measures to the patient:
- He must lie still during the procedure, which may last from 30 to 90 minutes.
- He must remove any metal, such as jewelry, before the procedure.
- If he becomes claustrophobic during the test, mild sedation may be ordered.

Ultrasonography

Ultrasonography uses a focused beam of high-frequency sound waves to create echoes, which then appear as spikes and dots on an oscilloscope. Echoes vary with tissue density. The test helps differentiate between obstructive and nonobstructive jaundice and diagnoses cholelithiasis, cholecystitis, and certain metastases and hematomas. When used with liver-spleen scanning, it can clarify the nature of cold spots, such as tumors, abscesses, and cysts. The technique also aids diagnosis of pancreatitis, pseudocysts, pancreatic cancer, ascites, and splenomegaly.

Ultrasonography aids diagnosis of pancreatitis and pancreatic cancer, among other things.

Nursing considerations

Explain these measures to the patient:
• If having pelvic ultrasonography, he'll need a full bladder; therefore, he must drink three or four glasses of water before the test and must avoid urinating until after the test.
• For gallbladder evaluation, he shouldn't eat solid food for 12 hours before the test.
• For pancreas, liver, or spleen evaluation, he should fast for 8 hours.
• Sound waves can't penetrate barium; therefore, if he's scheduled for a barium enema or an upper GI series, make sure it occurs after abdominal ultrasonography.

Radiographic tests

Radiographic tests include abdominal X-rays, CT scans, various contrast medium studies, and virtual colonoscopy.

On X-ray, I'm white, air is black, and adipose tissue is gray. Of course, I look fabulous in any color, but white is my signature color.

Abdominal X-rays

An abdominal X-ray, also called *flat plate of the abdomen* or *kidney-ureter-bladder radiography*, helps detect and evaluate tumors, kidney stones, abnormal gas collection, and other abdominal disorders. The test consists of two plates: one taken with the patient supine and the other taken while he stands. On X-ray, air appears black, adipose tissue appears gray, and bone appears white.

Compare and contrast

Although a routine X-ray won't reveal most abdominal organs, it will show the contrast between air and fluid. For example, intestinal blockage traps large amounts of detectable fluids and air inside organs. When an intestinal wall tears, air leaks into the abdomen and becomes visible on X-ray.

Nursing considerations

• Radiography requires no special pretest or posttest care. Explain the procedure to the patient.
• X-ray interpretation involves locating normal anatomic structures, discerning any abnormal images, and correlating findings with assessment data.

Computed tomography scan

In CT scanning, a computer translates the action of multiple X-ray beams into three-dimensional oscilloscope images of the biliary tract, liver, and pancreas. The test can be done with or without a contrast medium, but contrast is preferred unless the patient is allergic to contrast medium. This test:
• helps distinguish between obstructive and nonobstructive jaundice
• identifies abscesses, cysts, hematomas, tumors, and pseudocysts
• can help evaluate the cause of weight loss
• detects occult malignancy
• can help diagnose and evaluate pancreatitis.

Nursing considerations

Explain these measures to the patient:
• He should restrict food and fluids after midnight before the test, but continue any drug regimen, as ordered.
• During the test, he should lie still, relax, breathe normally, and remain quiet because movement will blur the X-ray picture and prolong the test.
• If the doctor orders an I.V. contrast medium, the patient may experience discomfort from the needle puncture and a localized feeling of warmth on injection.
• If the patient has a seafood or dye allergy, a pretest preparation kit containing prednisone, cimetidine, and diphenhydramine may be given to him. He should immediately report any adverse reactions, such as nausea, vomiting, dizziness, headache, and urticaria. Assure him that reactions are rare.
• He may resume his normal diet after the test.

Contrast radiography

Some X-ray tests require contrast media to more accurately assess the GI system because the media accentuate differences among densities of air, fat, soft tissue, and bone. These tests include barium enema, barium swallow test, cholangiography, endoscopic retrograde cholangiopancreatography (ERCP), small-bowel series and enema, and upper GI series.

X-ray tests using contrast media accentuate differences among densities of air, fat, soft tissue, and bone.

Barium below

The barium enema is most commonly used to evaluate suspected lower intestinal disorders. It helps diagnose inflammatory disorders, colorectal cancer, polyps, diverticula, and large-intestine structural changes such as intussusception.

Barium above

The barium swallow test allows examination of the pharynx and esophagus to detect strictures, ulcers, tumors, polyps, diverticula, hiatal hernia, esophageal webs, gastroesophageal reflux disease (GERD), motility disorders and, sometimes, achalasia.

Cholangiography clues

In cholangiography (percutaneous and postoperative), a contrast agent is injected into the biliary tree through a flexible needle. In percutaneous transhepatic cholangiography (PTHC), a radiopaque dye is injected directly into the liver through the eighth or ninth midaxillary intercostal space. If done postoperatively, the dye is injected by way of a T tube. In an oral cholangiogram, the patient is given the contrast medium by mouth. These tests are used to determine the cause of upper abdominal pain that persists after cholecystectomy, to evaluate jaundice, and to determine the location, extent and, usually, the cause of mechanical obstructions.

Down endoscope

In ERCP, the doctor passes an endoscope into the duodenum and injects dye through a cannula inserted into the ampulla of Vater. This test helps to determine the cause of jaundice; evaluate tumors and inflammation of the pancreas, gallbladder, or liver; and locate obstructions in the pancreatic duct and hepatobiliary tree.

Shorter series or better distender

Results of a small-bowel series or enema, which follow the contrast agent through the small intestine, may suggest sprue, obstruction, motility disorders, malabsorption syndrome, Hodgkin's disease, lymphosarcoma, ischemia, bleeding, inflammation, or Crohn's disease of the small intestine. Although the enema study is longer and more uncomfortable than the small-bowel series, it better distends the bowel, making lesion identification easier.

I spy with an upper GI

In an upper GI series, the doctor follows the barium's passage from the esophagus to the stomach. Usually combined with a small-bowel series, the upper GI series helps diagnose gastritis, cancer, hiatal hernia, diverticula, strictures, and (most commonly) gastric and duodenal ulcers. It may also suggest motility disorders.

A small-bowel enema makes identifying lesions easier because it distends the bowel better than a small-bowel series.

Nursing considerations

Tell the patient where and when the test will take place. Also, explain these measures:

• The test will take only 30 to 40 minutes for a barium swallow or enema, but up to 6 hours for an upper GI or small-bowel series.

• He must maintain a low-residue diet for 2 to 3 days and must restrict food, fluids, and smoking after midnight before the test. He'll receive a clear liquid diet for 12 to 24 hours before the test. As ordered, he's to stop taking medications for up to 24 hours before the test.

• Unless he's undergoing a barium swallow test, the patient will receive a laxative the afternoon before the test and up to three cleaning enemas the evening before or the morning of the test. Explain that the presence of food or fluid may obscure details of the structures being studied.

• If having a barium enema, the patient will lie on his left side and the doctor will insert a small, lubricated tube into his rectum. Instruct the patient to keep his anal sphincter tightly contracted against the tube to hold it in position and help prevent barium leakage. Stress the importance of retaining the barium.

Eliminating barium

• After the test, the patient may resume his normal diet and medication, as ordered, and will receive a laxative to help expel the barium. Stress the importance of barium elimination because retained barium may harden, causing obstruction or impaction. The barium will lighten the color of his stools for 24 to 72 hours after the test.

• If the patient is having an oral cholangiogram, explain that, if ordered, he'll eat a meal containing fat at noon the day before the test and a fat-free meal that evening. After the evening meal, he can have only water, but should continue any drug regimen, as ordered.

• He'll be given a cleansing enema and, 2 to 3 hours before the test, he'll be asked to swallow six tablets, one at a time, at 5-minute intervals. The enema and tablets help outline the gallbladder on the X-ray film. He should report immediately any adverse reactions from the tablets, such as diarrhea, nausea, vomiting, abdominal cramps, and dysuria.

• He'll be asked to swallow barium several times during the test. Describe barium's thick consistency and chalky taste.

Virtual colonoscopy

Virtual colonoscopy is a nonsurgical approach to evaluate the colon. Air is introduced into the colon using a soft-tipped catheter, while a three-dimensional CT scan is performed. The scan takes

Virtual colonoscopy is still in development, but may be useful for patients who refuse colonoscopy.

about 10 minutes. Images are assembled in a computer program that can be viewed on a screen. Although this test is still in the developmental stage, it may be useful for the patient who refuses colonoscopy.

Nursing considerations

Explain these measures to the patient:
- He may feel discomfort when air is introduced into the colon.
- He'll have to remain still while images are taken.
- He'll have no restrictions after the test, but he may feel bloated from the air introduced into the colon.

Treatments

GI dysfunction presents many treatment challenges. After all, it stems from various pathophysiologic mechanisms that may exist separately or simultaneously. These mechanisms include tumors, hyperactivity and hypoactivity, malabsorption, infection and inflammation, vascular disorders, intestinal obstruction, and degenerative disease. Treatments for these disorders include drug therapy, surgery, and related measures that allow you to provide effective nursing care.

Drug therapy

The most commonly used GI drugs include antacids, digestants, histamine-2 (H_2) receptor antagonists, proton pump inhibitors, anticholinergics, antidiarrheal agents, laxatives, emetics, and antiemetics. Some of these drugs, such as antacids and antiemetics, provide relief immediately. Other drugs, such as laxatives and H_2-receptor antagonists, may take several days or longer to solve the problem.

Surgery

The patient who has undergone GI surgery usually needs special postoperative support because he may have to make permanent and difficult changes in his lifestyle. For example, besides teaching a colostomy patient about stoma care, you'll also have to help him adjust to changes in his body image and personal relationships. Another patient may have to endure a bowel training program for weeks or even months, which can be a frustrating and embarrassing experience. You'll have to draw on your own emotional strengths to help the patient overcome these feelings. Still

Treatments for GI dysfunction include drug therapy, surgery, and related measures.

another patient may have great difficulty complying with dietary restrictions. He'll need to be convinced of the firm link between such measures and a full recovery.

Esophageal surgeries

Surgery may be necessary to manage an emergency, such as acute constriction, or to provide palliative care for an incurable disease such as advanced esophageal cancer. Major esophageal surgeries include cardiomyotomy, cricopharyngeal myotomy, Nissen fundoplication, esophagectomy, esophagogastrostomy, and esophagomyotomy. The surgical approach is through the neck, chest, or abdomen, depending on the location of the problem.

Patient preparation

Explain the procedure to the patient, including these measures:
• When he awakes from the anesthetic, he'll probably have an NG tube in place to aid feeding and relieve abdominal distention.
• Discuss possible postoperative complications and measures to prevent or minimize them.
• Warn him of the risk of pneumonia and the importance of good pulmonary hygiene during recovery to prevent it. Demonstrate coughing and deep-breathing exercises; show the patient how to splint his incision to protect it and minimize pain.

Monitoring and aftercare

After surgery, follow these steps:
• Place the patient in semi-Fowler's position to help minimize esophageal reflux.
• Provide antacids as needed for symptomatic relief.
• If surgery involving the upper esophagus produces hypersalivation, the patient may be unable to swallow the excess saliva. Control drooling with gauze wicks or suctioning. Allow the patient to spit into an emesis basin placed within his reach.
• To reduce the risk of aspiration pneumonia, elevate the head of the patient's bed and encourage him to turn frequently. Carefully monitor his vital signs and auscultate his lungs. Encourage coughing and deep-breathing exercises.
• Watch for developing mediastinitis, especially if surgery involved extensive thoracic invasion (as in esophagogastrostomy). Note and report fever, dyspnea, and complaints of substernal pain. If ordered, administer antibiotics to help prevent or correct this complication.
• Watch for signs of leakage at the anastomosis site. Check drainage tubes for blood, test for occult blood in stool and

I'll show you how to splint your incision to protect it and minimize pain while coughing and deep breathing.

drainage, and monitor hemoglobin levels for evidence of slow blood loss. If the patient has an NG tube in place, avoid handling the tube because this may damage the internal sutures or anastomoses. For the same reason, avoid deep suctioning in a patient who has undergone extensive esophageal repair.

Home care instructions

Provide these instructions to the patient:
• Advise him to sleep with his head elevated to prevent reflux. Suggest that he raise the head of his bed on blocks.
• If the patient smokes, encourage him to stop. Explain that nicotine adversely affects the LES. Advise the patient to avoid alcohol, aspirin, and effervescent over-the-counter products (such as Alka-Seltzer) because they may damage the tender esophageal mucosa.
• Advise the patient to avoid heavy lifting, straining, and coughing, which could rupture the weakened mucosa.
• Tell him to report any respiratory signs and symptoms, such as wheezing, coughing, and nocturnal dyspnea.

Gastric surgeries

If chronic ulcer disease doesn't respond to medication, diet, and rest, gastric surgery is used to remove diseased or malignant tissue, to prevent ulcers from recurring, or to relieve an obstruction or perforation. In an emergency, it may be performed to control severe GI hemorrhage or perforation. Surgery may also be necessary when laser endoscopic coagulation for control of severe GI bleeding isn't possible.

Gastric surgery can take various forms, depending on the location and extent of the disorder. For example, a partial gastrectomy reduces the amount of acid-secreting mucosa. A bilateral vagotomy relieves ulcer symptoms and eliminates vagal nerve stimulation of gastric secretions. A pyloroplasty improves drainage and prevents obstruction. Most commonly, however, two gastric surgeries are combined, such as vagotomy with gastroenterostomy or vagotomy with antrectomy. Although controversial in cases of morbid obesity, gastric reduction surgery may be performed to aid in weight loss. (See *Understanding common gastric surgeries.*)

Patient preparation

Before surgery, implement these measures:
• Evaluate and begin stabilizing the patient's fluid and electrolyte balance and nutritional status—both of which may be severely compromised by chronic ulcer disease or other GI disorders.
• Monitor intake and output, and draw serum samples for hematologic studies.
• Prepare the patient for abdominal X-rays.

Tell the patient to avoid alcohol, which may damage the tender esophageal mucosa.

Understanding common gastric surgeries

In addition to treating chronic ulcers, gastric surgeries help remove obstructions and malignant tumors. Names of gastric surgeries (other than vagotomy) usually refer to the stomach portion removed. Most procedures combine two surgery types.

Note: Keep in mind that *-ostomy* means "an opening into." If only one prefix precedes *-ostomy,* then the surgical opening is made from the exterior—for example, *gastrostomy.* Two prefixes indicate anastomosis—for example, *gastroenterostomy* means anastomosis of a stomach *(gastro-)* remnant with a small intestine *(entero-)* segment.

Make sure you're familiar with these commonly performed gastric surgeries.

Vagotomy with gastroenterostomy

In this procedure, the surgeon resects the vagus nerves and creates a stoma for gastric drainage. He'll perform selective, truncal, or parietal cell vagotomy, depending on the degree of decreased gastric acid secretion required.

Vagotomy with antrectomy

After resecting the vagus nerves, the surgeon removes the antrum. Then he anastomoses the remaining stomach segment to the jejunum and closes the duodenal stump.

Vagotomy with pyloroplasty

In this procedure, the surgeon resects the vagus nerves and refashions the pylorus to widen the lumen and aid gastric emptying.

Billroth I

In this partial gastrectomy with a gastroduodenostomy, the surgeon excises the distal one-third to one-half of the stomach and anastomoses the remaining stomach to the duodenum.

Billroth II

In this partial gastrectomy with a gastrojejunostomy, the surgeon removes the distal segment of the stomach and antrum. Then he anastomoses the remaining stomach and the jejunum and closes the duodenal stump.

• On the night before surgery, administer laxatives and enemas as necessary.
• On the morning of surgery, insert an NG tube, as ordered.

Monitoring and aftercare

Follow these steps after surgery:
• Place the patient in low or semi-Fowler's position. Either position will ease breathing and prevent aspiration if he vomits.
• Maintain tube feedings or total parenteral nutrition (TPN) and I.V. fluid and electrolyte replacement therapy, as ordered. Monitor blood studies daily. If you perform gastric suctioning, watch for signs of dehydration, hyponatremia, and metabolic alkalosis. Weigh the patient daily, and monitor and record intake and output, including NG tube drainage.
• Auscultate the abdomen frequently for bowel sounds. When they return, notify the doctor, who will order clamping or removal of the NG tube and gradual resumption of oral feeding. During NG tube clamping, watch for nausea and vomiting; if they occur, unclamp the tube immediately and reattach it to suction.
• Throughout recovery, have the patient cough, deep-breathe, and change position frequently. Encourage incentive spirometry. Teach the patient to splint his incision while coughing to help reduce pain. Assess his breath sounds frequently to detect atelectasis.
• Assess the patient for other complications, including vitamin B_{12} deficiency, anemia (especially common in patients who have undergone total gastrectomy), and dumping syndrome, a potentially serious digestive complication marked by weakness, nausea, flatulence, and palpitations within 30 minutes after a meal.

Home care instructions

Provide these instructions for the patient:
• Advise the patient to seek medical attention immediately if he develops any signs of life-threatening complications, such as hemorrhage, obstruction, and perforation.
• Explain dumping syndrome and how to avoid it. Advise the patient to eat small, frequent meals evenly spaced throughout the day. He should chew his food thoroughly and drink fluids between meals rather than with them. In his diet, he should decrease intake of carbohydrates and salt while increasing fat and protein. After a meal, he should lie down for 20 to 30 minutes. If the patient is being discharged on tube feedings, teach him and his family how to give the feeding.
• Tell the patient to avoid or limit foods high in fiber, such as fresh fruits and vegetables and whole grain breads. If the doctor has prescribed a GI anticholinergic to decrease motility and acid

Tell the patient to notify the doctor immediately if he develops any signs of life-threatening complications.

secretion, instruct the patient to take the drug 30 minutes to 1 hour before meals.
• Encourage the patient to avoid smoking because it alters pancreatic secretions that neutralize gastric acid in the duodenum.

Bowel surgery with ostomy

In bowel surgery with ostomy, the surgeon removes diseased colonic and rectal segments and creates a stoma on the outer abdominal wall to allow fecal elimination. This surgery is performed for such intestinal maladies as inflammatory bowel disease, familial polyposis, diverticulitis, and advanced colorectal cancer if conservative surgery and other treatments aren't successful or if the patient develops acute complications, such as obstruction, abscess, and fistula.

Take your pick

The surgeon can choose from several types of surgery, depending on the nature and location of the problem.
• Intractable obstruction of the ascending, transverse, descending, or sigmoid colon requires permanent colostomy and removal of the affected bowel segments.
• Cancer of the rectum and lower sigmoid colon commonly calls for abdominoperineal resection, which involves creation of a permanent colostomy and removal of the remaining colon, rectum, and anus.
• Perforated sigmoid diverticulitis, Hirschsprung's disease, rectovaginal fistula, and penetrating trauma commonly require temporary colostomy to interrupt the intestinal flow and allow inflamed or injured bowel segments to heal. After healing occurs (usually within 8 weeks), the divided segments are anastomosed to restore bowel integrity and function.
• In a double-barrel colostomy, the transverse colon is divided and both ends are brought out through the abdominal wall to create a proximal stoma for fecal drainage and a distal stoma leading to the nonfunctioning bowel.
• Loop colostomy, done to relieve acute obstruction in an emergency, involves creating proximal and distal stomas from a loop of intestine that has been pulled through an abdominal incision and supported with a plastic or glass rod.
• Severe, widespread colonic obstruction may require total or near-total removal of the colon and rectum and creation of an ileostomy from the proximal ileum. A permanent ileostomy requires that the patient wear a drainage pouch or bag over the stoma to receive the constant fecal drainage. In contrast, a continent, or Kock, ileostomy doesn't require an external pouch.

Patient preparation

Before surgery, implement these measures:
• Arrange for the patient to visit with an enterostomal therapist, who can provide more detailed information. The therapist can also help the patient select the best location for the stoma.

Sharing insights into reality

• Try to have the patient meet with an ostomy patient (from a group such as the United Ostomy Association), who can share his personal insights into the realities of living with and caring for a stoma.
• Evaluate his nutritional and fluid status. Typically, the patient will be receiving TPN to prepare him for the physiologic stress of surgery.
• Record the patient's fluid intake and output and weight daily, and watch for early signs of dehydration.
• Expect to draw periodic blood samples for hematocrit and hemoglobin determinations. Be prepared to transfuse blood if ordered.

> Before surgery, expect to draw periodic blood samples to measure hematocrit and hemoglobin and be prepared to administer a blood transfusion, if necessary.

Monitoring and aftercare

Follow these steps after surgery:
• Monitor intake and output, and weigh the patient daily. Maintain fluid and electrolyte balance, and watch for signs of dehydration (decreased urine output, poor skin turgor) and electrolyte imbalance.
• Provide analgesics, as ordered. Be especially alert for pain in the patient with an abdominoperineal resection because of the extent and location of the incisions.
• Note and record the color, consistency, and odor of fecal drainage from the stoma. If the patient has a double-barrel colostomy, check for mucus drainage from the inactive (distal) stoma. The nature of fecal drainage is determined by the type of ostomy surgery; generally, the less colon tissue that's removed, the more closely drainage will resemble normal stool. For the first few days after surgery, fecal drainage probably will be mucoid (and possibly slightly blood-tinged) and mostly odorless. Report excessive blood or mucus content, which could indicate hemorrhage or infection.

Searching for sepsis

• Observe the patient for signs of peritonitis or sepsis, caused by bowel contents leaking into the abdominal cavity. Remember that patients receiving antibiotics or TPN are at an increased risk for sepsis.

• Provide meticulous wound care, changing dressings often. Check dressings and drainage sites frequently for signs of infection (purulent drainage, foul odor) or fecal drainage. If the patient has had an abdominoperineal resection, irrigate the perineal area as ordered.

• Regularly check the stoma and surrounding skin for irritation and excoriation, and take corrective measures. Also observe the stoma's appearance. The stoma should look smooth, cherry red, and slightly edematous; immediately report any discoloration or excessive swelling, which may indicate circulatory problems that could lead to ischemia.

• During the recovery period, encourage the patient to express his feelings and concerns; reassure an anxious or depressed patient that these common postoperative reactions should fade as he adjusts to the ostomy. Continue to arrange for visits by an enterostomal therapist.

Home care instructions

Provide these instructions to the patient:

• If the patient has a colostomy, teach him or a caregiver how to apply, remove, and empty the pouch. When appropriate, teach him how to irrigate the colostomy with warm tap water to gain some control over elimination. Reassure him that he can regain continence with dietary control and bowel retraining.

• Instruct the colostomy patient to change the stoma appliance as needed, to wash the stoma site with warm water and mild soap every 3 days, and to change the adhesive layer. These measures help prevent skin irritation and excoriation.

• If the patient has an ileostomy, instruct him to change the drainage pouch only when leakage occurs. Also, emphasize meticulous skin care and use of a protective skin barrier around the stoma site.

• Discuss dietary restrictions and suggestions to prevent stoma blockage, diarrhea, flatus, and odor. Tell the patient to stay on a low-fiber diet for 6 to 8 weeks and to add new foods to his diet gradually. Suggest that the patient use an ostomy deodorant or an odorproof pouch if he includes odor-producing foods in his diet.

• Trial and error will help the patient determine which foods cause gas. Gas-producing fruits include apples, melons, avocados, and cantaloupe; gas-producing vegetables include beans, corn, and cabbage.

Reassure an anxious or depressed patient that such feelings are common and should fade as he adjusts to the ostomy.

Bring on the bouillon

• The patient is especially susceptible to fluid and electrolyte losses. He must drink plenty of fluids, especially in hot weather or

when he has diarrhea. Fruit juice and bouillon, which contain potassium, are particularly helpful.
• Warn the patient to avoid alcohol, laxatives, and diuretics, which will increase fluid loss and may contribute to an imbalance.
• Tell the patient to report persistent diarrhea through the stoma, which can quickly lead to fluid and electrolyte imbalance.
• If the patient had an abdominoperineal resection, suggest sitz baths to help relieve perineal discomfort. Recommend refraining from intercourse until the perineum heals.

Bowel resection and anastomosis

Resection of diseased intestinal tissue (colectomy) and anastomosis of the remaining segments helps treat localized obstructive disorders, including diverticulosis, intestinal polyps, bowel adhesions, and malignant or benign intestinal lesions. This is the preferred surgical technique for localized bowel cancer but not for widespread carcinoma, which usually requires massive resection and a temporary or permanent colostomy or an ileostomy.

Unlike the patient who undergoes total colectomy or more extensive surgery, the patient who undergoes simple resection and anastomosis usually retains normal bowel function.

Patient preparation

Before surgery, as ordered, administer antibiotics to reduce intestinal flora, and laxatives or enemas to remove fecal contents.

Monitoring and aftercare

Follow these steps after surgery:
• For the first few days after surgery, monitor the patient's intake, output, and weight daily. Maintain fluid and electrolyte balance through I.V. replacement therapy, and check regularly for signs of dehydration, such as decreased urine output and poor skin turgor.
• Keep the NG tube patent. Warn the patient that he should never attempt to reposition a dislodged tube himself because doing so could damage the anastomosis.
• Observe the patient for signs of peritonitis or sepsis caused by leakage of bowel contents into the abdominal cavity. He's at increased risk for sepsis if he's receiving antibiotics or TPN. Sepsis also may result from wicking of colonic bacteria up the NG tube to the oral cavity and can be prevented with frequent mouth and tube care.

For the first few days after surgery, monitor the patient's intake, output, and weight daily.

An attack of hot flashes

• Provide meticulous wound care, changing dressings when needed. Check dressings and drainage sites frequently for signs of infection (purulent drainage, foul odor) and fecal drainage. Also, watch for sudden fever, especially when accompanied by abdominal pain and tenderness.

• Regularly assess the patient for signs of postresection obstruction. Examine the abdomen for distention and rigidity, auscultate for bowel sounds, and note the passage of any flatus or stool.

• After the patient regains peristalsis and bowel function, help him avoid constipation and straining during defecation, both of which can damage the anastomosis. Encourage him to drink plenty of fluids, and administer a stool softener or other laxative, as ordered. Note and record the frequency and amount of all bowel movements as well as characteristics of the stool.

• Encourage regular coughing and deep breathing to prevent atelectasis; remind the patient to splint the incision site as necessary.

• Assess pain and provide analgesics, as ordered.

Home care instructions

Provide these instructions to the patient:

• Instruct the patient to record the frequency and character of bowel movements and tell the doctor if he notices any changes in his normal pattern. Warn him against using laxatives without consulting his doctor.

• Tell the patient to avoid abdominal straining and heavy lifting until the sutures are completely healed and the doctor gives permission to do so.

• Encourage the patient to maintain the prescribed semibland diet until his bowel has healed completely (usually 4 to 8 weeks after surgery). Stress the need to avoid carbonated beverages and gas-producing foods.

• Because extensive bowel resection may interfere with the patient's ability to absorb nutrients, emphasize the importance of taking prescribed vitamin supplements.

Appendectomy

With rare exception, the only effective treatment for acute appendicitis is to remove the inflamed vermiform appendix. A common emergency surgery, an appendectomy aims to prevent imminent rupture or perforation of the appendix. When completed before these complications occur, an appendectomy is usually effective and uneventful. If the appendix ruptures or perforates before surgery, its infected contents spill into the peritoneal cavity, possi-

An appendectomy is a common emergency procedure and virtually the only effective treatment for acute appendicitis.

bly causing peritonitis, which is the most common and fatal complication of appendicitis, with a mortality rate of 10%. Most appendectomies are now done laparoscopically, except in cases where rupture is suspected.

Patient preparation

Before surgery, implement these measures:
• Reduce the patient's pain by placing him in Fowler's position.
• Avoid giving analgesics, which can mask the pain that heralds rupture.
• Never apply heat to the abdomen, give cathartics or enemas, or palpate the abdomen; these measures could trigger rupture.

Monitoring and aftercare

Follow these steps after surgery:
• Carefully monitor vital signs and record intake and output for 2 days after surgery.
• Auscultate the abdomen for bowel sounds, which signal the return of peristalsis.
• Regularly check the wound dressing for drainage, and change it as necessary. If abdominal drains are in place, check and record the amount and nature of drainage, and maintain drain patency.
• Check drainage from the NG tube, and irrigate as needed.
• Encourage ambulation within 12 hours after surgery if possible. Assist the patient as needed.
• Encourage coughing, deep breathing, use of an incentive spirometer, and frequent position changes to prevent pulmonary complications.
• On the day after surgery, remove the NG tube and gradually resume oral foods and fluids, as ordered.
• Assess the patient closely for signs of peritonitis. Watch for and report continuing pain and fever, excessive wound drainage, hypotension, tachycardia, pallor, weakness, and other signs of infection and fluid and electrolyte loss. If peritonitis develops, expect to assist with emergency treatment, including GI intubation, parenteral fluid and electrolyte replacement, and antibiotic therapy.

Home care instructions

Provide these instructions to the patient:
• Tell the patient to watch for and immediately report fever, chills, diaphoresis, nausea, vomiting, or abdominal pain and tenderness.
• Instruct the patient to avoid strenuous activity (heavy lifting, stooping, and pushing or pulling) for up to 1 month following surgery.
• Encourage the patient to keep scheduled follow-up appointments to monitor healing and diagnose complications.

Gallbladder surgery

When gallbladder and biliary disorders fail to respond to drugs, diet therapy, and supportive treatments, surgery may be required to restore biliary flow from the liver to the small intestine. Gallbladder removal, or *cholecystectomy*, restores biliary flow in gallstone disease (cholecystitis or cholelithiasis). One of the most commonly performed surgeries, cholecystectomy relieves symptoms in 90% of patients with gallstone disease. Conventional cholecystectomy requires a large incision, produces considerable discomfort, and results in weeks of recovery time.

Laparoscope to the rescue

Laparoscopic laser cholecystectomy allows gallbladder removal without major abdominal surgery, thereby speeding recovery and reducing the risk of complications, such as infection and herniation. Patients are usually discharged from the hospital and are able to resume a normal diet after 24 to 36 hours. Typically, patients can return to the workplace within 10 days. Laparoscopic laser cholecystectomy is contraindicated in pregnancy, acute cholangitis, septic peritonitis, and severe bleeding disorders. (See *Understanding cholecystectomy*, page 440.)

A clean sweep

In patients who aren't good candidates for cholecystectomy, cholecystostomy (incision into the fundus of the gallbladder to remove and drain any retained gallstones or inflammatory debris) or choledochotomy (incision into the common bile duct to remove any gallstones or other obstructions) are sometimes performed.

Laparoscopic laser cholecystectomy speeds recovery and allows patients to resume a normal diet after 24 to 36 hours.

Patient preparation

Before laparoscopic surgery, implement these measures:
• Monitor and, if necessary, help stabilize the patient's nutritional status and fluid balance. Such measures may include vitamin K administration, blood transfusions, and glucose and protein supplements.
• For 24 hours before surgery, give the patient clear liquids only.
• As ordered, administer preoperative medications and insert an NG tube.

Monitoring and aftercare

Follow these steps after laparoscopic surgery:
• Check the small stab wounds; they will be closed with staples and may have small dressings.
• Monitor for anesthesia-related nausea and vomiting.

Understanding cholecystectomy

Gallbladder surgeries include abdominal cholecystectomy and laparoscopic laser cholecystectomy as well as several less commonly performed procedures. The two more common procedures are described here.

Abdominal cholecystectomy

Performed under general anesthesia, abdominal cholecystectomy begins with a right subcostal or paramedial incision. The surgeon then surveys the abdomen and uses laparotomy packs to isolate the gallbladder from the surrounding organs. After identifying biliary tract structures, he may use cholangiography or ultrasonography to help identify gallstones. Using a choledocoscope, he directly visualizes the bile ducts and inserts a balloon-tipped catheter to clear the ducts of stones.

　　The surgeon ligates and divides the cystic duct and artery and removes the entire gallbladder. Typically, he performs a choledochotomy—the insertion of a T tube into the common bile duct to decompress the biliary tree and prevent bile peritonitis during healing. He may also insert a drain into the ducts.

Laparoscopic laser cholecystectomy

Several small entry points (1 to 3 cm) are made on the abdomen—at the umbilicus (for the laparoscope and attached camera) and at the upper midline, right lateral line, and right midclavicular line (for various grasping and dissecting forceps). The abdomen is insufflated with carbon dioxide, which allows viewing of the structures. The attached camera transmits images to a television monitor, allowing the surgical team to view the procedure. The cystic duct and artery are clipped and divided. Laser or cautery is used to cut and coagulate during removal of the gallbladder from its liver bed. Needle aspiration of bile facilitates gallbladder removal through the stab wound at the umbilicus.

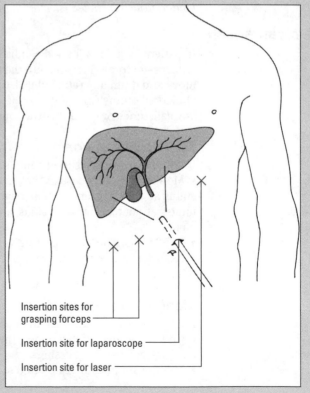

• Apply heat to the patient's shoulder to alleviate right shoulder pain caused by phrenic irritation from carbon dioxide under the diaphragm. To decrease discomfort, place the patient in semi-Fowler's position. Early ambulation also helps.
• Tell the patient a light meal is usually permitted the same evening.
• The day after discharge, place a follow-up phone call to the patient's home to check on his progress.

Conventional care cues

Follow these steps after conventional surgery:
• Place the patient in low Fowler's position. If an NG tube is being used, attach it to low intermittent suction. Monitor the amount and characteristics of drainage from the NG tube as well as from any abdominal drains. Check the dressing frequently, and change it as necessary.
• If the patient has a T tube in place, frequently assess the position and patency of the tube and drainage bag. Make sure the bag is level with the abdomen to prevent excessive drainage. Also note the amount and characteristics of drainage; bloody or blood-tinged bile usually occurs for only the first few hours after surgery. Provide meticulous skin care around the tube insertion site to prevent irritation.
• After a few days, expect to remove the NG tube and begin introducing foods: first liquids, then gradually soft solids. As ordered, clamp the T tube for an hour before and an hour after each meal to allow bile to travel to the intestine to aid digestion.
• Watch for signs of postcholecystectomy syndrome (such as fever, abdominal pain, and jaundice) and other complications involving obstructed bile drainage. For several days after surgery, monitor vital signs and record intake and output every 8 hours. Report unusual signs and symptoms to the doctor, and collect urine and stool specimens for laboratory analysis of bile content.

Many patients return to a normal activity within 10 days — before you can say laparoscopic laser cholecystectomy!

Home care instructions

After laparoscopic laser cholecystectomy, instruct the patient on the use of oral analgesics, how to clean the surgical stab sites, and when to call the doctor. Also, include these instructions in your teaching:
• Recommend activity, as tolerated, but tell the patient to avoid heavy lifting for about 2 weeks. Assure him that patients typically return to a normal schedule within 10 days.
• Tell the patient that he'll be given an appointment to see the doctor or return to the clinic within 7 days for removal of the staples. Assure him that scarring is usually minimal.

Teaching conventionally

After conventional surgery, give these instructions:
• If the patient is being discharged with a T tube in place, stress the need for the patient to practice meticulous tube care.
• Tell him to immediately report any signs or symptoms of biliary obstruction: fever, jaundice, pruritus, pain, dark urine, and clay-colored stools.
• Encourage the patient to maintain a diet low in fats and high in carbohydrates and protein. Tell him that his ability to digest fats will improve as bile flow to the intestine increases. As this occurs, usually within 6 weeks, he may gradually add fats to his diet.

Liver transplantation

For the patient with a life-threatening liver disorder that doesn't respond to treatment, a liver transplant may seem the last best hope. Even so, transplant surgery is used infrequently because of its risks, high cost, and shortage of suitable donor organs. Typically, it's used only in large teaching centers and is reserved for those terminally ill patients who have a realistic chance of surviving the surgery and withstanding postoperative complications. Candidates include patients with congenital biliary abnormalities, chronic hepatitis B or C, inborn errors of metabolism, or end-stage liver disease.

Meet the candidate

Careful identification of suitable candidates for referral to the transplant team is essential in the success of therapy. Criteria for referral for transplantation include:
• advanced hepatic failure with a predicted survival rate of less than 2 years
• unavailability of other medical or surgical therapies that offer long-term survival
• absence of contraindicated conditions, such as extrahepatic carcinoma, severe cardiac disease, and current active alcohol or drug addiction
• that the patient and his family must fully understand the physical, psychological, and financial aspects of the transplant process.

Waiting game

Many qualified transplant candidates are awaiting suitable donor organs, but few survive the wait. Also, even if a compatible healthy liver is located and transplantation performed, the patient faces many obstacles to recovery. Besides the complications accompanying extensive abdominal and vascular surgeries, liver transplantation carries a high risk of tissue rejection. Current 1-year survival rates range from 54% to 83%.

Current 1-year survival rates for liver transplant are 54% to 83%.

Patient preparation

Before surgery, implement these measures:
• As ordered, begin immunosuppressant therapy to decrease the risk of tissue rejection, using such drugs as cyclosporine and corticosteroids.
• Explain the need for lifelong therapy to prevent rejection.
• Address the patient's (and his family's) emotional needs. Discuss the typical stages of emotional adjustment to a liver transplant: overwhelming relief and elation at surviving the operation, followed by anxiety, frustration, and depression if complications occur.

Monitoring and aftercare

Focus your aftercare on four areas:
• maintaining immunosuppressant therapy to combat tissue rejection
• monitoring for early signs of rejection and other complications
• preventing opportunistic infections, which can lead to rejection
• providing emotional support to the patient throughout the prolonged recovery period.

Home care instructions

Teach the patient and his family to:
• watch for early indicators of tissue rejection, including fever, tachycardia, jaundice, changes in the color of urine or stool, and pain and tenderness in the right upper quadrant, right flank, or center of the back, and notify the doctor immediately if any of these signs or symptoms develop
• watch for and report any signs or symptoms of liver failure, such as abdominal distention, bloody stool or vomitus, decreased urine output, abdominal pain and tenderness, anorexia, and altered level of consciousness (LOC)

A wave instead of a handshake

• reduce the risk of tissue rejection by avoiding contact with any person who has or may have a contagious illness and report any early signs or symptoms of infection, including fever, weakness, lethargy, and tachycardia
• keep follow-up appointments, which will include regular liver function tests, complete blood count (CBC), and blood cyclosporin levels, to evaluate the integrity of the surgical site and continued tissue compatibility
• strictly comply with the prescribed immunosuppressive drug regimen because noncompliance can trigger rejection, even of a liver that has been functioning well for years

• be aware of potential adverse effects of immunosuppressive therapy, such as infection, fluid retention, acne, glaucoma, diabetes, and cancer
• seek psychological counseling, if necessary, to help the patient and his family cope with the effects of the patient's long and difficult recovery.

Liver resection or repair

Resection or repair of diseased or damaged liver tissue may be indicated for various hepatic disorders, including cysts, abscesses, tumors, and lacerations or crush injuries from blunt or penetrating trauma. Usually, surgery is performed only after conservative measures prove ineffective. For instance, if aspiration fails to correct a liver abscess, resection may be necessary.

Liver resection procedures include a partial or subtotal hepatectomy (excision of a portion of the liver) and lobectomy (excision of an entire lobe). Lobectomy is the surgery of choice for primary liver tumors, but partial hepatectomy may be effective for small tumors. Even so, because liver cancer is often advanced at diagnosis, few tumors are resectable. In fact, only single tumors confined to one lobe are usually considered resectable, and then only if the patient is free from complicating cirrhosis, jaundice, or ascites. Because of the liver's anatomic location, surgery is usually performed through a thoracoabdominal incision.

Surgery is performed only after conservative measures prove ineffective.

Patient preparation

Before surgery, implement these measures:
• Encourage rest and good nutrition and provide vitamin supplements, as ordered, to help improve liver function.
• Prepare the patient for additional diagnostic tests, which may include liver scan, CT scan, ultrasonography, percutaneous needle biopsy, hepatic angiography, and cholangiography.
• Explain postoperative care measures. Tell the patient he'll awaken from surgery with an NG tube, a chest tube, and hemodynamic monitoring lines in place. Tell him to expect frequent checks of vital signs, fluid and electrolyte balance, and neurologic status as well as I.V. fluid replacement and possible blood transfusions and TPN. If possible, allow the patient to visit and familiarize himself with the intensive care unit.
• To reduce the risk of postoperative atelectasis, encourage the patient to practice coughing and deep-breathing exercises, and teach him how to use an incentive spirometer.

Monitoring and aftercare

Follow these steps after surgery:
• Frequently assess for complications, such as hemorrhage and infection. Monitor the patient's vital signs and evaluate fluid status every 1 to 2 hours. Report any signs of volume deficit, which could indicate intraperitoneal bleeding. Keep an I.V. line patent for possible emergency fluid replacement or blood transfusion. Provide analgesics, as ordered.
• At least daily, check laboratory test results for hypoglycemia, increased PT, increased ammonia levels, azotemia (increased blood urea nitrogen [BUN] and creatinine levels), and electrolyte imbalances (especially potassium, sodium, and calcium imbalances). Promptly report adverse findings, and take corrective steps, as ordered. For example, give I.M. vitamin K to decrease PT, or infuse hypertonic glucose solution to correct hypoglycemia.

Pretend that it's a cow

• Check wound dressings often and change them as needed. Note and report excessive bloody drainage on the dressings or in the drainage tube. Also note the amount and characteristics of NG tube drainage; keep in mind that excessive drainage could trigger metabolic alkalosis. If the patient has a chest tube in place, maintain tube patency by milking it as necessary, and make sure the suction equipment is operating properly.
• Watch for symptoms of hepatic encephalopathy, including behavioral or personality changes, such as confusion, forgetfulness, lethargy or stupor, and hallucinations. Also observe for asterixis, apraxia, and hyperactive reflexes.

Home care instructions

Provide these instructions to the patient:
• Advise the patient that adequate rest and good nutrition conserve energy and reduce metabolic demands on the liver, thereby speeding healing. For the first 6 to 8 months after surgery, he should gradually resume normal activities, balance periods of activity and rest, and avoid overexertion.
• As ordered, instruct the patient to maintain a high-calorie, high-carbohydrate, and high-protein diet during this period to help restore the liver mass. However, if the patient had hepatic encephalopathy, advise him to follow a low-protein diet, with carbohydrates making up the balance of calorie intake.

If the patient had hepatic encephalopathy, advise him to follow a low-protein diet.

LeVeen shunt insertion

Intractable ascites resulting from chronic liver disease can be controlled by draining ascitic fluid from the abdominal cavity into the

How the LeVeen shunt works

The LeVeen peritoneovenous shunt consists of a peritoneal tube, a venous tube, and a one-way pressure-sensitive valve that controls fluid flow.

Operation is simple. As the patient inhales, pressure within his abdomen increases while pressure in his superior vena cava decreases. This pressure differential causes the shunt's valve to open, allowing ascitic fluid to drain from the abdominal cavity into the superior vena cava. When the patient exhales, superior vena cava pressure rises and intra-abdominal pressure falls; this pressure differential forces the valve shut, stopping fluid flow.

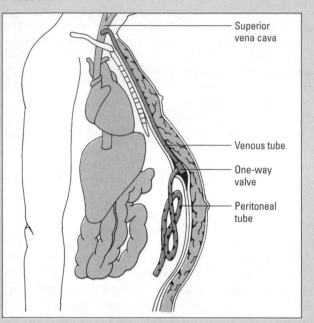

Superior
vena cava

Venous tube

One-way
valve

Peritoneal
tube

The valve's one-way design prevents blood from backing into the tubing, reducing the risk of clotting and shunt occlusion. It also prevents the valve from opening if superior vena cava pressure remains higher than intra-abdominal pressure, as may occur in patients with heart failure. This reduces the risk of fluid overload in the vascular system.

superior vena cava using the LeVeen peritoneovenous shunt. Commonly used with diuretic therapy, the LeVeen shunt provides an effective alternative to traditional treatments for ascites such as paracentesis.

Patient preparation
Before surgery, implement these measures:
• Show the shunt to the patient and describe how it works.
• Tell him that he'll receive a local anesthetic to prevent discomfort during shunt insertion.
• Measure and record the patient's weight and abdominal girth to serve as a baseline. (See *How the LeVeen shunt works*.)

Monitoring and aftercare
Follow these steps after surgery:

• After the patient returns from surgery, make him as comfortable as possible. Place him in low Fowler's or semi-Fowler's position, whichever he prefers, and administer analgesics, as ordered.
• Monitor vital signs frequently, and watch for hypervolemia or hypovolemia. As ordered, administer an I.V. or I.M. diuretic, such as furosemide, to reduce fluid retention. Check and record intake and output hourly for the first 24 hours after surgery, then daily until discharge. Measure abdominal girth and weight daily; compare the findings with baseline data to assess fluid drainage.
• As ordered, draw serum samples for a CBC; serum electrolyte, creatinine, albumin, and BUN levels; and other studies. Monitor the results of these tests, and notify the doctor of any abnormalities.
• Teach the patient to use the incentive spirometer four times daily, for at least 15 minutes each time. As ordered, apply an abdominal binder for the first 24 hours after surgery. Tell the patient that the incentive spirometer and binder raise intra-abdominal pressure and enhance ascitic fluid drainage.
• Regularly check the incision site for bleeding, swelling, inflammation, drainage, and hematoma, and change dressings as needed. Also be alert for signs of heart failure, disseminated intravascular coagulation, and GI bleeding.

Home care instructions

Provide these instructions to the patient:
• Encourage the patient to continue using the incentive spirometer four times per day, 15 minutes each time, for as long as the shunt is in place.
• Tell the patient to avoid putting pressure on the shunt to prevent clot formation and shunt occlusion.
• Instruct the patient to watch for and immediately report bleeding or drainage from the incision site as well as fever, chills, diaphoresis, or other signs or symptoms of infection.
• Encourage the patient to keep regular follow-up examination appointments to assess shunt patency and control ascites.

Endoscopic retrograde sphincterotomy

First used to remove retained gallstones from the common bile duct after cholecystectomy, endoscopic retrograde sphincterotomy (ERS) is now also used to treat high-risk patients with biliary dyskinesia and to insert biliary stents for draining malignant or benign strictures in the common bile duct. In this procedure, a fiberoptic endoscope is advanced through the stomach and duodenum to the ampulla of Vater. A papillotome is passed through the endoscope to make a small incision to widen the biliary sphincter. If the stone doesn't drop out into the duodenum on its own, the doc-

You don't have to be a judge to rule in favor of ERS. Any objection to a quicker, safer recovery is out of order.

tor may introduce a Dormia basket, a balloon, or a lithotriptor through the endoscope to remove or crush the stone.

Quick, painless, and safe

ERS allows treatment without general anesthesia or a surgical incision, ensuring a quicker and safer recovery. It may be performed on an outpatient basis for some patients, making it a cost-effective alternative to surgery.

Patient preparation

Explain the treatment to the patient, including these measures:
• His throat will be sprayed with an anesthetic to avoid discomfort during the insertion and he may also receive a sedative to help him relax. Reassure him that the procedure should cause little or no discomfort.
• He'll be positioned on the fluoroscopy table in a left side-lying position, with his left arm behind him. Encourage him to relax.

Monitoring and aftercare

Follow these steps after treatment:
• Instruct the patient to cough, deep-breathe, and expectorate regularly to avoid aspirating secretions. Keep in mind that the anesthetic's effects may hinder expectoration and swallowing.
• Withhold food and fluids until the anesthesia wears off and the patient's gag reflex returns.
• Check the patient's vital signs frequently and monitor carefully for signs of hemorrhage: hematemesis, melena, tachycardia, and hypotension. If any of these signs develop, notify the doctor immediately.

Home care instructions

Provide these instructions to the patient:
• Tell him to immediately report any signs of hemorrhage, sepsis, cholangitis, or pancreatitis.
• Encourage him to report any recurrence of the characteristic jaundice and pain of biliary obstruction. He may need repeat ERS to remove new stones or to replace a malfunctioning biliary stent.

Nursing diagnoses

Here are nursing diagnoses commonly used in patients with GI disorders. For each diagnosis, you'll also find nursing interventions with rationales.

Constipation

Related to inadequate intake of fluid and bulk, *Constipation* may pertain to all patients undergoing periods of restricted food or fluid intake.

Expected outcomes

- Patient expresses decreased feelings of constipation.
- Patient reports a more regular bowel elimination pattern.
- Patient identifies proper methods used to help promote a regular bowel pattern.

Nursing interventions and rationales

- Record intake and output accurately to ensure correct fluid replacement therapy.
- Note the color and consistency of stool and frequency of bowel movements to form the basis of an effective treatment plan.
- Promote ample fluid intake, if appropriate, to minimize constipation with increased intestinal fluid content.
- Encourage the patient to increase dietary intake of fiber to improve intestinal muscle tone and promote comfortable elimination.
- Discourage routine use of laxatives and enemas to avoid trauma to intestinal mucosa, dehydration, and eventual failure of defecation stimulus. (Bulk-adding laxatives aren't irritating and are usually permitted.)
- Encourage the patient to walk and exercise as much as possible to stimulate intestinal activity.
- Encourage the patient to take the time necessary each day to have a bowel movement to help promote a regular bowel pattern.

Encourage the patient to walk and exercise as much as possible to stimulate intestinal activity.

Diarrhea

Related to malabsorption, inflammation, or irritation of the bowel, *Diarrhea* may be associated with irritable bowel syndrome, colitis, Crohn's disease, and other conditions.

Expected outcomes

- Patient reports cessation of diarrhea as evidenced by formed stool.
- Patient identifies proper methods for treating diarrhea.

Nursing interventions and rationales

• Assess the patient's level of dehydration and electrolyte status. Fluid loss secondary to diarrhea can be life-threatening.
• Monitor the patient's weight daily to detect fluid loss or retention.
• Note color and consistency of stool and frequency of bowel movements to monitor treatment effectiveness.
• Test stool for occult blood, and obtain stool for culture to help evaluate factors contributing to diarrhea.
• Assess for fecal impaction. Liquid stool may seep around an impaction.

Diet changes, too

For acute diarrhea, provide the following dietary regimen:
• Give clear fluids, including glucose, electrolyte-containing beverages, and commercial rehydration preparations, orally. Clear fluids provide rapidly absorbed calories and electrolytes with minimal stimulation. After diarrhea has stopped for 24 to 48 hours, progress to a full fluid diet, then to a regular diet.
• Avoid milk, caffeine, and high-fiber foods for 1 week to avoid irritating the intestinal mucosa.
• In chronic diarrhea, encourage the patient to avoid foods and activities that may cause diarrhea. His awareness and self-regulation of contributing factors help manage chronic diarrhea.

Ineffective tissue perfusion: GI

Related to reduced blood flow, *Ineffective tissue perfusion: GI* may be associated with cirrhosis, hepatic failure, and other conditions.

Expected outcomes

• Patient maintains adequate blood flow to the intestinal mucosa.
• Patient identifies reportable symptoms.

Nursing interventions and rationales

• Assess the patient for bowel sounds, increasing abdominal girth, pain, nausea and vomiting, and electrolyte imbalance. Acute changes may indicate surgical emergency due to ischemia.
• If the patient has a chronic circulatory problem, provide small, frequent feedings of light, bland foods to promote digestion. Also, encourage rest after feedings to maximize blood flow available for digestion.

Bowel incontinence

Related to neuromuscular involvement, *Bowel incontinence* may be seen in patients who have had a hemorrhoidectomy, radical prostatectomy, or abdominal perineal resection.

Establish a bowel schedule for the patient with bowel incontinence — ½ hour after a meal is desirable for active peristalsis.

Expected outcomes

- Patient remains continent of stool.
- Patient identifies measures to help maintain bowel schedule.

Nursing interventions and rationales

- Establish a schedule for defecation — ½ hour after a meal is desirable for active peristalsis. A regular pattern encourages adaptation and routine physiologic function.
- Instruct the patient to use the bathroom or commode if possible to allow easy defecation without anxiety.
- If bedpan use is necessary, assist the patient to the most normal position possible for defecation to increase comfort and reduce anxiety.
- Instruct the patient to bear down or help him lean his trunk forward to increase intra-abdominal pressure.
- If necessary, use a glycerine suppository or gentle manual stimulation with a lubricated finger in the anal sphincter to encourage regular physiologic function, stimulate peristalsis, minimize infection, and promote comfort with elimination.
- Provide skin care to prevent infection and promote comfort.
- Refrain from commenting about "accidents" to avoid embarrassing the patient and help promote his self-image.

Common GI disorders

Here are several common GI disorders, along with their causes, pathophysiology, signs and symptoms, diagnostic test findings, treatments, and nursing interventions.

Although the appendix has no known function, it does regularly fill and empty itself of food.

Appendicitis

Appendicitis occurs when the appendix becomes inflamed. It's the most common major surgical emergency. More precisely, this disorder is an inflammation of the vermiform appendix, a small, fingerlike projection attached to the cecum just below the ileocecal valve. Although the appendix has no known function, it does regularly fill and empty itself of food.

What causes it

- Mucosal ulceration
- Fecal mass (fecalith)
- Stricture
- Barium ingestion
- Viral infection

Pathophysiology

Mucosal ulceration triggers inflammation, which temporarily obstructs the appendix. The obstruction blocks mucus outflow. Pressure in the now distended appendix increases, and the appendix contracts. Bacteria multiply, and inflammation and pressure continue to increase, restricting blood flow to the organ and causing severe abdominal pain.

Inflammation can lead to infection, clotting, tissue decay, and perforation of the appendix. If the appendix ruptures or perforates, the infected contents spill into the abdominal cavity, causing peritonitis, the most common and dangerous complication.

What to look for

Initially, the patient may manifest these signs and symptoms:
- abdominal pain, generalized or localized in the right upper abdomen, eventually localizing in the right lower abdomen (McBurney's point)
- anorexia
- nausea and vomiting
- boardlike abdominal rigidity
- retractive respirations
- increasingly severe abdominal spasms and rebound spasms. (Rebound tenderness on the opposite side of the abdomen suggests peritoneal inflammation.)

Later symptoms include:
- constipation (although diarrhea is also possible)
- fever of 99° to 102° F (37.2° to 38.9° C)
- tachycardia
- sudden cessation of abdominal pain (indicates perforation or infarction of the appendix).

What tests tell you

- White blood cell (WBC) count is moderately elevated, with increased immature cells.
- Ultrasound of the abdomen and pelvis can be helpful in diagnosing a nonperforated appendix. CT scan can help to identify abscess.

How it's treated

An appendectomy is the only effective treatment for appendicitis. If peritonitis develops, treatment involves GI intubation, parenteral replacement of fluids and electrolytes, and administration of antibiotics.

What to do

If appendicitis is suspected, or during preparation for an appendectomy, follow these guidelines:
• Administer I.V. fluids to prevent dehydration. Never administer cathartics or enemas because they may rupture the appendix.
• Give the patient nothing by mouth, and administer analgesics judiciously because they may mask symptoms of rupture.
• Place the patient in Fowler's position to reduce pain. (This is also helpful postoperatively.) Never apply heat to the lower right abdomen or perform palpation; these actions may cause the appendix to rupture.

After it's gone

After an appendectomy, follow these guidelines:
• Monitor the patient's vital signs and intake and output.
• Give analgesics, as ordered.
• Document bowel sounds, passing of flatus, or bowel movements—signs of peristalsis return. If these signs appear in a patient whose nausea and abdominal rigidity have subsided, he's ready to resume oral fluids.
• Watch closely for possible surgical complications. Continuing pain and fever may signal an abscess. The complaint that "something gave way" may mean wound dehiscence. If an abscess or peritonitis develops, incision and drainage may be necessary. Frequently assess the dressing for wound drainage.
• If peritonitis complicates appendicitis, an NG tube may be needed to decompress the stomach and reduce nausea and vomiting. If so, record drainage, and provide good mouth and nose care.
• Evaluate the patient. He should demonstrate appropriate activity restrictions, be able to resume a normal diet and bowel elimination pattern, and understand the importance of follow-up care. (See *Teaching the patient with appendicitis*.)

Administer I.V. fluids to prevent dehydration in suspected appendicitis or preparation for an appendectomy.

Education edge

Teaching the patient with appendicitis

• Explain what happens in appendicitis.
• Help the patient understand the required surgery and its possible complications. If time allows, provide preoperative teaching.
• Discuss postoperative activity limitations. Tell the patient to follow the doctor's orders for driving, returning to work, and resuming physical activity.

Gallbladder and biliary tract disorders

Gallbladder and biliary tract disorders, such as cholecystitis, cholelithiasis, choledocholithiasis, and cholangitis, are common, painful conditions that usually require surgery and may be life-threatening. They typically accompany calculus deposition and inflammation.

Understanding gallbladder and biliary tract disorders

There are five major disorders associated with the gallbladder and biliary tract. They are:

• *cholecystitis*—an acute or chronic inflammation of the gallbladder, usually associated with a gallstone impacted in the cystic duct, causing painful distention of the gallbladder. The acute form is most common during middle age; the chronic form, among elderly people. Prognosis is good with treatment.

• *cholangitis*—infection of the bile duct, commonly associated with choledocholithiasis, and may follow percutaneous transhepatic cholangiography. Widespread inflammation may cause fibrosis and stenosis of the common bile duct and biliary radicles. Prognosis for this rare condition is poor; stenosing or primary sclerosing cholangitis is almost always fatal.

• *cholelithiasis*—stones or calculi in the gallbladder (gallstones) resulting from changes in bile components. It's the leading biliary tract disease, affecting over 20 million Americans, and accounts for the third most common surgical procedure performed in the United States—cholecystectomy. Prognosis is usually good with treatment unless infection occurs, in which case prognosis depends on the infection's severity and response to antibiotics.

• *choledocholithiasis*—gallstones passed out of the gallbladder lodge in the common bile duct, causing partial or complete biliary obstruction. Prognosis is good unless infection develops.

• *gallstone ileus*—involves small-bowel obstruction by a gallstone. Typically, the gallstone travels through a fistula between the gallbladder and small bowel and lodges at the ileocecal valve. This condition is most common in elderly people. Prognosis is good with surgery.

What causes it

The exact cause of cholecystitis is unknown; risk factors include:
• a high-calorie, high-cholesterol diet, associated with obesity
• elevated estrogen levels from hormonal contraceptives, postmenopausal therapy, pregnancy, or multiparity
• the use of the antilipemic clofibrate
• diabetes mellitus, ileal disease, hemolytic disorders, liver disease, or pancreatitis
• genetic factors
• weight-reduction diets with severe calorie restriction and rapid weight loss.

Pathophysiology

Certain conditions (such as age, obesity, and estrogen imbalance) cause the liver to secrete bile that's abnormally high in cholesterol or that lacks the proper concentration of bile salts. Excessive water and bile salts are reabsorbed, making the bile less soluble. Cholesterol, calcium, and bilirubin then precipitate into gallstones. (See *Understanding gallbladder and biliary tract disorders* and *Understanding gallstone formation*.)

Age and estrogen imbalance can cause the liver to secrete bile that lacks the proper concentration of bile salts or is abnormally high in cholesterol.

Understanding gallstone formation

Abnormal metabolism of cholesterol and bile salts plays an important role in gallstone formation. Bile is made continuously by the liver and is concentrated and stored in the gallbladder until the duodenum needs it to help digest fat. Changes in the composition of bile may allow gallstones to form. Changes to the absorptive ability of the gallbladder lining may also contribute to gallstone formation.

Too much cholesterol

Certain conditions, such as age, obesity, and estrogen imbalance, cause the liver to secrete bile that's abnormally high in cholesterol or lacking the proper concentration of bile salts.

Liver

Gallbladder

Inside the gallbladder

When the gallbladder concentrates this bile, inflammation may or may not occur. Excessive water and bile salts are reabsorbed, making the bile less soluble. Cholesterol, calcium, and bilirubin precipitate into gallstones.

Fat entering the duodenum causes the intestinal mucosa to secrete the hormone cholecystokinin, which stimulates the gallbladder to contract and empty. If a stone lodges in the cystic duct, the gallbladder contracts but can't empty.

Contracting gallbladder

Obstructing gallstone

Jaundice, irritation, inflammation

If a stone lodges in the common bile duct, the bile flow into the duodenum becomes obstructed. Bilirubin is absorbed into the blood, causing jaundice.

Biliary narrowing and swelling of the tissue around the stone can also cause irritation and inflammation of the common bile duct.

Gallstones in the common bile duct

Up the biliary tree

Inflammation can progress up the biliary tree and cause infection of any of the bile ducts. This causes scar tissue, fluid accumulation, cirrhosis, portal hypertension, and bleeding.

Inflammation of the common bile duct

What to look for

In acute cholecystitis, acute cholelithiasis, and choledocholithiasis, look for:
• the classic attack with severe midepigastric or right upper quadrant pain radiating to the back or referred to the right scapula, commonly after meals rich in fats

- recurring fat intolerance
- belching that leaves a sour taste in the mouth
- flatulence
- indigestion
- diaphoresis
- nausea
- chills and low-grade fever
- possible jaundice and clay-colored stools with common duct obstruction.

Cholangitis gist

In cholangitis, look for:
- abdominal pain
- high fever and chills
- possible jaundice and related itching
- weakness and fatigue.

Ileus ailments

In gallstone ileus, look for:
- nausea and vomiting
- abdominal distention
- absent bowel sounds (in complete bowel obstruction)
- intermittent colicky pain over several days.

What tests tell you

- Ultrasonography reveals calculi in the gallbladder with 96% accuracy. PTHC distinguishes between gallbladder disease and cancer of the pancreatic head in patients with jaundice.
- CT scan may identify ductal stones.
- ERCP visualizes the biliary tree after endoscopic examination of the duodenum, cannulation of the common bile and pancreatic ducts, and injection of a contrast medium.
- Cholescintigraphy detects obstruction of the cystic duct.
- If stones are identified in the common bile duct by radiologic examination, a therapeutic ERCP may be performed before cholecystectomy to remove the stones.
- Oral cholecystography shows calculi in the gallbladder and biliary duct obstruction.
- Laboratory tests showing an elevated icteric index and elevated total bilirubin, urine bilirubin, and alkaline phosphatase levels support the diagnosis.
- WBC count is slightly elevated during a cholecystitis attack.
- Serum amylase levels distinguish gallbladder disease from pancreatitis.
- Serial enzyme tests and an electrocardiogram (ECG) should precede other diagnostic tests if heart disease is suspected.

Serial enzyme tests and ECG should precede other tests if heart disease is suspected.

How it's treated

• Surgery, usually elective, is the treatment of choice for gallbladder and duct disease. Procedures may include cholecystectomy, cholecystectomy with operative cholangiography and, possibly, exploration of the common bile duct.

• A low-fat diet is prescribed to prevent attacks as well as vitamin K for itching, jaundice, and bleeding tendencies caused by vitamin K deficiency.

• During an acute attack, treatment may include insertion of an NG tube and I.V. line as well as antibiotic administration.

• A nonsurgical treatment for choledocholithiasis involves insertion of a flexible catheter, formed around a T tube, through the sinus tract into the common bile duct. Guided by fluoroscopy, the doctor directs the catheter toward the stone. A Dormia basket is threaded through the catheter to entrap the calculi.

• Ursodiol, a drug that dissolves the solid cholesterol in gallstones, provides an alternative for patients who are poor surgical risks or who refuse surgery. However, use of ursodiol is limited by the need for prolonged treatment (2 years), the incidence of adverse reactions, and the frequency of calculi reformation after treatment.

• Lithotripsy, the ultrasonic breakup of gallstones, is usually unsuccessful and has a significant recurrence rate. The relative ease, short length of stay, and cost-effectiveness of laparoscopic cholecystectomy have made dissolution and lithotripsy less viable options.

What to do

• For information on preoperative and postoperative care of surgical patients, see "Gallbladder surgery," page 439.

• Evaluate the patient. He should return to normal nutrition and hydration status, be free from complications, be able to tolerate normal activity, and follow diet restrictions. (See *Teaching the patient with a gallbladder or biliary tract disorder.*)

Education edge

Teaching the patient with a gallbladder or biliary tract disorder

• If a low-fat diet is prescribed, suggest ways to implement it. If necessary, ask the dietitian to reinforce your instructions. Make sure the patient understands how dietary changes help to prevent biliary colic.

• Reinforce the doctor's explanation of the ordered treatment, such as surgery, endoscopic retrograde cholangiopancreatography, or lithotripsy. Make sure the patient fully understands the possible complications, if any, associated with his treatment.

Cirrhosis

Cirrhosis, a chronic liver disease, is characterized by widespread destruction of hepatic cells, which are replaced by fibrous cells. This process is called *fibrotic regeneration.* Cirrhosis is a common cause of death in the United States and, among people ages 35 to 55, the fourth leading cause of death. It can occur at any age.

What causes it

There are many types of cirrhosis; causes differ with each type and include the following:

• Laënnec's cirrhosis (also known as portal, nutritional, or alcoholic cirrhosis), the most common type of cirrhosis, results from malnutrition, especially of dietary protein, and chronic alcohol ingestion.

• Biliary cirrhosis results from bile duct diseases.

• Pigment cirrhosis may stem from disorders such as hemochromatosis.

• Other causes of cirrhosis include drug- or toxin-induced heart failure and chronic right-sided heart failure.

• In about 10% of patients, cirrhosis has no known cause.

Pathophysiology

Cirrhosis is characterized by irreversible chronic injury of the liver, extensive fibrosis, and nodular tissue growth. These changes result from:

• liver cell death (hepatocyte necrosis)

• collapse of the liver's supporting structure (the reticulin network)

• distortion of the vascular bed (blood vessels throughout the liver)

• nodular regeneration of the remaining liver tissue.

Getting complicated

When the liver begins to malfunction, blood clotting disorders (coagulopathies), jaundice, edema, and many metabolic problems develop. Fibrosis and the distortion of blood vessels may impede blood flow in the capillary branches of the portal vein and hepatic artery, leading to portal hypertension (elevated pressure in the portal vein). Increased pressure may lead to the development of esophageal varices — enlarged, tortuous veins in the lower part of the esophagus where it meets the stomach. Esophageal varices may easily rupture and leak large amounts of blood into the upper GI tract.

Sometimes cirrhosis occurs when I lose my support. It's always important to maintain support.

What to look for

Cirrhosis affects many body systems. Assess the patient for these signs and symptoms:

• GI (usually early and vague) — anorexia, indigestion, nausea and vomiting, constipation or diarrhea, dull abdominal ache

• respiratory — pleural effusion, limited thoracic expansion

• central nervous system — progressive signs and symptoms of hepatic encephalopathy, including lethargy, mental changes,

slurred speech, asterixis (flapping tremor), peripheral neuritis, paranoia, hallucinations, extreme obtundation, coma
- hematologic — bleeding tendencies (nosebleeds, easy bruising, bleeding gums), anemia
- endocrine — testicular atrophy, menstrual irregularities, gynecomastia, loss of chest and axillary hair
- skin — severe pruritus, extreme dryness, poor tissue turgor, abnormal pigmentation, spider angiomas, palmar erythema, possibly jaundice
- hepatic — jaundice, hepatomegaly, ascites, edema of the legs
- miscellaneous — musty breath, enlarged superficial abdominal veins, muscle atrophy, pain in the right upper abdominal quadrant that worsens when the patient sits up or leans forward, palpable liver or spleen, temperature of 101° to 103° F (38.3° to 39.4° C), bleeding from esophageal varices.

What tests tell you

Liver biopsy, the definitive test for cirrhosis, reveals destruction and fibrosis of hepatic tissue. A liver scan shows abnormal thickening and a liver mass. These tests also help confirm cirrhosis:
- Cholecystography and cholangiography allow visualization of the gallbladder and the biliary duct system, respectively.
- Splenoportal venography allows visualization of the portal venous system.
- PTHC helps differentiate extrahepatic from intrahepatic obstructive jaundice and helps reveal hepatic disorders and gallstones.
- CT scan can show lobe enlargement, vascular changes, and nodules.
- WBC count, hematocrit, and hemoglobin, albumin, serum electrolyte, and cholinesterase levels are decreased.
- Globulin, serum ammonia, total bilirubin, alkaline phosphatase, alanine aminotransferase (ALT), aspartate aminotransferase (AST), and lactate dehydrogenase levels are increased.
- Anemia, neutropenia, and thrombocytopenia are present. PT and PTT are prolonged.
- Folic acid, iron levels, and vitamins A, B_{12}, C, and K are decreased.
- Glucose tolerance tests may be abnormal.
- Galactose tolerance and urine bilirubin tests are positive.
- Fecal and urine urobilinogen levels are elevated.

How it's treated

Therapy aims to remove or alleviate the underlying cause of cirrhosis, prevent further liver damage, and prevent or treat complications. In cases of active variceal bleeding, treatment is aimed at active control of blood loss through medication, surgery, or balloon tamponade. The patient may benefit from a high-protein diet,

In cases of active variceal bleeding, control of blood loss is attempted through medication, surgery, or balloon tamponade.

but this may be restricted by developing hepatic encephalopathy. Sodium is usually restricted to 200 to 500 mg/day and fluids to 1 to 1½ qt (1 to 1.5 L)/day.

If the patient's condition continues to deteriorate, he may need tube feedings or TPN. Other supportive measures include:
• supplemental vitamins — A, B complex, C, and K — to compensate for the liver's inability to store them
• vitamin B_{12}, folic acid, and thiamine for anemia
• rest and moderate exercise and avoiding exposure to infections and toxic agents
• antiemetics, such as trimethobenzamide and benzquinamide, for nausea (when absolutely necessary)
• vasopressin for esophageal varices
• diuretics, such as furosemide and spironolactone, for edema with careful monitoring because fluid and electrolyte imbalance may precipitate hepatic encephalopathy
• paracentesis and infusions of salt-poor albumin to alleviate ascites
• LeVeen peritoneovenous shunt
• surgical procedures, including endoscopic sclerotherapy (or banding of varices), splenectomy, esophagogastric resection, and surgical shunts to relieve portal hypertension
• liver transplantation for the patient with advanced disease
• programs for preventing cirrhosis, which usually emphasize avoiding alcohol.

What to do

• Check skin, gums, stool, and vomitus regularly for bleeding. Apply pressure to injection sites to prevent bleeding.
• Observe closely for signs of behavioral or personality changes. Report increasing stupor, lethargy, hallucinations, or neuromuscular dysfunction. Watch for asterixis, a sign of developing hepatic encephalopathy.
• To assess fluid retention, weigh the patient and measure abdominal girth daily, inspect his ankles and sacrum for dependent edema, and accurately record intake and output.
• To prevent skin breakdown associated with edema and pruritus, avoid using soap when you bathe the patient. Instead, use lubricating lotion or moisturizing agents. Handle him gently, and turn and reposition him frequently to keep skin intact.
• Evaluate the patient's response to therapy. Look for him to maintain normal nutrition and skin integrity. Note whether he has adapted his lifestyle and diet to his disorder and whether he understands the need for appropriate follow-up care. (See *Teaching the patient with cirrhosis.*)

Education edge

Teaching the patient with cirrhosis

• Warn the patient against taking aspirin, straining during defecation, and blowing his nose or sneezing too vigorously. Suggest using an electric razor and a soft toothbrush.
• Tell the patient that rest and good nutrition will conserve energy and decrease metabolic demands on the liver. Urge him to eat frequent, small meals.
• Stress the need to avoid infections and abstain from alcohol. Refer the patient to Alcoholics Anonymous if necessary.

Crohn's disease

An inflammatory disorder, Crohn's disease can affect any part of the GI tract (usually the terminal ileum), extending through all layers of the intestinal wall. It may also involve regional lymph nodes and the mesentery.

Crohn's disease is an inflammatory disorder that can affect any part of the GI tract through all layers of the intestinal wall.

What causes it

The exact cause of Crohn's disease is unknown. Possible causes include allergies, immune disorders, lymphatic obstruction, infection, and genetic factors. Crohn's disease is most prevalent in adults ages 20 to 40, but a second peak incidence occurs between ages 55 and 65.

Pathophysiology

In Crohn's disease, inflammation spreads slowly and progressively. Here's what happens:
• Lymph nodes enlarge and lymph flow in the submucosa is blocked.
• Lymphatic obstruction causes edema, mucosal ulceration, fissures, abscesses and, sometimes, granulomas. Mucosal ulcerations are called *skipping lesions* because they aren't continuous as in ulcerative colitis.
• Oval, elevated patches of closely packed lymph follicles — called *Peyer's patches* — develop on the lining of the small intestine.
• Fibrosis occurs, thickening the bowel wall and causing stenosis, or narrowing of the lumen. (See *Changes to the bowel in Crohn's disease*, page 462.)

What to look for

Clinical effects vary according to the location and extent of inflammation and at first may be mild and nonspecific.
• In acute disease, look for right lower abdominal quadrant pain, cramping, tenderness, flatulence, nausea, fever, diarrhea, and bleeding (usually mild but may be massive).
• In chronic disease, look for diarrhea, four to six stools per day, right lower quadrant pain, steatorrhea, marked weight loss, possible weakness and, rarely, clubbing of fingers.

What tests tell you

• Laboratory findings typically indicate increased WBC count and erythrocyte sedimentation rate (ESR), hypokalemia, hypocalcemia, hypomagnesemia, and decreased hemoglobin levels.

Changes to the bowel in Crohn's disease

As Crohn's disease progresses, fibrosis thickens the bowel wall and narrows the lumen. Narrowing—or *stenosis*—can occur in any part of the intestine and causes varying degrees of intestinal obstruction. At first, the mucosa may appear normal but, as the disease progresses, it takes on a "cobblestone" appearance, as shown here.

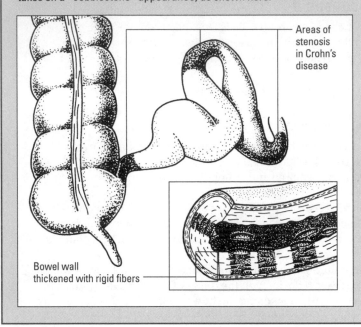

Areas of stenosis in Crohn's disease

Bowel wall thickened with rigid fibers

TPN helps maintain nutrition while resting the bowel of a debilitated patient.

• A barium enema showing the string sign (segments of stricture separated by normal bowel) supports this diagnosis.
• Sigmoidoscopy and colonoscopy may show patchy areas or inflammation, thus helping to rule out ulcerative colitis.
• Biopsy results confirm the diagnosis.
• Upper GI series with small bowel examination helps determine disease in the ileum.

How it's treated

• TPN to maintain nutrition while resting the bowel of a debilitated patient.
• Surgery may be necessary to correct bowel perforation, massive hemorrhage, fistulas, or acute intestinal obstruction. The patient with extensive disease of the large intestine and rectum may require colectomy with ileostomy.

Take a pill

Effective drug therapy requires important changes in lifestyle: physical rest, a restricted-fiber diet (no fruit or vegetables), and elimination of dairy products for lactose intolerance. Drug therapy may include:

- anti-inflammatory corticosteroids and antibacterials, such as sulfasalazine and 5-aminosalicylic acid
- metronidazole
- opium tincture and diphenoxylate to help combat diarrhea (contraindicated in patients with significant intestinal obstruction)
- immunosuppressants, such as azathioprine, cyclosporin, and 6-mercaptopurine, for patients who can't be controlled on steroid therapy
- infliximab, a tumor necrosis factor-alpha, to promote closure of fissures and treat refractory Crohn's disease flare-ups, given in a monitored setting by I.V. infusion in a cycle of three treatments (at weeks 1, 2, and 6).

What to do

- Record fluid intake and output (including the amount of stool), and weigh the patient daily.
- Watch for dehydration and maintain fluid and electrolyte balance.
- Be alert for signs of intestinal bleeding (bloody stool). Check stool daily for occult blood.
- If the patient is receiving steroids, watch for adverse reactions such as GI bleeding. Remember that steroids can mask signs of infection. Check hemoglobin level and hematocrit regularly. Also check the WBC count if the patient is on immunomodulators. Give iron supplements, blood transfusions, and analgesics, as ordered.
- Watch for fever and pain on urination, which may signal bladder fistula. Abdominal pain, fever, and a hard, distended abdomen may indicate intestinal obstruction.
- Before ileostomy, arrange for a visit by an enterostomal therapist. For postoperative care, see "Bowel surgery with ostomy," page 433.
- Evalate the patient. After successful treatment for Crohn's disease, he will maintain optimal nutrition, hydration, and skin integrity. He'll use positive coping mechanisms to deal with a changed body image. He should be able to identify and avoid foods likely to cause distress. Make sure he can demonstrate proper care of an ostomy, if required, and uses appropriate support groups. Evaluate his understanding of the need for follow-up care and when to seek immediate attention. (See *Teaching the patient with Crohn's disease.*)

Education edge

Teaching the patient with Crohn's disease

- Teach stoma care to the patient and his family. Realize that ileostomy changes the patient's body image; offer reassurance and emotional support.
- Stress the need for a severely restricted diet and bed rest, which may be difficult, particularly for the young patient. Encourage the patient to try to reduce tension. If stress is clearly an aggravating factor, refer him for counseling. Teach the patient to follow a low-residue diet, exercise, and seek family support.

Diverticular disease

In diverticular disease, bulging, pouchlike herniations (diverticula) in the GI wall push the mucosal lining through the surrounding muscle. Diverticula occur most commonly in the sigmoid colon, but they may develop anywhere, from the proximal end of the pharynx to the anus. Other typical sites are the duodenum, near the pancreatic border or the ampulla of Vater, and the jejunum.

Diverticular disease of the stomach is rare and is usually a precursor of peptic or neoplastic disease. Diverticular disease of the ileum (Meckel's diverticulum) is the most common congenital anomaly of the GI tract.

Diverticular disease has two clinical forms:
• diverticulosis—diverticula present but produces no symptoms
• diverticulitis—inflamed diverticula; may cause potentially fatal obstruction, infection, and hemorrhage.

Diverticular disease of the stomach is rare. Phew!

What causes it

The exact cause is unknown, but it may result from:
• diminished colonic motility and increased intraluminal pressure
• defects in colon wall strength.

Pathophysiology

Diverticula probably result from high intraluminal pressure on an area of weakness in the GI wall where blood vessels enter. Diet may be a contributing factor because insufficient fiber reduces fecal residue, narrows the bowel lumen, and leads to high intra-abdominal pressure during defecation.

In diverticulitis, undigested food and bacteria accumulate in the diverticular sac. This hard mass cuts off the blood supply to the thin walls of the sac, making them more susceptible to attack by colonic bacteria. Inflammation follows and may lead to perforation, abscess, peritonitis, obstruction, or hemorrhage. Occasionally, the inflamed colon segment adheres to the bladder or other organs and causes a fistula.

What to look for

• Meckel's diverticulum usually produces no symptoms.
• In diverticulosis, recurrent left lower abdominal quadrant pain is relieved by defecation or passage of flatus. Constipation and diarrhea alternate.
• In diverticulitis, the patient may have moderate left lower abdominal quadrant pain, mild nausea, gas, irregular bowel habits, low-grade fever, leukocytosis, rupture of the diverticuli (in severe diverticulitis), and fibrosis and adhesions (in chronic diverticulitis).

What tests tell you

• An upper GI series confirms or rules out diverticulosis of the esophagus and upper bowel.
• Barium enema confirms or rules out diverticulosis of the lower bowel. Biopsy rules out cancer; however, a colonoscopic biopsy isn't recommended during acute diverticular disease because of the strenuous bowel preparation it requires.
• Blood studies may show an elevated ESR in diverticulitis, especially if the diverticula are infected.

How it's treated

Diverticulosis that produces no symptoms usually doesn't require treatment. Treatment for diverticular disease depends on the type.
• Intestinal diverticulosis with pain, mild GI distress, constipation, or difficult defecation may respond to a liquid or bland diet, stool softeners, and occasional doses of mineral oil. These measures relieve symptoms, minimize irritation, and lessen the risk of progression to diverticulitis. After pain subsides, the patient also benefits from a high-residue diet and bulk-forming laxatives such as psyllium.

Colonoscopic biopsy isn't recommended during acute diverticular disease because of the strenuous bowel preparation required.

War on pathogens

• Treatment of mild diverticulitis without signs of perforation must prevent constipation and combat infection. It may include bed rest, a liquid diet, stool softeners, a broad-spectrum antibiotic, meperidine to control pain and relax smooth muscle, and an antispasmodic, such as dicyclomine or hyoscyamine, to control muscle spasms.
• Diverticulitis unresponsive to medical treatment requires a colon resection to remove the involved segment.
• Complications that accompany diverticulitis may require a temporary colostomy to drain abscesses and rest the colon, followed by later anastomosis.
• Patients who hemorrhage need blood replacement and careful monitoring of fluid and electrolyte balance. Such bleeding usually stops spontaneously. If it continues, angiography for catheter placement and infusion of vasopressin into the bleeding vessel is effective. Rarely, surgery may be required.

What to do

If the patient with diverticulosis is hospitalized, observe his stool carefully for frequency, color, and consistency; keep accurate pulse and temperature charts because changes in pulse or temperature may signal developing inflammation or complications.

Management of diverticulitis depends on the severity of symptoms.

• In mild disease, administer medications, as ordered; explain diagnostic tests and preparations for such tests; observe stool carefully; and maintain accurate records of temperature, pulse rate, respiratory rate, and intake and output.

• Monitor carefully if the patient requires angiography and catheter placement for vasopressin infusion. Inspect the insertion site frequently for bleeding, check pedal pulses frequently, and keep the patient from flexing his legs at the groin.

• Watch for signs and symptoms of vasopressin-induced fluid retention (apprehension, abdominal cramps, seizures, oliguria, and anuria) and severe hyponatremia (hypotension; rapid, thready pulse; cold, clammy skin; and cyanosis).

• For postsurgical care, see "Bowel resection and anastomosis," page 436.

• Evaluate the patient. After successful treatment and appropriate teaching, the patient will observe and report character of stool, modify his diet as needed, understand the need for follow-up care, and know when to seek immediate attention. (See *Teaching the patient with diverticular disease.*)

Gastroesophageal reflux disease

GERD is the backflow of gastric or duodenal contents, or both, past the LES, into the esophagus, without associated belching or vomiting. Reflux may or may not cause symptoms or abnormal changes. Persistent reflux may cause reflux esophagitis (inflammation of the esophageal mucosa).

What causes it

Reflux occurs when LES pressure is deficient or when pressure within the stomach exceeds LES pressure. Predisposing factors include:

• pyloric surgery (alteration or removal of the pylorus), which allows reflux of bile or pancreatic juice

• long-term NG intubation (more than 5 days)

• any agent that decreases LES pressure, such as food, alcohol, cigarettes, anticholinergics (atropine, belladonna, propantheline), and other drugs (morphine, diazepam, and meperidine)

• hiatal hernia (especially in children)

• any condition or position that increases intra-abdominal pressure.

Education edge

Teaching the patient with diverticular disease

• Explain what diverticula are as well as how they form.

• Make sure the patient understands the importance of dietary fiber and the harmful effects of constipation and straining at stool. Encourage increased intake of foods high in digestible fiber. Advise the patient to relieve constipation with stool softeners or bulk-forming laxatives, but caution against taking bulk-forming laxatives without plenty of water.

• As needed, teach colostomy care, and arrange for a visit by an enterostomal therapist.

Pathophysiology

Normally, the LES maintains enough pressure around the lower end of the esophagus to close it and prevent reflux. Typically, the sphincter relaxes after each swallow to allow food into the stomach. In GERD, the sphincter doesn't remain closed (usually due to deficient LES pressure or pressure within the stomach exceeding LES pressure), and stomach contents flow into the esophagus. The high acidity of the stomach contents causes pain and irritation in the esophagus, and stricture or ulceration can occur. If the gastric contents enter the throat and are aspirated, chronic pulmonary disease may result.

What to look for

Gastroesophageal reflux doesn't always cause symptoms, and in patients showing clinical effects, physiologic reflux isn't always confirmable. The most common feature of gastroesophageal reflux is heartburn, which may become more severe with vigorous exercise, bending, or lying down and may be relieved by antacids or sitting upright. The pain of esophageal spasm resulting from reflux esophagitis tends to be chronic and may mimic angina pectoris, radiating to the neck, jaws, and arms. Other symptoms include:
• odynophagia, which may be followed by a dull substernal ache from severe, long-term reflux
• dysphagia from esophageal spasm, stricture, or esophagitis and bleeding (bright red or dark brown)
• rarely, nocturnal regurgitation wakes the patient with coughing, choking, and a mouthful of saliva.

Hold your breath

Pulmonary symptoms, which result from reflux of gastric contents into the throat and subsequent aspiration, include:
• chronic pulmonary disease or nocturnal wheezing
• bronchitis
• asthma
• morning hoarseness and cough.

What tests tell you

• In children, barium esophagography under fluoroscopic control can show reflux. Recurrent reflux after age 6 weeks is abnormal.
• An acid perfusion (Bernstein) test can show that reflux is the cause of symptoms.
• Endoscopy and biopsy allow visualization and confirmation of any abnormal changes in the mucosa.

Endoscopy allows visualization of abnormal changes in the mucosa from GERD.

How it's treated

• Effective management relieves symptoms by reducing reflux through gravity, strengthening the LES with drug therapy, neutralizing gastric contents, and reducing intra-abdominal pressure.
• To reduce intra-abdominal pressure, the patient should sleep in a reverse Trendelenburg position (with the head of the bed elevated) and should avoid lying down after meals and late-night snacks. In uncomplicated cases, positional therapy is especially useful in infants and children.
• Antacids given 1 hour and 3 hours after meals and at bedtime are effective for intermittent reflux. A nondiarrheal antacid containing aluminum carbonate or aluminum hydroxide (rather than magnesium) may be preferred, depending on the patient's bowel status.
• Proton pump inhibitors are now a mainstay of therapy for GERD and erosive esophagitis. Metoclopramide and H_2-blockers have also been used with beneficial results.
• If possible, NG intubation shouldn't be continued for more than 5 days because the tube interferes with sphincter integrity and itself allows reflux, especially when the patient lies flat.
• Surgery may be necessary to control severe and refractory symptoms, such as pulmonary aspiration, hemorrhage, obstruction, severe pain, perforation, incompetent LES, and associated hiatal hernia. Surgery is also preferred in some young patients with severe GERD (rather than a lifetime of pharmacologic therapy).

What to do

After surgery using a thoracic approach, follow these steps:
• Carefully watch and record chest tube drainage and respiratory status.
• If needed, give chest physiotherapy and oxygen.
• Position the patient with an NG tube in semi-Fowler's position to help prevent reflux.
• Evaluate the patient; assess for optimal hydration and nutritional levels, diet modification, positioning, activity levels as needed, and increased comfort as the patient complies with therapy. (See *Teaching the patient with GERD*.)

Hepatic encephalopathy

Hepatic encephalopathy, also known as *portosystemic encephalopathy* or *hepatic coma*, is a neurologic syndrome that develops as a complication of chronic liver disease. It commonly occurs in patients with cirrhosis, resulting primarily from cerebral ammonia intoxication. It may be acute and self-limiting or chronic and progressive. In advanced stages, the prognosis is poor despite vigorous treatment.

What causes it

Rising blood ammonia levels may result from:
- cirrhosis
- excessive protein intake
- sepsis
- constipation or GI hemorrhage, resulting in excessive accumulation of nitrogenous body wastes
- bacterial action on protein and urea to form ammonia.

Pathophysiology

Hepatic encephalopathy follows rising blood ammonia levels. Normally, the protein breakdown in the bowel is metabolized to urea in the liver. When portal blood shunts past the liver, ammonia directly enters the systemic circulation and is carried to the brain. Such shunting may result from the collateral venous circulation that develops in portal hypertension or from surgically created portosystemic shunts.

What to look for

Clinical manifestations of hepatic encephalopathy vary (depending on the severity of neurologic involvement) and develop in four stages:

prodromal stage. Early symptoms are usually overlooked because they're subtle. They include slight personality changes (disorientation, forgetfulness, slurred speech), sleep disturbance, diminished affect, and slight tremor.

impending stage. Tremor progresses into asterixis, the hallmark of hepatic coma. Asterixis is characterized by quick, irregular extensions and flexions of the wrists and fingers when the wrists are held out straight and the hands flexed upward. Lethargy, aberrant behavior, and apraxia also occur.

stuporous stage. Hyperventilation occurs and the patient is stuporous, but noisy and abusive when aroused.

comatose stage. Signs include hyperactive reflexes, a positive Babinski's sign, fetor hepaticus (musty, sweet breath odor), and coma.

All the world's a stage, but hepatic encephalopathy develops in only four stages.

What tests tell you

• Elevated venous and arterial ammonia levels, clinical features, and a positive history of liver disease confirm the diagnosis.
• Arterial blood gas (ABG) analysis shows respiratory alkalosis with central hyperventilation.
• EEG shows slow waves as the disease progresses.
• Other test results that suggest the disorder include elevated serum bilirubin levels and prolonged PT.

How it's treated

• Treatment is aimed at improving hepatic function and correcting underlying liver disease.
• Adequate calorie intake (1,800 to 2,400 cal/day) in the form of glucose or carbohydrates is needed to prevent protein catabolism. Protein may be restricted to 40 g/day and advanced to up to 100 g/day as symptoms improve.
• Correction of electrolyte imbalances and management of GI bleeding are also essential.
• Effective treatment stops advancing encephalopathy by reducing blood ammonia levels. Ammonia-producing substances are removed from the GI tract by administering neomycin to suppress bacterial ammonia production, using sorbitol to induce catharsis to produce osmotic diarrhea, continuously aspirating blood from the stomach, reducing dietary protein intake, and administering lactulose to reduce blood ammonia levels.
• Potassium supplements are given to correct alkalosis (from increased ammonia levels), especially if the patient is taking diuretics.
• Hemodialysis may temporarily clear toxic blood. Exchange transfusions may provide dramatic but temporary improvement; however, these require a particularly large amount of blood.
• Salt-poor albumin may be used to maintain fluid and electrolyte balance, replace depleted albumin levels, and restore plasma.

What to do

• Frequently assess and record the patient's LOC.
• Continually orient him to place and time.
• Keep a daily record of the patient's handwriting to monitor progression of neurologic involvement.
• Monitor intake, output, and fluid and electrolyte balance. Check daily weight and measure abdominal girth.
• Watch for, and immediately report, signs of anemia (decreased hemoglobin levels), infection, alkalosis (increased serum bicarbonate levels), and GI bleeding (melena, hematemesis).

Salt-poor albumin may be used to maintain fluid and electrolyte balance, replace depleted albumin levels, and restore plasma.

• Provide the specified low-protein diet, with carbohydrates supplying most of the calories. Provide good mouth care.
• Promote rest, comfort, and a quiet atmosphere. Discourage stressful exercise.
• Protect the comatose patient's eyes from corneal injury by using artificial tears or eye patches.
• Provide emotional support for the patient's family in the terminal stage of hepatic coma.
• Evaluate the patient. He should have adequate hydration and intact skin. His family should have adequate support to deal with his condition. (See *Teaching the patient with hepatic encephalopathy*.)

Hepatitis, nonviral

Nonviral hepatitis is an inflammation of the liver that usually results from exposure to certain chemicals or drugs. Most patients recover from nonviral hepatitis, although a few develop fulminating hepatitis or cirrhosis.

What causes it

• Hepatotoxic chemicals, such as carbon tetrachloride, trichloroethylene, and vinyl chloride
• Hepatotoxic drugs such as acetaminophen
• Poisonous mushrooms

Pathophysiology

After exposure to a hepatotoxin, hepatic cellular necrosis, scarring, Kupffer cell hyperplasia, and infiltration by mononuclear phagocytes occur with varying severity. Alcohol, anoxia, and pre-existing liver disease exacerbate the effects of some toxins.

Drug-induced hepatitis may begin with a hypersensitivity reaction unique to the individual, unlike toxic hepatitis, which appears to affect all exposed people indiscriminately. Symptoms usually manifest after 2 to 5 weeks of therapy.

What to look for

Look for these signs and symptoms:
• anorexia, nausea, and vomiting
• jaundice
• dark urine
• hepatomegaly
• possibly, abdominal pain
• possibly, clay-colored stools and pruritus (in cholestatic form).

Education edge

Teaching the patient with hepatic encephalopathy

• Teach the patient, if he's still able to understand, and his family about hepatic encephalopathy and its treatment. Repeat explanations of each treatment before you perform it. Be sure to explain all procedures even if the patient is comatose.
• If the patient has chronic encephalopathy, be sure that he and his family understand the mental and physical effects that the illness will eventually have on the patient. Alert them to signs of complications or worsening symptoms. Advise them when to notify the doctor.
• As the patient begins to recover, inform him about the low-protein diet. Emphasize that recovery from a severe illness takes time. Review how to use medications.

What tests tell you

Liver biopsy may help identify the underlying disorder, especially if it shows infiltration with WBCs and eosinophils. Other test results may show:
• elevated serum transaminase levels (ALT and AST)
• elevated total and direct serum bilirubin levels (with cholestasis)
• elevated alkaline phosphatase levels
• elevated WBC count
• increased eosinophil levels in drug-induced nonviral hepatitis.

How it's treated

• Effective treatment aims to remove the causative agent by lavage, catharsis, or hyperventilation, depending on the route of exposure.
• Dimercaprol may serve as an antidote for toxic hepatitis caused by gold or arsenic poisoning, but it doesn't prevent drug-induced hepatitis caused by other substances.
• Corticosteroids may be ordered for patients with the drug-induced type.
• Thioctic acid, an investigational drug, may alleviate mushroom poisoning.

What to do

• Monitor closely for complications of liver failure (bleeding and hepatic coma).
• Ensure adequate hydration and nutrition.
• Relieve the patient's nausea, pruritus, and abdominal pain.
• Evaluate the patient. He should be able to maintain normal nutrition and hydration, make lifestyle and dietary changes, and seek follow-up care as needed. (See *Teaching the patient with nonviral hepatitis.*)

Treatment for nonviral hepatitis depends on the causative agent and the route of exposure.

Education edge

Teaching the patient with nonviral hepatitis

• Instruct the patient about the proper use of drugs.
• Instruct the patient about proper handling of cleaning agents and solvents.

Hepatitis, viral

The viral form of hepatitis is an acute inflammation of the liver marked by liver-cell destruction, necrosis, and autolysis. In most patients, hepatic cells eventually regenerate with little or no residual damage. However, old age and serious underlying disorders make complications more likely. The prognosis is poor if edema and hepatic encephalopathy develop.

Types of hepatitis

Five major forms of viral hepatitis are currently recognized, each caused by a different virus:

 Type A is transmitted almost exclusively by the fecal-oral route, and outbreaks are common in areas of overcrowding and poor sanitation. Day-care centers and other institutional settings are common sources of outbreaks. The incidence is also increasing among homosexuals and in people with human immunodeficiency virus (HIV) infection.

 Type B, also increasing among HIV-positive people, accounts for 5% to 10% of posttransfusion hepatitis cases in the United States. Vaccinations are available and are now required for health care workers and school children in many states.

 Type C accounts for about 20% of all viral hepatitis as well as most cases that follow transfusion.

 Type D, in the United States, is confined to people frequently exposed to blood and blood products, such as I.V. drug users and hemophiliacs.

 Type E was formerly grouped with type C under the name non-A, non-B hepatitis. In the United States, this type mainly occurs in people who have visited an endemic area, such as India, Africa, Asia, or Central America. (See *Viral hepatitis from A to E*, page 474.)

In the U.S., type E hepatitis mainly occurs in people who have visited an endemic area, such as India, Africa, Asia, or Central America.

What causes it

All forms of viral hepatitis are caused by hepatitis viruses A, B, C, D, or E.

Pathophysiology

Despite the different causative viruses, changes to the liver are usually similar in each type of viral hepatitis. Varying degrees of liver cell injury and necrosis occur. These changes in the liver are completely reversible when the acute phase of the disease subsides.

A fairly common complication is chronic persistent hepatitis, which prolongs recovery up to 8 months. Some patients also suffer relapses. A few may develop chronic active hepatitis, which destroys part of the liver and causes cirrhosis. In rare cases, severe and sudden (fulminant) hepatic failure and death may result from massive tissue loss.

Viral hepatitis from A to E

This chart compares the features of each type of viral hepatitis.

Feature	Hepatitis A	Hepatitis B	Hepatitis C	Hepatitis D	Hepatitis E
Incubation	15 to 45 days	30 to 180 days	15 to 160 days	14 to 64 days	14 to 60 days
Onset	Acute	Insidious	Insidious	Acute and chronic	Acute
Age-group most affected	Children, young adults	Any age	More common in adults	Any age	Ages 20 to 40
Transmission	Fecal-oral, sexual (especially oral-anal contact), non-percutaneous (sexual, maternal-neonatal), percutaneous (rare)	Blood-borne; parenteral route, sexual, maternal-neonatal; virus is shed in all body fluids	Blood-borne; parenteral route	Parenteral route; most people infected with hepatitis D are also infected with hepatitis B	Primarily fecal-oral
Severity	Mild	Commonly severe	Moderate	Can be severe and lead to fulminant hepatitis	Highly virulent with common progression to fulminant hepatitis and hepatic failure, especially in pregnant patients
Prognosis	Generally good	Worsens with age and debility	Moderate	Fair; worsens in chronic cases; can lead to chronic hepatitis D and chronic liver disease	Good unless pregnant
Progression to chronicity	None	Occasional	10% to 50% of cases	Occasional	None

What to look for

In the preicteric phase, look for:
- fatigue, malaise, arthralgia, myalgia, photophobia, and headache
- loss of appetite, nausea, and vomiting
- altered sense of taste and smell
- fever, possibly with liver and lymph node enlargement.

Icteric in the middle

The icteric phase lasts 1 to 2 weeks. Signs and symptoms include:
• mild weight loss
• dark urine and clay-colored stools
• yellow sclera and skin
• continued hepatomegaly with tenderness.

Time to rest

The convalescent phase lasts 2 to 12 weeks or longer. Signs and symptoms include:
• continued fatigue
• flatulence, abdominal pain or tenderness, and indigestion.

What tests tell you

These results help confirm the diagnosis.
• The presence of hepatitis B surface antigens and hepatitis B antibodies confirms a diagnosis of type B hepatitis.
• Detection of an antibody to type A hepatitis confirms past or present infection with type A hepatitis.
• Detection of an antibody to type C confirms a diagnosis of type C hepatitis. Viral load is measured by quantitative polymerase chain reaction assay and is useful in determining need for treatment and monitoring therapy.
• PT is prolonged (more than 3 seconds longer than normal indicates severe liver damage).
• Serum transaminase levels (ALT and AST) are elevated.
• Serum alkaline phosphatase levels are slightly elevated.
• Serum and urine bilirubin levels are elevated (with jaundice).
• Serum albumin levels are low, and serum globulin levels are high.
• Liver biopsy and scan show patchy necrosis.

How it's treated

• The patient should rest in the early stages of the illness and combat anorexia by eating small meals high in calories and protein. (Protein intake should be reduced if signs of precoma—lethargy, confusion, mental changes—develop.) Large meals are usually better tolerated in the morning.
• Chronic hepatitis B with liver inflammation is treated with interferon alfa-2b for 16 weeks. Monitoring of blood counts is essential during treatment.
• Lamivudine is another therapy for hepatitis B to decrease the viral load of hepatitis B.

> In the early stages of hepatitis, the patient should combat anorexia by eating small meals high in calories and protein.

• Current therapy for hepatitis C includes interferon or a combined interferon and ribavirin therapy. Decision to treat the individual is made after laboratory tests and liver biopsy confirm hepatic inflammation or early cirrhosis. Treatment lasts from 6 to 18 months, based on the outcome and genotype of the virus. The patient needs instruction on self-injection and adverse effects.

• Laboratory tests—including CBC with differential, thyroid studies, liver function tests, and hepatitis quantitative studies—help determine the effectiveness of therapy and prevent complications during treatment. Drug dosages may be reduced if WBC count, hemoglobin level, or hematocrit drop below normal.

• Caution patients against becoming pregnant during the course of therapy or in the 6 months immediately following treatment.

• Adverse effects of medication include depression, flulike syndrome, fatigue, malaise, and GI disturbance.

• Patients need to be proactive in their treatment to properly monitor and succeed in taking their medication. Current eradication rates of combined therapy in patients with hepatitis C range from 30% to 40%.

• Antiemetics, such as trimethobenzamide or benzquinamide, may be given 30 minutes before meals to relieve nausea and prevent vomiting; phenothiazines have a cholestatic effect and should be avoided. If vomiting persists, the patient needs I.V. infusions.

• In severe hepatitis, corticosteroids may give the patient a sense of well-being and may stimulate the appetite while decreasing itching and inflammation; however, their use in hepatitis is controversial.

Caution patients against becoming pregnant during therapy or in the 6 months after treatment.

What to do

• Observe enteric and blood and body fluid precautions for all types of hepatitis. Inform visitors about isolation precautions.

• Give the patient plenty of fluids (at least 4,000 ml/day). Encourage the anorexic patient to drink fruit juices. Also, offer chipped ice and effervescent soft drinks to promote adequate hydration without inducing vomiting.

• Record weight daily, and keep accurate intake and output records.

• Observe the patient's stool for color, consistency, frequency, and amount.

• Watch for signs of hepatic coma, dehydration, pneumonia, vascular problems, and pressure ulcers.

• Report all cases of hepatitis to health officials. Ask the patient to name anyone he came in contact with recently.

• Evaluate the patient. He should be able to maintain adequate hydration and nutrition, follow appropriate isolation precautions, modify his diet and lifestyle as needed, and obtain appropriate follow-up care. His close contacts also should seek evaluation and possible vaccination. (See *Teaching the patient with viral hepatitis*.)

Intestinal obstruction

In an intestinal obstruction, the lumen of the small or large bowel becomes partly or fully blocked. Small-bowel obstruction is far more common (affecting 90% of patients) and usually more serious. Complete obstruction in any part of the bowel, if untreated, can cause death within hours from shock and vascular collapse. Intestinal obstruction is most likely to occur after abdominal surgery or in persons with congenital bowel deformities.

What causes it

Mechanical obstruction can result from:
• adhesions and strangulated hernias (usually small-bowel obstruction)
• carcinomas (usually large-bowel obstruction)
• foreign bodies (fruit pits, gallstones, worms)
• compression
• stenosis
• intussusception
• volvulus of the sigmoid or cecum
• tumors
• atresia.

From the inside

Nonmechanical obstruction can result from:
• electrolyte imbalances
• toxicity
• neurogenic abnormalities
• thrombosis or embolism of mesenteric vessels
• paralytic ileus. (See *Paralytic ileus*, page 478.)

Pathophysiology

Intestinal obstruction develops in three forms:

simple. Blockage prevents intestinal contents from passing, with no other complications.

strangulated. Blood supply to part or all of the obstructed section is cut off, in addition to blockage of the lumen.

Paralytic ileus

Paralytic ileus is a physiologic form of intestinal obstruction that usually develops in the small bowel after abdominal surgery. It causes decreased or absent intestinal motility that usually disappears spontaneously after 2 to 3 days.

Signs and symptoms
• Severe abdominal distention
• Extreme distress
• Vomiting
• Severe constipation
• Passage of flatus and small, liquid stools

Causes
• Trauma
• Toxemia
• Peritonitis
• Electrolyte deficiencies (especially hypokalemia)

• Drugs, such as ganglionic blocking agents and anticholinergics
• Vascular causes, such as thrombosis and embolism
• Excessive air swallowing (rarely lasts more than 24 hours from this factor alone)

Treatment
• Intubation for decompression and na-sogastric suctioning (if lasts longer than 48 hours)
• Miller-Abbott tube in the patient with severe abdominal distention (used with

caution to avoid additional trauma to the bowel)
• Cholinergic agents, such as neostig-mine and bethanechol (when resulting from surgical manipulation of the bowel)
• Patient teaching to explain effects of cholinergics, such as intestinal cramps and diarrhea
• Monitoring for cardiovascular adverse effects of neostigmine, such as brady-cardia and hypotension
• Frequent checks for returning bowel sounds

close-looped. Both ends of a bowel section are occluded, isolating it from the rest of the intestine.

Similar effects

The physiologic effects are similar in all three forms of obstruction. When intestinal obstruction occurs, fluid, air, and gas collect near the site. Peristalsis increases temporarily as the bowel tries to force its contents through the obstruction, injuring intestinal mucosa and causing distention at and above the site of the obstruction. Distention blocks the flow of venous blood and halts normal absorptive processes. As a result, the bowel begins to secrete water, sodium, and potassium into the fluid pooled in the lumen.

What to look for

To help detect small-bowel obstruction:
• Assess the patient for colicky pain, nausea, vomiting, and constipation.
• Auscultate for high-pitched, loud, musical, or tinkling quality bowel sounds; borborygmi; and rushes (occasionally loud enough to be heard without a stethoscope).

- Palpate for abdominal tenderness with moderate distention. Rebound tenderness may occur when obstruction has caused strangulation with ischemia.
- Assess for vomiting of fecal contents in complete obstruction.

Big bowel block

In large-bowel obstruction:
- Assess for constipation in the first few days.
- Other symptoms include colicky abdominal pain, nausea (usually without vomiting at first), and abdominal distention. Eventually, pain becomes continuous and the patient may vomit fecal contents.

Symptoms of large-bowel obstruction include colicky abdominal pain.

What tests tell you

- Abdominal X-rays confirm the diagnosis. They show the presence and location of intestinal gas or fluid. In small-bowel obstruction, a typical "stepladder" pattern emerges, with alternating fluid and gas levels apparent in 3 to 4 hours.
- CT scans are used to rule out obstruction or identify perforation or volvulus.
- In large-bowel obstruction, barium enema reveals a distended, air-filled colon or a closed loop of sigmoid with extreme distention (in sigmoid volvulus).
- Early in diagnosis, laboratory results might be normal.

Later labs don't lie

These laboratory results support this diagnosis:
- Sodium, chloride, and potassium levels are decreased (from vomiting).
- WBC count is slightly elevated (with necrosis, peritonitis, or strangulation).
- Serum amylase level is increased (possibly from irritation of the pancreas).
- ABG analysis determines acid-base balance.

How it's treated

- Preoperative treatment aims to correct fluid and electrolyte imbalances, decompress the bowel to relieve vomiting and distention, and alleviate shock and peritonitis.
- Strangulated obstruction usually requires blood replacement as well as I.V. fluid administration. Passage of a Levin tube, followed by use of the longer, weighted Miller-Abbott tube, usually accomplishes decompression, especially in small-bowel obstruction.
- Esophagogastroduodenoscopy may be performed to remove obstructive lesions.

• Close monitoring of the patient's condition determines duration of treatment. If the patient fails to improve or his condition deteriorates, surgery is necessary.

• In large-bowel obstruction, surgical resection with anastomosis, colostomy, or ileostomy commonly follows decompression with a Levin tube.

• TPN may be appropriate if the patient suffers a protein deficit from chronic obstruction, postoperative or paralytic ileus, or infection.

• Drug therapy includes analgesics or sedatives, such as meperidine or phenobarbital (not opiates, which inhibit GI motility), and antibiotics for peritonitis caused by bowel strangulation or infarction.

• For intussusception, hydrostatic reduction may be attempted by infusing barium into the rectum. If this fails, manual reduction or bowel resection is performed.

What to do

• Monitor the patient's vital signs frequently. Decreased blood pressure may indicate reduced circulating blood volume due to blood loss from a strangulated hernia. Remember, as much as 10 L of fluid can collect in the small bowel, drastically reducing plasma volume. Observe closely for signs of shock (such as pallor, decreased urine output, rapid pulse, and hypotension).

• Stay alert for signs and symptoms of metabolic alkalosis (including changes in sensorium, hypertonic muscles, tetany, and slow, shallow respirations) or acidosis (including shortness of breath on exertion, disorientation and, later, deep, rapid breathing, weakness, and malaise). Watch for signs and symptoms of secondary infection, such as fever and chills.

• Monitor urine output carefully to assess renal function and possible urine retention from bladder compression by the distended intestine. If you suspect bladder compression, catheterize the patient for residual urine immediately after he has voided. Also, measure abdominal girth frequently to detect progressive distention.

• Provide thorough mouth and nose care if the patient has undergone decompression by intubation or if he has vomited. Look for signs of dehydration (such as a thick, swollen tongue; dry, cracked lips; and dry oral mucous membranes).

• Record the amount and color of drainage from the decompression tube. Irrigate the tube, if necessary, with normal saline solution to maintain patency.

• If a weighted tube has been inserted, check periodically to make sure it's advancing. Help the patient turn from side to side (or walk around, if he can) to facilitate passage of the tube.

Decreased blood pressure may indicate reduced circulating blood volume from a strangulated hernia.

• Keep the patient in Fowler's position as much as possible to promote pulmonary ventilation and ease respiratory distress from abdominal distention.

• Auscultate for bowel sounds, and watch for signs of returning peristalsis (passage of flatus and mucus through the rectum).

• Evaluate the patient. He should have normal fluid and electrolyte status, adequate oral intake, normal bowel sounds, and regular bowel elimination patterns. He should also be free from abdominal distention and complications. (See *Teaching the patient with intestinal obstruction*.)

Education edge

Teaching the patient with intestinal obstruction

• Provide emotional support and positive reinforcement after surgery.

• Arrange for an enterostomal therapist to visit the patient who has had a colostomy.

Irritable bowel syndrome

Also referred to as *spastic colon* or *spastic colitis*, irritable bowel syndrome (IBS) is marked by chronic symptoms of abdominal pain, alternating constipation and diarrhea, excess flatulence, a sense of incomplete evacuation, and abdominal distention. IBS is a common, stress-related disorder. About 20% of patients never seek medical attention for this benign condition that has no anatomical abnormality or inflammatory component. It's twice as common in women as in men.

What causes it

IBS is usually associated with psychological stress, but may also result from physical factors, such as:

• ingestion of irritants (coffee, raw fruits or vegetables)
• lactose intolerance
• abuse of laxatives
• hormonal changes (menstruation).

Pathophysiology

IBS appears to reflect motor disturbances of the entire colon in response to stimuli. Some muscles of the small bowel are particularly sensitive to motor abnormalities and distention; others are particularly sensitive to certain foods and drugs. The patient may be hypersensitive to the hormones gastrin and cholecystokinin. The pain of IBS seems to be caused by abnormally strong contractions of the intestinal smooth muscle as it reacts to distention, irritants, or stress.

What to look for

These symptoms alternate with constipation or normal bowel function:

In addition to stress, IBS may result from ingestion of such irritants as coffee.

• lower abdominal pain (usually relieved by defecation or passage of gas)
• diarrhea (typically occurring during the day)
• small stools that contain visible mucus
• possible dyspepsia
• abdominal distention.

What tests tell you

Tests may include sigmoidoscopy, colonoscopy, barium enema, rectal biopsy, and stool examination for blood, parasites, and bacteria to rule out other disorders.

How it's treated

• Counseling helps the patient understand the relationship between stress and her illness.
• Strict dietary restrictions aren't beneficial, but food irritants should be investigated and the patient should be instructed to avoid them.
• Rest is helpful, as is judicious use of sedatives (such as phenobarbital) and antispasmodics (such as propantheline, diphenoxylate with atropine sulfate, hyoscyamine, or dicyclomine). With chronic use, however, the patient may become dependent on these drugs.
• If the cause of IBS is chronic laxative abuse, bowel retraining may help correct the condition.

What to do

Evaluate the patient. She should modify her diet and lifestyle to control or avoid symptoms, demonstrate a regular bowel elimination pattern, understand the need for follow-up care, and know when to seek immediate attention. However, because the patient with IBS isn't hospitalized, focus your care on patient teaching. (See *Teaching the patient with irritable bowel syndrome.*)

Education edge

Teaching the patient with irritable bowel syndrome

• Tell the patient to avoid irritating foods, and encourage her to develop regular bowel habits.
• Teach her to keep a food diary to identify food irritants.
• Help her deal with stress, and warn against dependence on sedatives or antispasmodics.

Pancreatitis

Pancreatitis — inflammation of the pancreas — occurs in acute and chronic forms and may result from edema, necrosis, or hemorrhage. The prognosis is good when pancreatitis follows biliary tract disease, but poor when it's a complication of alcoholism. Mortality reaches 60% when pancreatitis causes tissue destruction or hemorrhage.

A common cause of pancreatitis is alcoholism. So, ixnay on the inkdray!

What causes it

Most commonly caused by biliary tract disease and alcoholism, pancreatitis also results from:
- pancreatic cancer
- possibly, peptic ulcer, mumps, or hypothermia
- certain drugs, such as glucocorticoids, zidovudine, didanosine, sulfonamides, chlorothiazide, and azathioprine
- less commonly, from stenosis or obstruction of Oddi's sphincter, hyperlipidemia, metabolic and endocrine disorders, vascular disease, viral infections, mycoplasmal pneumonia, or pregnancy
- iatrogenic causes, including diagnostic or therapeutic ERCP, which increases the risk of pancreatitis by 3% to 6%.

Pathophysiology

Chronic pancreatitis is a persistent inflammation that produces irreversible changes in the structure and function of the pancreas. It sometimes follows an episode of acute pancreatitis. Here's what probably happens:
- Protein precipitates block the pancreatic duct and eventually harden or calcify.
- Structural changes lead to fibrosis and atrophy of the glands.
- Growths called *pseudocysts*, containing pancreatic enzymes and tissue debris, form.
- An abscess results if these growths become infected.

The acute angle

Acute pancreatitis occurs in two forms:

  edematous (interstitial), causing fluid accumulation and swelling

 necrotizing, causing cell death and tissue damage.

   The inflammation that occurs with both types is caused by premature activation of enzymes, which causes tissue damage. Normally, the acini in the pancreas secrete enzymes in an inactive form.

Interesting theories...

Two theories explain why enzymes become prematurely activated:

 A toxic agent, such as alcohol, alters the way the pancreas secretes enzymes. This agent increases pancreatic secretion, alters the metabolism of the acinar cells, and encourages duct obstruction by causing pancreatic secretory proteins to precipitate.

A reflux of duodenal contents containing activated enzymes enters the pancreatic duct, activating other enzymes and setting up a cycle of more pancreatic damage.

What to look for

Steady epigastric pain centered close to the umbilicus, radiating between the 10th thoracic and 6th lumbar vertebrae, and unrelieved by vomiting may be the first and only symptom of mild pancreatitis. A severe attack may cause:

- extreme pain
- persistent vomiting
- abdominal rigidity
- diminished bowel activity (suggesting peritonitis)
- crackles at lung bases
- left pleural effusion
- extreme malaise
- restlessness
- mottled skin
- tachycardia
- low-grade fever (100° to 102° F [37.8° to 38.9° C])
- cold, sweaty extremities
- possible ileus.

A severe attack of pancreatitis may cause crackles at lung bases.

What tests tell you

- Dramatically elevated serum amylase levels—commonly more than 500 Somogyi units/dl—confirm pancreatitis and rule out perforated peptic ulcer, acute cholecystitis, appendicitis, and bowel infarction or obstruction. Dramatic elevations of amylase levels also occur in urine, ascites, and pleural fluid. Characteristically, amylase levels return to normal 48 hours after the onset of pancreatitis, despite continuing symptoms.
- Serum lipase levels are increased, but rise more slowly than serum amylase levels.
- Serum calcium levels are low from fat necrosis and formation of calcium soaps.
- Glucose levels are elevated and may be as high as 900 mg/dl, indicating hyperglycemia.
- WBC counts range from 8,000 to 20,000/µl, with increased polymorphonuclear leukocyte levels.
- Hematocrit occasionally exceeds 50% concentrations.
- Abdominal X-rays may show dilation of the small or large bowel or calcification of the pancreas.
- GI series indicates extrinsic pressure on the duodenum or stomach caused by edema of the pancreas head.

- An ultrasound isn't usually helpful in providing diagnosis because the pancreas is poorly visualized.
- An abdominal CT scan can help distinguish between cholelithiasis and pancreatitis.

How it's treated

Treatment must maintain circulation and fluid volume, relieve pain, and decrease pancreatic secretions.
- Emergency treatment for shock (the most common cause of death in early-stage pancreatitis) consists of vigorous I.V. replacement of electrolytes and proteins. Metabolic acidosis secondary to hypovolemia and impaired cellular perfusion requires vigorous fluid volume replacement.
- Hypocalcemia requires infusion of 10% calcium gluconate; serum glucose levels greater than 300 mg/dl require insulin therapy.

One week on I.V. therapy
- After the emergency phase, continuing I.V. therapy for 5 to 7 days should provide adequate electrolytes and protein solutions that don't stimulate the pancreas.
- If the patient isn't ready to resume oral feedings by then, TPN may be necessary.
- Nonstimulating elemental gavage feedings may be safer because of the decreased risk of infection and overinfusion.
- In extreme cases, laparotomy to drain the pancreatic bed, 95% pancreatectomy, or a combination of cholecystostomy-gastrostomy, feeding jejunostomy, and drainage may be necessary.

What to do

- Give plasma or albumin, if ordered, to maintain blood pressure.
- Record fluid intake and output, check urine output hourly, and monitor electrolyte levels.
- For bowel decompression, maintain constant NG suctioning, and give nothing by mouth. Perform good mouth and nose care.
- Watch for signs of calcium deficiency—tetany, cramps, carpopedal spasm, and seizures. If you suspect hypocalcemia, keep airway and suction apparatus handy and pad side rails.
- Administer analgesics as needed to relieve the patient's pain and anxiety.

A case of dry mouth
- Don't confuse thirst caused by hyperglycemia (indicated by serum glucose levels of up to 350 mg/dl and glucose and acetone in urine) with dry mouth caused by NG intubation and anticholinergics.

After the emergency phase, I.V. therapy should be continued for 5 to 7 days with solutions that don't stimulate the pancreas.

• Watch for complications due to TPN, such as sepsis, hypokalemia, overhydration, and metabolic acidosis.
• Evaluate the patient. He should have normal nutrition and hydration levels, balanced electrolyte levels, and an improved comfort level. He also should understand the need for lifestyle modifications and adjust lifestyle factors that aggravate his disease. (See *Teaching the patient with pancreatitis.*)

Peptic ulcers

Appearing as circumscribed lesions in the gastric mucosal membrane, peptic ulcers can develop in the lower esophagus, stomach, pylorus, duodenum, or jejunum from contact with gastric juice (especially hydrochloric acid and pepsin). About 80% of all peptic ulcers are duodenal ulcers.

What causes it

The precise cause of peptic ulcer is unknown but may include:
• *H. pylori* infection
• use of NSAIDs or salicylates
• inadequate protection of mucous membranes
• pathologic hypersecretory disorders.

Factor in

Factors that predispose a person to peptic ulcer include:
• blood type (gastric ulcers and type A; duodenal ulcers and type O) and other genetic factors
• exposure to irritants, such as alcohol, coffee, and tobacco
• emotional stress
• physical trauma
• normal aging.

Pathophysiology

In a peptic ulcer due to *H. pylori*, acid adds to the effects of the bacterial infection. *H. pylori* releases a toxin that destroys the stomach's mucus coat, promoting mucosal inflammation and ulceration. Salicylates and other NSAIDs encourage ulcer formation by inhibiting the secretion of prostaglandins (substances that block ulceration). (See *A close look at peptic ulcers.*)

What to look for

Patients with duodenal ulcers may experience attacks about 2 hours after meals, whenever the stomach is empty, or after consuming orange juice, coffee, aspirin, or alcohol. Exacerbations

Education edge

Teaching the patient with pancreatitis

• Emphasize the importance of avoiding factors that precipitate acute pancreatitis, especially alcohol.
• Refer the patient and his family to a dietitian. Stress the need for a diet high in carbohydrates and low in protein and fats. Caution the patient to avoid beverages with caffeine and irritating foods.

Patients with duodenal ulcers may experience attacks about 2 hours after meals.

A close look at peptic ulcers

This illustration shows different degrees of peptic ulceration. Lesions that don't extend below the mucosal lining (epithelium) are called *erosions*. Lesions of acute and chronic ulcers can extend through the epithelium and may perforate the stomach wall. Chronic ulcers also have scar tissue at the base.

Note that acute and chronic ulcers extend beyond the mucosal lining.

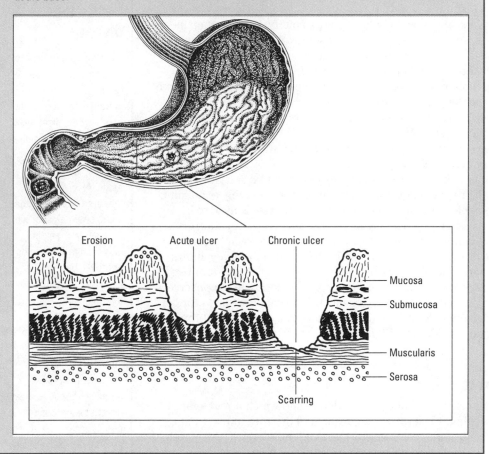

tend to recur several times a year, then fade into remission. Such patients may report heartburn and localized midepigastric pain, which is relieved after eating.

What tests tell you

- Upper GI tract X-rays show abnormalities in the mucosa.
- Gastric secretory studies show hyperchlorhydria.
- Upper GI endoscopy confirms the presence of an ulcer.

- Serologic or breath urea test shows presence of *H. pylori.*
- Biopsy rules out cancer.
- Stool may test positive for occult blood.

How it's treated

Treatment is essentially symptomatic and emphasizes drug therapy and rest.

- Antacids are given to reduce gastric acidity. Proton pump inhibitors, such as omeprazole or lansoprazole, or H_2-receptor antagonists, such as cimetidine or ranitidine, reduce gastric secretion in short-term therapy (up to 8 weeks).
- Anticholinergics, such as propantheline, inhibit the vagus nerve effect on the parietal cells and reduce gastrin production and excessive gastric activity in duodenal ulcers.
- Physical rest promotes healing.
- Gastroscopy can facilitate coagulation of the bleeding site by cautery or laser therapy.
- If GI bleeding occurs, emergency treatment begins with passage of an NG tube to allow for iced saline lavage, possibly containing norepinephrine. Sclerotherapy with epinephrine is used to ligate active vessels. Angiography facilitates placement of an intra-arterial catheter, followed by infusion of vasopressin to constrict blood vessels and control bleeding. This type of therapy allows postponement of surgery until the patient's condition stabilizes.
- Surgery is indicated for perforation unresponsive to conservative treatment and suspected cancer. Surgical procedures for peptic ulcers include vagotomy and pyloroplasty or distal subtotal gastrectomy. (For more information, see "Gastric surgeries," page 430.)

What to do

- Administer medications, as ordered, and watch for adverse effects of cimetidine (dizziness, rash, mild diarrhea, muscle pain, leukopenia, and gynecomastia) and anticholinergics (dry mouth, blurred vision, headache, constipation, and urine retention). Anticholinergics are usually most effective when given 30 minutes before meals. Give sedatives and tranquilizers as needed.
- Evaluate the patient. After successful treatment for peptic ulcers, he'll understand the disease process and comply with the treatment regimen. He'll recognize the need to avoid factors that may exacerbate his condition and modify his diet and lifestyle to do so. He should also understand the need for follow-up care and know when to seek immediate attention. (See *Teaching the patient with peptic ulcer disease.*)

Education edge

Teaching the patient with peptic ulcer disease

- Instruct the patient to take antacids 1 hour after meals. Advise the patient who has a history of cardiac disease or one who's on a sodium-restricted diet to take only low-sodium antacids. Also warn him that antacids may cause some changes in bowel habits (diarrhea with magnesium-containing antacids and constipation with aluminum-containing antacids).
- Warn the patient to avoid aspirin-containing drugs, nonsteroidal anti-inflammatory drugs, reserpine, and phenylbutazone because they irritate the gastric mucosa. Also warn him against excessive intake of coffee, exposure to stressful situations, and consumption of alcoholic beverages during exacerbations. Advise him to stop smoking and to avoid milk products because these stimulate gastric secretion.

Peritonitis

An acute or chronic inflammation, peritonitis may extend throughout the peritoneum, the membrane that lines the abdominal cavity and covers the visceral organs, or it may be localized as an abscess. Peritonitis commonly reduces intestinal motility and causes intestinal distention with gas. Mortality is 10%. Death usually results from bowel obstruction.

What causes it

• Peritonitis results from bacterial inflammation due to appendicitis, diverticulitis, peptic ulcer, ulcerative colitis, volvulus, a strangulated obstruction, an abdominal neoplasm, or a stab wound.
• It may also result from chemical inflammation, as in ruptured fallopian tubes or bladder, perforated gastric ulcer, or released pancreatic enzymes.

Pathophysiology

Although the GI tract normally contains bacteria, the peritoneum is sterile. When bacteria or chemical irritants invade the peritoneum due to inflammation and perforation of the GI tract, peritonitis is the result. In chemical and bacterial inflammation, accumulated fluids containing protein and electrolytes make the transparent peritoneum opaque, red, inflamed, and edematous. Because the peritoneal cavity is so resistant to contamination, infection is commonly localized as an abscess.

What to look for

The main symptom of peritonitis is sudden, severe, diffuse abdominal pain that tends to intensify and localize in the area of the underlying disorder. Also assess the patient for:
• weakness, pallor, excessive sweating, and cold skin
• decreased intestinal motility and paralytic ileus
• abdominal distention
• an acutely tender abdomen associated with rebound tenderness
• shallow breathing
• diminished movement by the patient to minimize pain
• hypotension, tachycardia, and signs of dehydration
• fever of 103° F (39.4° C) or higher
• possible shoulder pain and hiccups.

What tests tell you

• Abdominal X-rays showing edematous and gaseous distention of the small and large bowel support the diagnosis. With perfora-

First the peritoneum, then the world! Heh, heh, heh...

tion of a visceral organ, the X-ray shows air in the abdominal cavity.
• Chest X-ray may show an elevated diaphragm.
• Blood studies show leukocytosis (more than 20,000 leukocytes/µl).
• Paracentesis reveals bacteria, exudate, blood, pus, or urine.
• Laparotomy may be necessary to identify the underlying cause.

How it's treated

Early treatment of GI inflammatory conditions and preoperative and postoperative antibiotic therapy prevent peritonitis. After peritonitis develops, emergency treatment aims to stop infection, restore intestinal motility, and replace fluids and electrolytes:
• Massive antibiotic therapy usually includes administration of cefoxitin with an aminoglycoside, or penicillin G and clindamycin with an aminoglycoside, depending on the infecting organisms. Other agents used include cephalosporins and quinolones.
• To decrease peristalsis and prevent perforation, the patient should be given nothing by mouth and should receive supportive fluids and electrolytes parenterally.
• Supplementary treatment measures include preoperative and postoperative analgesics, such as meperidine; NG intubation to decompress the bowel; and possible use of a rectal tube to facilitate passage of flatus.
• When peritonitis results from perforation, surgery is performed as soon as the patient can tolerate it. Surgery aims to eliminate the infection source by evacuating the spilled contents and inserting drains.
• Occasionally, paracentesis may be needed to remove accumulated fluid.
• Irrigation of the abdominal cavity with antibiotic solutions during surgery may be appropriate.

What to do

• Regularly monitor vital signs, fluid intake and output, and the amount of NG drainage or vomitus.
• Place the patient in semi-Fowler's position to help him deep-breathe with less pain and thus prevent pulmonary complications.

After evacuation

After surgery to evacuate the peritoneum:
• Watch for signs and symptoms of dehiscence (the patient may complain that "something gave way") and abscess formation (continued abdominal tenderness and fever).

When peristalsis, temperature, and pulse are normal, gradually decrease parenteral fluids. Then I can take a vacation. Cal-i-forn-ya here I come...

• Frequently assess peristaltic activity by listening for bowel sounds and checking for gas, bowel movements, and a soft abdomen.

• When peristalsis returns and temperature and pulse rate are normal, gradually decrease parenteral fluids and increase oral fluids. If the patient has an NG tube in place, clamp it for short intervals. If neither nausea nor vomiting results, begin oral fluids as ordered and tolerated.

• Evaluate the patient by assessing for normal fluid and electrolyte balance, normal body temperature and WBC count, lack of bowel obstruction or other complications, and normal oral intake and bowel elimination patterns. (See *Teaching the patient with peritonitis*.)

Ulcerative colitis

An inflammatory, typically chronic disease, ulcerative colitis affects the mucosa and submucosa of the colon. It usually begins in the rectum and sigmoid colon and commonly extends upward into the entire colon. It rarely affects the small intestine, except for the terminal ileum. Severity ranges from a mild, localized disorder to a fulminant disease that may cause a perforated colon, progressing to potentially fatal peritonitis and toxemia.

What causes it

The cause of ulcerative colitis is unknown. Risk factors include a family history of the disease; bacterial infection; allergic reaction to food, milk, or other substances that release inflammatory histamine in the bowel; overproduction of enzymes that break down the mucous membranes; and emotional stress. Autoimmune disorders, such as rheumatoid arthritis, hemolytic anemia, erythema nodosum, and uveitis, may heighten the risk.

Pathophysiology

Ulcerative colitis damages the large intestine's mucosal and submucosal layers. Here's how it progresses:

Usually, the disease originates in the rectum and lower colon. Then it spreads to the entire colon.

The mucosa develops diffuse ulceration with hemorrhage, congestion, edema, and exudative inflammation. Unlike Crohn's disease, ulcerations are continuous.

Abscesses formed in the mucosa drain purulent pus, become necrotic, and ulcerate.

Education edge

Teaching the patient with peritonitis

• Teach the patient about peritonitis, its cause (in his case), and necessary treatments. If time allows before surgery, reinforce the doctor's explanation of the procedure and its possible complications. Tell him how long he can expect to be hospitalized; many patients remain hospitalized for 2 weeks or more after surgery.

• Review diet and activity limitations (depending on the type of surgery). Typically, the patient must avoid lifting for at least 6 weeks postoperatively.

Sloughing occurs, causing bloody, mucus-filled stools.

Close-up on the colon

As ulcerative colitis progresses, the colon undergoes changes:

 Initially, the colon's mucosal surface becomes dark, red, and velvety.

Abscesses form and coalesce into ulcers.

 Necrosis of the mucosa occurs.

As abscesses heal, scarring and thickening may appear in the bowel's inner muscle layer.

As granulation tissue replaces the muscle layer, the colon narrows, shortens, and loses its characteristic pouches (haustral folds).

What to look for

Recurrent bloody diarrhea and symptom-free remissions are the hallmark characteristics of ulcerative colitis. The stool typically contains pus and mucus. Assess the patient for other signs and symptoms, such as:
- spastic rectum and anus
- abdominal pain
- irritability
- weight loss
- weakness
- anorexia
- nausea and vomiting
- fever
- occasional constipation (in elderly patients).

What tests tell you

- Sigmoidoscopy shows increased mucosal friability, decreased mucosal detail, and thick inflammatory exudate. Biopsy during sigmoidoscopy helps confirm the diagnosis.
- Colonoscopy helps determine the extent of disease and evaluate strictured areas and pseudopolyps.
- Barium enema helps assess the extent of the disease and detect complications, such as strictures and carcinoma.
- A stool specimen may be analyzed for leukocytes, ova, and parasites.
- The ESR will be increased in relation to the severity of the attack.

Among other things, assess your patient for weight loss, a possible sign of ulcerative colitis.

• Decreased serum levels of potassium, magnesium, hemoglobin, and albumin as well as leukocytosis and increased PT support the diagnosis.

How it's treated

The goals of ulcerative colitis treatment are to control inflammation, replace nutritional losses and blood volume, and prevent complications.
• Supportive treatment includes bed rest, I.V. fluid replacement, and a clear liquid diet.
• For patients awaiting surgery or showing signs of dehydration and debilitation from excessive diarrhea, TPN is administered to rest the intestinal tract, decrease stool volume, and restore positive nitrogen balance. Blood transfusions or iron supplements may be needed to correct anemia.
• Drug therapy to control inflammation includes adrenocorticotropic hormone and adrenal corticosteroids, such as prednisone, prednisolone, hydrocortisone, and budesonide.
• If disease is limited to the left side of the colon, topical mesalamine suppositories or enemas or hydrocortisone enemas may be effective.
• Sulfasalazine, which has anti-inflammatory and antimicrobial properties, may also be used.

Don't be such a spaz

• Antispasmodics, such as tincture of belladonna, and antidiarrheals, such as diphenoxylate, are used only for patients whose ulcerative colitis is under control but who have frequent, troublesome diarrheal stools. These drugs may precipitate massive dilation of the colon (toxic megacolon) and are usually contraindicated.
• Immunomodulatory agents, such as azathioprine and 6-mercaptopurine, may be effective for patients who have frequent flareups of symptoms despite continuous steroid therapy. Patients with severe disease have also been treated with cyclosporine. These medications require careful monitoring along with serial CBC with differential counts.
• Surgery is the treatment of last resort if the patient has toxic megacolon, fails to respond to drugs and supportive measures, or finds symptoms unbearable. The most common surgical technique is proctocolectomy with ileostomy. Total colectomy with ileorectal anastomosis is done less often because of its associated mortality (2% to 5%).
• In pouch ileostomy, a pouch is created from a small loop of the terminal ileum and a nipple valve formed from the distal ileum.

Supportive treatment for ulcerative colitis includes I.V. fluid replacement, a clear liquid diet, and plenty of bed rest.

The resulting stoma opens just above the pubic hairline; the pouch empties through a catheter inserted in the stoma several times each day.
• Colectomy to prevent colon cancer is controversial in treatment for ulcerative colitis. (For more information, see "Bowel surgery with ostomy," page 433.)

What to do

• Accurately record intake and output, particularly the frequency and volume of stools. Watch for signs of dehydration (poor skin turgor, furrowed tongue) and electrolyte imbalances, especially signs of hypokalemia (muscle weakness, paresthesia) and hypernatremia (tachycardia, flushed skin, fever, dry tongue).
• Monitor hemoglobin level and hematocrit and give blood transfusions as ordered.
• Provide good mouth care for the patient who's allowed nothing by mouth.
• After each bowel movement, thoroughly clean the skin around the rectum.
• Provide an air mattress or a sheepskin to help prevent skin breakdown.
• Watch for adverse effects of prolonged corticosteroid or immunomodulator therapy (hyperglycemia, hypertension, hirsutism, edema, gastric irritation). Be aware that such therapy may mask infection.
• Watch closely for signs of complications, such as a perforated colon and peritonitis (fever, severe abdominal pain, abdominal rigidity and tenderness, cool, clammy skin) and toxic megacolon (abdominal distention, decreased bowel sounds).
• Do a bowel preparation, as ordered. This usually involves keeping the patient on a clear liquid diet, using cleansing enemas, and administering antimicrobials such as neomycin.
• Evaluate the patient. He should maintain optimal nutrition and hydration, report his feelings about his changed body image, identify and avoid foods likely to cause distress, demonstrate proper ostomy care, use appropriate support groups, understand the need for follow-up care, and know when to seek immediate attention. (See *Teaching the patient with ulcerative colitis*.)

Education edge

Teaching the patient with ulcerative colitis

• Prepare the patient for surgery and inform him about ileostomy. Encourage him to verbalize his feelings and provide emotional support.
• After a proctocolectomy and ileostomy, teach good stoma care. After a pouch ileostomy, also teach the patient how to insert the catheter.
• Instruct the patient about his disease, and teach him to watch for signs of increased activity and flare-ups. Discuss adverse effects of medications, especially immunomodulators.
• Include instruction on self-administration of enemas and topical creams.
• Include the importance of a healthy, low-residue diet and an adequate intake of protein, calcium, folate, and vitamin D.
• Encourage the patient to have regular physical examinations because he's at risk for developing colorectal cancer.

Quick quiz

1. When performing an abdominal assessment, do the four basic steps in which order?

    A.   Inspection, percussion, palpation, auscultation
    B.   Inspection, auscultation, percussion, palpation
    C.   Palpation, inspection, percussion, auscultation
    D.   Percussion, auscultation, palpation, inspection

Answer: B. In an abdominal assessment, auscultation is performed before percussion and palpation because the latter can alter intestinal activity.

2. When performing a urine bilirubin test or a urobilinogen test, the specimen must be tested within:

    A.   5 minutes.
    B.   10 minutes.
    C.   30 minutes.
    D.   1 hour.

Answer: C. Both tests must be conducted within 30 minutes of specimen collection before the specimen deteriorates.

3. Your patient has severe midepigastric or right upper quadrant pain radiating to the back or referred to the right scapula, belching that leaves a sour taste in the mouth, and flatulence. She most likely has:

    A.   appendicitis.
    B.   acute cholecystitis, acute cholelithiasis, or choledocholithiasis.
    C.   diverticular disease.
    D.   acute gastritis.

Answer: B. These signs and symptoms suggest your patient has acute cholecystitis, acute cholelithiasis, or choledocholithiasis.

4. In a patient with suspected appendicitis, which of these interventions are appropriate?

    A.   Give I.V. fluids, give the patient nothing by mouth, and apply heat to his abdomen for comfort.
    B.   Give I.V. fluids, give the patient nothing by mouth, and give an enema to clean his bowel before surgery.
    C.   Give I.V. fluids; give the patient nothing by mouth, but give analgesics judiciously; and place him in Fowler's position to reduce pain.
    D.   Give clear liquids only along with heat applied to the abdomen for comfort.

Answer: C. Never apply heat to the right lower abdomen or give cathartics or enemas as they may cause the appendix to rupture. Give analgesics judiciously because they may mask symptoms of rupture.

5. Which statement about hepatitis is true?
   A. Type A hepatitis can lead to fulminant hepatitis.
   B. Type B hepatitis is transmitted via blood products, urine, and other body fluids.
   C. Type C hepatitis is transmitted via the fecal-oral route only.
   D. Type D hepatitis is mild in severity.

Answer: B. Type B hepatitis is transmitted via serum, blood, blood products, and all other body fluids. Type A hepatitis is mild in severity and won't lead to fulminant hepatitis. Type C hepatitis is transmitted via blood and other parenteral means. Type D hepatitis can be severe and lead to fulminant hepatitis.

Scoring

☆☆☆ If you answered all five items correctly, excellent! You've fully digested this GI information.

☆☆ If you answered three or four items correctly, super! You're full steam ahead in your knowledge of the alimentary canal.

☆ If you answered fewer than three items correctly, relax. Chew on this chapter a bit more, and it should go down smoothly.

Endocrine disorders

Just the facts

In this chapter, you'll learn:

♦ about hormones and how they affect the body

♦ how to assess the endocrine system

♦ causes, pathophysiology, diagnostic tests, and nursing
interventions for common disorders of the endocrine
system.

Endocrine disorders alter a patient's health and self-image. These
disorders may affect the patient's growth and development, reproductive system, energy level, metabolic rate, or ability to adapt to
stress. Some disorders, such as Cushing's syndrome and goiter,
disfigure the body. Others, such as diabetes mellitus, require the
patient to follow a stringent drug regimen and meal plan.

Anatomy and physiology

The endocrine system consists of three major components:

 glands, which are specialized cell clusters or organs

 hormones, which are chemical substances secreted by glands
in response to stimulation

 receptors, which are protein molecules that trigger specific
physiologic changes in a target cell in response to hormonal stimulation.

Glands

The major glands of the endocrine system are:
• pituitary gland

Endocrine system components

Endocrine glands secrete hormones directly into the bloodstream to regulate body function. This illustration shows the location of the major endocrine glands (except the gonads).

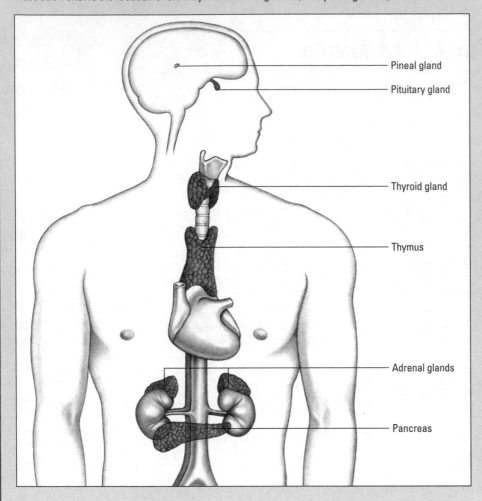

Pineal gland

Pituitary gland

Thyroid gland

Thymus

Adrenal glands

Pancreas

- thyroid gland
- parathyroid glands
- adrenal glands
- pancreas
- thymus
- pineal gland
- gonads (ovaries and testes). (See *Endocrine system components.*)

Pituitary gland

The pituitary gland rests in the sella turcica, a depression in the sphenoid bone at the base of the brain. This pea-size gland has two regions. The posterior pituitary lobe stores and releases oxytocin and antidiuretic hormone, which are produced by the hypothalamus. The largest, the anterior pituitary lobe, produces at least six hormones:

 growth hormone (GH), or somatotropin

 thyroid-stimulating hormone (TSH), or thyrotropin

 corticotropin

 follicle-stimulating hormone (FSH)

 luteinizing hormone (LH)

prolactin.

I keep my pituitary gland in my sella, my sella turcica, that is!

Thyroid gland

The thyroid gland lies directly below the larynx, partially in front of the trachea. Its two lateral lobes—one on either side of the trachea—join with a narrow tissue bridge, called the *isthmus*, to give the gland its butterfly shape. The two lobes of the thyroid function as one unit to produce the hormones:

• triiodothyronine (T_3) and thyroxine (T_4), collectively referred to as thyroid hormone, which is the body's major metabolic hormone
• calcitonin, which maintains the blood calcium level by inhibiting the release of calcium from bone.

Parathyroid glands

Four parathyroid glands lie embedded on the posterior surface of the thyroid, one in each corner. Like the thyroid lobes, the parathyroid glands work together as a single gland, producing parathyroid hormone (PTH), which helps regulate the blood's calcium balance.

Adrenal glands

The two adrenal glands sit atop the two kidneys. Each gland contains two distinct structures—the adrenal cortex and the adrenal medulla—that function as separate endocrine glands. The adrenal medulla, the inner portion, produces catecholamines. Because catecholamines play an important role in the autonomic nervous system, the adrenal medulla is considered a neuroendocrine structure.

I have an adrenal gland on my head. I like to refer to it as a beret — it makes me seem continental. The ladies dig it.

Zone in on the outer layer

The adrenal cortex is the large outer layer. It has three zones, or cell layers:
• zona glomerulosa, the outermost zone, which produces mineralocorticoids, primarily aldosterone
• zona fasciculata, the middle and largest zone, which produces the glucocorticoids cortisol (hydrocortisone), cortisone, and corticosterone as well as small amounts of the sex hormones androgen and estrogen
• zona reticularis, the innermost zone, which produces mainly glucocorticoids and some sex hormones.

Pancreas

The pancreas is nestled in the curve of the duodenum, stretching horizontally behind the stomach and extending to the spleen. The islets of Langerhans, which perform the endocrine function of this gland, contain alpha, beta, and delta cells. Alpha cells produce glucagon; beta cells, insulin; and delta cells, somatostatin.

Thymus

The thymus is located below the sternum and contains lymphatic tissue. Although this gland produces the hormones thymosin and thymopoietin, its major role seems related to the immune system; it produces T cells, which are important in cell-mediated immunity.

Pineal gland

The tiny pineal gland lies at the back of the third ventricle of the brain. It produces the hormone melatonin, which may play a role in the neuroendocrine reproductive axis as well as other widespread actions.

Gonads

The gonads include the ovaries (in females) and the testes (in males). The ovaries promote development and maintenance of the female sex characteristics, regulate the menstrual cycle, maintain the uterus for pregnancy and, along with other hormones, prepare the mammary glands for lactation. The testes produce spermatozoa and the male sex hormone testosterone. Testosterone stimulates and maintains male sex characteristics.

Testosterone stimulates and maintains male sex characteristics.

Yeah, but can it find the remote?

Hormones

Structurally, hormones can be classified into three types:

 amines

 polypeptides

 steroids.

Amenable amines

Amines are derived from tyrosine, an essential amino acid found in most proteins. They include the thyroid hormones (T_3 and T_4) and the catecholamines (epinephrine, norepinephrine, and dopamine).

Poly want a peptide?

Polypeptides are protein compounds made of many amino acids that are connected by peptide bonds. They include anterior pituitary hormones (GH, TSH, corticotropin, FSH, LH, interstitial-cell-stimulating hormone, and prolactin), posterior pituitary hormones (antidiuretic hormone [ADH] and oxytocin), PTH, and pancreatic hormones (insulin and glucagon).

Steroid secretions

Steroids, derived from cholesterol, include the adrenocortical hormones secreted by the adrenal cortex (aldosterone and cortisol) and the sex hormones (estrogen and progesterone in females and testosterone in males) secreted by the gonads.

Hormonal release and transport

Although all hormone release results from endocrine gland stimulation, their release patterns vary greatly. For example:
• corticotropin (secreted by the anterior pituitary) and cortisol (secreted by the adrenal cortex) are released in irregular spurts in response to body rhythm cycles, with levels peaking in the early morning.
• secretion of PTH (by the parathyroid gland) and prolactin (by the anterior pituitary) occurs fairly evenly throughout the day.
• secretion of insulin by the pancreas has both steady and sporadic release patterns.

Hormonal action

When a hormone reaches its target site, it binds to a specific receptor on the cell membrane or within the cell. Polypeptides and some amines bind to membrane receptor sites. The smaller,

When a hormone reaches its target site, it binds to a specific receptor on or in the cell.

more lipid-soluble steroids and thyroid hormones diffuse through the cell membrane and bind to intracellular receptors.

Right on target!

After binding occurs, each hormone produces unique physiologic changes, depending on its target site and its specific action at that site. A particular hormone may have different effects at different target sites.

Hormonal regulation

A complex feedback mechanism involving hormones, the central nervous system (CNS), and blood chemicals and metabolites helps maintain the body's delicate equilibrium by regulating hormone synthesis and secretion. Feedback refers to information sent to endocrine glands that signals the need for changes in hormone levels, either increasing or decreasing hormone production and release. (See *The feedback loop.*)

Assessment

To thoroughly assess the endocrine system, you must take an accurate health history and conduct a physical examination.

History

Because the endocrine system interacts with all other body systems, it's important to ask patients about their overall patterns of health and illness.

Current health status

Ask the patient to describe his chief complaint. Common complaints associated with endocrine disorders include fatigue, weakness, weight changes, mental status changes, polyuria, polydipsia, and abnormalities of sexual maturity and function.

Ask the question

Conduct a complete body systems review. Such questions may include:
• Have you noticed changes in your skin?
• Do you bruise more easily than you used to?
• Have you noticed a change in the amount or distribution of your body hair?
• Do your eyes burn or feel "gritty" when you close them?
• How good is your sense of smell?

Information about current and previous health, family history, and lifestyle provide clues you need for a thorough assessment.

The feedback loop

This diagram shows the negative feedback mechanism that helps regulate the endocrine system.

From simple...

Simple feedback occurs when the level of one substance regulates the secretion of hormones (simple loop). For example, a low serum calcium level stimulates the parathyroid gland to release parathyroid hormone (PTH). PTH, in turn, promotes resorption of calcium. A high serum calcium level inhibits PTH secretion.

...to complex

When the hypothalamus receives negative feedback from target glands, the mechanism is more complicated (complex loop). *Complex feedback* occurs through an axis established between the hypothalamus, pituitary gland, and target organ. For example, secretion of corticotropin-releasing hormone from the hypothalamus stimulates release of corticotropin by the pituitary, which in turn stimulates cortisol secretion by the adrenal gland (the target organ). A rise in serum cortisol levels inhibits corticotropin secretion by decreasing corticotropin-releasing hormone.

Simple feedback occurs when the level of one substance regulates the secretion of hormones.

Complex feedback occurs through an axis established between the hypothalamus, pituitary gland, and target organ.

Previous health status

Ask about the patient's medical history. You may identify insidious and vague symptoms of endocrine dysfunction by asking if the patient has had a skull fracture, surgery, complications of surgery, or brain infection, such as meningitis or encephalitis.

Family history

Ask about family history because certain endocrine disorders are inherited or have strong familial tendencies, such as diabetes mellitus, thyroid disease, and hypertension.

Lifestyle patterns

Ask the patient about temperature intolerance, which may indicate certain thryoid disorders. For example, intolerance to cold may indicate hypothyroidism, and intolerance to warmth, hyperthyroidism.

Physical examination

Your physical examination should include a total body evaluation and a complete neurologic assessment because the hypothalamus plays an important role in regulating endocrine function through the pituitary gland. Begin by measuring the patient's vital signs, height, and weight. Compare the findings with normal expected values and the patient's baseline measurements, if available. Then inspect, palpate, and auscultate the patient to obtain the most objective findings.

Inspection

Systematically inspect the patient's overall appearance and examine all areas of his body.

Appearances are revealing

Assess the patient's physical appearance and mental and emotional status. Note such factors as overall affect, speech, level of consciousness (LOC) and orientation, appropriateness and neatness of dress and grooming, and activity level. Evaluate general body development, including posture, body build, proportionality of body parts, and distribution of body fat.

What big nails you have

Assess the patient's overall skin color and inspect his skin and mucous membranes for lesions or areas of increased, decreased, or absent pigmentation. As you do so, be sure to consider racial and ethnic variations. In a dark-skinned patient, color variations are best assessed in the sclera, conjunctiva, mouth, nail beds, and palms. Next, assess the patient's skin texture and hydration.

Inspect the hair for amount, distribution, condition, and texture. Observe scalp and body hair for abnormal patterns of growth or hair loss. Again, remember to consider normal racial and ethnic—as well as gender—differences in hair growth and texture. Next, check the patient's fingernails for cracking, peeling, separation from the nail bed (onycholysis), or clubbing; observe the toenails for fungal infection, ingrown nails, discoloration, length, and thickness.

Remember to consider racial, ethnic, and gender differences in hair growth and texture. Boy, I guess I could use some conditioner.

Head for the head

Assess the patient's face for overall color and the presence of erythematous areas, especially in the cheeks. Note facial expression. Is it pained and anxious, dull and flat, or alert and interested? Note the shape and symmetry of his eyes and look for eyeball protrusion, incomplete eyelid closure, or periorbital edema. Have the patient extend his tongue, and inspect it for color, size, lesions, positioning, and tremors or unusual movements.

While standing in front of the patient, examine his neck—first with it held straight, then slightly extended, and finally while the patient swallows water. Check for neck symmetry and midline positioning and for symmetry of the trachea. Use tangential lighting directed downward from the patient's chin to help you see the thyroid gland. An enlarged thyroid may be diffuse and asymmetrical.

Test the chest

Evaluate the overall size, shape, and symmetry of the patient's chest, noting deformities. In females, assess the breasts for size, shape, symmetry, pigmentation (especially on the nipples and in skin creases), and nipple discharge (galactorrhea). In males, observe for bilateral or unilateral breast enlargement (gynecomastia) and nipple discharge.

Gentle check

Inspect the patient's external genitalia—particularly the testes and clitoris—for normal development.

Extreme inspection

Inspect the patient's extremities. Check the arms and hands for tremors. To do so, have the patient hold both arms outstretched in front with the palms down and fingers separated. Place a sheet of paper on the outstretched fingers and watch for trembling. Note any muscle wasting, especially in the upper arms, and have the patient grasp your hands to assess the strength and symmetry of his grip.

Next, inspect the legs for muscle development, symmetry, color, and hair distribution. Then assess muscle strength by having the patient sit on the edge of the examination table and extend his legs horizontally. A patient who can maintain this position for 2 minutes exhibits normal strength. Examine the feet for size, and note lesions, corns, calluses, or marks from socks or shoes. Inspect the toes and the spaces between them for maceration and fissures.

Have the patient grasp your hands to assess grip strength and symmetry.

Palpation

Palpate the thyroid gland and testes, the only endocrine glands accessible to palpation. You won't be able to palpate the thyroid gland in every patient. However, when you can examine the gland, it should be smooth, finely lobulated, nontender, and either soft or firm. You should be able to feel the gland's sections. (See *Palpating the thyroid.*)

A thyroid nodule feels like a knot, protuberance, or swelling; a firm, fixed nodule may be a tumor. Be careful not to confuse thick neck musculature with an enlarged thyroid or a goiter.

The testes should be firm to palpation and about ¾″ (2 cm) long before puberty. By age 16, the testes should be about 1¾″ (4.5 cm) long (normal range is 1⅜″ to 2⅛″ [3.5 to 5.5 cm]). Palpate the spermatic cord while the patient is standing.

Attempt to elicit Chvostek's sign and Trousseau's sign if you suspect a patient has hypocalcemia (low serum calcium levels) related to deficient or ineffective PTH secretion from hypoparathyroidism or surgical removal of the parathyroid glands. To elicit Chvostek's sign, tap the facial nerve in front of the ear with a finger; if the facial muscles contract toward the ear, the test is positive for hypocalcemia. To elicit Trousseau's sign, place a blood pressure cuff on the arm and inflate it above the patient's systolic pressure. In a positive test, the patient will exhibit carpal spasm (ventral contraction of the thumb and digits) within 3 minutes.

Auscultation

If you palpate an enlarged thyroid, auscultate the gland for systolic bruits, a sign of hyperthyroidism. Bruits occur when accelerated blood flow through the thyroid arteries produces vibrations. To auscultate for bruits, place the bell of the stethoscope over one of the lateral lobes of the thyroid and then listen carefully for a

Palpating the thyroid

To palpate the thyroid from the front, as shown, stand in front of the patient and place your index and middle fingers below the cricoid cartilage on both sides of the trachea. Palpate for the thyroid isthmus as he swallows. Then ask the patient to flex his neck toward the side being examined as you gently palpate each lobe. In most cases, you'll feel only the isthmus connecting the two lobes. However, if the patient has a thin neck, you may feel the whole gland. If he has a short, stocky neck, you may have trouble palpating even an enlarged thyroid.

Right lobe location
To locate the right lobe, use your right hand to displace the thyroid cartilage slightly to your left. Hook your left index and middle fingers around the sternocleidomastoid muscle to palpate for thyroid enlargement. Then examine the left lobe, using your left hand to displace the thyroid cartilage and your right hand to palpate the lobe.

Palpating the right lobe, from the front

Sternocleidomastoid muscles

Thyroid gland

Thyroid cartilage

Isthmus

Trachea

Auscultate for bruits by placing the stethoscope's bell over one of the thyroid's lateral lobes and listening for a low, soft, rushing sound.

low, soft, rushing sound. To ensure that tracheal sounds don't obscure bruits, have the patient hold his breath while you auscultate.

To distinguish a bruit from a venous hum, first listen for the rushing sound; then gently occlude the jugular vein with your fingers on the side you're auscultating and listen again. A venous hum (produced by jugular blood flow) disappears during venous compression; a bruit doesn't.

Diagnostic tests

Endocrine function is tested by direct, indirect, provocative, and radiographic studies.

Direct testing

The most common method, direct testing, measures hormone levels in the blood or urine. However, accurate measurement requires special techniques because the body contains only minute hormone amounts. (See *Methods of direct testing*.)

Methods of direct testing

Methods of direct testing used to measure hormone levels in the blood or urine are:
- immunoradiometric assays (IRMAs)
- radioimmunoassay (RIA)
- 24-hour urine testing.

Immunoradiometric assays
IRMAs are used to measure levels of peptide and protein hormones. These tests use a receptor antiserum labeled with radioiodine. Immunochemiluminometric assays (ICMAs) use a chemical reagent that emits a specific light wavelength when activated by a particular substance. IRMAs and ICMAs are more specific, stable, precise, and easier than RIAs. Tests called *radioreceptor assays* measure the activity of a hormone.

Radioimmunoassay
RIA, the technique used to determine many hormone levels, incubates blood or urine (or a urine extract) with the hormone's antibody and a radiolabeled hormone tracer (antigen). Antibody-tracer complexes are then measured. For example, charcoal absorbs and removes a hormone not bound to its antibody-antigen complex. Measuring the remaining radiolabeled complex indicates the extent to which the sample hormone blocks binding, compared with a standard curve showing reactions with known hormone quantities. Although the RIA method provides reliable results, it doesn't measure every hormone.

24-hour urine testing
A 24-hour urine test measures hormones and their metabolites. Metabolite measurement helps evaluate hormones excreted in virtually undetectable amounts. The patient's health care provider usually orders 24-hour urine tests to confirm adrenal, renal, and gonadal disorders.

Nursing considerations
For all types of direct testing, hormone measurement may include serum or urine collection. Tell the patient:
- that a venipuncture will be done to collect blood, when it will be done, and who will do it
- accurate testing may require several blood samples taken at different times of the day, because physiologic factors—such as stress, diet, episodic secretions, and body rhythms—can alter circulating hormone levels
- urine is collected for 24 hours with the appropriate collection device provided and that if a specimen is accidentally discarded, the collection must be restarted.

Indirect testing

Indirect testing measures the substance a particular hormone controls but not the hormone itself. For instance, glucose measurements help evaluate insulin, and calcium measurements help assess PTH activity. Although radioimmunoassays measure these substances directly, indirect testing is easier and less costly.

Glucose levels obtained indirectly will accurately reflect insulin's effectiveness, but various factors unrelated to an endocrine problem may affect calcium levels. For example, abnormal protein levels can lead to seemingly abnormal calcium levels because nearly one-half of calcium binds to plasma proteins. Therefore, rule out other possibilities before you assume that an abnormal calcium level reflects a PTH imbalance.

Rule out other possibilities before you assume that abnormal calcium levels reflect a PTH imbalance.

Provocative testing

Provocative testing helps determine an endocrine gland's reserve function when other tests show borderline hormone levels or can't quite pinpoint the abnormality's site. For instance, an abnormally low cortisol level may indicate adrenal hypofunction or indirectly reflect pituitary hypofunction.

Provocative testing works on this principle: Stimulate an underactive gland and suppress an overactive gland, depending on the patient's suspected disorder. A hormone level that doesn't increase with stimulation confirms primary hypofunction. Hormone secretion that continues after suppression confirms hyperfunction.

Radiographic studies

Radiographic studies are done with or after other tests. Computed tomography (CT) scans and magnetic resonance imaging (MRI) studies assess an endocrine gland by providing high-resolution, tomographic, three-dimensional images of the gland's structure, whereas nuclear imaging studies help determine the cause of hyperthyroidism.

Routine X-rays help evaluate how an endocrine dysfunction affects body tissues, although they don't reveal endocrine glands. For example, a bone X-ray, routinely ordered for a suspected parathyroid disorder, can show the effects of a calcium imbalance.

Provocative testing helps determine endocrine function when other tests can't pinpoint the abnormality's site.

Treatments

Here is practical information about treatments for patients with endocrine disorders. You'll play a crucial role in preparing these patients for treatment, monitoring them during and after treatment, and teaching various aspects of self-care.

Drug therapy

Commonly used drugs to treat endocrine disorders include:
• corticosteroids for inflammation and adrenal insufficiency
• antidiabetics to lower blood glucose levels for type 1 and type 2 diabetes mellitus and diabetic ketoacidosis
• glucagon for hypoglycemia
• drugs that affect calcium levels for Paget's disease and hypocalcemia
• pituitary hormones for some forms of diabetes insipidus and pituitary growth hormone deficiency
• thyroid hormone antagonists for hyperthyroidism
• thyroid hormone for hypothyroidism.

Nonsurgical treatments

Nonsurgical treatments for endocrine disorders include meal planning for diabetes and radioactive iodine (^{131}I) administration.

Diabetic meal planning

Diabetes specialists regard meal planning as the cornerstone of diabetes care because it directly controls the body's major glucose source. Your patient's food intake can be carefully controlled to prevent widely fluctuating blood glucose levels. If he's taking insulin or sulfonylureas, he'll have to adhere to his meal plan even more carefully to avoid hypoglycemia.

In balance

Your patient's nutritional requirements include a well-balanced diet containing all the necessary nutrients. However, to avoid wide blood glucose variations, he needs to closely regulate his protein, fat and, especially, carbohydrate intake. Currently, the American Dietetic Association and the American Diabetes Association recommend an individual nutritional assessment to determine appropriate medical nutrition therapy.

Your patient's nutritional requirements include a well-balanced diet containing all the necessary nutrients.

Carbohydrate and protein composition will vary, depending on therapeutic goals, and fat should be less than 30% of total calories. The relatively low fat content may help reduce the risk of cardiovascular disease.

Patient preparation

• Explain to the patient that he'll require a special meal plan to help control his blood glucose levels.
• Take a thorough dietary history, keeping in mind that difficulty with the diabetic meal plan may result from unnecessarily limiting the patient's food preferences and habits. Considering not only what he eats but also when he eats will help you and the patient to set up appropriate meal and snack times.
• Determine what your patient knows about diabetic meal planning. If using the exchange system, explain that he needs to keep track of all the foods he eats and categorize them according to food exchanges. Mention that no foods can be exempted — even so-called dietetic foods.

Lowdown on sweets

• Make sure you discuss concentrated sweets (foods high in simple sugars) with the patient. Old-fashioned diabetic diets forbid such foods as ice cream, cookies, candies, and pastries. Studies that categorize foods according to their glycemic index (the blood glucose level after ingestion) show that complete restriction may not be necessary. Baked potatoes, for instance, have a higher glycemic index than ice cream. Findings such as these challenge researchers to investigate diabetic meal plans more closely. However, encourage your patient not to abandon caution regarding concentrated sweets, particularly if weight loss is a goal. It may be prudent to avoid them unless his diabetes is well controlled.
• Arrange for a dietitian to teach your patient how to plan his meals. The dietitian may recommend the food exchange system. This method, based on the carbohydrate, fat, and protein content of six basic food groups, allows greater flexibility in meal planning. Exchange groups include milk products, vegetables, fruits, breads, meats, and fats.

Monitoring and aftercare

If your patient has newly diagnosed diabetes with extremely high blood glucose levels, he may require hospitalization while his blood glucose levels are monitored and insulin therapy is initiated. During his stay:
• Monitor him for signs of hypoglycemia, such as nervousness, diaphoresis, tremors, dizziness, fatigue, faintness and, possibly, seizures or coma.

• Also watch for signs of hyperglycemia, such as polyuria, poly-dipsia, and dehydration.
• Finally, be on guard for signs of ketoacidosis, such as a fruity breath odor, dehydration, weak and rapid pulse, and Kussmaul's respirations. Be sure to monitor urine ketones if his blood glucose levels are over 400 mg/dl.

Home care instructions
• Teach the patient how to adjust his meal plan when he engages in extra activity or exercise. If he eats many meals in restaurants, have the dietitian show him how to select a meal that fits his plan. If appropriate, tell him how to obtain nutrient composition lists from fast-food restaurants.
• For an overweight patient, implement weight-reduction measures as ordered, and explain the reduced-calorie meal plan. Suggest a support group, such as Weight Watchers and Overeaters Anonymous, if necessary.

^{131}I administration

A form of radiation therapy, the administration of ^{131}I treats hyperthyroidism, particularly Graves' disease, and is an adjunctive treatment of thyroid cancer. It shrinks functioning thyroid tissue, decreasing circulating thyroid hormone levels and destroying malignant cells. After oral ingestion, ^{131}I is rapidly absorbed and concentrated in the thyroid as if it were normal iodine, resulting in acute radiation thyroiditis and gradual thyroid atrophy. ^{131}I causes symptoms to subside after about 3 weeks and exerts its full effect only after 3 to 6 months.

Patient preparation
• Before ^{131}I administration, explain the procedure and check the patient's history for allergies to iodine.
• Unless contraindicated, instruct the patient to stop thyroid hormone antagonists 4 to 7 days before ^{131}I administration because these drugs reduce the sensitivity of thyroid cells to radiation.
• Tell the patient to fast overnight because food may delay ^{131}I absorption.
• Make sure the patient isn't taking lithium carbonate, which may interact with ^{131}I to cause hypothyroidism.
• Inform the patient that ^{131}I won't be administered if he develops severe vomiting or diarrhea because these conditions reduce absorption.

^{131}I doesn't exert its full effect until 3 to 6 months after therapy.

Monitoring and aftercare

After ^{131}I administration, the patient is usually discharged with appropriate instructions. However, he may stay in the hospital for monitoring if he received an unusually large dose or if treatment was for cancer. In such cases, observe radiation precautions for 3 days.

Home care instructions

Instruct the patient to:
- drink plenty of fluids for 48 hours to speed excretion of ^{131}I
- urinate into a lead-lined container for 48 hours
- use disposable eating utensils, and avoid close contact with young children and pregnant women for 7 days after therapy (If you're pregnant, arrange for another nurse to care for this patient.)
- dispose of urine, saliva, and vomitus properly because urine and saliva will be slightly radioactive for 24 hours and vomitus will be highly radioactive for 6 to 8 hours after therapy
- expect to see improvement in several weeks, although the maximum effects won't occur for up to 3 months
- report pain, swelling, fever, and other signs and symptoms that could result from radiation treatment because these signs and symptoms are easily treated when reported
- avoid conception for several months after therapy (if patient is a female of childbearing age).

Surgery

Surgical treatment of endocrine disorders includes adrenalectomy, hypophysectomy, pancreatectomy, parathyroidectomy, and thyroidectomy.

Adrenalectomy

Adrenalectomy — the resection or removal of one or both adrenal glands — is the treatment of choice for adrenal hyperfunction and hyperaldosteronism. It's also used to treat adrenal tumors, such as adenomas and pheochromocytomas, and has been used to aid treatment of breast and prostate cancer. The prognosis is good when adrenalectomy is used to treat adrenal adenomas. However, it's less favorable for adrenal carcinomas.

Patient preparation

- Expect to give oral or I.V. potassium supplements to correct low serum potassium levels. Monitor for muscle twitching and a positive Chvostek's sign (indications of alkalosis).

Adrenalectomy is the treatment of choice for adrenal hyperfunction and hyperaldosteronism.

- Keep the patient on a low-sodium, high-potassium diet as ordered to help correct hypernatremia.
- Give aldosterone antagonists as ordered for blood pressure control.
- Explain to the patient that surgery may cure his hypertension if it results from an adenoma.
- The patient with adrenal hyperfunction needs emotional support and a controlled environment to offset his emotional lability. If ordered, give a sedative to help him rest.
- Expect to administer medications to control his hypertension, edema, diabetes, and cardiovascular symptoms as well as his increased tendency to develop infections.
- As ordered, give glucocorticoids the morning of surgery to help prevent acute adrenal insufficiency during surgery.

Monitoring and aftercare

- Monitor vital signs carefully, observing for indications of shock from hemorrhage.
- Keep in mind that postoperative hypertension is common because handling the adrenal glands stimulates catecholamine release.
- Watch for weakness, nausea, and vomiting, which may signal hyponatremia.
- Use sterile technique when changing dressings to minimize the risk of infection.
- Administer analgesics for pain, and give replacement steroids as ordered.
- Remember, glucocorticoids from the adrenal cortex are essential to life and must be replaced to prevent adrenal crisis until the hypothalamic, pituitary, and adrenal axis resumes functioning.
- If the patient had primary hyperaldosteronism, he'll have had preoperative renin suppression with resulting postoperative hypoaldosteronism. Monitor his serum potassium levels carefully; he may develop hyperkalemia if he's receiving spironolactone, a potassium-sparing diuretic for control of postoperative hypertension. Fludrocortisone may be indicated.

Home care instructions

- Explain the importance of taking prescribed medications as directed. If the patient had a unilateral adrenalectomy, explain that he may be able to taper his medications in a few months, when his remaining gland resumes function and his pituitary resumes secreting corticotropin.
- Make sure the patient understands that sudden withdrawal of steroids can precipitate adrenal crisis and that he needs continued medical follow-up to adjust his steroid dosage appropriately during stress or illness.

Explain the importance of taking prescribed medications as directed.

Read the signs

• Describe the signs of adrenal insufficiency, and make sure the patient understands how this can progress to adrenal crisis if not treated. Explain that he should consult his doctor if he develops such adverse reactions as weight gain, acne, headaches, fatigue, and increased urinary frequency, which can indicate steroid overdose. Advise him to take his steroids with meals or antacids to minimize gastric irritation.

• If the patient had adrenal hyperfunction, explain that he'll see a reversal of the physical characteristics of his disease over the next few months. However, caution him that his improved physical appearance doesn't mean he can stop his medications.

• Advise the patient to wear medical identification jewelry to ensure adequate medical care in an emergency.

Hypophysectomy

Microsurgical techniques have dramatically reversed the high mortality previously associated with removal of pituitary and sella turcica tumors. Transsphenoidal hypophysectomy is now the treatment of choice for pituitary tumors, which can cause acromegaly, gigantism, and Cushing's disease. The surgery is also a palliative measure for patients with metastatic breast or prostate cancer to relieve pain and reduce the hormonal secretions that spur neoplastic growth.

Subfrontal or sphenoidal

Hypophysectomy may be performed subfrontally (approaching the sella turcica through the cranium) or transsphenoidally (entering from the inner aspect of the upper lip through the sphenoid sinus). (See *Transsphenoidal hypophysectomy,* page 516.) The subfrontal approach carries a high risk of mortality or complications, such as loss of smell and taste and permanent, severe diabetes insipidus. As a result, this approach is used only rarely — in cases where a tumor causes marked subfrontal or subtemporal extension and with optic chiasm involvement.

Patient preparation

• Tell the patient that he'll receive a general anesthetic and may go to the intensive care unit (ICU) postoperatively for up to 48 hours for careful monitoring.

• Mention that he'll have a nasal catheter and packing in place for at least 1 day after surgery as well as an indwelling urinary catheter.

• Arrange for appropriate tests and examinations as ordered. For example, if the patient has acromegaly, he'll need a thorough car-

Transsphenoidal hypophysectomy

When a pituitary tumor is confined to the sella turcica, the doctor performs transsphenoidal hypophysectomy. For the procedure, the patient is placed in a semirecumbent position and given a general anesthetic. The doctor incises the upper lip's inner aspect so that he can enter the sella turcica through the sphenoid sinus to remove the tumor.

Sphenoid sinus entry to sella turcica
Sella turcica
Anterior pituitary lobe
Pituitary gland
Posterior pituitary lobe
Sphenoid sinus

Many patients undergoing hypophysectomy receive I.V. hydrocortisone preoperatively and postoperatively.

diac evaluation because he may have incipient myocardial ischemia. If he has Cushing's disease, he'll need blood pressure and serum potassium level checks.

• Arrange visual field tests to serve as a baseline for all patients.
• Review the patient's preoperative medication regimen if appropriate. If he has hypothyroidism, he may need hormone replacement therapy (HRT). Many patients receive I.V. hydrocortisone preoperatively and postoperatively.

Monitoring and aftercare

• Keep the patient on bed rest for 24 hours after surgery and then encourage ambulation.
• Keep the head of his bed elevated to avoid placing tension or pressure on the suture line.
• Tell him not to sneeze, cough, blow his nose, or bend over for several days to avoid disturbing the suture line.
• Give mild analgesics, as ordered, for headache caused by cerebrospinal fluid loss during surgery or for paranasal pain. Paranasal pain typically subsides when the catheters and packing are removed — usually 24 to 72 hours after surgery.

- Anticipate that the patient may develop transient diabetes insipidus, usually 24 to 48 hours after surgery. Be alert for increased thirst and increased urine volume with a low specific gravity.
- If diabetes insipidus occurs, replace fluids and administer aqueous vasopressin, or give sublingual desmopressin acetate, as ordered. With these measures, diabetes insipidus usually resolves within 72 hours.
- Arrange for visual field testing as soon as possible because vision defects can indicate hemorrhage.
- Collect a serum sample to measure pituitary hormone levels and evaluate the need for hormone replacement.

Home care instructions

- Instruct the patient to report signs of diabetes insipidus immediately. Explain that he may need to limit fluid intake or take prescribed medications.
- Tell the patient with hyperprolactinemia that he'll need follow-up visits for several years because relapse is possible. Explain that he may be placed on bromocriptine (inhibits secretion of prolactin) if relapse occurs.
- Advise the patient not to brush his teeth for 2 weeks to avoid suture line disruption. Mention that he can use a mouthwash.
- He may need HRT as a result of decreased pituitary secretion of tropic hormones. If he needs cortisol or thyroid hormone replacement, teach him to recognize the signs of excessive or insufficient dosage.
- Advise him to wear medical identification jewelry.

Thyroidectomy

Thyroidectomy (removal of all or part of the thyroid gland) is performed to treat hyperthyroidism, respiratory obstruction from goiter, and thyroid cancer. Subtotal thyroidectomy, which reduces secretion of thyroid hormone, is used to correct hyperthyroidism when drug therapy fails or radiation therapy is contraindicated. It may also effectively treat diffuse goiter. After surgery, the remaining thyroid tissue usually supplies enough thyroid hormone for normal function, although hypothyroidism may occur later.

Patient preparation

- Explain to the patient that thyroidectomy will remove diseased thyroid tissue or, if necessary, the entire gland.
- Tell him that he'll have an incision in his neck and a drain and dressing in place after surgery and that he may experience some hoarseness and a sore throat from

After thyroidectomy, remaining thyroid tissue usually supplies enough thyroid hormone for normal function.

intubation and anesthesia. Reassure him that he'll receive analgesics to relieve his discomfort.
• Make sure that the patient has followed his preoperative drug regimen, which will render the gland euthyroid (having a normally functioning thyroid gland) to prevent thyrotoxicosis during surgery. He probably will have received either propylthiouracil or methimazole, usually starting 4 to 6 weeks before surgery.
• Expect him to receive iodine for 10 to 14 days before surgery to reduce the gland's vascularity and thus prevent excess bleeding. He may also take propranolol to reduce excess sympathetic effects. Notify the doctor immediately if the patient hasn't followed his medication regimen.
• If necessary, arrange for an electrocardiogram (ECG) to evaluate cardiac status.

Monitoring and aftercare
• Keep the patient in high semi-Fowler's position to promote venous return from the head and neck and to decrease oozing into the incision.
• Check for laryngeal nerve damage by asking the patient to speak as soon as he wakes from anesthesia.
• Watch for signs of respiratory distress. Tracheal collapse, mucus accumulation in the trachea, laryngeal edema, and vocal cord paralysis can all cause respiratory obstruction with sudden stridor and restlessness. Keep a tracheostomy tray at the patient's bedside for 24 hours after surgery and be prepared to assist with emergency tracheotomy if necessary.

Round-the-clock drainage
• Assess for signs of hemorrhage, which may cause shock, tracheal compression, and respiratory distress. Check the patient's dressing and palpate the back of his neck, where drainage tends to flow. Expect about 50 ml of drainage in the first 24 hours; if you find no drainage, check for drain kinking or the need to reestablish suction. Expect only scant drainage after 24 hours.
• As ordered, administer a mild analgesic to relieve a sore neck or throat. Reassure the patient that his discomfort should resolve within a few days.
• Assess for hypocalcemia, which may occur when bones depleted of calcium from hyperthyroidism begin to heal, rapidly taking up calcium from the blood, or if the parathyroid glands are injured or destroyed. Test for positive Chvostek's and Trousseau's signs, indicators of neuromuscular irritability from hypocalcemia. Keep calcium gluconate available for emergency I.V. administration.
• Be alert for signs of thyroid storm (a sudden and dangerous increase of the symptoms of thyrotoxicosis), a rare but serious com-

plication. In thyroid storm pulse and respirations rise to dangerous levels and temperature increases rapidly.

Home care instructions

• If the patient has had a subtotal or total thyroidectomy, or if the parathyroid glands are injured or destroyed, explain the importance of regularly taking his prescribed thyroid hormone replacement. Teach him to recognize and report signs of hypothyroidism and hyperthyroidism.

• If parathyroid damage occurred during surgery, explain to the patient that he may need to take calcium supplements. Teach him to recognize the warning signs of hypocalcemia.

• Tell the patient to keep the incision site clean and dry.

• Help the patient cope with concerns about appearance. Suggest loosely buttoned collars, high-necked blouses and shirts, jewelry, or scarves, which can hide the incision until it heals. The health care provider may recommend a mild body lotion to soften the healing scar and improve its appearance.

• Arrange follow-up appointments as necessary, and explain to the patient that the doctor needs to check the incision and serum thyroid hormone levels.

Be alert for signs of thyroid storm, a rare but serious complication.

Nursing diagnoses

When caring for patients with endocrine disorders, you'll typically use several nursing diagnoses. These nursing diagnoses appear below, along with appropriate nursing interventions and rationales.

Imbalanced nutrition: More than body requirements

Related to increased appetite, high calorie intake, inability to use nutrients, and inactivity, *Imbalanced nutrition: More than body requirements* is associated with many disorders, including Cushing's syndrome and diabetes mellitus.

Expected outcomes

• Patient expresses feelings about weight.
• Patient plans menus appropriate to prescribed diet.
• Patient adheres to prescribed diet.

Nursing interventions and rationales

• Obtain the patient's dietary history. Permanent weight change begins with examination of contributing factors. Provide the patient with a written copy of a calorie-based meal plan. Obtain dietary consultation as needed. Evaluate the patient's eating habits and include preferred foods in his meal plan.

• Provide support and encouragement as the patient attempts to change his calorie intake. Encouragement provides positive reinforcement and reduces frustration.

• Encourage activity and exercise based on the patient's physical ability and limitations. In addition to helping the patient lose weight, exercise reduces stress and helps curb stress-related eating.

• Refer the patient to community resources as needed and available.

Encourage activity and exercise based on the patient's physical ability and limitations.

Disturbed sleep pattern

Related to anxiety or hormone imbalance, *Disturbed sleep pattern* is associated with such disorders as hyperthyroidism, diabetes insipidus, and diabetes mellitus.

Expected outcomes

• Patient identifies factors that prevent or disrupt sleep.
• Patient sleeps ___ hours per night.
• Patient expresses a feeling of being well-rested.

Nursing interventions and rationales

• Promote usual sleep and rest practices. Decrease environmental stimuli. Provide a quiet, darkened, private room.
• Encourage frequent, short periods of ambulation.
• Administer antihormone medications as ordered and sedatives as needed.
• Instruct the patient and his family to eliminate caffeine-containing foods — such as coffee, tea, cola, and chocolate — from his diet.
• Provide and encourage quiet diversionary activities to promote rest and sleep.

Common endocrine disorders

Endocrine dysfunction takes one of two forms: hyperfunction, which results in excessive hormone production or response, or hypofunction, which results from a relative or absolute hormone deficiency. Hormonal imbalance can also be classified according to the disease site. Disease within an endocrine gland causes *primary dysfunction*. Disease caused by dysfunction outside a particular endocrine gland, but affecting that gland or its hormone or hormones, is termed *secondary dysfunction.*

Addison's disease

Addison's disease, the most common form of adrenal hypofunction, occurs when more than 90% of the adrenal gland is destroyed. With early diagnosis and adequate replacement therapy, the prognosis for adrenal hypofunction is good. Acute adrenal insufficiency, or adrenal crisis (addisonian crisis), is a medical emergency requiring immediate, vigorous treatment.

What causes it

In addition to autoimmune causes, which are the most common, Addison's disease can result from:
- tuberculosis
- bilateral adrenalectomy
- hemorrhage into the adrenal gland
- neoplasms
- fungal infections.
    Secondary adrenal hypofunction can be caused by:
- hypopituitarism
- abrupt withdrawal of long-term corticosteroid therapy
- removal of a nonendocrine, corticotropin-secreting tumor.

Autoimmune causes are the most common in Addison's disease.

Pathophysiology

In the autoimmune process of Addison's disease, circulating antibodies react specifically against the adrenal tissue, leading to decreased secretion of androgens, glucocorticoids, and mineralocorticoids. Adrenal hypofunction may also be caused by a disorder outside the gland, in which case aldosterone secretion commonly continues. In a patient with adrenal hypofunction, adrenal crisis occurs when the body's stores of glucocorticoids are exhausted by trauma, infection, surgery, or other physiologic stressors.

What to look for

When trying to determine the presence of Addison's disease, look for:
- weakness or fatigue
- anorexia and weight loss
- nausea and vomiting
- chronic constipation or diarrhea
- conspicuous bronze skin coloration, especially in hand creases and over the metacarpophalangeal joints, elbows, and knees

- darkening of scars and areas of vitiligo (absence of pigmentation)
- increased pigmentation of the mucous membranes, especially the buccal mucosa
- cardiovascular abnormalities, such as orthostatic hypotension, decreased heart size and cardiac output, and a weak, irregular pulse
- decreased tolerance for even minor stress
- poor coordination
- fasting hypoglycemia
- a craving for salty food
- amenorrhea.

The clinical effects of secondary adrenal hypofunction resemble those of Addison's disease but without hyperpigmentation, hypotension, and electrolyte abnormalities. Adrenal crisis is characterized by profound weakness and fatigue, shock, severe nausea and vomiting, hypotension, dehydration and, occasionally, high fever.

What tests tell you
- Adrenal hypofunction is confirmed if plasma cortisol and serum sodium levels are decreased and corticotropin, serum potassium, and blood urea nitrogen (BUN) levels are increased.
- Metyrapone and corticotropin stimulation tests are special provocative studies that determine whether adrenal hypofunction is primary or secondary.

How it's treated
- Corticosteroid replacement, usually with cortisone or hydrocortisone (both also have a mineralocorticoid effect), is the primary lifelong treatment for patients with primary or secondary adrenal hypofunction.
- Drug therapy may also include fludrocortisone, which acts as a mineralocorticoid to prevent dehydration and hypotension.
- Adrenal crisis requires prompt administration of dexamethasone, hydrocortisone, or both. Later doses of hydrocortisone are given I.V. until the patient's condition stabilizes. With proper treatment, the crisis usually subsides quickly, blood pressure stabilizes, and fluid and sodium levels return to normal. Subsequent oral maintenance doses of hydrocortisone preserve stability.

What to do
- In an adrenal crisis, monitor vital signs carefully for hypotension, volume depletion, and other signs of shock (decreased LOC

Hmmm. Decreased plasma cortisol and serum sodium and increased corticotropin, serum potassium, and BUN. I suspect adrenal hypofunction!

and urine output). Watch for hyperkalemia before treatment and for hypokalemia after treatment (from excessive mineralocorticoid effect).

• If the patient also has diabetes, check blood glucose levels periodically because steroid replacement may necessitate changing the insulin dosage. Carefully record weight and intake and output, because the patient may have volume depletion. Force fluids to replace excessive fluid loss until the onset of mineralocorticoid effects.

• Arrange for a diet that maintains sodium and potassium balance. If the patient is anorectic, suggest six small meals per day to increase calorie intake. Ask the dietitian to provide a diet high in protein and carbohydrates.

• Observe the patient receiving steroids for cushingoid signs such as fluid retention around the eyes and face. Watch for fluid and electrolyte imbalance, especially if the patient receives mineralocorticoids.

• Evaluate the patient. He should maintain a proper diet; maintain normal serum sodium, potassium, and plasma cortisol levels; understand the need to take his medication routinely; and make necessary adjustments in times of stress. (See *Addison's disease teaching tips*.)

Cushing's syndrome

Cushing's syndrome, a disorder of adrenal hyperfunction, results from excessive levels of adrenocortical hormones (particularly cortisol) or related corticosteroids and, to a lesser extent, androgens and aldosterone. Its unmistakable signs include adiposity of the face (moon face), neck, and trunk and purple striae on the skin, especially the abdomen. Cushing's syndrome is most common in females. Prognosis depends on the underlying cause; it's poor in untreated persons and in those with untreatable ectopic corticotropin-secreting carcinoma or metastatic adrenal carcinoma.

What causes it

Adrenal hyperfunction can be caused by:
• pituitary hypersecretion of corticotropin (Cushing's disease)
• corticotropin-secreting tumor in another organ (particularly bronchogenic or pancreatic carcinoma)
• administration of synthetic glucocorticoids
• adrenal tumor, which is usually benign in adults (less common cause).

Education edge

Addison's disease teaching tips

• Explain that lifelong cortisone replacement therapy is necessary.
• Advise the patient of symptoms of overdose and underdose, and that he'll need to increase the dosage during times of stress (when he has a cold, for example).
• Warn that infection, injury, or profuse sweating in hot weather may precipitate a crisis.
• Instruct the patient to always carry a medical identification card and wear a bracelet stating the name and dosage of the steroid he takes.
• Teach the patient how to give himself a hydrocortisone injection.
• Tell him to keep an emergency kit containing hydrocortisone in a prepared syringe for use in times of stress.
• Warn that he may need additional cortisone to prevent a crisis after any type of stress.

Pathophysiology

A loss of normal feedback inhibition by cortisol occurs in Cushing's syndrome. Elevated levels of cortisol don't suppress hypothalamic and anterior pituitary secretion of corticotropin-releasing hormone and corticotropin. The result is excessive levels of circulating cortisol.

What to look for

If your patient has some or all of these signs, he might have Cushing's syndrome:
- weight gain
- muscle weakness
- fatigue
- buffalo hump
- thinning extremities with muscle wasting and fat mobilization
- thin, fragile skin
- moon face and ruddy complexion
- hirsutism
- truncal obesity
- broad purple striae
- bruising
- impaired wound healing.

Buffalo hump is a sign of Cushing's syndrome — in humans, that is.

What tests tell you

- A low-dose (overnight) dexamethasone suppression test, elevated 24-hour urinary free cortisol levels, and high nighttime cortisol levels (indicating loss of circadian rhythm) confirm the diagnosis of Cushing's syndrome.
- A plasma corticotropin test and high-dose dexamethasone suppression test can determine the cause of Cushing's syndrome.
- With an adrenal tumor, corticotropin levels aren't detectable and steroid levels aren't suppressed. Ectopic corticotropin syndrome shows elevated corticotropin or unsuppressed steroid levels. Normal to elevated corticotropin with steroid suppressed to less than 50% of baseline indicates Cushing's disease.
- Ultrasonography, CT scan, or angiography localizes adrenal tumors.
- CT scan or MRI of the head helps localize pituitary tumors.

How it's treated

Radiation, drug therapy, or surgery may be necessary to restore hormone balance and reverse Cushing's syndrome. For example:
• Transsphenoidal resection of the corticotropin-secreting pituitary microadenoma is the therapy of choice for Cushing's disease.
• Adrenal tumor is treated by unilateral adrenalectomy with good prognosis, but the patient will require glucocorticoid therapy perioperatively and postoperatively.
• Nonendocrine corticotropin-secreting tumors require excision. Drug therapy with aminoglutethimide, etomidate, ketoconazole, metyrapone, mitotane, or trilostane decreases cortisol levels if symptoms persist or the tumor is inoperable.
• Aminoglutethimide, etomidate, and cyproheptadine decrease cortisol levels. Aminoglutethimide alone or in combination with metyrapone may also be useful in metastatic adrenal carcinoma.
• Before surgery, the patient with cushingoid signs and symptoms needs special management to control hypertension, edema, diabetes, and cardiovascular manifestations and to prevent infection. Glucocorticoid administration on the morning of surgery can help prevent acute adrenal insufficiency during surgery.

What to do

Patients with Cushing's syndrome require painstaking assessment and supportive care. Implement these measures:
• Frequently monitor vital signs, especially blood pressure. Carefully observe the hypertensive patient who also has cardiac disease.
• Check laboratory reports for hypernatremia, hypokalemia, hyperglycemia, and glycosuria.
• Because the cushingoid patient is likely to retain sodium and water, check for edema and carefully monitor daily weight, intake, and output. To minimize weight gain, edema, and hypertension, ask the dietitian to provide a diet high in protein and potassium but low in calories, carbohydrates, and sodium.
• Watch for infection—a significant problem in Cushing's syndrome.
• Carefully perform passive range-of-motion exercises for patients who have osteoporosis and are bedridden.
• Cushing's syndrome produces emotional lability. Record incidents that upset the patient, and try to prevent such situations if possible. Help him get the physical and mental rest he needs—by sedation if necessary. Offer emotional support throughout the difficult testing period.

Patients with Cushing's syndrome require painstaking assessment and supportive care.

526

• Evaluate the patient. After successful therapy, the patient will take his medication as prescribed, recognize signs of steroid underdose and overdose, and carry medical identification. His fluid, electrolyte, and plasma cortisol levels will be within normal limits and he'll seek counseling for stress as needed. (See *Cushing's syndrome teaching tips.*)

Diabetes insipidus

Diabetes insipidus results from a deficiency of circulating ADH, or vasopressin. It's an uncommon condition but occurs equally in men and women. The prognosis is good with uncomplicated diabetes insipidus and, with adequate water replacement, patients usually lead normal lives. The prognosis varies in cases complicated by an underlying disorder such as metastatic cancer.

What causes it

Diabetes insipidus may be familial, acquired, or idiopathic. It can be acquired as the result of intracranial neoplastic or metastatic lesions. Other causes may include:
• hypophysectomy or other neurosurgery
• head trauma, which damages the neurohypophyseal structures
• infection
• granulomatous disease
• vascular lesions
• autoimmune disorders.

Pathophysiology

Normally, ADH is synthesized in the hypothalamus and then stored by the posterior pituitary gland. When it's released into the general circulation, ADH increases the water permeability of the distal and collecting tubules of the kidneys, causing water reabsorption. If ADH is absent, the filtered water is excreted in the urine instead of being reabsorbed, and the patient excretes large quantities of dilute urine.

What to look for

The cardinal sign of diabetes insipidus is extreme polyuria — usually 4 to 16 L/day of dilute urine but sometimes as much as 30 L/day, with a low specific gravity (less than 1.005). Other symptoms include:
• polydipsia, particularly for cold, iced drinks
• nocturia
• fatigue (in severe cases)

Education edge

Cushing's syndrome teaching tips

• Advise the patient to take replacement steroids with antacids or meals to minimize gastric irritation. (It can help to take two-thirds of the dose in the morning and the remaining one-third in the late afternoon to mimic diurnal adrenal secretion.)
• Instruct him to use I.M. cortisol when he's ill and can't keep food down, and provide guidelines for when he should contact his doctor.
• Have the patient carry medical identification and have him immediately report physiologically stressful situations, which require increased dosage.
• Instruct him to recognize signs and symptoms of steroid underdose (fatigue, weakness, dizziness) and overdose (severe edema, weight gain).
• Warn him that discontinuing steroid dosage abruptly may produce a fatal adrenal crisis.

• dehydration, characterized by weight loss, poor tissue turgor, dry mucous membranes, constipation, muscle weakness, dizziness, tachycardia, and hypotension.

What tests tell you

• Urinalysis reveals almost colorless urine of low osmolality (less than 200 mOsm/kg) and low specific gravity (less than 1.005).
• A water deprivation test confirms the diagnosis by demonstrating renal inability to concentrate urine (evidence of ADH deficiency).
• Subcutaneous injection of 5 U of vasopressin produces decreased urine output with increased specific gravity if the patient has central diabetes insipidus.

How it's treated

Until the cause of diabetes insipidus can be identified and eliminated, administering various forms of vasopressin or a vasopressin stimulant controls fluid balance and prevents dehydration. Thiazide diuretics may be prescribed to reduce urine volume by creating mild salt depletion.

> Until the cause of diabetes insipidus can be identified, vasopressin or a vasopressin stimulant helps control fluid balance and prevent dehydration.

What to do

• Record fluid intake and output carefully. Maintain fluid intake to prevent severe dehydration.
• Watch for signs of hypovolemic shock, and monitor blood pressure and heart and respiratory rates regularly, especially during the water deprivation test.
• Check weight daily.
• Remember to keep the bed's side rails up and assist with walking if the patient is dizzy or has muscle weakness.
• Monitor urine specific gravity between doses. Watch for decreased specific gravity with increased urine output, indicating an inability to concentrate urine and the need for the next dose or a dosage increase.
• Add more bulk foods and fruit juices to the diet if constipation develops. If necessary, obtain an order for a mild laxative such as milk of magnesia.
• Provide meticulous skin and mouth care, and apply a lubricant to cracked or sore lips.
• Make sure caloric intake is adequate and the meal plan is low in sodium.
• Watch for decreased urine output and increased specific gravity between doses of medication.

• Monitor laboratory values for hyponatremia.
• Evaluate the patient. He should maintain an adequate fluid volume and electrolyte balance and resume his normal elimination pattern. If diabetes insipidus hasn't been eliminated, the patient should also know how to administer his medication correctly and how to record his intake and output; preferably he'll self-medicate while still an inpatient. He should wear medication identification jewelry and carry a wallet identification card, and schedule regular follow-up appointments. (See *Diabetes insipidus teaching tips.*)

Diabetes mellitus

Diabetes mellitus is characterized by disturbances in carbohydrate, protein, and fat metabolism. A leading cause of death in North America, diabetes is a major risk factor for myocardial infarction (MI), stroke, renal failure, and peripheral vascular disease. It's also the leading cause of blindness in adults.

Taking form

Two forms exist: type 1 and the more prevalent type 2 diabetes mellitus. Type 1 diabetes usually occurs before age 30 (although it may occur at any age); the patient is usually thin and will require exogenous insulin and dietary management to achieve control. Conversely, type 2 most commonly occurs in obese adults after age 40; it's usually treated with exercise, meal planning, and antidiabetic drugs. Treatment may include insulin therapy. An increasing number of adolescents and young people are being diagnosed with type 2 diabetes.

In hyperosmolar hyperglycemic nonketotic syndrome (HHNS), dehydration may cause hypovolemia and shock. Long-term diabetes may lead to retinopathy, nephropathy, atherosclerosis, and peripheral and autonomic neuropathy. Peripheral neuropathy usually affects the legs and may cause numbness.

What causes it

Type 1 is an autoimmune disease strongly associated with human leukocyte antigens DR 3 and 4. It may also be associated with certain viral infections.

Type 2 may result from:
• impaired insulin secretion
• peripheral insulin resistance
• increased basal hepatic glucose production.
Other associated factors include:
• obesity

Education edge

Diabetes insipidus teaching tips

• Teach the patient to monitor fluid intake and output and restrict sodium in his meal plan if he's taking a thiazide diuretic.
• Instruct him to administer desmopressin by nasal insufflation or by mouth. Advise the patient about possible adverse drug effects such as headaches. Tell him to report weight gain because it may mean the dosage is too high. Recurrence of polyuria, as reflected on the intake and output sheet, indicates that the dosage is too low.
• Advise the patient to wear medical identification jewelry and carry his medication with him at all times.
• Provide written instructions on how and when to use his medication and what signs and symptoms he should report to his doctor.

- insulin antagonists (such as excess counter-regulatory hormones and phenytoin)
- hormonal contraceptives
- pregnancy.

Pathophysiology

The effects of diabetes mellitus result from insulin deficiency or resistance to endogenous insulin. Normally, insulin allows glucose transport into the cells for use as energy or storage as glycogen. Insulin also stimulates protein synthesis and free fatty acid storage in adipose tissue. Insulin deficiency compromises the body tissues' access to essential nutrients for fuel and storage.

Insulin stimulates protein synthesis and free fatty acid storage in adipose tissue.

What to look for

Assess the patient for:
- fatigue
- polyuria related to hyperglycemia
- polydipsia
- nocturia
- dry mucous membranes
- poor skin turgor
- weight loss
- blurred vision
- polyphagia.

What tests tell you

- Two fasting plasma glucose tests above 126 mg/dl or, with normal fasting glucose, two blood glucose levels above 200 mg/dl during a 2-hour glucose tolerance test confirm the diagnosis.
- Ophthalmologic examination may show diabetic retinopathy.
- Other tests include plasma insulin level determination, urine testing for glucose and acetone, and glycosylated hemoglobin (hemoglobin A_{1C} [Hb A_{1C}]) determination.

How it's treated

Meal planning, exercise and, sometimes, insulin or oral antidiabetic agents are prescribed to normalize carbohydrate, fat, and protein metabolism and avert long-term complications while avoiding hypoglycemia.

All about food

All types of diabetes require strict adherence to carefully planned meals to meet nutritional needs, control blood glucose levels, and reach and maintain appropriate body weight. The American Diabetes Association recommends an individualized nutritional assessment and medical nutrition therapy to achieve therapeutic goals. It's helpful if the patient consistently follows the meal plan. In addition, aerobic exercise is generally prescribed at least three times per week for a minimum of 45 to 60 minutes. Patients are asked to exercise five or six times per week when weight loss is a therapeutic goal.

Absolute deficiency

Patients with type 1 diabetes must take insulin daily because of their absolute insulin deficiency. Patients with type 2 diabetes may require insulin to control blood glucose levels unresponsive to diet and oral antidiabetic agents, or during periods of acute stress. Patients with other types of diabetes commonly require daily insulin therapy to achieve blood glucose control. (See *Insulin therapy*.)

Insulin therapy

Administer insulin as prescribed, usually by subcutaneous (S.C.) injection with a standard insulin syringe. S.C. insulin can also be given with a penlike insulin injector device that uses a disposable needle and replaceable insulin cartridges, eliminating the need to draw insulin into a syringe. Jet-injection devices are expensive and require special cleaning procedures, but they disperse insulin more rapidly and speed absorption. These devices draw up insulin from standard containers (which allows the patient to mix insulins, if necessary, but requires a special procedure for drawing up) and deliver it into the subcutaneous tissue with a pressure jet.

Pump it up
Multiple-dose regimens may use an insulin pump to deliver insulin continuously into subcutaneous tissue. The infusion rate selector automatically releases about one-half of the total daily insulin requirement evenly over 24 hours. The patient releases the remainder in bolus amounts before meals and snacks.

Ready, set, rotate!
When administering insulin injections S.C., rotate the injection sites. Because absorption rates differ at each site, diabetic educators recommend rotating the injection site within a specific area such as the abdomen.

Only I.V. or I.M.
Regular insulin or insulin lispro may also be administered I.M. or I.V. during severe episodes of hyperglycemia. Never administer any other type of insulin by these routes.

Grand experiment
Two newer methods of insulin administration are the intranasal delivery method and the programmable implantable medication system (PIMS); both are still experimental. Intranasal administration uses aerosolized insulin combined with a surfactant; it's administered as a nasal spray. Because nasal solutions are less potent than S.C. insulin, dosages are higher.

Now undergoing clinical trials, the PIMS has an implantable infusion pump unit that holds and delivers the insulin and a delivery catheter that feeds insulin directly into the peritoneal cavity. The pump, encased in a titanium shell, contains a tiny computer to regulate dosages and runs on a battery with a 5-year life span. The patient uses a handheld external radio transmitter to control insulin release. Because the PIMS has no built-in blood glucose sensor, the patient must monitor his glucose levels several times per day.

Diet and exercise plus drugs

Patients with type 2 diabetes who can't achieve their target blood glucose levels with meal planning and exercise may require antidiabetic medications. Used in combination with one another or with insulin, these medications help patients with type 2 diabetes maintain normal glucose levels. Several types of medications are used to treat type 2 diabetes:
• Insulin secretagogues enhance pancreatic insulin secretion and include the sulfonylureas, acetohexamide, chlorpropamide, tolazamide, tolbutamide (first generation), and glyburide, glipizide, and glimepiride (second generation). In addition, repaglinide enhances insulin secretion but acts more quickly.
• Biguanides (metformin is the only one currently available) prevent inappropriate hepatic gluconeogenesis.
• Alpha-glucosidase inhibitors acarbose and miglitol delay the intestinal absorption of carbohydrates.
• Thiazolidinedione insulin sensitizers pioglitazone and rosiglitazone enhance the sensitivity of peripheral cells to insulin.

Patients with type 2 diabetes may need antidiabetic drugs in addition to meal planning and exercise.

What to do

• Emphasize that adherence to the treatment plan is essential. It's crucial to bring the patient's blood glucose level within an acceptable range (usually less than 120 mg/dl before a meal and 180 mg/dl between meals) and alleviate or prevent diabetic ketoacidosis (DKA) or hypoglycemia.
• For the patient with unstable diabetes who isn't experiencing DKA or HHNS, monitor blood glucose levels several times per day as prescribed until they stabilize.
• Administer insulin as prescribed and keep the doctor informed until blood glucose levels are under control. Then expect to begin the patient on an insulin regimen.
• If the patient has type 2 diabetes, he may need an oral antidiabetic or a trial period with diet therapy.

Dinner is at 6 sharp

• Make sure meals are on time for patients receiving insulin or an insulin secretagogue.
• Monitor the patient closely for signs and symptoms of DKA or HHNS as well as for hypoglycemia (caused by too rapid reduction in blood glucose level). Suspect DKA or HHNS if your patient begins to exhibit Kussmaul's respirations, develops a fruity odor to his breath, and shows signs and symptoms of severe dehydration. If these indications are evident, immediately notify the doctor.
• If the patient has DKA or HHNS, treatment may include fluid and electrolyte replacement, increased insulin therapy, and thera-

py to reduce acidosis. Administer doses of I.V. insulin as prescribed. Monitor the patient's blood glucose levels frequently during insulin infusion. Alert the doctor when the glucose level reaches 250 to 300 mg/dl, so the insulin dosage can be decreased to prevent hypoglycemia. Typically, insulin decreases blood glucose levels by about 75 to 100 mg/dl each hour. Patients with HHNS have a greater insulin sensitivity than patients with DKA, so expect to give less insulin.

• After the crisis, expect to resume the patient's usual insulin regimen. Infuse I.V. fluids rapidly at the prescribed rate. Hypotonic or isotonic saline solution will be administered, depending on the patient's condition. When the glucose level is slightly above normal, the doctor may switch to a glucose solution to prevent hypoglycemia and reduce the risk of cerebral edema.

Preserving potassium

• Monitor an elderly patient closely for evidence of fluid overload. Monitor the patient's electrolyte levels closely and administer potassium replacement therapy as ordered. Patients with an extremely low pH level may require bicarbonate therapy to treat acidosis, but fluid and insulin replacement alone usually correct metabolic acidosis.

• The meal plan is the cornerstone of diabetes care because it directly controls the body's major glucose source. Your patient can prevent widely fluctuating blood glucose levels by controlling his food intake. If he takes insulin or sulfonylureas, he'll need to adhere to his meal plan even more carefully to avoid hypoglycemia.

• Monitor the patient for complications related to insulin therapy, which include hypoglycemia, the dawn phenomenon (early morning rise in blood glucose), insulin lipodystrophy (usually caused by continually using the same injection site), insulin allergy, and insulin resistance.

• Administer oral antidiabetics as prescribed. Check the patient's history for conditions, such as pregnancy, breast-feeding, stressful situations or illnesses that increase insulin requirements, and known allergies to sulfa agents. Monitor the patient for adverse reactions.

Catching ketone

• If necessary, check your patient's urine for ketones. Urine testing is sometimes used to monitor blood glucose control, but it's rapidly being replaced with blood glucose monitoring. Despite their convenience, urine tests don't always reflect blood glucose levels accurately. However, only urine testing can detect ketone bodies—particularly important for ketosis-prone patients with type 1 diabetes.

The meal plan is the cornerstone of diabetes care.

• Demonstrate to the patient how to check his blood glucose. Because blood glucose changes may cause misleading signs and symptoms — or none at all — the patient with diabetes must measure his glucose level often. Capillary blood glucose monitoring allows the patient (and the nurse) to determine metabolic status quickly, receive feedback on problems with the diet or medication regimen, and make immediate adjustments. It's especially useful for the patient on a tightly controlled regimen. Recent research shows that good glycemic control, Hb A_{1C} level less than 7%, reduces the risk of long-term complications from diabetes.

• Blood glucose monitoring equipment varies greatly, so it's important to carefully follow the manufacturer's instructions. The health care provider may order blood glucose testing before meals, after meals, and at bedtime, or less frequently for a patient who has established stable control.

• Monitor the patient's Hb A_{1C} as ordered to assess long-term diabetes control. The amount of glycosylation directly correlates with blood glucose levels. Ideally, the patient's Hb A_{1C} should measure no more than $1\frac{1}{2}$ times the normal level, which ranges from 3% to 6%. A high Hb A_{1C} value with any blood glucose level suggests hyperglycemia over several weeks; a low value coupled with a high blood glucose level suggests recent onset of hyperglycemia.

Vital records

• Keep accurate records of vital signs, weight, fluid intake, urine output, and caloric intake in addition to monitoring serum glucose and urine ketone levels.

• Monitor the patient closely for signs and symptoms of hyperglycemia and hypoglycemia. If a hypoglycemic reaction occurs, obtain a blood glucose level and immediately give carbohydrates in the form of fruit juice, hard candy, or honey. Give glucagon or I.V. dextrose if the patient is unconscious. Notify the doctor of a significant change in the patient's blood glucose levels.

• Provide meticulous skin care, especially to the feet and legs, to avert problems associated with peripheral vascular disease and neuropathy. Even a tiny skin break can produce complications that lead to amputation. Avoid constricting hose, slippers, or bed linens. Refer the patient to a podiatrist if indicated.

• Evaluate the patient. He should have normal blood glucose levels, maintain an adequate nutritional intake, understand his drug regimen, monitor himself for complications of the disease, and obtain medical identification jewelry and a wallet identification card. (See *Diabetes mellitus teaching tips*.)

Education edge

Diabetes mellitus teaching tips

• Review the prescribed meal plan, and teach the patient how to adjust his diet when engaged in extra activity. Teach him how to select restaurant meals and how to obtain nutrient composition lists from fast-food restaurants.

• Advise the patient about aerobic exercise programs. Explain how exercise affects blood glucose levels, and provide safety guidelines.

• Instruct the patient on insulin administration, if prescribed, including type, peak times, dosage, drawing up the insulin, mixing (if applicable), administration technique, and site rotation.

• Instruct the patient on oral antidiabetic therapy, if prescribed.

• Tell the patient about the Internet as a source of information and about the American Diabetes Association Web site, *www.diabetes.org*.

Hyperparathyroidism

Hyperparathyroidism is characterized by excess activity of one or more of the four parathyroid glands, resulting in excessive secretion of PTH. Such hypersecretion of PTH promotes bone resorption and leads to hypercalcemia and hypophosphatemia. Increased renal and GI absorption of calcium also occurs.

What causes it

Primary hyperparathyroidism may result from a single adenoma, a genetic disorder, or multiple endocrine neoplasias. Secondary hyperparathyroidism may be caused by rickets, vitamin D deficiency, chronic renal failure, or phenytoin or laxative abuse.

Pathophysiology

Hyperparathyroidism may be primary or secondary. In primary hyperparathyroidism, one or more of the parathyroid glands enlarge, leading to increased PTH secretion and elevated serum calcium levels.

A close second

In secondary hyperparathyroidism, a hypocalcemia-producing abnormality outside the parathyroid gland doesn't respond to the metabolic action of PTH, leading to excessive compensatory production of PTH.

What to look for

Hyperparathyroidism may produce symptoms. Secondary hyperparathyroidism may produce the same clinical features as primary hyperparathyroidism, with possible skeletal deformities of the long bones (for example, rickets) as well as other symptoms of the underlying disease. Symptoms include:
• *CNS*—psychomotor and personality disturbances, loss of memory for recent events, depression, overt psychosis, stupor and, possibly, coma
• *GI*—anorexia, nausea, vomiting, dyspepsia, and constipation
• *neuromuscular*—fatigue; marked muscle weakness and atrophy, particularly in the legs
• *renal*—symptoms of recurring nephrolithiasis, which may lead to renal insufficiency
• *skeletal and articular*—chronic lower back pain and easy fracturing from bone degeneration, bone tenderness, and joint pain
• *other*—skin pruritus, vision impairment from cataracts, and subcutaneous calcification.

What tests tell you

• Immunoradiometric assay reveals elevated serum PTH levels. Along with increased serum calcium and decreased phosphorus levels, these findings confirm the diagnosis of hyperparathyroidism.
• X-rays may show diffuse demineralization of bones, bone cysts, outer cortical bone resorption, and subperiosteal erosion of the radial aspect of the middle fingers.
• Laboratory tests reveal elevated urine and serum calcium, chloride, and alkaline phosphatase levels and decreased serum phosphorus levels.
• Secondary hyperparathyroidism is confirmed when serum calcium levels are normal or slightly decreased, with variable serum phosphorus and bicarbonate levels.

How it's treated

Treatment varies, depending on the cause of the disease. Surgery to remove the adenoma or all but one-half of one gland (the remaining part of the gland is needed to maintain normal PTH levels) is commonly the treatment of choice. Although surgery can relieve bone pain within 3 days, the patient's renal damage may be irreversible.

Less invasive treatments are used to decrease calcium levels preoperatively or when surgery isn't an option. These include:
• forcing fluids
• limiting dietary calcium intake
• promoting sodium and calcium excretion through forced diuresis
• using normal saline solution (up to 6 L in life-threatening situations)
• furosemide, or ethacrynic acid
• administering oral sodium or potassium phosphate, calcitonin, or plicamycin.

Get down to it

Treatment for secondary hyperparathyroidism must correct the underlying cause of parathyroid hypertrophy. It includes vitamin D therapy or aluminum hydroxide for hyperphosphatemia in the patient with renal disease. In the patient with chronic secondary hyperparathyroidism, the enlarged glands may not revert to normal size and function even after calcium levels have been controlled; if so, they should be surgically removed.

What to do

Nursing care aims to prevent complications from the underlying disease and its treatment. Implement these measures:

- Record intake and output as the patient receives hydration to reduce serum calcium levels.
- Strain urine to check for calculi.
- Monitor sodium, potassium, and magnesium levels frequently.
- Auscultate for breath sounds often, and be alert for pulmonary edema in the patient receiving large amounts of I.V. saline solution—especially in the presence of pulmonary or cardiac disease.
- Take precautions to avoid falls because the patient is predisposed to pathologic fractures.
- Evaluate the patient. He should understand the need for regular serum calcium level studies, the signs and symptoms of hypercalcemia and hypocalcemia and what are reportable ones, the reasons for drug therapy and adequate hydration, and possible adverse drug effects. (See *Hyperparathyroidism teaching tips*.)

Hypoparathyroidism

Hypoparathyroidism stems from a deficiency of PTH. Because PTH primarily regulates calcium balance, hypoparathyroidism leads to hypocalcemia and produces neuromuscular symptoms ranging from paresthesia to tetany. The clinical effects are usually correctable with replacement therapy. However, some complications of this disorder, such as cataracts and basal ganglion calcifications, are irreversible.

What causes it

The three major causes of hypoparathyroidism are:
- congenital absence or malfunction of the parathyroid glands
- autoimmune destruction
- removal of or injury to one or more parathyroid glands during neck surgery.

Other causes include:
- ischemic infarction of the parathyroids during surgery or from disease, such as amyloidosis or neoplasms
- suppression of normal gland function caused by hypercalcemia (reversible)
- hypomagnesemia-induced impairment of hormone secretion (reversible)
- massive thyroid radiation therapy (rare).

Pathophysiology

PTH usually maintains serum calcium levels by increasing bone resorption and by stimulating renal conversion of vitamin D to its active form, which enhances GI absorption of calcium and bone

Education edge

Hyperparathyroidism teaching tips

- Teach the patient about the possible adverse effects of drug therapy.
- Emphasize the need for periodic follow-up through laboratory blood tests.
- If hyperparathyroidism isn't corrected surgically, warn the patient to avoid prolonged periods of immobilization, to maintain adequate hydration, and to avoid calcium-containing antacids and thiazide diuretics.
- Also instruct the patient to contact his doctor if he experiences significant diarrhea or vomiting.

resorption. PTH also maintains the inverse relationship between serum calcium and phosphate levels by inhibiting phosphate reabsorption in the renal tubules and enhancing calcium reabsorption. Abnormal PTH production in hypoparathyroidism disrupts this delicate balance.

What to look for

Hypoparathyroidism may not produce symptoms in mild cases. Otherwise, signs and symptoms include:
- neuromuscular irritability
- increased deep tendon reflexes
- positive Chvostek's and Trousseau's signs
- dysphagia
- paresthesia
- psychosis.

Other indications include tetany; seizures; arrhythmias; cataracts; abdominal pain; dry, lusterless hair; spontaneous hair loss; brittle fingernails that develop ridges or fall out; possibly dry, scaly skin; and weakened tooth enamel that may cause teeth to stain, crack, and decay easily.

What tests tell you

- Test results that confirm hypoparathyroidism include decreased PTH and serum calcium levels and elevated serum phosphorus levels.
- X-rays reveal increased bone density.
- ECG shows prolonged QT intervals and QRS-complex and ST-segment changes that are caused by hypocalcemia and may be mistaken for acute MI or conduction abnormalities.

X-rays reveal increased bone density in the patient with hypoparathyroidism.

How it's treated

Therapy includes vitamin D, usually with supplemental calcium. Such therapy is usually lifelong, except for patients with the reversible form of the disease. Types of vitamin D given include dihydrotachysterol if renal function is adequate and calcitriol if renal function is severely compromised.

Acute angle

Acute life-threatening tetany calls for immediate I.V. administration of calcium to raise serum calcium levels. Sedatives and anticonvulsants are given to control spasms until calcium levels rise. Chronic tetany calls for vitamin D and possibly oral calcium supplements to maintain normal serum calcium levels.

What to do

- While awaiting diagnosis of hypoparathyroidism in a patient with a history of tetany, maintain a patent I.V. line and keep 10% calcium gluconate solution available.
- Institute seizure precautions because the patient is at risk for seizures.
- Keep a tracheostomy tray and an endotracheal tube at the bedside because laryngospasm may result from hypocalcemia.
- Monitor for Chvostek's and Trousseau's signs.
- For the patient with tetany, prepare to administer 10% calcium gluconate by slow I.V. infusion and maintain a patent airway. Prepare the patient for transport to the ICU per facility policy as the patient may also require intubation and sedation with I.V. diazepam. Monitor vital signs often especially if I.V. diazepam was given to make sure blood pressure and heart rate return to normal.
- When caring for the patient with hypoparathyroidism, stay alert for minor muscle twitching (especially in the hands) and for signs of laryngospasm (respiratory stridor or dysphagia). These effects may signal the onset of tetany.
- Because the patient with chronic disease has prolonged QT intervals on an ECG, watch for heart block and signs of decreased cardiac output. Closely monitor the patient who receives digoxin and calcium because calcium potentiates the effect of digoxin. Watch for signs and symptoms of digoxin toxicity (arrhythmias, nausea, fatigue, changes in vision).
- Evaluate the patient. He shouldn't develop tetany, and his serum calcium levels should be normal. The patient should understand the symptoms of hypocalcemia and hypercalcemia and state reportable ones; identify high-calcium, low-phosphorus foods; and understand the importance of good nail grooming and the need for emollient creams to soften the skin. (See *Hypoparathyroidism teaching tips.*)

Education edge

Hypoparathyroidism teaching tips

- Instruct the patient with scaly skin to use creams to soften his skin.
- Tell him to keep his nails trimmed to prevent them from splitting.
- Advise him to follow a high-calcium, low-phosphorus diet, and tell him which foods are permitted.
- If he's on drug therapy, emphasize the importance of checking serum calcium levels at least three times per year. Instruct him to watch for signs of hypercalcemia and to keep medications away from light.

Hyperthyroidism

Hyperthyroidism is a metabolic imbalance that results from excessive thyroid hormone. The most common form of hyperthyroidism is Graves' disease (thyrotoxicosis), which increases T_4 production, enlarges the thyroid gland (goiter), and causes multisystem changes. With treatment, most patients can lead normal lives. However, thyroid storm — an acute exacerbation of hyperthyroidism — is a medical emergency that may lead to heart failure. (See *Understanding forms of hyperthyroidism.*)

Understanding forms of hyperthyroidism

In addition to Graves' disease, hyperthyroidism occurs in several other forms, including:

• *Toxic multinodular goiter*—a small, benign nodule in the thyroid gland that secretes thyroid hormone—is the second most common cause of hyperthyroidism. The cause of this type of goiter is unknown; incidence is highest among elderly patients. Clinical effects are essentially similar to those of Graves' disease, but they're milder and may have cardiovascular predominance. This condition doesn't induce ophthalmopathy, pretibial myxedema, or acropachy. Toxic multinodular goiter is confirmed by radioactive iodine (^{131}I) uptake and thyroid scan, which shows at least one hyperfunctioning nodule that may suppress the rest of the gland. Treatment includes ^{131}I therapy or surgery to remove the goiter after antithyroid drugs achieve a euthyroid state.

• *Thyrotoxicosis factitia* results from chronic ingestion of thyroid hormone for thyrotropin suppression in patients with thyroid carcinoma, or from thyroid hormone abuse by persons who are trying to lose weight.

• *Functioning metastatic thyroid carcinoma* is a rare disease that causes excess production of thyroid hormone.

• *Thyroid-stimulating hormone-secreting pituitary tumor* causes overproduction of thyroid hormone.

• *Subacute thyroiditis* is a virus-induced granulomatous inflammation of the thyroid, producing transient hyperthyroidism associated with fever, pain, pharyngitis, and tenderness in the thyroid gland.

• *Silent thyroiditis* is a self-limiting, transient form of hyperthyroidism with histologic thyroiditis but no inflammatory symptoms.

What causes it

Graves' disease is an autoimmune disease and is usually familial. Thyroid receptor antibodies occur in most patients with this disorder.

Pathophysiology

In Graves' disease, thyroid-stimulating antibodies bind to and stimulate the TSH receptors of the thyroid gland. The trigger for this autoimmune response is unclear. Graves' disease is also associated with the production of several autoantibodies formed because of a defect in suppressor T-lymphocyte function.

What to look for

Classic signs and symptoms of Graves' disease include:
• diffusely enlarged thyroid
• nervousness
• heat intolerance
• weight loss despite increased appetite
• sweating
• diarrhea
• tremor
• palpitations
• possibly exophthalmos.

Weathering the storm

In thyroid storm, these signs and symptoms can be accompanied by extreme irritability, hypertension, tachycardia, vomiting, temperature up to 106° F (41.1° C), delirium, and coma. Other signs and symptoms include:

• *cardiovascular system* — tachycardia; full, bounding pulse; wide pulse pressure; cardiomegaly; increased cardiac output and blood volume; a visible point of maximal impulse; paroxysmal supraventricular tachycardia and atrial fibrillation (found especially in elderly patients); occasionally, a systolic murmur at the left sternal border

• *CNS* — difficulty concentrating, excitability or nervousness, fine tremor, shaky handwriting, clumsiness, and mood swings ranging from occasional outbursts to overt psychosis

• *eyes* — exophthalmos; occasional inflammation of conjunctivae, corneas, or eye muscles; diplopia; increased tearing; lid lag; lid retraction

• *GI* — increased appetite but occasional anorexia, especially in elderly patients; increased defecation; soft stools or, with severe disease, diarrhea; liver enlargement

• *musculoskeletal system* — weakness, fatigue, and proximal muscle atrophy; periodic paralysis, especially in Asian and Latino males; occasional acropachy (soft-tissue swelling), accompanied by underlying bone changes where new bone formation occurs

• *reproductive system* — in females, oligomenorrhea or amenorrhea, decreased fertility, higher incidence of spontaneous abortions; in males, gynecomastia

• *respiratory system* — dyspnea on exertion and, possibly, at rest

• *skin, hair, and nails* — smooth, warm, flushed paper thin skin; pretibial myxedema (dermopathy), producing thickened skin, accentuated hair follicles, and raised red patches of skin that are itchy and sometimes painful, with occasional nodule formation; fine, soft hair; premature graying and increased hair loss in both sexes; friable nails and Plummer's nails (distal nail separated from the bed).

What tests tell you

• Radioimmunoassay test shows elevated T_4 levels.
• Thyroid scan reveals increased ^{131}I uptake. Immunometric assay shows suppressed sensitive TSH levels.
• Orbital sonography and CT scan show subclinical ophthalmopathy.

How it's treated

The primary forms of treatment of hyperthyroidism are antithyroid drugs, ^{131}I, beta-adrenergic blockers, sedation, and surgery. Appropriate treatment depends on the size of the

Primary treatment of hyperthyroidism includes drugs and surgery.

goiter, the causes, the patient's age and parity, and how long surgery (if planned) will be delayed. Treatment includes:

• Antithyroid drug therapy with propylthiouracil (PTU) and methimazole blocks thyroid hormone synthesis. It's used for pregnant women and patients who refuse surgery or ^{131}I treatment.

PTU for pregnancy

• During pregnancy, PTU is the preferred therapy. Limit antithyroid medication to the minimum dosage required to keep maternal thyroid function testing at high-normal or slightly elevated levels. About 1% of the infants born to mothers receiving antithyroid medication will be hypothyroid.

• Another major form of therapy for hyperthyroidism is a single oral dose of [131]I. After ablative treatment with ^{131}I or surgery, patients require regular, frequent medical supervision for the rest of their lives. They usually develop hypothyroidism, sometimes several years after treatment.

• Partial thyroidectomy is indicated for the patient with a very large goiter, whose hyperthyroidism has repeatedly relapsed after drug therapy. Subtotal thyroidectomy removes part of the thyroid gland, decreasing its size and capacity for hormone production and storage.

• Before surgery, the patient may receive iodides (Lugol's solution or saturated solution of potassium iodide), antithyroid drugs, or high doses of propranolol, a beta-adrenergic blocker, to help prevent thyroid storm (uncontrolled hyperthyroidism caused by release of increased amounts of thyroid hormones into the bloodstream). If euthyroidism isn't achieved, surgery is delayed and propranolol is administered to decrease systemic effects (such as cardiac arrhythmias) caused by hyperthyroidism.

Steroid injections

• Therapy for hyperthyroid ophthalmopathy includes local applications of topical medications but may also require high doses of corticosteroids given systemically or, in severe cases, injected into the retrobulbar area.

• A patient with severe exophthalmos that causes pressure on the optic nerve may require surgical decompression to lessen pressure on the orbital contents.

• Treatment for thyroid storm includes an antithyroid drug such as PTU; I.V. propranolol to block sympathetic effects; a corticosteroid to replace depleted cortisol levels; and an iodide to block release of thyroid hormone. Supportive measures include nutrients, vitamins, fluid administration, and sedation, as necessary.

• If iodine is part of the treatment, mix it with water or juice to prevent GI distress, and administer it through a straw to prevent tooth discoloration.

What to do

Patients with hyperthyroidism require vigilant care to prevent acute exacerbations and complications. Implement these measures:

• Record vital signs and weight.
• Monitor serum electrolyte levels, and check periodically for hyperglycemia and glycosuria.
• Carefully monitor cardiac function.
• Check LOC and urine output.
• If the patient is in her first trimester of pregnancy, report signs of spontaneous abortion (spotting and occasional mild cramps) to the doctor immediately.
• Remember, extreme nervousness may produce bizarre behavior. Reassure the patient and his family that such behavior subsides with treatment. Provide sedatives as necessary.
• To promote weight gain, provide a high-protein, high-calorie diet, with six meals per day and vitamin supplements. Suggest a low-sodium diet for the patient with edema.

Storm watch

• Watch for signs of thyroid storm. Check intake and output carefully to ensure adequate hydration and fluid balance. Closely monitor blood pressure, cardiac rate and rhythm, and body temperature. If the patient has a high fever, reduce it with appropriate hypothermic measures (sponging, hypothermia blankets, and acetaminophen); avoid aspirin because it raises T_4 levels. Maintain an I.V. line and give drugs, as ordered.
• Thyroidectomy requires meticulous postoperative care to prevent complications.
• Evaluate the patient. He should maintain adequate fluid volume and electrolyte balance, normal cardiac function, normal body temperature, and weight (preferably, he'll gain weight); his eyes should be as comfortable as possible and be free from corneal damage; thyroid storm should be prevented. He will understand the need for regular medical follow-up and will schedule return appointments. If he takes an antithyroid drug or is on ^{131}I therapy, he'll know which signs and symptoms to report to his doctor and will have a sheet that lists them. (See *Hyperthyroidism teaching tips*.)

Hypothyroidism

A state of low serum thyroid hormone levels or cellular resistance to thyroid hormone, hypothyroidism results from hypothalamic, pituitary, or thyroid insufficiency. Hypothyroidism is most prevalent in women and can progress to life-threatening myxedema

Hyperthyroidism teaching tips

• If the patient has exophthalmos or another ophthalmopathy, suggest sunglasses or eye patches to protect his eyes from light. Moisten the conjunctivae often with artificial tears. Warn the patient with severe lid retraction to avoid sudden physical movements that might cause the lid to slip behind the eyeball. Elevate the head of the bed to reduce periorbital edema.
• Stress the importance of regular medical follow-up after discharge because hypothyroidism may develop from 2 to 4 weeks postoperatively. Drug therapy and ^{131}I therapy require careful monitoring and comprehensive patient teaching.
• If the patient is pregnant, tell her to watch closely during the 1st trimester for signs of spontaneous abortion (spotting, occasional mild cramps) and to report such signs to the doctor immediately.

coma—usually precipitated by infection, exposure to cold, or sedatives.

What causes it

Hypothyroidism in adults may result from:
- thyroidectomy
- radiation therapy
- chronic autoimmune thyroiditis (Hashimoto's disease)
- inflammatory conditions, such as amyloidosis and sarcoidosis
- pituitary failure to produce TSH
- hypothalamic failure to produce thyrotropin-releasing hormone (TRH)
- inborn errors of thyroid hormone synthesis
- inability to synthesize thyroid hormone because of iodine deficiency (usually dietary)
- use of antithyroid medications such as PTU.

Hypothyroidism is most prevalent in women.

Pathophysiology

In primary hypothyroidism, a decrease in thyroid hormone production is a result of the loss of thyroid tissue. This results in an increased secretion of TSH that leads to a goiter. In secondary hypothyroidism, typically the pituitary fails to synthesize or secrete adequate amounts of TSH, or target tissues fail to respond to normal blood levels of thyroid hormone. Either type may progress to myxedema, which is clinically more severe and considered a medical emergency. (See *Managing myxedema coma*, page 544.)

What to look for

Signs and symptoms of hypothyroidism include:
- weakness, fatigue
- forgetfulness
- cold intolerance
- unexplained weight gain
- constipation
- goiter
- slow speech
- decreasing mental stability
- cool, dry, coarse, flaky, inelastic skin
- puffy face, hands, and feet; periorbital edema
- dry, sparse hair
- thick, brittle nails.

Other indications include a slow pulse rate, anorexia, abdominal distention, menorrhagia, decreased libido, infer-

Either type of hypothyroidism may progress to myxedema, a medical emergency.

What do I do?

Managing myxedema coma

Myxedema coma is a medical emergency that commonly has a fatal outcome. Progression is usually gradual, but when stress aggravates severe or prolonged hypothyroidism, coma may develop abruptly. Examples of severe stress are infection, exposure to cold, and trauma. Other precipitating factors include thyroid medication withdrawal and the use of sedatives, narcotics, or anesthetics.

Patients in myxedema coma have significantly depressed respirations, so their partial pressure of carbon dioxide in arterial blood may increase. Decreased cardiac output and worsening cerebral hypoxia may also occur. The patient is stuporous and hypothermic, and her vital signs reflect bradycardia and hypotension.

Lifesaving interventions

If the patient becomes comatose, begin these interventions as soon as possible:
• Maintain airway patency with ventilatory support if necessary.
• Maintain circulation through I.V. fluid replacement.

• Provide continuous electrocardiogram monitoring.
• Monitor arterial blood gas measurements to detect hypoxia and metabolic acidosis.
• Warm the patient by wrapping her in blankets. Don't use a warming blanket because it might increase peripheral vasodilation, causing shock.
• Monitor the patient's body temperature until stable with a low-reading thermometer.
• Replace thyroid hormone by administering large I.V. levothyroxine doses as ordered. Monitor vital signs because rapid correction of hypothyroidism can cause adverse cardiac effects.
• Monitor intake and output and daily weight. With treatment, urine output should increase and body weight should decrease; if not, report this to the doctor.
• Replace fluids and other substances such as glucose. Monitor serum electrolyte levels.
• Administer corticosteroids as ordered.
• Check for possible sources of infection, such as blood, sputum, or urine, which may have precipitated coma. Treat infections or other underlying illnesses.

tility, ataxia, intention tremor, nystagmus, and delayed reflex relaxation time (especially in the Achilles tendon).

Clinical effects of myxedema coma include progressive stupor, hypoventilation, hypoglycemia, hyponatremia, hypotension, and hypothermia.

What tests tell you

• Radioimmunoassay tests showing low T_3, and T_4 levels indicate hypothyroidism.
• The TSH level increases with primary hypothyroidism and decreases in secondary hypothyroidism. The TRH level is decreased in hypothalamic insufficiency.
• Serum cholesterol, carotene, alkaline phosphatase, and triglyceride levels are increased.
• In myxedema coma, laboratory tests may also show low serum sodium levels and decreased pH and increased partial pressure of carbon dioxide in arterial blood, indicating respiratory acidosis.

How it's treated

Therapy for hypothyroidism consists of gradual thyroid replacement with levothyroxine. Effective treatment of myxedema coma supports vital functions while restoring euthyroidism. To support blood pressure and pulse rate, the patient receives I.V. levothyroxine, plus hydrocortisone in cases of pituitary or adrenal insufficiency. Hypoventilation requires oxygenation and vigorous respiratory support. Other supportive measures include careful fluid replacement and antimicrobial medications for infection.

What to do

 • Provide a high-bulk, low-calorie diet and encourage activity.
• Administer cathartics and stool softeners, as needed.
• After thyroid replacement therapy begins, watch for signs of hyperthyroidism, such as restlessness, sweating, and excessive weight loss.
• Advise the patient how to obtain medical identification jewelry.
• Evaluate the patient. She should have a normal bowel elimination pattern and adequate cardiac function, know which cardiac symptoms to report, and understand the need for lifelong thyroid replacement and regular medical care to monitor replacement therapy. She should have medical identification jewelry and a wallet identification card. She should show signs of adequate cardiac output and function, including blood pressure and pulse rate; adequate urine output; intact skin; adequate fluid volume and electrolyte balance; and adequate gas exchange. (See *Hypothyroidism teaching tips.*)

Hypothyroidism teaching tips

• Tell the patient to report signs of aggravated cardiovascular disease, such as chest pain and tachycardia.
• To prevent myxedema coma, tell the patient to continue his course of antithyroid medication even if his symptoms subside.
• Instruct the patient to report infection immediately and to make sure any health care provider who prescribes drugs for him knows about his hypothyroidism.

Quick quiz

1. After ^{131}I administration, urine and saliva will be slightly radioactive for how many hours?
    A.   Fewer than 2 hours
    B.   6 to 8 hours
    C.   24 hours
    D.   36 hours

Answer: C. Urine and saliva will be slightly radioactive for 24 hours and vomitus will be highly radioactive for 6 to 8 hours after therapy.

2. Which statement should be stressed in home care instructions after adrenalectomy?

    A.   The patient can stop taking his medication when his physical appearance improves.

    B.   The patient should take his steroids on an empty stomach.

    C.   The patient should take prescribed medications as directed and continue medical follow-up for dosage adjustment.

    D.   The patient can take his medication any time he chooses.

Answer: C. The patient should take his prescribed medication as directed. Sudden withdrawal of steroids can precipitate adrenal crisis.

3. An adrenal crisis is characterized by all of these signs and symtoms except:

    A.   weakness and fatigue.

    B.   nausea and vomiting.

    C.   hypotension.

    D.   sodium and fluid retention.

Answer: D. Sodium and fluid retention are characteristics of Cushing's syndrome; adrenal crisis causes decreased sodium levels and hypotension.

4. Which statement about diabetes mellitus is false?

    A.   Type 2 diabetes commonly occurs in adults after age 40.

    B.   Type 1 diabetes usually occurs before age 30.

    C.   Type 1 diabetes is treated with exercise, meal planning and antidiabetic drugs.

    D.   An increasing number of adolescents are being diagnosed with type 2 diabetes.

Answer: C. Type 1 diabetes is treated with insulin and dietary management.

Scoring

☆☆☆ If you answered all four items correctly, zowee! You've got all the energy you need to master endocrine disorders.

☆☆ If you answered three items correctly, yahoo! Your receptors are doing a great job of triggering correct endocrine information.

☆ If you answered fewer than three items correctly, don't stress! With a quick infusion of endocrine information, you'll achieve a regular release of correct answers.

Renal and urologic disorders

Just the facts

In this chapter, you'll learn:

♦ the role of the renal system and its effect on other body systems

♦ history and physical assessment techniques that target renal function

♦ appropriate treatments to promote a healthy renal system

♦ causes, signs and symptoms, diagnostic tests, and nursing interventions for common renal and urologic disorders.

The renal system retains useful materials and excretes foreign or excessive materials and waste. Through this basic function, the renal system profoundly affects other body systems and the patient's overall health.

Anatomy and physiology

The renal system consists of two kidneys, two ureters, one bladder, and one urethra. Working together, these structures remove wastes from the body, regulate acid-base balance by retaining or excreting hydrogen ions, and regulate fluid and electrolyte balance. (See *Renal system*, page 548.)

The kidneys

The kidneys are:
• bean-shaped
• highly vascular
• located retroperitoneally on either side of the vertebral column, between the 12th thoracic and 3rd lumbar vertebrae

Ooh, I'm highly vascular. That sounds impressive.

Renal system

As this frontal view suggests, the kidneys constitute the major portion of the renal system. These bean-shaped organs lie near and on either side of the spine at the small of the back, with the left kidney positioned slightly higher than the right. The *adrenal glands,* perched atop the kidneys, influence blood pressure as well as sodium and water retention by the kidneys.

Filtration station

The kidneys receive waste-filled blood from the *renal artery,* which branches off the *aorta.* After passing through a complicated network of smaller blood vessels and nephrons, the fil-

tered blood recirculates through the *renal vein,* which empties into the *inferior vena cava.*

Excrete to complete

Waste products that the nephrons remove from the blood are excreted by the kidneys, along with other fluids that constitute the formed urine. Urine passes, by peristalsis, through the *ureters* to the *urinary bladder.* As the bladder fills, nerves in the bladder wall relax the *sphincter* (an action known as the *micturition reflex);* then a voluntary stimulus occurs, and the urine passes into the urethra and is expelled from the body.

Inferior vena cava

Right adrenal gland

Right kidney

Right renal artery

Right renal vein

Right ureter

Urinary bladder

Left adrenal gland

Left kidney

Left renal artery

Left renal vein

Abdominal aorta

Left ureter

• protected by abdominal contents, muscles attached to the vertebral column, and a perirenal fat layer
• made up of the renal cortex, central renal medulla, internal calyces, and renal pelvis as well as the nephron, which serves as the kidney's functional unit. (See *A close look at the kidney*, page 550.)

More system structures

The structures of the renal system, extending downward from the kidneys, include:
• *ureters* — tubes that act as ducts channeling urine to the bladder via peristaltic waves that occur about one to five times per minute; they measure about 10″ to 12″ (25.5 to 30.5 cm) in adults and have a diameter varying from 2 to 8 mm, with the narrowest portion being at the ureteropelvic junction
• *urinary bladder* — a hollow, spherical, muscular organ in the pelvis that serves to store urine delivered by the ureters; bladder capacity ranges from 500 to 600 ml in a normal adult (less in children and elderly people)
• *urethra* — a small duct that channels urine outside the body from the bladder; it has an exterior opening known as the *urinary (urethral) meatus*; in the female, the urethra ranges from 1″ to 2″ (2.5 to 5 cm) long, with the urethral meatus located anterior to the vaginal opening; in the male, the urethra is about 8″ (20 cm) long, with the urethral meatus located at the end of the glans penis; the male urethra serves as a passageway for semen as well as urine.

Urine formation

The kidneys collect and eliminate wastes from the body in a three-step process:

glomerular filtration — filtering the blood that flows through the kidney's blood vessels, or glomeruli (see *Understanding the GFR*, page 551)

tubular reabsorption — reabsorbing filtered fluid through the minute canals (tubules) that make up the kidney

tubular secretion — release of the filtered substance by the tubules.

Results may vary

Varying with fluid intake and climate, total daily urine output averages 720 to 2,400 ml. For example, after a patient drinks a large volume of fluid, urine

> Total daily urine output varies with fluid intake and climate.

A closer look

A close look at the kidney

Illustrated here is a kidney along with an enlargement of a nephron, the kidney's functional unit. Major structures of the kidney include:
• medulla — inner portion of the kidney, made up of renal pyramids and tubular structures
• renal artery — supplies blood to the kidney
• renal pyramid — channels output to renal pelvis for excretion
• renal calyx — channels formed urine from the renal pyramids to the renal pelvis
• renal vein — about 99% of filtered blood is circulated through the renal vein back to the general circulation; the remaining 1%, which contains waste products, undergoes further processing in the kidney
• renal pelvis — after blood that contains waste products is processed in the kidney, formed urine is channeled to the renal pelvis
• ureter — tube that terminates in the urinary bladder; urine then enters the urethra for excretion
• cortex — outer layer of the kidney.

Note the nephron

The nephron is the functional and structural unit of the kidney. Each kidney contains about 1 million nephrons. The nephron's two main activities are selective reabsorption and secretion of ions and mechanical filtration of fluids, wastes, electrolytes, and acids and bases.

Components of the nephron include:
• glomerulus — a network of twisted capillaries that acts as a filter for the passage of protein-free and red blood cell-free filtrate to the proximal convoluted tubules
• Bowman's capsule — contains the glomerulus and acts as a filter for urine
• proximal convoluted tubule — site of reabsorption of glucose, amino acids, metabolites, and electrolytes from filtrate; reabsorbed substances return to circulation
• loop of Henle — a U-shaped nephron tubule located in the medulla and extending from the proximal convoluted tubule to the distal convoluted tubule, site for further concentration of filtrate through reabsorption
• distal convoluted tubule — site from which filtrate enters the collecting tubule
• collecting tubule — releases urine.

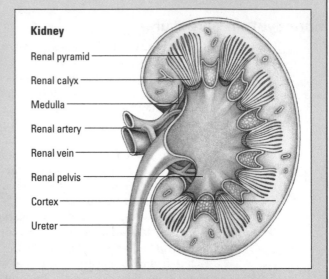

Kidney

Renal pyramid
Renal calyx
Medulla
Renal artery
Renal vein
Renal pelvis
Cortex
Ureter

Nephron

Proximal convoluted tubule
Glomerulus
Bowman's capsule
Collecting tubule
Loop of Henle

Understanding the GFR

The glomerular filtration rate (GFR) is the rate at which the glomeruli filter blood. The normal GFR is about 120 ml/minute. GFR depends on:
- permeability of capillary walls
- vascular pressure
- filtration pressure.

GFR and clearance

Clearance is the complete removal of a substance from the blood. The most accurate measure of glomerular filtration is creatinine clearance because creatinine is filtered by the glomeruli but not reabsorbed by the tubules.

Equal to, greater than, or less than

Here's more about how the GFR affects clearance measurements for a substance in the blood:
- If the tubules neither reabsorb nor secrete the substance—as happens with creatinine—clearance equals the GFR.
- If the tubules reabsorb the substance, clearance is less than the GFR.
- If the tubules secrete the substance, clearance exceeds the GFR.
- If the tubules reabsorb and secrete the substance, clearance may be less than, equal to, or greater than the GFR.

output increases as the body rapidly excretes excess water. If a patient restricts water intake or has an excessive intake of such solutes as sodium, urine output declines as the body retains water to maintain normal fluid concentration.

Hormones and the kidneys

Two hormones help regulate tubular reabsorption and secretion:

Antidiuretic hormone (ADH), which is produced by the pituitary gland, acts in the distal tubule and collecting ducts to increase water reabsorption and urine concentration. ADH deficiency decreases water reabsorption, causing dilute urine.

Aldosterone, which is produced by the adrenal gland, affects tubular reabsorption by regulating sodium retention and helping control potassium secretion by tubular epithelial cells.

Those other hormones

Other hormonal functions of the kidneys include:
- *secretion of the hormone erythropoietin.* In response to low arterial oxygen tension, the kidneys produce erythropoietin, which travels to the bone marrow and stimulates red blood cell (RBC) production.
- *regulation of calcium and phosphorus balance.* To help regulate calcium and phosphorus balance, the kidneys filter and reabsorb about one-half of unbound serum calcium and activate vitamin D_3, a compound that promotes intestinal calcium absorption and regulates phosphate excretion.

Renin's role

The kidneys help regulate blood pressure by producing and secreting the enzyme renin in response to an actual or perceived decline in extracellular fluid volume. Renin, in turn, forms angiotensin I, which is converted to the more potent angiotensin II.

Potassium regulation

The distal tubules of the kidneys regulate potassium excretion. Responding to an elevated serum potassium level, the adrenal cortex increases aldosterone secretion. Through a poorly understood mechanism, aldosterone also affects the potassium secreting capacity of distal tubular cells.

Assessment

Assessing the urinary system may uncover clues to problems in any body system.

Assessing the urinary system may uncover clues to problems in any body system.

History

Begin your assessment with a thorough history, including current and past health, family history, and lifestyle patterns.

Current health status

To determine the patient's chief complaint, ask "What made you seek medical help?" Document the reason for seeking care in the patient's own words. When a patient has a renal disorder, expect these common complaints:
- urinary frequency and urgency
- pain on urination
- difficulty urinating
- flank pain.

Previous health status

Explore all of the patient's previous major illnesses, recurrent minor illnesses, accidents or injuries, surgical procedures, and allergies. Ask about a history of urologic-related disorders such as hypertension.

A complete sexual history helps you identify your patient's knowledge deficits and expectations. This information may suggest a need for psychological or sexual therapy. It can also guide treatment decisions. For example, pain or discomfort associated with intercourse or diminished sexual desire may reflect disease progression or depression.

Other questions to ask include:
- Have you ever had a urinary infection?
- Are you taking prescription, over-the-counter, or illicit drugs?
- Are you allergic to drugs, foods, or other products? If yes, describe the reaction you experienced.
- Have you ever had a sexually transmitted disease (STD)?

Family history

For clues to risk factors, ask if blood relatives have ever been treated for renal or cardiovascular disorders, diabetes, cancer, or other chronic illness.

Lifestyle patterns

Investigate psychosocial factors that may affect the way the patient deals with his condition. Marital problems, poor living conditions, job insecurity, and other stresses can strongly affect how he feels.

Also, find out how the patient views himself. A disfiguring genital lesion or an STD can alter self-image. Try to determine what concerns he has about his condition. For example, does he fear that the disease or therapy will affect his sex life? If he can express his fears and concerns, you can develop appropriate nursing interventions more easily.

Investigate psychosocial factors that may affect the way the patient deals with his condition.

Physical examination

Begin the physical examination by documenting baseline vital signs and weighing the patient. Ask the patient to urinate into a specimen cup. Assess the specimen for color, odor, and clarity. Because the renal system affects many body functions, a thorough assessment includes examination of multiple related body systems using inspection, auscultation, percussion, and palpation techniques.

Inspection

Renal system inspection includes examination of the abdomen and urethral meatus.

Abdomen

Help the patient assume a supine position with his arms relaxed at his sides. Expose the patient's abdomen from the xiphoid process to the symphysis pubis and inspect the abdomen for gross en-

554

Percussing the urinary organs

Percuss the kidneys and bladder using the techniques described below.

Kidney percussion

With the patient sitting upright, percuss each costovertebral angle (the angle over each kidney whose borders are formed by the lateral and downward curve of the lowest rib and the vertebral column). To perform mediate percussion, place your left palm over the costovertebral angle and gently strike it with your right fist. To perform immediate percussion, gently strike your fist over each costovertebral angle. Usually, the patient will feel a thudding sensation or pressure during percussion.

Bladder percussion

Using mediate percussion, percuss the area over the bladder, beginning 2″ (5 cm) above the symphysis pubis. To detect differences in sound, percuss toward the bladder's base. Percussion usually produces a tympanic sound. (Over a urine-filled bladder, it produces a dull sound.)

12th rib

Costovertebral angle

---

largements or fullness by comparing the left and right sides, noting asymmetric areas. In a normal adult, the abdomen is smooth, flat or scaphoid (concave), and symmetrical. Ask about scars, lesions, bruises, or discolorations found on abdominal skin.

Urethral meatus

Help the patient feel more at ease during your inspection by examining the urethral meatus last and by explaining beforehand how you'll assess this area. Be sure to wear gloves.

Auscultation

Auscultate the renal arteries in the left and right upper abdominal quadrants by pressing the stethoscope bell lightly against the abdomen and instructing the patient to exhale deeply. Begin auscultating at the midline and work to the left. Then return to the mid-

Palpating the urinary organs

In a normal adult, the kidneys usually aren't palpable because they're located deep within the abdomen. However, they may be palpable in a thin patient or in one with reduced abdominal muscle mass, and the right kidney, slightly lower than the left, may be easier to palpate altogether. Keep in mind that both kidneys descend with deep inhalation. An adult's bladder may not be palpable either. However, if it's palpable, it usually feels firm and relatively smooth. When palpating urinary organs, use bimanual palpation, beginning on the patient's right side and proceeding as follows.

Kidney palpation

Help the patient to a supine position, and expose the abdomen from the xiphoid process to the symphysis pubis. Standing at the right side, place your left hand under the back, midway between the lower costal margin and the iliac crest.

Next, place your right hand on the patient's abdomen, directly above your left hand. Angle this hand slightly toward the costal margin. To palpate the right lower edge of the right kidney, press your right fingertips about 1½" (3.5 cm) above the right iliac crest at the midinguinal line; press your left fingertips upward into the right costovertebral angle.

Instruct the patient to inhale deeply so that the lower portion of the right kidney can move down between your hands. If it does, note its shape and size. Usually, it feels smooth, solid, and firm, yet elastic. Ask the patient if palpation causes tenderness. (*Note:* Avoid using excessive pressure to palpate the kidney because this may cause intense pain.)

To assess the left kidney, move to the patient's left side, and position your hands as described above, but with this change: Place your right hand 2" (5 cm) above the left iliac crest. Then apply pressure with both hands as the patient inhales. If the left kidney can be palpated, compare it with the right kidney; it should be the same size.

Bladder palpation

Before palpating the bladder, make sure the patient has voided. Then locate the edge of the bladder by pressing deeply in the midline 1" to 2" (2.5 to 5 cm) above the symphysis pubis. As the bladder is palpated, note its size and location, and check for lumps, masses, and tenderness. The bladder normally feels firm and relatively smooth. During deep palpation, the patient may report the urge to urinate—a normal response.

line and work to the right. Systolic bruits (whooshing sounds) or other unusual sounds are potentially significant abnormalities.

Percussion

After auscultating the renal arteries, percuss the patient's kidneys to detect any tenderness or pain, and percuss the bladder to evaluate its position and contents. (See *Percussing the urinary organs*, page 554.)

Palpation

Palpation of the kidneys and bladder is next. Through palpation, you can detect any lumps, masses, or tenderness. To achieve optimal results, ask the patient to relax his abdomen by taking deep breaths through his mouth. (See *Palpating the urinary organs*, page 555.)

Auscultate the renal arteries by pressing the bell lightly against the abdomen and telling the patient to exhale deeply.

Diagnostic tests

With the help of advanced technology, including improved computer processing and imaging techniques, renal and urologic problems that were previously detectable only by invasive techniques can now be evaluated. These diagnostic tests can help evaluate the patient's renal and urologic status.

Blood studies

When considered with urinalysis findings, blood studies help the doctor diagnose genitourinary disease and evaluate kidney function. Blood studies include blood urea nitrogen (BUN) and serum creatinine.

BUN

Urea, the chief end product of protein metabolism, constitutes 40% to 50% of the blood's nonprotein nitrogen. It's formed from ammonia in the liver, filtered by the glomeruli, reabsorbed (to a limited degree) in the tubules, and finally excreted. Insufficient urea excretion elevates the BUN level.

Normal BUN levels range from 8 to 16 mg/dl. For the most accurate interpretation of test results, examine BUN levels in conjunction with serum creatinine levels and in light of the patient's underlying condition.

When considered with urinalysis findings, blood studies evaluate my function.

Nursing considerations

- Tell the patient that the test requires a blood sample.
- Check the patient's medication history for drugs that may influence BUN levels. (Chloramphenicol may depress levels; aminoglycosides, amphotericin B, and methicillin can elevate levels.)
- If a hematoma develops at the venipuncture site, apply warm soaks.

Serum creatinine

Creatinine, another nitrogenous waste, results from muscle metabolism of creatine. Normal serum creatinine values for males range from 0.8 to 1.2 mg/dl; for females, 0.6 to 0.9 mg/dl. Diet and fluid intake don't affect serum creatinine levels.

This test measures renal damage more reliably than BUN level measurements because severe, persistent renal impairment is virtually the only reason that creatinine levels rise significantly. Creatinine levels greater than 1.5 mg/dl indicate 66% or greater loss of renal function; levels greater than 2 mg/dl indicate renal insufficiency.

Nursing considerations

- Tell the patient that the test requires a blood sample.
- Check the patient's medication history for drugs that may influence serum creatinine levels (ascorbic acid, barbiturates, and diuretics may raise serum creatinine levels).
- If a hematoma develops at the venipuncture site, apply warm soaks.

Clearance tests

Clearance tests for filtration, reabsorption, and secretion permit a precise evaluation of renal function. These tests measure the volume of plasma that can be cleared of a substance (such as creatinine) per unit of time, thus helping evaluate urine-forming mechanisms. They also measure renal blood flow, which renal disease may reduce.

Creatinine clearance

The creatinine clearance test, commonly used to assess glomerular filtration rate (GFR), determines how efficiently the kidneys clear creatinine from the blood. Normal values depend on the patient's age.

Yawn... I was up late cramming for my clearance tests. I hope I pass. Get it? Pass? I'm such a punster.

Nursing considerations

- Tell the patient the test requires a timed urine specimen and at least one blood sample.
- A high-protein diet before the test and strenuous physical exercise during the collection period may increase creatinine excretion. Inform the patient that he shouldn't eat an excessive amount of meat before the test and should avoid strenuous physical exercise during the collection period.

Urea clearance

The urea clearance test measures urine levels of urea, the chief end product of protein metabolism and the chief nitrogenous component of urine.

The urea clearance rate usually ranges from 64 to 100 ml/minute at a urine flow rate of 2 ml/minute or more. At flow rates of less than 2 ml/minute, the normal range decreases to 40 to 70 ml/minute.

Nursing considerations

- Tell the patient that the test requires two timed urine specimens and one blood sample.
- Instruct him to fast after midnight before the test and to abstain from exercise before and during the test.

Radiologic and imaging studies

Noninvasive radiologic and imaging studies help screen for renal and urologic abnormalities. These studies include computed tomography (CT) scan, excretory urography, kidney-ureter-bladder (KUB) radiography, magnetic resonance imaging (MRI), radionuclide renal scans, renal angiography, ultrasonography, and voiding cystourethrography.

CT scan

In a renal CT scan, the image's density reflects the amount of radiation absorbed by renal tissue, thus permitting identification of masses and other lesions.

Nursing considerations

- If contrast enhancement isn't scheduled, inform the patient that he need not restrict food or fluids. If a contrast medium will be used, instruct him to fast for 4 hours before the test.

Radiologic and imaging studies screen for renal and urologic abnormalities.

- Inform the patient that he'll be positioned on an X-ray table and that a scanner will take films of his kidneys. Warn him that he may hear loud, clacking sounds as the scanner rotates around his body.
- Just before the procedure, instruct the patient to put on a hospital gown and to remove any metallic objects that could interfere with the scan.

Excretory urography

After I.V. administration of a contrast medium, this common procedure (also known as *I.V. pyelography*) allows visualization of the renal parenchyma, calyces, pelvises, ureters, bladder and, in some cases, the urethra. In the 1st minute after injection (the nephrographic stage), the contrast medium delineates the size and shape of the kidneys. After 3 to 5 minutes (the pyelographic stage), the contrast medium moves into the calyces and pelvises, allowing visualization of cysts, tumors, and other obstructions.

Nursing considerations

- Check the patient's history for hypersensitivity to iodine, iodine-containing foods, or contrast media containing iodine.
- Ensure that the patient is well hydrated, and instruct him to fast for 8 hours before the test.
- Inform the patient that he may experience a transient burning sensation and metallic taste when the contrast medium is injected.

KUB radiography

KUB radiography is the main radiologic study used for the urinary system. The KUB study, consisting of plain, contrast-free X-rays, shows kidney size, position, and structure as well as calculi and other lesions. Before performing a renal biopsy, the doctor may use this test to determine kidney placement. For diagnostic purposes, however, the KUB study provides limited information.

Nursing considerations

- Inform the patient that he need not restrict food or fluids before the test.
- No specific posttest care is necessary.

MRI

MRI provides tomographic images that reflect the differing hydrogen densities of body tissues. Physical, chemical, and cellular microenvironments modify these densities, as do the fluid characteristics of tissues. MRI can provide precise images of anatomic detail and important biochemical infor-

For diagnostic purposes, the KUB study provides limited information.

mation about the tissue examined and can efficiently visualize and
stage kidney, bladder, and prostate tumors.

Nursing considerations

• Before the patient enters the MRI chamber, make sure he has
removed all metal objects, such as earrings, watch, necklace,
bracelets, and rings. Patients with internal metal objects, such as
pacemakers or aneurysm clips, can't undergo MRI testing.
• If you're accompanying the patient, be sure to remove metal objects from your pockets, such as scissors, forceps, a penlight, metal pens, and your credit cards (the magnetic field will erase the
numerical information in the code strips).
• Tell the patient that he must remain still throughout the test,
which takes about 45 minutes. If the patient complains of claustrophobia, reassure him and provide emotional support.

If you're
accompanying the
patient for an MRI, be
sure to remove metal
objects from your
pockets as well as
your credit cards.

Radionuclide renal scan

A radionuclide renal scan, which may be substituted for excretory
urography in patients who are hypersensitive to contrast media,
involves I.V. injection of a radionuclide, followed by scintiphotog-
raphy. Observation of the uptake concentration and radionuclide
transit during the procedure allows assessment of renal blood
flow, nephron and collecting system function, and renal structure.

Nursing considerations

• Inform the patient that he'll receive an injection of a radionuclide and may experience transient flushing and nausea. Emphasize that he'll receive only a small amount of radionuclide, which
is usually excreted within 24 hours.
 • After the test, instruct the patient to flush the toilet immediately
every time he urinates for 24 hours as a radiation precaution.

Renal angiography

Renal angiography permits radiographic examination of the renal
vasculature and parenchyma after arterial injection of a contrast
medium. Renal venography (angiography of the veins) may be performed to detect renal vein thrombosis and venous extension of
renal cell carcinoma.

Nursing considerations

• Check the patient's history for hypersensitivity to iodine-based
contrast media or iodine-containing foods such as shellfish.
• Instruct him to fast for 8 hours before the test and drink extra
fluids the day before the test and after the test to maintain adequate hydration (or start an I.V. line if needed).

• Keep the patient flat in bed after the procedure; keep the leg on the affected side straight for at least 6 hours or as ordered.

Ultrasonography

Ultrasonography uses high-frequency sound waves to reveal internal structures. The pulse-echo transmission technique of this test determines the kidney's size, shape, and position. It also reveals internal structures and perirenal tissue and helps the doctor diagnose complications after kidney transplantation.

Nursing considerations

• Tell the patient that he'll either be prone (renal examination position) or supine during the test.
• Explain that a technician will spread coupling oil or gel on the patient's skin and then press a probe or transducer against the skin and move it across the area being tested.

Voiding cystourethrography

In voiding cystourethrography, a urinary catheter allows instillation of a contrast medium into the bladder by gentle syringe pressure or gravity. Fluoroscopic films or overhead radiographs demonstrate bladder filling and then show excretion of the contrast medium as the patient voids.

Nursing considerations

• Check the patient's history for hypersensitivity to contrast media or iodine-containing foods such as shellfish.
• Inform the patient that a catheter will be inserted into his bladder and a contrast medium will be instilled through the catheter. Tell him he may experience a feeling of fullness and an urge to void when the contrast is instilled.
• After the test, instruct the patient to drink lots of fluids to reduce burning on urination and to flush out any residual contrast dye.
• Monitor for chills and fever related to extravasation of contrast material or urinary sepsis.

Urine studies

Urine studies, such as urinalysis and urine osmolality, can indicate urinary tract infection (UTI) and other disorders.

Urinalysis

Performed on a urine specimen of at least 10 ml, urinalysis can indicate urinary or systemic disorders, warranting further investigation.

Nursing considerations

• Collect a random urine specimen, preferably the first-voided morning specimen. Send the specimen to the laboratory immediately.
• Refrigerate the specimen if analysis will be delayed longer than 1 hour.

Urine osmolality

Urine osmolality evaluates the diluting and concentrating ability of the kidneys. It may aid in the differential diagnosis of polyuria, oliguria, or syndrome of inappropriate antidiuretic hormone secretion. To obtain additional information about the patient's renal function, compare the urine specific gravity with urine osmolality.

Refrigerate the urine specimen if analysis will be delayed longer than 1 hour.

Nursing considerations

• Obtain a random specimen of preservative-free urine. If possible, obtain a first-voided morning specimen.
• Usually, urine osmolality ranges from 50 to 1,400 mOsm/kg, with the average being 300 to 800 mOsm/kg.

Other tests

Additional diagnostic tests may be used to evaluate urologic structure and function. These include cystometry, percutaneous renal biopsy, and uroflowmetry.

Cystometry

Cystometry, which helps determine the cause of bladder dysfunction, assesses the bladder's neuromuscular function by measuring the efficiency of the detrusor muscle reflex, intravesicular pressure and capacity, and the bladder's reaction to thermal stimulation. Abnormal test results may indicate a lower urinary tract obstruction.

Nursing considerations

• Explain to the patient the different steps of the test and what will happen in each. A urinary catheter will need to be inserted.

• Tell the patient that, if no more tests are needed, the catheter will be removed after the test. Warn the patient that he may experience transient burning or urinary frequency after the test, but that a sitz bath may alleviate discomfort.

Percutaneous renal biopsy

Histologic examination can help differentiate glomerular from tubular renal disease, monitor the disorder's progress, and assess the effectiveness of therapy. It can also reveal a malignant tumor such as Wilms' tumor. Histologic studies can help the doctor diagnose disseminated lupus erythematosus, amyloid infiltration, acute and chronic glomerulonephritis, renal vein thrombosis, and pyelonephritis. (See *Assisting with percutaneous renal biopsy*.)

Histologic examination can help differentiate glomerular from tubular renal disease. Oy, there's a mixed blessing.

Assisting with percutaneous renal biopsy

To prepare a patient for percutaneous renal biopsy, position him on his abdomen. To stabilize his kidneys, place a sandbag beneath his abdomen as shown.

After administering a local anesthetic, the doctor instructs the patient to hold his breath and remain immobile. Then the doctor inserts a needle with the obturator between the patient's last rib and the iliac crest as shown below. After asking the patient to breathe deeply, the doctor removes the obturator and inserts cutting prongs, which gather blood and tissue samples. This test is commonly performed in the radiology department so that special radiographic procedures may be used to help guide the needle.

Nursing considerations

• Instruct the patient to restrict food and fluids for 8 hours before the test. Inform him that he'll receive a mild sedative before the test to help him relax.
• After the test, tell him that pressure will be applied to the biopsy site to stop superficial bleeding and then a pressure dressing will be applied.
• Instruct the patient to lie flat on his back without moving for at least 12 hours to prevent bleeding.

Uroflowmetry

Uroflowmetry measures the volume of urine expelled from the urethra in milliliters per second (urine flow rate) and determines the urine flow pattern. This test is performed to evaluate lower urinary tract function and demonstrate bladder outlet obstruction. Normal flow rate for males is 20 to 25 ml/second; for females, 25 to 30 ml/second.

Nursing considerations

• Advise the patient not to urinate for several hours before the test and to increase his fluid intake so that he'll have a full bladder and a strong urge to void.

Treatments

If uncorrected, renal and urologic disorders can adversely affect virtually every body system. Treatments for these disorders include drug therapy, dialysis, nonsurgical procedures, and surgery.

Drug therapy

Ideally, drug therapy should be effective and not impair renal function. However, because renal disorders alter the chemical composition of body fluids and the pharmacokinetic properties of many drugs, standard regimens of some drugs may require adjustment. For instance, dosages of drugs that are mainly excreted by the kidneys unchanged or as active metabolites may require adjustment to avoid nephrotoxicity. In renal failure, potentially toxic drugs should be used cautiously and sparingly.

Drug therapy for renal and urologic disorders can include:
• antibiotics

> Renal disorders can alter chemical composition of body fluids and pharmacokinetic properties of drugs, so many drug regimens require adjustment.

- urinary tract antiseptics
- electrolytes and replacements
- diuretics.

Dialysis

Depending on the patient's condition and, at times, his preference, dialysis may take the form of hemodialysis or peritoneal dialysis.

Hemodialysis

Hemodialysis removes toxic wastes and other impurities from the blood of a patient with renal failure. In this technique, the blood is removed from the body through a surgically created access site, pumped through a dialyzing unit to remove toxins, and then returned to the body. The extracorporeal dialyzer works through a combination of osmosis, diffusion, and filtration. By extracting by-products of protein metabolism—notably urea and uric acid—as well as creatinine and excess water, hemodialysis helps restore or maintain acid-base and electrolyte balance and prevent the complications associated with uremia. (See *How hemodialysis works*, page 566.)

Hemodialysis extracts by-products of protein metabolism, creatinine, and excess water.

Patient preparation
- If the patient is undergoing hemodialysis for the first time, explain its purpose and what to expect during and after treatment. Explain that he first will undergo surgery to create vascular access.
- Assess the access site for the presence of a bruit and thrill and keep the vascular access site supported and resting on a sterile drape or sterile barrier shield.

Monitoring and aftercare
- After completion of hemodialysis, monitor the vascular access site for bleeding. If bleeding is excessive, maintain pressure on the site and notify the doctor.
- To prevent clotting or other problems with blood flow, make sure that the arm used for vascular access isn't used for any other procedure, including I.V. line insertion, blood pressure monitoring, and venipuncture.
- At least four times per day, assess circulation at the access site by auscultating for the presence of bruits and palpating for thrills. Unlike most other circulatory assessments, bruits and thrills should be present here. Lack of a bruit at a venous access site for dialysis may indicate a blood clot requiring immediate surgical attention.

How hemodialysis works

Within the dialyzer, the patient's blood flows between coils, plates, or hollow fibers of semipermeable material, depending on the machine being used. Simultaneously, the dialysis solution is pumped around the other side under hydrostatic pressure.

Pressure and concentration

Pressure and concentration gradients between blood and the dialysis solution remove toxic wastes and excess water. The dialysis solution is an aqueous solution typically containing low concentrations of sodium, potassium, calcium, and magnesium cations and chloride anions as well as high concentrations of acetate (which the body readily converts to bicarbonate) and glucose. Because blood has higher concentrations of hydrogen ions and other electrolytes than dialysis solution, these solutes diffuse across the semipermeable material into the solution. Conversely, glucose and acetate are more highly concentrated in the dialysis solution and so diffuse back across the semipermeable material into the blood. Through this mechanism, hemodialysis removes excess water and toxins, reverses acidosis, and amends electrolyte imbalances.

Dialyzer

Dialysis solution

Hollow fiber

Waste products

Blood

Home care instructions

Instruct the patient to:
- care for his vascular access site by keeping the incision clean and dry
- notify the doctor of pain, swelling, redness, or drainage in the accessed arm
- use a stethoscope to auscultate for bruits
- refuse treatments or procedures on the accessed arm, including blood pressure monitoring or needle punctures
- avoid putting excessive pressure on the arm (such as sleeping on it, wearing constricting clothing on it, and lifting heavy objects or straining with it), showering, bathing, or swimming for several hours after dialysis.

Peritoneal dialysis

Like hemodialysis, peritoneal dialysis removes toxins from the blood of a patient with acute or chronic renal failure that doesn't respond to other treatments. Unlike hemodialysis, it uses the patient's peritoneal membrane as a semipermeable dialyzing membrane. In this technique, a hypertonic dialyzing solution (dialysate) is instilled through a catheter inserted into the peritoneal cavity. Then, by diffusion, excessive concentrations of electrolytes and uremic toxins in the blood move across the peritoneal membrane into the dialysis solution. Next, through osmosis, excessive water in the blood does the same. After an appropriate dwelling time, the dialysate is drained, taking toxins and wastes with it.

Unlike hemodialysis, peritoneal dialysis uses the patient's peritoneal membrane as a semipermeable dialyzing membrane.

Patient preparation

• For the first-time peritoneal dialysis patient, explain the purpose of the treatment and what he can expect during and after the procedure.
• Tell him that first the doctor will insert a catheter into his abdomen to allow instillation of dialysate. Explain the appropriate insertion procedure. (See *Comparing catheters for peritoneal dialysis*, page 568.)

Monitoring and aftercare

• Using sterile technique, change the catheter dressing every 24 hours or whenever it becomes soiled or wet.
• Watch closely for developing complications. Peritonitis can cause fever, persistent abdominal pain and cramping, slow or cloudy dialysis drainage, swelling and tenderness around the catheter, and increased white blood cell (WBC) count.

Home care instructions

Instruct the patient to:
• participate in a training program before beginning treatment on his own
• wear medical identification jewelry or carry a card identifying him as a dialysis patient and keep the phone number of the dialysis center on hand at all times in case of an emergency
• watch for and report signs of infection and fluid imbalance
• follow up with the doctor and dialysis team to evaluate the success of treatment and detect any problems.

Tell the patient to watch for and report signs of infection and fluid imbalance.

Comparing catheters for peritoneal dialysis

The first step in any type of peritoneal dialysis is the insertion of a catheter to allow instillation of dialyzing solution. The surgeon may insert one of three different catheters, as described below.

Tenckhoff catheter

The Tenckhoff catheter is the most commonly used peritoneal catheter. To implant a Tenckhoff catheter, the surgeon inserts the first 6¾" (17.1 cm) of the catheter into the patient's abdomen. The next 2¾" (7-cm) segment, which has a Dacron cuff at each end, is imbedded subcutaneously. Within a few days of insertion, the patient's tissues grow around these Dacron cuffs, forming a tight barrier against bacterial infiltration. The remaining 3⅞" (9.8 cm) of the catheter extends outside of the abdomen and is equipped with a metal adapter at the tip to allow connection to dialyzer tubing.

- Skin
- Fat
- Muscle
- Dacron cuff
- Peritoneum
- Bowel

Swan-neck catheter

The Swan-neck catheter has an inverted U-shaped arc (170 to 180 degrees) between the deep and superficial cuffs. This arc allows the catheter to exit the skin pointing downward. At the same time, the catheter enters the peritoneum pointing toward the pelvis. This catheter must be implanted in a tunnel the same shape as the catheter.

- Cuff
- Skin
- Flanged collar
- Fat
- Muscle
- Peritoneum
- Bowel

TWH catheter

The Toronto-Western Hospital (TWH) catheter has silicone discs perpendicular to the catheter. The discs' purpose is to hold the omentum and the bowel away from the exit holes and maintain their position in the pelvis, minimizing catheter tip migration. This catheter is more difficult to insert and remove than the Tenckhoff catheter.

- Skin
- Fat
- Muscle
- Dacron cuff
- Abdominal entry port
- Implant disk
- Peritoneum
- Bowel

Nonsurgical procedures

Several nonsurgical procedures may be employed to treat renal or urologic disorders, including calculi basketing, catheterization, and extracorporeal shock-wave lithotripsy (ESWL).

Calculi basketing

When ureteral calculi are too large for normal elimination, removal with a basketing instrument is the treatment of choice, helping to relieve pain and prevent infection and renal dysfunction. In this technique, a basketing instrument is inserted through a cystoscope or ureteroscope into the ureter to capture the calculus and then is withdrawn to remove it.

Patient preparation

• Tell the patient that after calculi removal, he'll have an indwelling urinary catheter inserted to ensure normal urine drainage; the catheter will probably remain in place for 24 to 48 hours.
• Tell him that he'll receive I.V. fluids during and immediately after the procedure to maintain urine output and prevent complications, such as hydronephrosis and pyelonephritis.

Monitoring and aftercare

• Promote fluids to maintain a urine output of 3 to 4 L/day. Observe the color of urine drainage from the indwelling urinary catheter; it should be slightly blood-tinged at first, gradually clearing within 24 to 48 hours. Irrigate the catheter as ordered using sterile technique.
• Administer analgesics as ordered.
• Observe for and report any signs or symptoms of septicemia, which may result from ureteral perforation during basketing.

Home care instructions

Instruct the patient to:
• follow prescribed dietary and medication regimens to prevent recurrence of calculi
• drink 3 to 4 qt (3 to 4 L) of fluid per day, unless contraindicated
• take prescribed analgesics as needed
• immediately report signs and symptoms of recurrent calculi (such as flank pain, hematuria, nausea, fever, and chills) or acute ureteral obstruction (such as severe pain and inability to void).

Tell the patient to drink 3 to 4 quarts of fluid per day unless contraindicated.

Catheterization

The insertion of a drainage device into the urinary bladder, catheterization may be intermittent or continuous. Intermittent catheterization drains urine remaining in the bladder after voiding. It's used for patients with urinary incontinence, urethral strictures, cystitis, prostatic obstruction, neurogenic bladder, or other disorders that interfere with bladder emptying. It may also be used postoperatively.

Catheterization helps relieve bladder distention caused by such conditions as urinary tract obstruction and neurogenic bladder. It allows continuous urine drainage in patients with a urinary meatus swollen from local trauma or childbirth as well as from surgery. Catheterization also can provide accurate monitoring of urine output when normal voiding is impaired.

Patient preparation

• Thoroughly review the procedure with the patient and reassure him that although catheterization may produce slight discomfort, it shouldn't be painful. Explain that you'll stop the procedure if he experiences severe discomfort.
• Assemble the necessary equipment, preferably a sterile catheterization package.

Monitoring and aftercare

• During catheterization, note the difficulty or ease of insertion, any patient discomfort, and the amount and nature of urine drainage.
• During urine drainage, monitor the patient for pallor, diaphoresis, and painful bladder spasms. If these occur, clamp the catheter tubing and call the doctor.
• Frequently assess the patient's intake and output. Encourage fluid intake to maintain continuous urine flow through the catheter and decrease the risk of infection and clot formation.
• Maintain good catheter care throughout the course of treatment. Clean the urinary meatus and catheter junction at least daily, more often if you note a buildup of exudate.
• To help prevent infection, avoid separating the catheter and tubing unless absolutely necessary. Throughout treatment, remain alert for signs and symptoms of UTI and for signs of catheter obstruction.

Home care instructions

Instruct the patient to:
• drink at least 2 qt (2 L) of water per day, unless the doctor orders otherwise

• perform daily periurethral care to minimize the risk of infection
• perform thorough hand washing before and after handling the catheter and collection system
• take showers but avoid tub baths while the catheter is in place
• notify the doctor if he notices urine leakage around the catheter or any signs and symptoms of UTI, such as fever, chills, flank or urinary tract pain, and cloudy or foul-smelling urine.

ESWL

A noninvasive technique for removing obstructive renal calculi, ESWL uses high-energy shock waves to break up calculi and allow their normal passage.

ESWL uses high-energy shock waves to break up calculi and allow their normal passage.

Patient preparation
• Tell the patient that he may receive a general or epidural anesthetic, depending on the type of lithotriptor and the intensity of shock waves needed.
• Tell the patient that he'll have an I.V. line and an indwelling urinary catheter in place after ESWL.

Monitoring and aftercare
• Encourage ambulation as early as possible after treatment and increase fluid intake as ordered to aid passage of calculi fragments.
• Strain all urine for calculi fragments and send these to the laboratory for analysis.
• Remember that slight hematuria usually occurs for several days after ESWL. However, notify the doctor if you detect frank or persistent bleeding.

Home care instructions
Instruct the patient to:
• drink 3 to 4 qt (3 to 4 L) of fluid each day for about 1 month after treatment.
• strain all urine for the 1st week after treatment, save all fragments in the container provided, and bring the container with him on his first follow-up doctor's appointment
• report severe, unremitting pain, persistent hematuria, inability to void, fever and chills, or recurrent nausea and vomiting
• resume normal activities, including exercise and work, as soon as he feels able (unless, of course, the doctor instructs otherwise)
• comply with any special dietary or drug regimen designed to reduce the risk of new calculi formation.

Surgery

Surgery may be necessary when conservative treatments fail to control the patient's renal or urologic disorder. Common surgeries include cystectomy, kidney transplantation, nephrectomy, suprapubic catheterization, transurethral resection of the bladder, and urinary diversion.

Surgery may be necessary when conservative treatments fail to control the patient's disorder.

Cystectomy

Partial or total removal of the urinary bladder and surrounding structures may be necessary to treat advanced bladder cancer or, rarely, other bladder disorders such as interstitial cystitis. In most patients with bladder cancer, the combined use of chemotherapy, radiation therapy, and surgery yields the best results. In metastatic bladder cancer, cystectomy and radiation therapy may provide palliative benefits and prolong life.

Three types

Cystectomy may be partial, simple, or radical.

Partial, or segmental, cystectomy involves resection of cancerous bladder tissue. Typically preserving bladder function, this surgery is most commonly indicated for a single, easily accessible tumor.

Simple, or total, cystectomy involves resection of the entire bladder, with preservation of surrounding structures. It's indicated for multiple or extensive carcinoma, advanced interstitial cystitis, and related disorders.

Radical cystectomy is usually indicated for muscle-invading, primary bladder carcinoma. In men, the bladder, prostate, and seminal vesicles are removed. In women, the bladder, urethra and, usually, the uterus, fallopian tubes, ovaries, and a segment of the vaginal wall are excised. This procedure may involve bilateral pelvic lymphadenectomy. Because this surgery is so extensive, it typically produces impotence in men and sterility in women. A permanent urinary diversion is needed in both radical and simple cystectomy.

Patient preparation
• If the patient will be undergoing simple or radical cystectomy, reassure him that such diversion need not interfere with his normal activities and arrange for a visit by an enterostomal therapist, who can provide additional information.

• If the patient is scheduled for radical cystectomy, you'll need to address concerns about the loss of sexual or reproductive function. As appropriate, refer the patient for psychological and sexual counseling.

• Explain to the patient that he'll awaken in an intensive care unit after surgery.

• About 4 days before surgery, begin full bowel preparation to help prevent infection. Maintain a low-residue diet for 3 days and then infuse high-calorie fluids on the 4th day. As ordered, administer antibiotics for 24 hours before surgery. On the night before surgery, administer an enema to clear fecal matter from the bowel.

> Begin full bowel preparation about 4 days before surgery. Maintain a low-residue diet for 3 days, and infuse high-calorie fluids on the 4th day.

Monitoring and aftercare

• Periodically inspect the stoma and incision for bleeding and observe urine drainage for frank hematuria and clots. Slight hematuria commonly occurs for several days after surgery but should clear thereafter.

• Observe the wound site and all drainage for signs or symptoms of infection. Change abdominal dressings frequently, using sterile technique.

• Periodically ask the patient about incisional pain and, if he has had a partial cystectomy, ask about bladder spasms. Provide analgesics and an antispasmodic such as oxybutynin as ordered.

• To prevent pulmonary complications associated with prolonged immobility, encourage frequent position changes, coughing and deep breathing and, if possible, early ambulation.

Home care instructions

Instruct the patient to:

• watch for and report signs or symptoms of UTI and persistent hematuria

• learn how to care for his stoma and where to obtain needed supplies

• contact the local chapter of the United Ostomy Association for support

• follow up with the doctor as recommended.

Kidney transplantation

Ranking among the most commonly performed and most successful of all organ transplantations, kidney transplantation represents an attractive alternative to dialysis for many patients with otherwise unmanageable end-stage renal disease. It also may be necessary to sustain life in a patient who has suffered traumatic loss of

Kidney transplantation site and vascular connections

With kidney transplantation, the donated organ is implanted in the iliac fossa. The organ's vessels are then connected to the internal iliac vein and internal iliac artery, as shown below.

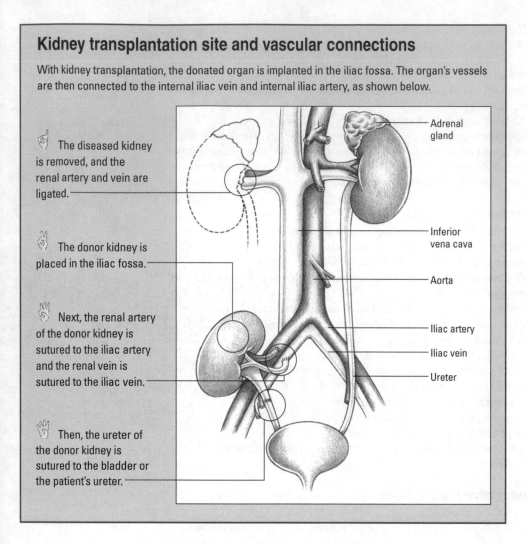

The diseased kidney is removed, and the renal artery and vein are ligated.

The donor kidney is placed in the iliac fossa.

Next, the renal artery of the donor kidney is sutured to the iliac artery and the renal vein is sutured to the iliac vein.

Then, the ureter of the donor kidney is sutured to the bladder or the patient's ureter.

Adrenal gland

Inferior vena cava

Aorta

Iliac artery

Iliac vein

Ureter

kidney function or for whom dialysis is contraindicated. (See *Kidney transplantation site and vascular connections.*)

Patient preparation

• The patient will understandably find the prospect of kidney transplantation confusing and frightening. Help him cope with such emotions by preparing him thoroughly for transplantation and a prolonged recovery period and by offering ongoing emotional support.

• Describe the routine preoperative measures. Point out that he may need dialysis for a few days after surgery if his transplanted kidney doesn't start functioning immediately.

- Review the transplantation procedure itself, supplementing and clarifying the doctor's explanations as necessary.
- Discuss the immunosuppressant drugs he'll be taking and explain their possible adverse effects. Point out that these drugs increase his susceptibility to infection; as a result, he'll be kept temporarily isolated after surgery.

Monitoring and aftercare

- First and foremost, take special precautions to reduce the risk of infection. For instance, use strict sterile technique when changing dressings and performing catheter care. Also, limit the patient's contact with staff, other patients, and visitors and have all people in the patient's room wear surgical masks for the first 2 weeks after surgery.

Have all people in the transplant patient's room wear surgical masks for the first 2 weeks after surgery.

- Throughout the recovery period, watch for signs and symptoms of tissue rejection. Observe the transplantation site for redness, tenderness, and swelling.
- Carefully monitor urine output; promptly report output of less than 100 ml/hour. A sudden decrease in urine output could indicate thrombus formation at the renal artery anastomosis site.

Home care instructions

Instruct the patient to:
- carefully measure and record intake and output to monitor kidney function
- weigh himself at least twice per week and report any rapid gain (any gain of 2½ lb [1.1 kg] or more in a single day)
- watch for and promptly report any signs and symptoms of infection or transplant rejection, including redness, warmth, tenderness, or swelling over the kidney; fever; decreased urine output; and elevated blood pressure
- avoid crowds and contact with people with known or suspected infections for at least 3 months after surgery
- continue immunosuppressant therapy for as long as he has the transplanted kidney to prevent rejection.

Nephrectomy

Nephrectomy, the surgical removal of a kidney, represents the treatment of choice for advanced renal cell carcinoma that's refractory to chemotherapy and radiation. It's also used to harvest a healthy kidney for transplantation. When conservative treatments fail, nephrectomy may be used to treat renal trauma, infection, hypertension, hydronephrosis, and inoperable renal calculi.

One side or both

Nephrectomy may be unilateral or bilateral. Unilateral nephrectomy, the more commonly performed procedure, usually doesn't interfere with renal function as long as one healthy kidney remains. However, bilateral nephrectomy (or the removal of a lone kidney) requires lifelong dialysis or transplantation to support renal function.

Four major types of nephrectomy are performed:

Other than being a little lonely, I can still maintain function after unilateral nephrectomy.

✌ *partial nephrectomy* — involving resection of only a portion of the kidney

✌ *simple nephrectomy* — removal of the entire kidney

✌ *radical nephrectomy* — resection of the entire kidney and the surrounding fat tissue

✌ *nephroureterectomy* — removal of the entire kidney, the perinephric fat, and the entire ureter.

Patient preparation
• If the patient is having unilateral nephrectomy, reassure him that one healthy kidney is all he'll need for adequate function.
• If the surgery is bilateral or will remove the patient's only kidney, prepare him for radical changes in his lifestyle, most notably the need for regular dialysis.

Monitoring and aftercare
• Carefully monitor the rate, volume, and type of I.V. fluids. Keep in mind that mistakes in fluid therapy can be particularly devastating for a patient who has only one kidney.
• Check the patient's dressing and drain every 4 hours for the first 24 to 48 hours, then once every shift to assess the amount and nature of drainage. Maintain drain patency.

Home care instructions
Instruct the patient to:
• monitor intake and output and explain how this helps assess renal function
• follow the doctor's guidelines on fluid intake and dietary restrictions
• attend follow-up examinations to evaluate kidney function and assess for possible complications
• notify the doctor immediately if he detects any significant decrease in urine output, fever, chills, hematuria, or flank pain
• avoid strenuous exercise or heavy lifting and sexual activity until his doctor grants permission.

Suprapubic catheterization

Suprapubic catheterization is a type of urinary diversion connected to a closed drainage system that involves transcutaneous insertion of a catheter through the suprapubic area into the bladder. Typically, suprapubic catheterization provides temporary urinary diversion after certain gynecologic procedures, bladder surgery, or prostatectomy and relieves obstruction from calculi, severe urethral strictures, or pelvic trauma. Less commonly, it may be used to create a permanent urinary diversion, thereby relieving obstruction from an inoperable tumor.

Patient preparation
• Tell the patient that the doctor will insert a soft plastic tube through the skin of the abdomen and into the bladder and then connect the tube to an external collection bag.
• Explain that the procedure is done under local anesthesia, causes little or no discomfort, and takes 15 to 45 minutes.

Monitoring and aftercare
• To ensure adequate drainage and tube patency, check the suprapubic catheter at least hourly for the first 24 hours after insertion. Make sure the collection bag is below bladder level to enhance drainage and prevent backflow, which can lead to infection.
• Tape the catheter securely in place on the abdominal skin to reduce tension and prevent dislodgment. To prevent kinks in the tube, curve it gently but don't bend it.
• Check dressings often and change them at least once per day or as ordered. Observe the skin around the insertion site for signs of infection and encrustation.

Home care instructions
Instruct the patient to:
• change the dressing, and empty and reattach the collection bag
• drink plenty of fluids
• follow up with the doctor as recommended
• meet with the enterostomal therapist to help manage the urinary diversion
• notify the doctor promptly of signs of infection or encrustation, such as discolored or foul-smelling discharge, impaired drainage, and swelling, redness, and tenderness at the tube insertion site.

Transurethral resection of the bladder

A relatively quick and simple procedure, transurethral resection of the bladder (TURB) involves insertion of a resectoscope through

Suprapubic catheterization provides temporary or, less commonly, permanent urinary diversion.

the urethra and into the bladder to remove lesions. (It can also be performed using an Nd:YAG laser.) Most commonly performed to treat superficial and early bladder carcinoma, TURB may also be used to remove benign papillomas or to relieve fibrosis of the bladder neck. This treatment isn't indicated for large or infiltrating tumors or for metastatic bladder cancer.

Patient preparation
• Tell the patient that he'll receive a local anesthetic and be awake during treatment.
• Inform him that he'll have an indwelling urinary catheter in place for 1 to 5 days after the procedure to ensure urine drainage.

Monitoring and aftercare
• Maintain adequate fluid intake and provide meticulous catheter care, including frequent irrigation. (The doctor may prescribe continuous or intermittent irrigation, especially if the removal of a large vascular lesion has compromised hemostasis).
• Observe urine drainage for blood. Remember that slight hematuria usually occurs directly after TURB. However, notify the doctor immediately of any frank bleeding or if the hematuria seems excessive.
• Assess for signs and symptoms of bladder perforation, including abdominal pain and rigidity, fever, and decreased urine output despite adequate hydration.

Home care instructions
Instruct the patient to:
• report bleeding or hematuria that lasts longer than several weeks, fever, chills, or flank pain, which may indicate UTI
• drink plenty of water (10 glasses daily) and to void every 2 to 3 hours to reduce the risk of clot formation, urethral obstruction, and UTI
• heed the urge to urinate
• refrain from sexual or other strenuous activity, avoid lifting anything heavier than 10 lb (4.5 kg), and continue taking a stool softener or other laxative until the doctor orders otherwise
• follow up with the doctor as recommended.

Urinary diversion

A urinary diversion provides an alternate route for urine excretion when a disorder or abnormality impedes normal flow through the bladder. Most commonly performed in patients who have under-

> You'll receive a local anesthetic and you'll be awake during treatment.

Common urinary diversions

Various urinary diversions may be done for bladder cancer patients. Two of the most commonly performed types are the continent vesicostomy and the ileal conduit.

Continent vesicostomy

Also referred to as a Kock pouch, continent vesicostomy is an alternative to the ileal conduit. It allows urine to be diverted to a reservoir that has been reconstructed from part of the bladder wall. One end of the tube, formed from part of the bladder wall, is brought to the abdominal surface to form the stoma, through which the reservoir is emptied. At the internal end of this tube, a nipple valve is created from the bladder wall. The urethral neck is then sutured closed. Accumulated urine can be drained by inserting a catheter through the stoma into the bladder pouch.

Ileal conduit

An ileal conduit is the preferred procedure for diverting urine through a segment of the ileum to a stoma on the abdomen (as shown). In this procedure, a segment of the ileum is excised, and the two ends of the ileum that result from the excision of the segment are sutured closed. Then the ureters are dissected from the bladder and anastomosed to the ileal segment. One end of the ileal segment is closed with sutures; the opposite end is brought through the abdominal wall, thereby forming a stoma. Because urine empties continuously, the patient must wear a collecting device (or pouch).

Stoma

Restructured bladder pouch

Kidney

Ureter

Ileal conduit

Stoma

Anastomosis of ileum

gone total or partial cystectomy, diversion surgery may also be performed in patients with a congenital urinary tract defect or a severe, unmanageable UTI that threatens renal function; an injury to the ureters, bladder, or urethra; an obstructive malignant tumor; or a neurogenic bladder.

Several types of urinary diversion surgery can be performed. The two most common are ileal conduit and continent vesicostomy. (See *Common urinary diversions*.)

Patient preparation

• Prepare the patient for the appearance and general location of the stoma. If he's scheduled for an ileal conduit, explain that the stoma will be located somewhere in the lower abdomen, probably below the waistline. If he's scheduled for a cutaneous ureterosto-

my, explain that the exact stoma site is commonly chosen during surgery, based on the length of the patent ureter available.
• Review the enterostomal therapist's explanation of the urine collection device that the patient will use after surgery.

Monitoring and aftercare

• Carefully check and record urine output. Report any decrease, which could indicate obstruction from postoperative edema or ureteral stenosis.
• Perform routine ostomy maintenance. Make sure the collection device fits tightly around the stoma; allow no more than a ⅛″ (0.3 cm) margin of skin between the stoma and the device's faceplate. Regularly check the appearance of the stoma and peristomal skin.

Home care instructions

Instruct the patient to:
• properly perform stoma care or ostomy self-catheterization
• watch for and report signs and symptoms of complications, such as fever, chills, abdominal pain, and pus or blood in the urine
• keep scheduled follow-up appointments with the doctor and enterostomal therapist to evaluate stoma care and make any necessary changes in equipment
• contact a support group such as the United Ostomy Association.

Nursing diagnoses

When caring for patients with renal or urologic disorders, you'll find that several nursing diagnoses can be commonly used. These nursing diagnoses appear here, along with appropriate nursing interventions and rationales.

Deficient fluid volume

Related to actual loss, *Deficient fluid volume* can be associated with dialysis, ingestion of large amounts of diuretics, renal failure, or metabolic acidosis.

Expected outcomes

• Patient exhibits normal skin color and temperature.
• Patient produces adequate urine volume.
• Patient's urine specific gravity remains between 1.005 and 1.030.

Nursing interventions and rationales

• Monitor and record vital signs every 2 hours, or as often as necessary until stable. Then monitor and record vital signs every 4 hours. Tachycardia, dyspnea, or hypotension may indicate deficient fluid volume or electrolyte imbalance.
• Measure intake and output every 1 to 4 hours. Record and report significant changes. Include urine, stools, vomitus, wound drainage, and any other output. Low urine output and high specific gravity indicate hypovolemia.
• Administer fluids, blood or blood products, or plasma expanders to replace fluids and whole blood loss and to facilitate fluid movement into vascular space. Monitor and record effectiveness and any adverse effects.
• Weigh the patient at the same time daily to give more accurate and consistent data. Weight loss or gain is a good indicator of fluid status.
• Assess skin turgor and oral mucous membranes every 8 hours to check for dehydration. Give meticulous mouth care every 4 hours to avoid dehydrating mucous membranes.

Monitor and record vital signs every 2 hours, or as often as necessary until stable.

Excess fluid volume

Related to compromised regulatory mechanisms, *Excess fluid volume* can be associated with acute glomerulonephritis, acute or chronic renal failure, pyelonephritis, or other renal diseases.

Expected outcomes

• Patient's blood pressure is no lower than ____ mm Hg and no higher than ____ mm Hg.
• Patient demonstrates no signs of hyperkalemia on electrocardiogram (ECG).
• Patient maintains fluid intake of no more than ____ ml and output of no less than ____ ml.

Nursing interventions and rationales

• Monitor blood pressure, pulse rate, cardiac rhythm, temperature, and breath sounds at least once every 4 hours; record and report changes. Changed parameters may indicate altered fluid or electrolyte status.
• Carefully monitor intake, output, and urine specific gravity at least once every 4 hours. Intake greater than output and elevated specific gravity may indicate fluid retention or overload.

• Monitor BUN, creatinine, electrolyte, and hemoglobin (Hb) levels, and hematocrit (HCT). BUN and creatinine levels indicate renal function; electrolyte levels, Hb levels, and HCT help to indicate fluid status.

• Weigh the patient daily before breakfast, as ordered, to provide consistent readings. Check for signs of fluid retention, such as dependent edema, sacral edema, or ascites.

• Give fluids as ordered. Monitor I.V. flow rate carefully because excess I.V. fluids can worsen the patient's condition.

• If oral fluids are allowed, help the patient create a schedule for fluid intake. Patient involvement encourages compliance.

• Assess skin turgor to monitor for dehydration.

Monitor I.V. flow rate carefully because excess I.V. fluids can worsen the patient's condition.

Urge urinary incontinence

Related to decreased bladder capacity, *Urge urinary incontinence* may be associated with such conditions as acute bladder infection, bladder obstruction, and interstitial cystitis.

Expected outcomes

• Patient has decreased frequency of incontinence episodes.
• Patient states increased comfort.
• Patient demonstrates skill in managing incontinence.

Nursing interventions and rationales

• Observe voiding pattern and document intake and output to ensure correct fluid replacement therapy and provide information about the patient's ability to void adequately.

• Provide appropriate care for existing urologic conditions, monitor progress, and report the patient's responses to treatment. The patient should receive adequate and qualified care as well as understand and participate in care as much as possible.

• Unless contraindicated, maintain fluid intake of 3 qt (2.8 L)/day to moisten mucous membranes and ensure hydration; limit the patient to 5 oz (150 ml) after supper to reduce the need to void at night.

• Explain the urologic condition to the patient and his family; include instructions on preventive measures and the established bladder schedule. Patient education begins with educational assessment and depends on the nurse's establishment of a therapeutic relationship with the patient and his family.

Common renal and urologic disorders

This section discusses the most common renal and urologic disorders, including their causes, assessment findings, diagnostic tests, treatment, nursing interventions, patient-teaching recommendations, and evaluation criteria.

Acute poststreptococcal glomerulonephritis

Acute poststreptococcal glomerulonephritis is a bilateral inflammation of the glomeruli, commonly following a streptococcal infection. It's most common in boys ages 3 to 10 but can occur at any age. Up to 95% of children and up to 70% of adults fully recover; the rest may progress to chronic renal failure within months.

Acute poststreptococcal glomerulonephritis is most common in boys ages 3 to 10 but can occur at any age.

What causes it

- Streptococcal infection of the respiratory tract
- Impetigo
- Immunoglobulin (Ig) A nephropathy (Berger's disease)
- Lipoid nephrosis.

Pathophysiology

Acute poststreptococcal glomerulonephritis results from entrapment and collection of antigen-antibody complexes in the glomerular capillary membranes after infection with group A hemolytic streptococci. The antigens stimulate the formation of antibodies. Circulating antigen-antibody complexes become lodged in the glomerular capillaries.

Glomerular injury occurs when complexes initiate the release of immunologic substances that break down cells and increase membrane permeability. The severity of glomerular damage and renal insufficiency is related to the size, number, location, duration of exposure, and type of antigen-antibody complexes.

What to look for

Typically, this disorder begins within 1 to 3 weeks after untreated pharyngitis. The most common symptoms are:
- mild to moderate edema
- azotemia
- hematuria (smoke- or coffee-colored urine)
- oliguria (less than 400 ml/day)
- fatigue

- mild to severe hypertension
- sodium or water retention.

What tests tell you

These tests are used to diagnose acute poststreptococcal glomeru-lonephritis:
- Blood studies reveal elevated electrolyte, BUN, and creatinine levels.
- Urine studies reveal RBCs, WBCs, mixed cell casts, and protein.
- Elevated antistreptolysin-O titers (in 80% of patients), elevated streptozyme and anti-DNase B titers, and low serum complement levels verify recent streptococcal infection.
- A throat culture may also show group A beta-hemolytic strepto-cocci.
- KUB X-rays show bilateral kidney enlargement.

How it's treated

The goals of treatment are the relief of symptoms and the preven-tion of complications. Vigorous supportive care includes bed rest, fluid and dietary sodium restrictions as well as correction of electrolyte imbalances (possibly with dialysis, although this is rarely necessary). Therapy may include di-uretics such as furosemide to reduce extracellular fluid overload and an antihypertensive such as hy-dralazine. The use of antibiotics to prevent sec-ondary infection or transmission to others is con-troversial.

> Vigorous supportive care includes bed rest, sodium restrictions, and correction of electrolyte imbalances.

What to do

Because this disorder usually resolves within 2 weeks, patient care is primarily supportive:
- Promote bed rest during the acute phase. Allow the patient to resume normal activities gradually as symptoms subside.
- Monitor vital signs, electrolyte values, intake and output, and daily weight.
- Assess renal function daily through serum creatinine and BUN levels, and urine creatinine clearance.
- Watch for and immediately report signs of acute renal failure (such as oliguria, azotemia, and acidosis).
- Consult the dietitian to provide a diet high in calories and low in protein, sodium, potassium, and fluids.
- Evaluate the patient. After successful treatment, the patient has normal serum creatinine and BUN levels and a normal urine crea-tinine clearance and is free from complications. He's prepared to

follow a diet high in calories and low in protein and obtain the necessary follow-up examination. (See *Acute poststreptococcal glomerulonephritis teaching tips.*)

Acute pyelonephritis

One of the most common renal diseases, acute pyelonephritis is a sudden bacterial inflammation. It primarily affects the interstitial area, the renal pelvis and, less commonly, the renal tubules. With treatment and continued follow-up care, the prognosis is good. Extensive permanent damage is rare. (See *Understanding chronic pyelonephritis.*)

What causes it

Causes of chronic pyelonephritis include:
- infection
- hematogenous or lymphatic spread.

Risk increasers

Risk factors include:
- diagnostic and therapeutic use of instruments, as in catheterization, cystoscopy, or urologic surgery
- inability to empty the bladder
- urinary stasis
- urinary obstruction
- sexual activity (in women)

Understanding chronic pyelonephritis

Chronic pyelonephritis, or persistent inflammation of the kidneys, can scar the kidneys and may lead to chronic renal failure. Its cause may be bacterial, metastatic, or urogenous. This disease occurs most commonly in patients who are predisposed to recurrent acute pyelonephritis, such as those with urinary obstructions or vesicoureteral reflux.

Signs and symptoms
Patients with chronic pyelonephritis may have a childhood history of unexplained fevers or bed-wetting. Signs and symptoms include flank pain, anemia, low urine specific gravity, pro-

teinuria, leukocytes in urine and, especially in late stages, hypertension. Uremia rarely develops from chronic pyelonephritis, unless structural abnormalities exist in the urinary system. Bacteriuria may be intermittent. When no bacteria are found in the urine, diagnosis depends on excretory urography (where the renal pelvis may appear small and flattened) and renal biopsy.

Treatment
Treatment requires control of hypertension, elimination of the existing obstruction (when possible), and long-term antimicrobial therapy.

Education edge

Acute post-streptococcal glomerulonephritis teaching tips

- Stress the need for regular blood pressure, urine protein, and renal function assessments during the convalescent months to detect recurrence.
- Tell the patient that follow-up examinations are necessary to detect chronic renal failure. After the disorder resolves, hematuria may recur during nonspecific viral infections; abnormal urinary findings may persist for years.
- Advise the patient with a history of chronic upper respiratory tract infections to report immediately signs of infection (such as fever or sore throat).
- Encourage a pregnant woman with a history of the disorder to have frequent medical evaluations because pregnancy further stresses the kidneys and increases the risk of chronic renal failure.

- use of diaphragms and condoms with spermicidal gel
- pregnancy
- diabetes
- other renal diseases.

Pathophysiology

Typically, the infection spreads from the bladder to the ureters, then to the kidneys. Bacteria refluxed to intrarenal tissues may create colonies of infection within 24 to 48 hours.

What to look for

Signs and symptoms of pyelonephritis include:
- urinary urgency and frequency
- burning during urination
- dysuria, nocturia, hematuria
- cloudy urine with an ammonia or fish odor
- temperature of 102° F (38.9 C) or higher
- shaking chills
- flank pain
- anorexia
- general fatigue.

What tests tell you

- Urinalysis reveals pyuria and, possibly, a few RBCs; low specific gravity and osmolality; slightly alkaline pH; and, possibly, proteinuria, glycosuria, and ketonuria.
- Urine culture reveals more than 100,000 organisms/μl of urine.
- KUB radiography may reveal calculi, tumors, or cysts in the kidneys and the urinary tract.
- Excretory urography may show asymmetrical kidneys.

How it's treated

Therapy centers on antibiotic therapy appropriate to the specific infecting organism, after identification by urine culture and sensitivity studies. When the infecting organism can't be identified, therapy usually consists of a broad-spectrum antibiotic. If the patient is pregnant, antibiotics must be prescribed cautiously. Urinary analgesics, such as phenazopyridine, are also appropriate.

Symptoms may disappear after several days of antibiotic therapy. Although urine usually becomes sterile within 48 to 72 hours, the course of such therapy is 10 to 14 days. Follow-up treatment includes reculturing urine 1 week after drug therapy stops, then periodically for the next year to detect residual or recurring infection. Most patients with uncomplicated infections respond well to therapy and don't suffer reinfection.

Infection from obstruction or vesicoureteral reflux may be less responsive to antibiotics. Treatment may then necessitate surgery to relieve the obstruction or correct the anomaly. Patients at high risk for recurring UTIs and kidney infections, such as those using an indwelling urinary catheter for a prolonged period and those on maintenance antibiotic therapy, require long-term follow-up care.

What to do

• Administer antipyretics for fever.
• Encourage increased fluid intake to achieve a urine output of more than 2,000 ml (2 qt)/day. Don't encourage intake of more than 2 to 3 qt (2 to 3 L) because this may decrease the effectiveness of antibiotics.
• Evaluate the patient. The recovering patient has a normal temperature, has no urinary discomfort or flank pain, forces fluids, and takes antibiotics as prescribed. (See *Acute pyelonephritis teaching tips*.)

Acute renal failure

Acute renal failure (ARF) is the sudden interruption of kidney function from obstruction, reduced circulation, or renal parenchymatous disease. It's usually reversible with treatment. Otherwise, it can progress to end-stage renal disease, uremic syndrome, or death.

What causes it

ARF may be classified as prerenal, intrarenal, or postrenal. Each type has separate causes. (See *Causes of ARF,* page 588.)

Pathophysiology

Prerenal failure results from conditions that damage blood flow to the kidneys (hypoperfusion). When renal blood flow is interrupted, so is oxygen delivery. The ensuing hypoxemia and ischemia can rapidly and irreversibly damage the kidney. The tubules are most susceptible to the effects of hypoxemia.

Intrarenal failure results from damage to the filtering structures of the kidneys. Causes of intrarenal failure are classified as nephrotoxic, inflammatory, or ischemic. When the damage is caused by nephrotoxicity or inflammation, the delicate layer un-

Education edge

Acute pyelonephritis teaching tips

• Teach proper technique for collecting a clean-catch urine specimen. Tell the patient to be sure to refrigerate a urine specimen within 30 minutes of collection to prevent overgrowth of bacteria.
• Stress the need to complete the prescribed antibiotic therapy even after symptoms subside.
• Advise routine checkups for a patient with chronic urinary tract infections. Teach the patient to recognize signs and symptoms of infection, such as cloudy urine, burning on urination, and urinary urgency and frequency, especially when accompanied by a low-grade fever.
• Encourage long-term follow-up care for high-risk patients.

Causes of ARF

Acute renal failure (ARF) is classified as prerenal, intrarenal, or postrenal. All conditions that lead to prerenal failure impair blood flow to the kidneys (renal perfusion), resulting in decreased glomerular filtration rate and increased tubular reabsorption of sodium and water. Intrarenal failure results from damage to the kidneys themselves; postrenal failure, from obstructed urine flow. This table shows the causes of each type of ARF.

Prerenal failure

Cardiovascular disorders
- Arrhythmias
- Cardiac tamponade
- Cardiogenic shock
- Heart failure
- Myocardial infarction

Hypovolemia
- Burns
- Dehydration
- Diuretic overuse
- Hemorrhage
- Hypovolemic shock
- Trauma

Peripheral vasodilation
- Antihypertensive drugs
- Sepsis

Renovascular obstruction
- Arterial embolism
- Arterial or venous thrombosis
- Tumor

Severe vasoconstriction
- Disseminated intravascular coagulation
- Eclampsia
- Malignant hypertension
- Vasculitis

Intrarenal failure

Acute tubular necrosis
- Ischemic damage to renal parenchyma from unrecognized or poorly treated prerenal failure
- Nephrotoxins, including anesthetics such as methoxyflurane, antibiotics such as gentamicin, and heavy metals, such as lead, radiographic contrast media, and organic solvents
- Obstetric complications, such as eclampsia, postpartum renal failure, septic abortion, and uterine hemorrhage
- Pigment release, such as crush injury, myopathy, sepsis, and transfusion reaction

Other parenchymal disorders
- Acute glomerulonephritis
- Acute interstitial nephritis
- Acute pyelonephritis
- Bilateral renal vein thrombosis
- Malignant nephrosclerosis
- Papillary necrosis
- Periarteritis nodosa (inflammatory disease of the arteries)
- Renal myeloma
- Sickle cell disease
- Systemic lupus erythematosus
- Vasculitis

Postrenal failure

Bladder obstruction
- Anticholinergic drugs
- Autonomic nerve dysfunction
- Infection
- Tumor

Ureteral obstruction
- Blood clots
- Calculi
- Edema or inflammation
- Necrotic renal papillae
- Retroperitoneal fibrosis or hemorrhage
- Surgery (accidental ligation)
- Tumor
- Uric acid crystals

Urethral obstruction
- Prostatic hyperplasia or tumor
- Strictures

der the epithelium (the basement membrane) becomes irreparably damaged, typically leading to chronic renal failure. Severe or prolonged lack of blood flow by ischemia may lead to renal damage (ischemic parenchymal injury) and excess nitrogen in the blood (intrinsic renal azotemia).

Postrenal failure is a consequence of bilateral obstruction of urine outflow. The cause may be in the bladder, ureters, or urethra.

What to look for

Signs and symptoms of acute renal failure include:
- oliguria (usually the earliest sign)
- anorexia
- nausea and vomiting
- diarrhea or constipation
- stomatitis
- GI bleeding
- hematemesis
- dry mucous membranes
- uremic breath
- hypotension.

Oliguria is usually the earliest sign of acute renal failure.

What tests tell you

- Blood studies reveal elevated BUN, creatinine, and potassium levels as well as low pH, bicarbonate levels, Hb levels, and HCT.
- Urine specimens show casts, cellular debris, decreased specific gravity and, in glomerular diseases, proteinuria and urine osmolality close to serum osmolality. Urine sodium level is less than 20 mEq/L if oliguria results from decreased perfusion; greater than 40 mEq/L if it results from an intrinsic problem.
- Creatinine clearance test measures the GFR and is used to estimate the number of remaining functioning nephrons.
- Other studies include ultrasonography of the kidneys, renal scan, CT scan, retrograde pyelography, MRI, and plain films of the abdomen, kidneys, ureters, and bladder.

How it's treated

The major goals for ARF are to reestablish effective renal function, if possible, and to maintain the constancy of the internal environment despite transient renal failure. Supportive measures include a diet high in calories and low in protein, sodium, and potassium, with supplemental vitamins and restricted fluids. Meticulous electrolyte monitoring is essential to detect hyperkalemia.

If hyperkalemia occurs, acute therapy may include dialysis, sodium bicarbonate, and hypertonic glucose and insulin infusions, all administered I.V. Sodium polystyrene sulfonate can be administered by mouth or by enema to remove potassium from the body.

If these measures fail to control uremic symptoms, hemodialysis or peritoneal dialysis may be necessary.

What to do

• Measure and record intake and output, including all body fluids, such as wound drainage, nasogastric output, and diarrhea. Weigh the patient daily.
• Assess HCT and Hb level and replace blood components as ordered. Don't use whole blood if the patient is prone to heart failure and can't tolerate extra fluid volume.
• Monitor vital signs.
• Watch for and report any signs or symptoms of pericarditis (such as pleuritic chest pain, tachycardia, and pericardial friction rub), inadequate renal perfusion (such as hypotension), or acidosis.
• Maintain the patient's nutritional status. Provide a high-calorie, low-protein, low-sodium, and low-potassium diet, with vitamin supplements. Give the anorectic patient small, frequent meals.

Days with malaise

• Maintain electrolyte balance. Strictly monitor potassium levels. Watch for symptoms of hyperkalemia (such as malaise, anorexia, paresthesia, and muscle weakness) and ECG changes (including tall, peaked T waves, widening QRS segment, and disappearing P waves) and report them immediately. Avoid administering medications containing potassium.
• Assist with peritoneal dialysis or hemodialysis as needed.
• Evaluate the patient. After successful treatment, the patient has no weight gain, has stable vital signs, exhibits no complications or signs of infection, talks openly about his illness, and has normal blood values. The patient is prepared to follow his diet and any necessary medical regimen at home. (See *ARF teaching tips*.)

Education edge

ARF teaching tips

• Instruct the patient to follow a high-calorie, low-protein, low-sodium, and low-potassium diet with vitamin supplements.
• If the patient requires dialysis, explain what equipment is used during treatment and the monitoring that's involved with any type of dialysis.
• Explain the importance of fluid restriction and the need for daily weight measurements.

Chronic glomerulonephritis

Chronic glomerulonephritis, a slowly progressive, noninfectious disease, is characterized by inflammation of the renal glomeruli. It remains subclinical until the progressive phase begins. By the time it produces symptoms, it's usually irreversible. It results in eventual renal failure.

What causes it

• Membranoproliferative glomerulonephritis
• Membranous glomerulopathy

By the time symptoms of chronic glomerulonephritis appear, it's usually irreversible. Ugh.

- Focal glomerulosclerosis
- Poststreptococcal glomerulonephritis

Blame the system

Systemic causes include:
- lupus erythematosus
- Goodpasture's syndrome
- hemolytic uremic syndrome.

Pathophysiology

The inflammation of the glomeruli that occurs with this condition results in sclerosis, scarring, and eventual renal failure.

What to look for

This disease usually develops insidiously and without producing symptoms, commonly over many years. At any time, however, it may suddenly become progressive. The initial stage includes:
- nephrotic syndrome
- hypertension
- proteinuria
- hematuria.

Late-stage findings include azotemia, nausea, vomiting, pruritus, dyspnea, malaise, fatigability, mild to severe anemia, and severe hypertension, which may cause cardiac hypertrophy, leading to heart failure.

What tests tell you

- Urinalysis reveals proteinuria, hematuria, cylindruria, and RBC casts.
- Blood tests reveal rising BUN and serum creatinine levels, indicating advanced renal insufficiency.
- X-ray or ultrasound examination shows small kidneys.

How it's treated

Treatment is essentially nonspecific and symptomatic. The goals are to control hypertension with antihypertensives and a sodium-restricted diet, correct fluid and electrolyte imbalances through restrictions and replacement, reduce edema with diuretics such as furosemide, and prevent heart failure. Treatment may also include antibiotics (for symptomatic UTIs), dialysis, or transplantation.

I'll take the low-sodium special, please!

What to do

Patient care is primarily supportive, focusing on continual observation and sound patient teaching:

• Monitor vital signs, intake and output, and daily weight to evaluate fluid retention. Observe for signs of fluid, electrolyte, and acid-base imbalances.

• Consult the dietitian to plan low-sodium, high-calorie meals with adequate protein.

• Administer medications as ordered, and provide good oral hygiene and skin care (because of pruritus and edema).

• Evaluate the patient. After successful treatment, the patient has normal vital signs and hasn't gained weight after complying with his diet and medication regimen. He shows no signs of complications, is prepared to follow dietary and medical regimens at home, verbalizes openly regarding his illness, and exhibits good understanding of necessary procedures. (See *Chronic glomerulonephritis teaching tips*.)

Chronic renal failure

Typically the result of a gradually progressive loss of renal function, chronic renal failure occasionally results from a rapidly progressive disease of sudden onset. Few symptoms develop until after more than 75% of glomerular filtration is lost. Then the remaining normal parenchyma deteriorate progressively, and symptoms worsen as renal function decreases. If this condition continues unchecked, uremic toxins accumulate and produce potentially fatal physiologic changes in all major organ systems.

What causes it

Causes of chronic renal failure include:

• chronic glomerular disease such as glomerulonephritis

• chronic infections, such as chronic pyelonephritis and tuberculosis

• congenital anomalies such as polycystic kidney disease

• vascular diseases, such as renal nephrosclerosis and hypertension

• obstructive processes such as calculi

• collagen diseases such as systemic lupus erythematosus

• nephrotoxic agents such as long-term aminoglycoside therapy

• endocrine diseases such as diabetic neuropathy

• acute renal failure that fails to respond to treatment.

Education edge

Chronic glomerulonephritis teaching tips

• Instruct the patient to continue taking prescribed antihypertensives as scheduled, even if he's feeling better, and to report any adverse effects.

• Advise the patient to take diuretics in the morning so that sleep won't be disrupted to void. Teach the patient how to assess ankle edema.

• Warn the patient to report signs of infection, particularly urinary tract infection, and to avoid contact with infectious people.

• Urge follow-up examinations to assess renal function. Help the patient adjust to this illness by encouraging him to express his feelings.

• Explain all necessary procedures beforehand and answer the patient's questions about them.

Pathophysiology

Nephron damage is progressive. When nephrons are damaged, they can't function. Healthy nephrons compensate for damaged nephrons by enlarging and increasing their clearance capacity. The kidneys can maintain relatively normal function until about 75% of the nephrons are nonfunctional.

Eventually, the healthy glomeruli are so overburdened they become sclerotic and stiff, leading to their destruction as well. If this condition continues unchecked, toxins accumulate and produce potentially fatal changes in all major organ systems.

What to look for

The degree of renal failure partly determines the frequency and severity of clinical manifestations. (See *Effects of chronic renal failure*, page 594.)

What tests tell you

- Creatinine clearance tests can identify the stage of chronic renal failure. Reduced renal reserve occurs when the creatinine clearance GFR is 40 to 70 ml/minute. Renal insufficiency occurs at a GFR of 20 to 40 ml/minute, renal failure at a GFR of 10 to 20 ml/minute, and end-stage renal disease at a GFR of less than 10 ml/minute.
- Blood studies show elevated BUN, creatinine, and potassium levels; decreased arterial pH and bicarbonate levels; and low Hb level and HCT.
- Urine specific gravity becomes fixed at 1.010; urinalysis may show proteinuria, glycosuria, erythrocytes, leukocytes, and casts, depending on the cause.
- X-ray studies include KUB films, excretory urography, nephrotomography, renal scan, and renal arteriography.
- Kidney biopsy allows histologic identification of the underlying abnormality.

How it's treated

The major goal of treatment early in the disease is to preserve existing kidney function and to correct specific symptoms. Conservative measures include a low-protein diet to reduce the production of end products of protein metabolism that the kidneys can't excrete. However, a patient receiving continuous peritoneal dialysis should have a high-protein diet. A high-calorie diet prevents ketoacidosis and the negative nitrogen balance that results in catabolism and tissue atrophy. Such a diet also restricts sodium and

Effects of chronic renal failure

Here are effects of chronic renal failure by body system.

Renal and urologic system
- Initially, hypotension, dry mouth, loss of skin turgor, listlessness, fatigue, and nausea from salt wasting and consequent hyponatremia
- Later, somnolence and confusion
- Salt retention and overload due to the decrease in functioning nephrons and the kidneys' subsequent inability to excrete sodium
- Muscle irritability, then weakness from accumulation of potassium
- Fluid overload from sodium retention and metabolic acidosis from loss of bicarbonate
- Decreased urine output with dilute urine that contains casts and crystals

Cardiovascular system
- Hypertension
- Arrhythmias (including life-threatening ventricular tachycardia and fibrillation)
- Cardiomyopathy
- Uremic pericarditis
- Pericardial effusion with possible cardiac tamponade
- Heart failure and peripheral edema

Respiratory system
- Reduced pulmonary macrophage activity
- Increased susceptibility to infection, pulmonary edema, pleuritic pain, pleural friction rub and effusions, uremic pleuritis and uremic lung (or uremic pneumonitis), dyspnea from heart failure, and Kussmaul's respirations as a result of acidosis

GI system
- Inflammation and ulceration of GI mucosa causing stomatitis, gum ulceration and bleeding and, possibly, parotitis, esophagitis, gastritis, duodenal ulcers, lesions on the small and large bowel, uremic colitis, pancreatitis, and proctitis
- Metallic taste in the mouth
- Uremic fetor (ammonia smell on breath)
- Anorexia
- Nausea and vomiting

Skin
- Typically, pallid, yellowish bronze, dry, and scaly
- Severe itching
- Purpura
- Ecchymoses
- Petechiae
- Uremic frost (usually in critically ill or terminally ill patients)
- Thin, brittle fingernails with characteristic lines
- Dry, brittle hair that may change color and fall out easily

Neurologic system
- Restless leg syndrome, one of the first signs of peripheral neuropathy, causing pain, burning, and itching in the legs and feet, which may be relieved by voluntarily shaking, moving, or rocking
- Eventually, paresthesia and motor nerve dysfunction (usually bilateral footdrop) unless dialysis is initiated
- Muscle cramping and twitching
- Shortened memory and attention span
- Apathy, drowsiness, irritability, confusion

- Coma
- Seizures
- EEG changes that indicate metabolic encephalopathy

Endocrine system
- Stunted growth patterns in children (even with elevated growth hormone levels)
- Infertility and decreased libido in both sexes
- Amenorrhea and cessation of menses in women
- Impotence and decreased sperm production in men
- Increased aldosterone secretion
- Impaired carbohydrate metabolism

Hematopoietic system
- Anemia
- Decreased red blood cell survival time
- Blood loss from dialysis and GI bleeding
- Mild thrombocytopenia
- Platelet defects
- Increased bleeding and clotting disorders, demonstrated by purpura, hemorrhage from body orifices, easy bruising, ecchymoses, and petechiae

Musculoskeletal system
- Muscle and bone pain, skeletal demineralization, pathologic fractures, and calcifications in the brain, eyes, gums, joints, myocardium, and blood vessels caused by calcium-phosphorus imbalance and consequent parathyroid hormone imbalances
- Coronary artery disease due to arterial calcification
- Renal osteodystrophy in children

potassium. Maintaining fluid balance requires careful monitoring of vital signs, weight changes, and urine output.

Send in the drugs

Drug therapy commonly relieves associated symptoms, but dosages may need to be adjusted in medications excreted by the kidneys. If antacids are used, avoid those that are magnesium-based. Antacids and laxatives containing magnesium must be avoided to prevent magnesium toxicity. Drugs commonly used to treat chronic renal failure include:
• antipruritics, such as diphenhydramine to relieve itching, and calcium carbonate to lower serum phosphate levels.
• vitamin supplements (particularly B vitamins and vitamin D) and essential amino acids to relieve deficiencies caused by inadequate intake (from anorexia or dietary restrictions), altered metabolism (from uremia and medications), or increased losses of vitamins during dialysis.
• loop diuretics, such as furosemide (if some renal function remains), along with fluid restriction to reduce fluid retention
• digoxin to mobilize edema fluids
• antihypertensives to control blood pressure and associated edema
• antiemetics taken before meals to relieve nausea and vomiting
• famotidine or nizatidine to decrease gastric irritation
• docusate to help prevent constipation.

Anemia and related troubles

Anemia necessitates iron and folate supplements; severe anemia requires infusion of fresh frozen packed cells or washed packed cells. Even so, transfusions only temporarily relieve anemia. Epoetin alfa may be administered to increase RBC production. Treatment may also include cleansing enemas to remove blood from the GI tract detected through regular stool analysis (guaiac test).

Dialysis dilemmas

Hemodialysis or peritoneal dialysis—particularly such techniques as continuous ambulatory peritoneal dialysis and continuous cyclic peritoneal dialysis—can help control most manifestations of end-stage renal disease. Altering dialyzing bath fluids can correct fluid and electrolyte disturbances. However, anemia, peripheral neuropathy, cardiopulmonary and GI complications, sexual dysfunction, and skeletal defects may persist. In addition, maintenance dialysis may produce complications, such as protein wast-

> Maintaining fluid balance requires careful monitoring of vital signs, weight changes, and urine output.

ing, refractory ascites, dialysis dementia, and hepatitis B from numerous blood transfusions.

What to do

• Monitor potassium levels.
• Assess hydration status carefully. Check for jugular vein distention and auscultate the lungs for crackles. Measure daily intake and output carefully. Record daily weight and the presence or absence of thirst, axillary sweat, dry tongue, hypertension, and peripheral edema.
• Observe for signs of bleeding.
• If the patient requires dialysis, explain the procedure fully and watch for complications during and after the procedure.
• Evaluate the patient. After successful therapy, the patient verbalizes an understanding of the disease process and medical regimen, exhibits no signs of complications, and has his symptoms controlled by dialysis or transplantation. He has normal BUN, creatinine, and electrolyte levels and maintains a satisfactory diet with normal bowel function. (See *Chronic renal failure teaching tips*.)

Lower UTIs

Lower UTIs commonly respond readily to treatment, but recurrence and resistant bacterial flare-up during therapy are possible. Lower UTIs are nearly 10 times more common in women than in men and affect 1 in 5 women at least once. Lower UTIs also occur in relatively large percentages in sexually active teenage girls. Lower UTIs fall into two types:

 cystitis, which is an inflammation of the bladder that usually results from an ascending infection

urethritis, which is an inflammation of the urethra.

What causes it

• Infection by gram-negative enteric bacteria, such as *Escherichia coli*, *Klebsiella*, *Proteus*, *Enterobacter*, *Pseudomonas*, or *Serratia*
• Simultaneous infection with multiple pathogens in a patient with neurogenic bladder
• Indwelling urinary catheter

Lower UTIs are nearly 10 times more common in women than in men.

• Fistula between the intestine and bladder

Pathophysiology

Recent studies suggest that infection results from a breakdown in local defense mechanisms in the bladder that allows bacteria to invade the bladder mucosa and multiply. These bacteria can't be readily eliminated by normal micturition.

What to look for

Characteristic signs and symptoms include:
• urinary urgency and frequency
• dysuria
• bladder cramps or spasms
• itching
• feeling of warmth during urination
• nocturia
• possibly hematuria
• fever
• urethral discharge in males.

   Other common features include lower back pain, malaise, confusion, nausea, vomiting, abdominal pain or tenderness over the bladder, chills, and flank pain.

Urine specimen revealing a bacterial count of more than 100,000/ml confirms UTI.

What tests tell you

• Microscopic urinalysis showing RBC and WBC levels greater than 10/high-power field points to UTI. A clean midstream urine specimen revealing a bacterial count of more than 100,000/ml confirms it. Sensitivity testing suggests the appropriate therapeutic antimicrobial agent.
• A blood test or stained smear rules out venereal disease.
• Voiding cystourethrography or excretory urography may detect congenital anomalies.

How it's treated

A 7-day to 10-day course of an appropriate antibiotic usually represents the treatment of choice for initial lower UTI. After 3 days of antibiotic therapy, urine culture should show no organisms. If the urine isn't sterile, bacterial resistance has probably occurred, making the use of a different antimicrobial necessary. Single-dose antibiotic therapy with amoxicillin or co-trimoxazole may be effective in women with acute noncomplicated UTI. A urine culture taken 1 to 2 weeks later indicates whether the infection has been eradicated.

It's back

Recurrent infections caused by renal calculi, chronic prostatitis, or a structural abnormality may require surgery. If there are no predisposing conditions, long-term, low-dose antibiotic therapy is preferred.

What to do

• Collect all urine specimens for culture and sensitivity testing carefully and promptly.
• Watch for GI disturbances from antibiotic therapy. Nitrofurantoin macrocrystals, taken with milk or a meal, prevent such distress.
• Evaluate the patient. After successful treatment, the patient can explain the relation between personal hygiene and UTIs. She can describe hygiene practices to prevent UTIs and has completed the prescribed course of antibiotic therapy. (See *Lower UTI teaching tips.*)

Nephrotic syndrome

Nephrotic syndrome (NS) is a condition characterized by marked proteinuria, hypoalbuminemia, hyperlipidemia, and edema. Although NS isn't a disease itself, it results from a specific glomerular defect and indicates renal damage.

What causes it

• Primary (idiopathic) glomerulonephritis (affecting children and adults)
• Diabetes mellitus
• Collagen vascular disorders
• Circulatory diseases
• Nephrotoxins
• Allergic reactions
• Infection
• Pregnancy
• Hereditary nephritis
• Multiple myeloma and other neoplastic diseases

Pathophysiology

Regardless of the cause, the injured glomerular filtration membrane allows the loss of plasma proteins, especially albumin and immunoglobulin. Hypoalbuminemia results not only from urine loss but also from decreased hepatic synthesis of replacement albumin. Hypoalbuminemia stimulates the liver to synthesize lipoprotein (with consequent hyperlipidemia) and clotting factors. Decreased dietary intake (as with anorexia, malnutrition, or concomitant disease) further contributes to decreased plasma albumin levels. Loss of immunoglobulin also increases susceptibility to infection.

Runnin' on empty

Extensive proteinuria (more than 3.5 g/day) and a low serum albumin level lead to low serum colloid osmotic pressure and edema. The low serum albumin level also leads to hypovolemia and compensatory salt and water retention. Consequent hypertension may precipitate heart failure in compromised patients. (See *What happens in nephrotic syndrome.*)

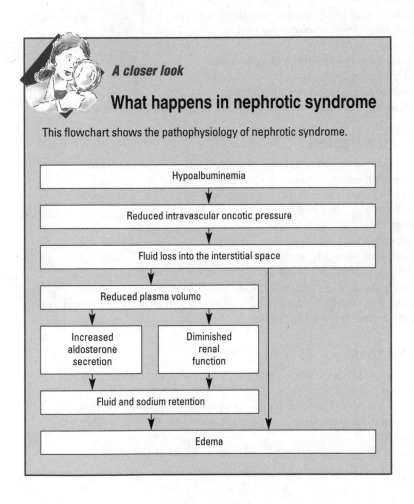

A closer look

What happens in nephrotic syndrome

This flowchart shows the pathophysiology of nephrotic syndrome.

Hypoalbuminemia

↓

Reduced intravascular oncotic pressure

↓

Fluid loss into the interstitial space

↓

Reduced plasma volume

↓

| Increased aldosterone secretion | Diminished renal function |

↓

Fluid and sodium retention

↓

Edema

What to look for

The dominant clinical feature in NS is mild to severe dependent edema of the ankles or sacrum or periorbital edema, especially in children. It may lead to ascites, pleural effusion, and swollen external genitalia. Other signs and symptoms include:

- foamy urine
- orthostatic hypotension
- lethargy
- anorexia
- depression
- pallor.

The dominant clinical feature of nephrotic syndrome is dependent edema of the ankles or sacrum.

What tests tell you

- Urine testing that reveals consistent proteinuria in excess of 3.5 g/day; an increased number of hyaline, granular, and waxy, fatty casts; and oval fat bodies strongly suggests NS.
- Increased cholesterol, phospholipid, and triglyceride levels and decreased albumin levels support the diagnosis.
- Histologic identification of the lesion requires kidney biopsy.

How it's treated

Effective treatment necessitates correction of the underlying cause if possible. Supportive treatment consists of:

- protein replacement with a nutritional diet of 1 g of protein per kilogram of body weight
- restricted sodium intake
- diuretics for edema
- antibiotics for infection.

Some patients respond to an 8-week course of corticosteroid therapy (such as prednisone), followed by a maintenance dose. Others respond better to a combination course of prednisone and azathioprine or cyclophosphamide.

What to do

- Frequently check urine for protein. (Urine that contains protein appears frothy.)
- Measure blood pressure while the patient is supine and while he's standing; immediately report a drop in blood pressure that exceeds 20 mm Hg.
- Monitor intake and output and check weight at the same time each morning.

• Ask the dietitian to plan a moderate-protein, low-sodium diet.
• Provide good skin care because the patient with NS usually has edema.
• To avoid thrombophlebitis, encourage activity and exercise and provide antiembolism stockings as ordered.
• To prevent GI complications, administer steroids with an antacid or with cimetidine or ranitidine.
• Evaluate the patient. After successful therapy, the patient is prepared to follow dietary and medical regimens at home, has no proteinuria, and exhibits no signs of complications. (See *Nephrotic syndrome teaching tips*.)

Education edge

Nephrotic syndrome teaching tips

• Watch for and teach the patient and his family how to recognize adverse effects of drug therapy, such as bone marrow toxicity from cytotoxic immunosuppressants and cushingoid symptoms from long-term steroid therapy.
• Because a steroid crisis may occur if the drug is discontinued abruptly, explain that steroid-related adverse effects will subside when therapy stops.
• Refer the patient and his family to appropriate counseling and support groups.

Neurogenic bladder

Neurogenic bladder refers to any bladder dysfunction caused by an interruption of normal bladder innervation. Other names for this disorder include neuromuscular dysfunction of the lower urinary tract, neurologic bladder dysfunction, and neuropathic bladder.

What causes it

Neurogenic bladder appears to stem from a host of underlying conditions, including:
• interstitial cystitis, cerebral disorders (such as stroke), brain tumor (such as meningioma and glioma), Parkinson's disease, multiple sclerosis, dementia, and incontinence from aging
• spinal cord disease or trauma (such as spinal stenosis and arachnoiditis), cervical spondylosis, myelopathies from hereditary disorders or nutritional deficiencies and, rarely, tabes dorsalis
• disorders of peripheral innervation, including autonomic neuropathies resulting from endocrine disturbances such as diabetes mellitus (most common)
• metabolic disturbances such as hypothyroidism
• acute infectious diseases such as Guillain-Barré syndrome
• heavy metal toxicity
• chronic alcoholism
• collagen diseases such as lupus erythematosus
• vascular diseases such as atherosclerosis
• distant effects of cancer such as primary oat cell carcinoma of the lung
• herpes zoster.

Pathophysiology

An upper motor neuron lesion (at or above T12) causes spastic neurogenic bladder. A lower motor neuron lesion (at or below S2 to S4) affects the spinal reflex that controls voiding, with a resulting flaccid neurogenic bladder. Mixed neurogenic bladder results from an incomplete upper motor neuron, the result of cortical damage from some disorder or trauma.

What to look for

Neurogenic bladder produces a wide range of clinical effects depending on the underlying cause and its effect on the structural integrity of the bladder. All types of neurogenic bladder are associated with:
• some degree of incontinence
• changes in initiation or interruption of micturition
• an inability to empty the bladder completely.
  Vesicoureteral reflux, deterioration or infection in the upper urinary tract, and hydroureteral nephrosis may also result.

Spastic characteristics

Spastic neurogenic bladder symptoms depend on the site and extent of the spinal cord lesion. They may include:
• involuntary, frequent, scant urination without a feeling of bladder fullness
• spontaneous spasms of the arms and legs
• increased anal sphincter tone
• voiding and spontaneous contractions of the arms and legs with tactile stimulation of the abdomen, thighs, or genitalia
• severe hypertension, bradycardia, and headaches, with bladder distention if cord lesions are in the upper thoracic (cervical) level.

Spastic neurogenic bladder symptoms depend on the site and extent of the spinal cord lesion.

Flaccid features

Clinical features of flaccid neurogenic bladder include:
• overflow incontinence
• diminished anal sphincter tone
• greatly distended bladder (evident on percussion or palpation) without the accompanying feeling of bladder fullness because of sensory impairment.

In the mix

Symptoms of mixed neurogenic bladder include:
• dulled perception of bladder fullness and a diminished ability to empty the bladder
• urgency to void without control of the bladder.

What tests tell you

Because the causes of neurogenic bladder vary, diagnosis includes various tests:

• Cerebrospinal fluid analysis showing increased protein levels may indicate cord tumor; increased gamma globulin levels may indicate multiple sclerosis.
• Skull and vertebral column X-rays show fracture, dislocation, congenital anomalies, or metastasis.
• Myelography may show spinal cord compression.
• EEG may be abnormal if a brain tumor exists.
• Electromyelography confirms peripheral neuropathy.
• Brain and CT scans localize and identify brain masses.

Check the bladder

Other tests assess bladder function:
• Cystometry evaluates bladder nerve supply and detrusor muscle tone.
• A urethral pressure profile determines urethral function.
• Uroflowmetry shows diminished or impaired urine flow.
• Retrograde urethrography reveals strictures and diverticula.
• Voiding cystourethrography evaluates bladder neck function and continence.
• Postvoid residual determination test measures the amount of urine remaining in the bladder using a catheter or bladder ultrasonography.

How it's treated

Bladder evacuation, drug therapy, surgery or, less commonly, neural blocks and electrical stimulation aim to maintain the integrity of the upper urinary tract, control infection, and prevent urinary incontinence.

Drug therapy may include oxybutynin, bethanechol, and phenoxybenzamine to facilitate bladder emptying and propantheline, methantheline, flavoxate, dicyclomine, and imipramine to facilitate urine storage. When drug therapy fails, structural impairment may be repaired through transurethral resection of the bladder neck, urethral dilation, external sphincterotomy, or urinary diversion procedures. Implantation of an artificial urinary sphincter may be necessary if permanent incontinence follows surgery.

What to do

• Watch for signs of infection (such as fever and cloudy or foul-smelling urine).
• Encourage the patient to drink plenty of fluids to prevent calculus formation and infection from urinary stasis. Try to keep the patient as mobile as possible.

Treatment of neurogenic bladder aims to maintain upper urinary tract integrity, control infection, and prevent urinary incontinence.

• If a urinary diversion procedure is to be performed, arrange for consultation with an enterostomal therapist and coordinate the plans of care.

• Evaluate the patient. After successful therapy, the patient is free from infection, is continent, and verbalizes an understanding of his condition and the treatment techniques. (See *Neurogenic bladder teaching tips*.)

Renal calculi

Renal calculi may form anywhere in the urinary tract but usually develop in the renal pelvis or calyces. Such formation follows precipitation of substances normally dissolved in the urine (calcium oxalate, calcium phosphate, magnesium ammonium phosphate or, occasionally, urate or cystine). Renal calculi vary in size and may be solitary or multiple. They may remain in the renal pelvis or enter the ureter and may damage renal parenchyma. Large calculi cause pressure necrosis. In certain locations, calculi cause obstruction (with resultant hydronephrosis) and tend to recur. (See *A close look at renal calculi*.)

What causes it

Renal calculi may result from:

• *dehydration.* Decreased urine production concentrates calculus-forming substances.

• *infection.* Infected, damaged tissue serves as a site for calculus development. Infected calculi (usually magnesium ammonium phosphate or staghorn calculi) may develop if bacteria serve as the nucleus in calculus formation. Such infections may promote destruction of renal parenchyma.

• *changes in urine pH.* Consistently acidic or alkaline urine provides a favorable medium for calculus formation.

• *obstruction.* Urinary stasis (as in immobility from spinal cord injury) allows calculus constituents to collect and adhere, forming calculi. Obstruction also promotes infection which, in turn, compounds the obstruction.

• *diet.* Increased intake of calcium or oxalate-rich foods encourage calculus formation.

• *immobilization.* Immobility from spinal cord injury or other disorders allows calcium to be released into the circulation and, eventually, filtered by the kidneys.

• *metabolic factors.* Hyperparathyroidism, renal tubular acidosis, elevated uric acid levels (usually with gout), defective metabolism of oxalate, genetically defective metabolism of cystine, and excessive intake of vitamin D, protein, or dietary calcium may predispose a patient to renal calculi.

Education edge

Neurogenic bladder teaching tips

• Assure the patient that the lengthy diagnostic process is necessary to identify the most effective treatment plan.

• Explain the treatment plan to the patient in detail and teach him and his family bladder evacuation techniques.

• Counsel the patient regarding sexual activities. Remember, the incontinent patient feels embarrassed and distressed. Provide emotional support.

Renal calculi vary in size and may be solitary or multiple. What, this? No, this is an orange for my lunch break!

A close look at renal calculi

Renal calculi vary in size and type. Small calculi may remain in the renal pelvis or pass down the ureter as shown below. A staghorn calculus, shown in the second illustration, is a cast of the innermost part of the kidney—the calyx and renal pelvis. A staghorn calculus may develop from a calculus that stays in the kidney.

Multiple small calculi

Staghorn calculus

Pathophysiology

Calculi form when substances normally dissolved in the urine, such as calcium oxalate and calcium phosphate, precipitate. Large, rough calculi may occlude the opening to the ureteropelvic junction. The frequency and force of peristaltic contractions increase, causing pain.

What to look for

Clinical effects vary with size, location, and cause of the calculus. Pain is the key symptom. The pain of classic renal colic travels from the costovertebral angle to the flank, the suprapubic region, and the external genitalia. The pain fluctuates in intensity and may be excruciating at its peak. If calculi are in the renal pelvis and calyces, pain may be more constant and dull. Back pain occurs from calculi that produce an obstruction within a kidney. Nausea and vomiting usually accompany severe pain.

Other symptoms include:
- abdominal distention
- fever and chills
- hematuria, pyuria and, rarely, anuria.

Pain is the key symptom of renal calculi.

What tests tell you

- KUB X-rays reveal most renal calculi.
- Calculus analysis shows mineral content.
- Excretory urography confirms the diagnosis and determines the size and location of calculi.
- Renal ultrasonography may detect obstructive changes such as hydronephrosis.
- Urine culture of a midstream specimen may indicate UTI.
- Urinalysis results may be normal or may show increased specific gravity and acid or alkaline pH suitable for different types of calculus formation. Other urinalysis findings include hematuria (gross or microscopic), crystals (urate, calcium, or cystine), casts, and pyuria with or without bacteria and WBCs. A 24-hour urine collection is evaluated for calcium oxalate, phosphorus, and uric acid excretion levels.
- Other laboratory results support the diagnosis. Serial blood calcium and phosphorus levels detect hyperparathyroidism and show increased calcium levels in proportion to normal serum protein levels. Blood protein levels determine free calcium unbound to protein. Blood chloride and bicarbonate levels may show renal tubular acidosis. Increased blood uric acid levels may indicate gout as the cause.

How it's treated

Because 90% of renal calculi are smaller than 5 mm in diameter, treatment usually consists of measures to promote their natural passage. Along with vigorous hydration, such treatment includes antimicrobial therapy (varying with the cultured organism) for infection; analgesics, such as meperidine and ketorolac (Toradol), for pain; and diuretics to prevent urinary stasis and further calculus formation (thiazide diuretics decrease calcium excretion into the urine, which reduces calculus formation).

Prophylaxis to prevent calculus formation includes a low-calcium diet for absorptive hypercalciuria, parathyroidectomy for hyperparathyroidism, allopurinol for uric acid calculi, and daily administration of ascorbic acid by mouth to acidify the urine.

A calculus that's too large for natural passage may require surgical removal, percutaneous ultrasonic lithotripsy and ESWL, or chemolysis.

What to do

- Strain all urine through gauze or a tea strainer and save the solid material recovered for analysis.

Because 90% of renal calculi are smaller than 5 mm, treatment usually consists of measures to promote their natural passage.

• Promote sufficient intake of fluids to maintain a urine output of 3 to 4 L/day (urine should be very dilute and colorless). If the patient can't drink the required amount of fluid, supplemental I.V. fluids may be given. Record intake and output and daily weight to assess fluid status and renal function.

• If surgery is necessary, reassure the patient by supplementing and reinforcing what the surgeon has told him about the procedure. Explain preoperative and postoperative care.

• Evaluate the patient. A successfully treated and counseled patient is free from pain, has recovered the calculus, and exhibits no signs of complications. He's prepared to follow dietary and medical regimens, if necessary. He verbalizes a good understanding of his illness and the diagnostic procedures. (See *Renal calculi teaching tips*.)

Education edge

Renal calculi teaching tips

• Before discharge, teach the patient and his family the importance of following the prescribed dietary and medication regimens to prevent recurrence of calculi.

• Encourage increased fluid intake.

• Tell the patient to immediately report symptoms of acute obstruction (such as pain and inability to void).

Quick quiz

1. Glomerular filtration is the process of:
    A. filtering the blood that flows through the kidney's blood vessels, or glomeruli.
    B. removing renal calculi from the ureters.
    C. measuring creatinine in the blood.
    D. reabsorbing filtered fluid.

Answer: A. Glomerular filtration is the filtering of the blood that flows through the kidney's blood vessels, or glomeruli.

2. The laboratory tests most specific to renal function are:
    A. potassium and sodium measurements.
    B. chloride and bicarbonate measurements.
    C. BUN and creatinine measurements.
    D. blood glucose and ketone measurements.

Answer: C. Although serum creatinine levels indicate renal damage more reliably than BUN levels do, you need both for a complete view of kidney function. Their simultaneous rise is the key to diagnosing kidney disease.

3. Prerenal failure results from:
    A. bilateral obstruction of urine outflow.
    B. conditions that diminish blood flow to the kidneys.
    C. damage to the kidneys themselves.
    D. any preexisting condition that contributed to renal dysfunction.

Answer: B. Prerenal failure is renal failure due to diminished blood flow to the kidneys. Prerenal azotemia accounts for 40% to 80% of all cases of acute renal failure.

4.   A risk factor for developing a lower UTI is:
A.   frequent urination.
B.   elevated potassium level.
C.   presence of renal calculi.
D.   ingestion of a large amount of caffeine.

Answer: C. A narrowed ureter or calculi lodged in the ureter or bladder can obstruct urine flow. Slowed urine flow allows bacteria to multiply.

5.   Which of the following factors can contribute to the formation of renal calculi?
A.   Hypocalcemia
B.   Heart failure
C.   Hypothyroidism
D.   Changes in urine pH

Answer: D. Urine that's consistently acidic or alkaline provides a favorable medium for calculus formation.

Scoring

☆☆☆   If you answered all five items correctly, excellent! There's no obstruction to your passage of knowledge.

☆☆   If you answered three or four items correctly, wow! You're headed for perfect filtration of information.

☆   If you answered fewer than three items correctly, don't get spastic! Just review the chapter and try again.

Reproductive disorders

Just the facts

In this chapter, you'll learn:

♦ anatomy and physiology of the female and male reproductive systems

♦ assessment techniques

♦ tests to diagnose reproductive disorders

♦ treatments, including drugs and surgery

♦ typical nursing diagnoses

♦ common reproductive disorders, including causes, pathophysiology, signs and symptoms, test results, treatments, nursing interventions, and patient teaching.

A look at reproductive disorders

Because of the misinformation and cultural taboos surrounding the reproductive system, reproductive disorders present a special nursing challenge. Problems such as impotence, abnormal uterine bleeding, and infertility strike at a patient's deepest sense of self. Besides needing expert health care, each patient requires sensitive counseling and straightforward teaching.

Anatomy and physiology review

To meet the patient's needs, you'll need a clear understanding of the female and male reproductive systems.

Cultural taboos can make discussing reproductive disorders quite a challenge.

Female reproductive system

Major female external genitalia include the vulva, which contains the mons pubis, clitoris, labia majora, labia minora, and adjacent structures (Bartholin's glands, Skene's glands, and the urethral meatus). Major internal genitalia include the vagina, uterus, ovaries, and fallopian tubes. (See *Reviewing the female genitalia.*)

Love those hormones!

Hormonal influences determine the development and function of external and internal female genitalia and affect fertility, childbearing, and the ability to experience sexual pleasure.

Hormones and the menstrual cycle

The hypothalamus, ovaries, and pituitary gland secrete hormones that affect the buildup and shedding of the uterine lining during the menstrual cycle. Ovulation occurs through a network of positive and negative feedback loops that run from the hypothalamus, to the pituitary, to the ovaries, and back to the hypothalamus and pituitary.

The menstrual cycle consists of three phases: menstrual (preovulatory), proliferative (follicular), and luteal (secretory). These phases correspond to the phases of ovarian function. (See *Understanding the menstrual cycle*, page 613.)

Supply exhausted

Cessation of menses usually occurs between ages 40 and 55. Although the pituitary gland still releases follicle-stimulating hormone (FSH) and luteinizing hormone (LH), the body has exhausted the supply of ovarian follicles that respond to these hormones, so menstruation no longer occurs. A woman is considered to have reached menopause after menses are absent for 1 year.

Male reproductive system

The two major organs of the male reproductive system are the penis and testes. This system supplies male sex cells through sperm formation or spermatogenesis and is involved in male sex hormone secretion. (See *Reviewing the male reproductive system*, pages 614 and 615.)

Reviewing the female genitalia

External and internal structures make up the female genitalia.

External genitalia

The vulva contains the external female genitalia that are visible on inspection. The mons pubis is the cushion of adipose and connective tissue covered by skin and coarse, curly hair in a triangular pattern over the symphysis pubis (the joint formed by union of the pubic bones anteriorly).

The labia majora border the vulva laterally from the mons pubis to the perineum (muscle, fascia, and ligaments between the anus and vulva). The labia minora, two moist lesser mucosal folds, darker pink to red, lie within and alongside the labia majora.

The clitoris is the small, protuberant organ located just beneath the arch of the mons pubis. The clitoris contains erectile tissue, venous cavernous spaces, and specialized sensory corpuscles that are stimulated during coitus.

When the labia are spread, the introitus (vaginal orifice) and the urethral meatus are visible. Less easily visible are the multiple orifices of Skene's glands, mucus-producing glands located on both sides of the urethral opening.

Openings of the two mucus-producing Bartholin's glands are located laterally and posteriorly on either side of the inner vaginal orifice. The hymen, a tissue membrane varying in size and thickness, may completely or partially cover the vaginal orifice. A disrupted hymen appears as remnants of uneven mucosal tissue tags, called *myrtiform caruncles*.

View of external genitalia in lithotomy position

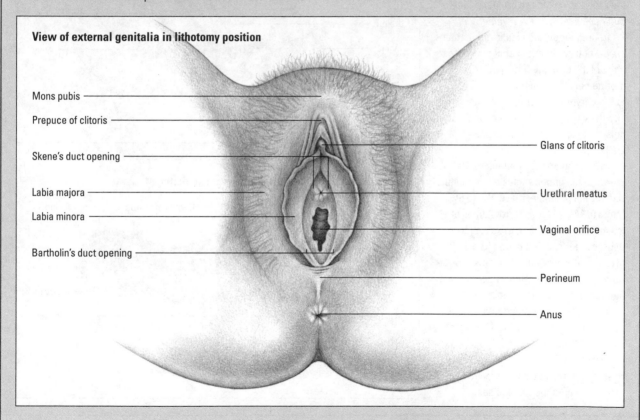

Mons pubis

Prepuce of clitoris

Skene's duct opening

Labia majora

Labia minora

Bartholin's duct opening

Glans of clitoris

Urethral meatus

Vaginal orifice

Perineum

Anus

(continued)

Reviewing the female genitalia *(continued)*

Internal genitalia

The vagina, a highly elastic muscular tube, is located between the urethra and the rectum. Between 2½″ and 2¾″ (6.5 to 7 cm) long anteriorly and 3½″ (9 cm) long posteriorly, the vagina lies at a 45-degree angle to the long axis of the body.

The uterus, a small, firm, pear-shaped, muscular organ, rests between the bladder and the rectum and usually lies at almost a 90-degree angle to the vagina. However, other locations may be normal. The mucous membrane lining the uterus is called the *endometrium*; the muscular layer, the *myometrium*.

In pregnancy, the elastic, upper uterine portion (the fundus) accommodates most of the growing fetus until term. The uterine neck (isthmus) joins the fundus to the cervix, the uterine part extending into the vagina. The fundus and the isthmus make up the corpus, the main uterine body.

Two fallopian tubes attach to the uterus at the upper angles of the fundus. Usually nonpalpable, these 2¾″ to 5½″ (7-cm to 14-cm) long, narrow tubes of muscle fibers have fingerlike projections, called *fimbriae*, on the free ends that partially surround the ovaries. Fertilization of the ovum usually occurs in the outer one-third of the fallopian tube.

Palpable, oval, almond-shaped organs measuring 1¼″ to 1½″ (3 to 4 cm) long, ¾″ (2 cm) wide, and ¼″ to ½″ (0.5 to 1 cm) thick, the ovaries usually lie near the lateral pelvic walls, a little below the anterosuperior iliac spine.

Lateral view of internal genitalia

Anterior cross-sectional view of internal genitalia

Understanding the menstrual cycle

The average menstrual cycle usually occurs over 28 days, although the normal cycle may range from 22 to 34 days. The cycle is regulated by fluctuating hormone levels that, in turn, are regulated by negative and positive feedback mechanisms.

Menstrual (preovulatory) phase

The cycle starts with menstruation (cycle day 1), which usually lasts 5 days. As the cycle begins, low estrogen and progesterone levels in the bloodstream stimulate the hypothalamus to secrete gonadotropin-releasing hormone (GnRH). In turn, this substance stimulates the anterior pituitary to secrete follicle-stimulating hormone (FSH) and luteinizing hormone (LH). When the FSH level rises, LH output increases.

Proliferative (follicular) phase and ovulation

The proliferative phase lasts from days 6 through 14 of the cycle. During this phase, LH and FSH act on the ovarian follicle (mature ovarian cyst containing the ovum), causing estrogen secretion, which in turn stimulates the buildup of the endometrium. Late in the proliferative phase, estrogen levels peak, FSH secretion declines, and LH secretion increases, surging at midcycle (around day 14). Then, estrogen production decreases, the follicle matures, and ovulation occurs. Typically, one folli-

cle matures during the ovulatory process and is released from the ovary during each cycle.

Luteal (secretory) phase

During the luteal phase, which lasts about 14 days, FSH and LH levels drop. Estrogen levels decline initially, then increase along with progesterone levels as the corpus luteum (progesterone-producing, yellow structure that develops after the follicle ruptures) begins functioning. During this phase, the endometrium responds to progesterone stimulation by becoming thick and secretory in preparation for implantation of a fertilized ovum.

Between 10 and 12 days after ovulation, the corpus luteum begins to diminish as do estrogen and progesterone levels, until the hormone levels are insufficient to sustain the endometrium in a fully developed secretory state. Then the endometrial lining is shed (menses).

Decreasing estrogen and progesterone levels stimulate the hypothalamus to produce GnRH, and the cycle begins again.

Spermatogenesis

Sperm formation begins when a male reaches puberty and usually continues throughout life. Stimulated by male sex hormones, mature sperm cells are formed continuously within the seminiferous tubules.

Sperm on the move

Newly mature sperm pass from the seminiferous tubules through the vasa recta into the epididymis. Only a small number of sperm can be stored in the epididymis; most of them move into the vas deferens, where they're stored until sexual stimulation triggers emission. Sperm cells retain their potency in storage for many weeks. After ejaculation, sperm survive for 24 to 72 hours at body temperature.

I can survive for 24 to 72 hours ... I gotta get movin'!

Reviewing the male reproductive system

The male reproductive system consists of the penis, the scrotum and its contents, the prostate gland, and the inguinal structures.

Penis

Internally, the cylindrical penile shaft consists of three columns of erectile tissue bound together by heavy fibrous tissue. Two corpora cavernosa form the major part of the penis; on the underside, the corpus spongiosum encases the urethra.

The penile shaft terminates distally in the glans penis, a cone-shaped expansion of the corpus spongiosum that's highly sensitive to sexual stimulus. The expanded lateral margin of the glans forms a ridge of tissue known as the *corona*.

Thin, loose skin covers the penile shaft. In an uncircumcised male, a skin flap—the foreskin, or prepuce—covers the corona and much of the glans. The urethral meatus opens through the glans to allow urination and ejaculation.

Scrotum

The penis meets the scrotum, or scrotal sac, at the penoscrotal junction. The scrotum consists of a thin layer of skin overlying a tighter, musclelike layer, which in turn overlies the tunica vaginalis, a serous membrane covering the internal scrotal cavity.

Externally, the median raphe (seam of union of the two halves) continues from the penis to superficially bisect the scrotal skin. Internally, a septum divides the scrotum into two sacs, each containing a testis, an epididymis, and a spermatic cord. Each testis measures about 2″ (5 cm) long by 1″ (2.5 cm) wide and weighs about ½ oz (14 g). The testes contain the seminiferous tubules, where spermatogenesis takes place.

A complex duct system conveys sperm from the testes to the ejaculatory ducts near the bladder. From the seminiferous tubules, newly formed sperm travel to the epididymis—a tubular reservoir for sperm storage and maturation that curves over the posterolateral surface and upper end of the testes.

Mature sperm then move from the epididymis to the vas deferens. This duct begins at the end of the epididymis, passes up through the external inguinal canal, and descends near the bladder fundus, where it enters the ejaculatory duct inside the prostate gland. The vas deferens is enclosed within the spermatic cord, a compact bundle of vessels, nerves, and muscle fibers.

Prostate gland

Lying under the bladder and surrounding the urethra, the walnut-size (about 1½″ [4 cm] in diameter) prostate gland consists of three lobes—the left and right lateral lobes and the median lobe. The prostate continuously secretes prostatic fluid—a thin, milky alkaline fluid. During sexual activity, prostatic fluid adds volume to the semen and enhances sperm motility and possibly fertility by neutralizing the acidity of the urethra and of the woman's vagina.

Inguinal structures

The spermatic cord travels from the testis through the inguinal canal, exiting the scrotum through the external inguinal ring and entering the abdominal cavity through the internal inguinal ring. The external inguinal ring is located just above and lateral to the pubic tubercle; the internal ring, about ½″ (1 cm) above the midpoint of the inguinal ligament, between the pubic tubercle of the symphysis pubis and the anterior superior iliac spine.

Between the two rings lies the inguinal canal. Lymph nodes from the penis, scrotal surface, and anus drain into the inguinal lymph nodes. Lymph nodes from the testes drain into the lateral aortic and preaortic lymph nodes in the abdomen.

Hormones and sexual development

Male sex hormones (androgens) are produced in the testes and the adrenal glands. Leydig's cells are located in the testes between the seminiferous tubules. These cells secrete testosterone, the most significant male sex hormone. They proliferate during puberty and remain abundant throughout life. Testosterone is responsible for the development and maintenance of male sex organs and

Male pelvic organs

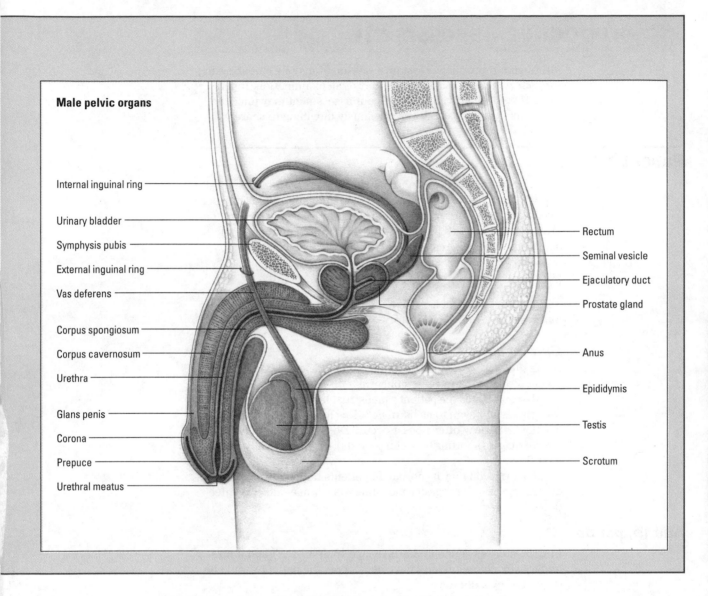

- Internal inguinal ring
- Urinary bladder
- Symphysis pubis
- External inguinal ring
- Vas deferens
- Corpus spongiosum
- Corpus cavernosum
- Urethra
- Glans penis
- Corona
- Prepuce
- Urethral meatus

- Rectum
- Seminal vesicle
- Ejaculatory duct
- Prostate gland
- Anus
- Epididymis
- Testis
- Scrotum

secondary sex characteristics. It's also required for spermatogenesis.

    Male sexuality is also affected by other hormones. Two of these—LH, also known as *interstitial cell-stimulating hormone,* and FSH—directly affect testosterone secretion.

Reproductive assessment

Although a reproductive system assessment may be embarrassing for your patient, it's an essential part of an examination. If performed with sensitivity and tact, your assessment may uncover concerns that the patient was previously unwilling to share.

Patient history

Begin your assessment by obtaining a detailed reproductive health history. Establish a good rapport to help the patient relax and confide in you. Ask your questions in a comfortable environment that protects the patient's privacy. Leave time for the patient to ask questions about his reproductive organs or sexual activity.

Female patients

Ask the patient about her chief complaint, reproductive history, family history, and social history.

Current illness

Using the PQRST method, help the patient describe her chief complaint, along with any other concerns.

Also ask about the patient's menstrual history. How old was she when she began to menstruate? How long does her period usually last? How often does it occur? Does she have cramps, metrorrhagia (spotting between periods), or an unusually heavy or light flow?

Metrorrhagia may be normal in patients taking low-dose oral contraceptives or progesterone; otherwise, it may indicate infection or cancer.

Age 15, period

In girls, menses generally starts by age 15. If it hasn't and if no secondary sex characteristics have developed, the patient should be evaluated by a doctor.

Reproductive history

Ask the patient if she has ever been pregnant. If so, how many times? How many times did she give birth? If she gave birth, did she have a vaginal or cesarean delivery? What kind of birth control, if any, does she use? If the patient is sexually active, talk to her about the importance of safer sex and the prevention of sexually transmitted diseases (STDs).

Family history

Because some reproductive problems tend to be familial, ask about family history. Ask the patient if she or anyone in her family ever had reproductive problems, hypertension, diabetes mellitus (including gestational diabetes mellitus), obesity, heart disease, or gynecologic surgery.

Social history

Ask the patient if she's sexually active. If so, ask her when she had intercourse last and if she has more than one partner. Ask if her sexual partner or partners have any signs or symptoms of infection, such as genital sores, warts, dysuria, or penile discharge.

Male patients

The most common complaints about the male reproductive system are penile discharge, impotence, infertility, and scrotal or inguinal masses, pain, and tenderness.

Current illness

Analyze the patient's chief complaint. Also ask him if he's circumcised. If he isn't, can he retract and replace the prepuce easily? Inquire whether he has noticed sores, lumps, or ulcers on his penis. These can signal an STD. Does he have scrotal swelling? This can indicate an inguinal hernia, a hematocele, epididymitis, or a testicular tumor. Ask whether he has penile discharge or bleeding.

Reproductive history

If the patient had reproductive system problems in the past or had problems in other body systems, this may affect his current reproductive function. Be sure to ask these questions:
• Have you fathered any children? If so, how many and how old are they? Have you ever had a problem with infertility? If so, is it a current concern?
• Have you ever been diagnosed with an STD or other infection in the genitourinary tract? If so, what was the specific problem and were there any complications? How long did the problem last? What treatment was provided?
• Do you have a history of undescended testes or an endocrine disorder? Have you ever had mumps? If so, did the disease affect your testes?

Past problems in other body systems may affect current reproductive function.

Family history

Questions about family health history can provide clues to disorders with known familial tendencies. Ask the patient if anyone in his family has had infertility problems, a hernia, or cancer of the reproductive tract.

Social history

Obtain information about the patient's lifestyle and relationships with others. Ask the patient if he's sexually active and if he has more than one partner. If he's sexually active, ask what precautions he takes to prevent contracting an STD or acquired immunodeficiency syndrome (AIDS). If he's experiencing sexual difficulty, is it affecting his emotional and social relationships?

Wearing me helps protect against STDs!

Physical examination

Physical assessment of the female patient involves inspection and palpation. You may examine only the external genitalia or perform a complete gynecologic examination, which includes examination of both the external and internal genitalia.

For the male patient, physical assessment involves inspecting and palpating the groin, penis, and scrotum. If the patient is age 50 or over or has a high likelihood of prostate problems, you should also palpate the prostate gland.

Examining the female patient

You may assist a doctor or nurse practitioner with a gynecologic assessment or perform the assessment yourself. Before the examination, ask the patient to void to prevent discomfort and inaccurate findings during palpation. Have her disrobe and put on an examination gown. Then wash your hands and put on gloves. Have the patient lie in the supine position, and drape all areas not being examined. Make sure you explain the procedure to her.

Begin by examining the external genitalia; then move to the internal genitalia.

Inspecting the external genitalia

If the patient complains of sores or itching, you may only need to inspect her external genitalia to determine the origin of the problem. In any case, uncover the pubic area, and inspect pubic hair for amount and pattern. It's usually thick and appears on the mons pubis as well as the inner aspects of the upper thighs.

Male patients age 50 and older should have a prostate examination.

Checking further

Using your index finger and thumb, gently spread the labia majora and look for the labia minora. Both labia should be pink and moist with no lesions.

Check for cervical discharge. Normal discharge varies in color and consistency. It's clear and stretchy before ovulation, white and opaque after ovulation, and usually odorless and nonirritating to the mucosa. No other discharge should be present.

Palpating the external genitalia
Next, spread the labia with one hand and palpate with the other. The labia should feel soft. Note swelling, hardness, or tenderness. If you detect a mass or lesion, palpate it to determine its size, shape, and consistency.

Main squeeze

If you find swelling or tenderness, see if you can palpate Bartholin's glands, which usually aren't palpable. To do this, insert your index finger carefully into the patient's posterior introitus, and place your thumb along the lateral edge of the swollen or tender labium. Gently squeeze the labium. If discharge from the gland results, culture it.

Examining the internal genitalia
If you practice in a facility specializing in women's health care, you may perform complete gynecologic assessments. As part of this assessment, obtain a Papanicolaou (Pap) smear after inspecting the cervix. (Obtain the smear before touching the cervix in any manner.) Also obtain other specimens if an abnormal cervical or vaginal discharge indicates infection.

Examining the male patient
Before examining the reproductive system of a male patient, put on gloves. Make the patient as comfortable as possible, and explain what you're doing every step of the way. This helps the patient feel less embarrassed.

Inspection
Inspect the penis, scrotum, and testicles as well as the inguinal and femoral areas.

Penis
First, evaluate the color and integrity of the penile skin. It should be loose and wrinkled over the shaft and taut and smooth over the glans penis. The skin should be pink to light brown in whites, light to dark brown in blacks, and free from scars, lesions, ulcers, or breaks of any kind.

Retract and replace

Ask an uncircumcised patient to retract his prepuce, or foreskin, to expose the glans penis. Inspect the glans for ulcers or lesions. Then ask the patient to replace the foreskin over the glans. He should be able to retract and replace the foreskin easily.

The urethral meatus, a slitlike opening, is normally located at the tip of the glans. There should be no discharge from it.

Scrotum

First, evaluate the amount, distribution, color, and texture of pubic hair. Hair should cover the symphysis pubis and scrotum.

Scrutinizing scrotal skin

Next, inspect the scrotal skin for lesions, ulcerations, induration (hardness), or reddened areas, and evaluate the scrotal sac for symmetry and size. The scrotal skin should be coarse and more deeply pigmented than the body skin. The left testis usually hangs slightly lower than the right.

Inguinal area

Check the inguinal area for obvious bulges — a sign of hernias. Then ask the patient to bear down as you inspect again. This maneuver increases intra-abdominal pressure, which pushes a herniation downward and makes it more easily visible. Also check for enlarged lymph nodes, a sign of infection.

Palpation

After inspection, palpate the penis and scrotum for structural abnormalities; then palpate the inguinal area for hernias.

Penis

To palpate the penis, gently grasp the shaft between the thumb and first two fingers and palpate along its entire length, noting any indurated, tender, or lumpy areas. The flaccid penis should feel soft and have no nodules.

Scrotum

Like the penis, the scrotum can be palpated using the thumb and first two fingers. Begin by feeling the scrotal skin for nodules, lesions, or ulcers.

Into the sack

Next, palpate the scrotal sac. Typically, the right and left halves of the sac have identical contents and feel the same. You should feel the testes as separate, freely movable oval masses low in the scrotal sac. Their surface should feel smooth and even in contour.

Slight compression of the testes should elicit a dull, aching sensation that radiates to the patient's lower abdomen. This pressure–pain sensation shouldn't occur when the other structures are compressed. No other pain or tenderness should be present.

Posterolateral palpation

Palpate the epididymis on the posterolateral surface by grasping each testis between your thumb and forefinger and feeling from the epididymis to the spermatic cord or vas deferens up to the inguinal ring. The epididymis should feel like a ridge of tissue lying vertically on the testicular surface.

The vas deferens should feel like a smooth cord and be freely movable. The arteries, veins, lymph vessels, and nerves, which are located next to the vas deferens, may feel like indefinite threads.

Inguinal area

Palpate the inguinal area for hernias. A hernia will feel like a small bulge or mass.

Diagnostic tests

Diagnostic testing can help you assess reproductive organs and associated structures for abnormalities, detect cancers, or determine the cause of infertility or sexual dysfunction. Diagnostic procedures include endoscopic tests, radiographic and ultrasound studies, and tissue analyses.

Endoscopic tests

Endoscopic tests are invasive procedures that allow examination of internal reproductive structures to assess lesions, cancers, or infections or to perform various therapeutic procedures. Such tests include colposcopy and laparoscopy.

Colposcopy

During colposcopy, the examiner studies the vulva, cervix, and vagina with a colposcope, an instrument that contains a magnifying lens and a light. The areas to be studied are first bathed in white vinegar (5% acetic acid), which causes abnormal areas to turn white.

Tissue analysis can help detect cancers or abnormalities.

Coping with a colposcope

Although originally used to screen for cancer, colposcopy is now used to:

• evaluate abnormal cytologic specimens or grossly suspicious lesions

• examine the cervix and vagina to confirm cancer after a positive Pap test result

• monitor patients whose mothers took diethylstilbestrol during pregnancy.

During the examination, a biopsy may be performed and photographs taken of suspicious lesions using the colposcope and its attachments.

Nursing considerations

Take these measures:

• Tell the patient that she doesn't need to restrict food or fluids before the test.

• Explain that the test takes 10 to 15 minutes. A biopsy may be performed during the examination, and this may cause cramping and pain for a short time as well as minimal, easily controlled bleeding.

• Warn the patient to abstain from intercourse after the biopsy and not to insert anything into her vagina (except a tampon) until the doctor confirms healing of the biopsy site.

• Instruct the patient to call the doctor if she begins to bleed more heavily than during a period. She should also call the doctor if she has signs and symptoms of infection—such as discharge, pain, and fever. Reassure her that abstaining from douching, sexual intercourse, and tub baths will help prevent these complications.

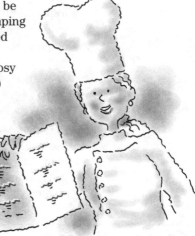

Tell the patient that she doesn't need to worry about restricting food or fluids before the test.

Laparoscopy

Laparoscopy allows the doctor to inspect the organs in the peritoneal cavity by inserting a small fiber-optic telescope (laparoscope) through the anterior abdominal wall.

A scope for all reasons

This test is used to:

• detect abnormalities, such as cysts, adhesions, fibroids, and infection

• identify the cause of pelvic pain

• diagnose endometriosis, ectopic pregnancy, or pelvic inflammatory disease (PID)

• evaluate pelvic masses or the fallopian tubes of infertile patients.
• stage cancer.

Therapeutic uses of this procedure include lysis of adhesions, tubal sterilization, removal of foreign bodies, and fulguration of endometriotic implants.

Nursing considerations

Take these measures:
• Instruct the patient to fast after midnight before the test or at least 8 hours before surgery.
• Assure the patient that she'll receive either a local or general anesthetic, and tell her that the procedure will require either an outpatient visit or overnight hospitalization Warn her that she may experience pain at the puncture site and in her shoulders.
• Check the patient's history to make sure she isn't hypersensitive to the anesthetic. Make sure that all laboratory work is completed and results reported before the test.
• During the procedure, check for proper drainage of the catheter, and monitor vital signs and urine output. Report sudden changes immediately — they may indicate complications. After administration of a general anesthetic, check for allergic reactions. Monitor electrolyte and hemoglobin levels and hematocrit as ordered.
• After recovery, help the patient walk, as ordered. Instruct her to restrict activity for 2 to 7 days as ordered. Reassure her that some abdominal and shoulder pain is normal and should disappear in 24 to 36 hours. Provide pain medication as ordered.

Radiographic and ultrasound studies

Radiographic and ultrasound studies are noninvasive tests that use X-rays and high-frequency sound waves to inspect internal reproductive structures.

Hysterosalpingography

Hysterosalpingography allows the doctor to visually inspect the uterine cavity, fallopian tubes, and peritubal area. A contrast medium is injected through a cannula that's inserted through the cervix. Fluoroscopic X-rays are taken as the contrast medium flows through the uterus and the fallopian tubes.

Long name, lotsa uses

This test is usually performed as part of an infertility study to confirm tubal abnormalities, such as adhesions and occlusion, and uterine abnormalities, such as foreign bodies, congenital malformations, and traumatic injuries.

A doctor may also order this test to evaluate repeated fetal loss or to follow up after surgery, especially uterine unification procedures and tubal reanastomosis.

Nursing considerations

Take these measures:
• Warn the patient that she may have moderate cramping, nausea, and dizziness during or after the procedure but that she may receive a mild sedative such as diazepam beforehand to relax her. Reassure her that these reactions are transient.
• When monitoring the patient, watch for an allergic reaction to the contrast medium (such as hives, itching, or hypotension) and for signs and symptoms of infection (such as fever, pain, increased pulse rate, malaise, and muscle aches).

Don't worry about a thing — If you need me, I'll help you to relaxxxxx...

Pelvic ultrasonography

During pelvic ultrasonography, a crystal generates high-frequency sound waves that are reflected to a transducer. The transducer then converts sound energy into electrical energy and forms images of the interior pelvic area on an oscilloscope screen. This test is most commonly used to:
• evaluate symptoms that suggest pelvic disease to confirm a tentative diagnosis
• determine fetal viability, position, gestational age, and growth rate during pregnancy.

Nursing considerations

Take these measures:
• Reassure the pregnant patient that ultrasonography won't harm the fetus, and provide emotional support during the test.
• Instruct the patient that the test requires a full bladder, so she may have to drink several glasses of water beforehand. A full bladder is used as a landmark to define the pelvic organs.
• Explain that a water enema may be necessary to produce a better outline of the large intestine.
• Allow the patient to empty her bladder immediately after the test.

Tissue analysis

Analysis of cervical material may be useful for detecting cancers and infections.

Pap test

A Pap test screens for cancer in women who have no symptoms or findings suggesting cancer. It's widely used for:
• early detection of cervical cancer
• detection of inflammatory tissue changes
• detection of viral, fungal, and, occasionally, parasitic invasion
• assessment of the patient's response to chemotherapy and radiation therapy.

Scrape, spread, slide

To perform a Pap test, the examiner scrapes secretions from the patient's cervix and spreads them on a slide. After the slide is immersed in a fixative, it's sent to the laboratory for cytologic analysis.

Alternatively, the Thin Prep Pap test may be used, in which the collection device is rinsed in a vial of preservative solution and sent to the laboratory.

Paps all around

The American Cancer Society recommends this schedule for Pap tests:
• women who are or who have been sexually active and for all women age 18 or older: annually
• women ages 30 to 70 with three or more consecutive examinations with normal findings: every 2 to 3 years
• women age 70 and older with three or more consecutive normal examinations and no abnormal Pap tests in the last 10 years: screening may stop.

Nursing considerations

Take these measures:
• Explain to the patient that the Pap test allows cervical cells to be studied. Stress the test's importance in detecting cancer at a stage when it commonly produces no symptoms and is still curable.
• Explain that the test shouldn't be scheduled during menses. The best time is 1 week before or after menses, when there are more cervical cells and less mucus.
• Instruct the patient not to have intercourse for 24 hours before the test and not to douche or insert vaginal medications for 72 hours before the test. These activities can wash away cellular deposits and change the vaginal pH.
• Obtain an accurate patient history, and note any pertinent data on the laboratory request.

The best time to perform a Pap test is 1 week before or after the patient's menses.

• If the patient is anxious, be supportive and tell her that test results should be available within a few days.
• Just before the test, ask the patient to empty her bladder.
• Preserve the slides immediately. A delay in fixing a specimen allows the cells to dry, destroys the effectiveness of the nuclear stain, and makes cytologic interpretation difficult.
• Make sure that you aspirate and scrape the specimen from the cervix. Aspiration of the posterior fornix of the vagina can supplement a cervical specimen but shouldn't replace it.
• If vaginal or vulval lesions are present, take scrapings directly from the lesion.
• If the patient's uterus is involuted or atrophied from age, use a small pipette, if necessary, to aspirate cells from the squamo-columnar junction and the cervical canal.

Treatments

To provide effective care for the patient with a reproductive disorder, you'll need a working knowledge of current drug therapy, surgery, and related treatments.

All stressed out

Keep in mind that many of these disorders place your patient under enormous social and psychological stress, so your ability to maintain a caring, nonjudgmental attitude will prove especially valuable.

Drug therapy

Drugs are the treatment of choice for many reproductive disorders. For example, estrogens are prescribed for several disorders associated with estrogen deficiency and for inoperable prostatic cancer, breast cancer, and hypogonadism. Gonadotropins are used to treat certain forms of infertility as well as undescended testes in males.

Surgery

Women with gynecologic disorders may need surgery. Gynecologic surgeries include dilatation and curettage (D&C), dilatation and evacuation (D&E), and hysterectomy. Such surgery may cause an altered body image. Therefore, you must consistently provide these patients with strong emotional support.

For men only

Men with erectile dysfunction may benefit from penile prosthesis implantation.

D&C and D&E

During a D&C or D&E—the most common gynecologic procedures—the doctor expands or dilates the cervix to access the endocervix and uterus. In D&C, he uses a curette to scrape endometrial tissue. In D&E, he applies suction to extract the uterine contents.

D&C is used to treat an incomplete abortion, to control abnormal uterine bleeding, and to obtain an endometrial or endocervical tissue specimen for cytologic study. D&E is also a treatment for an incomplete abortion. In addition, it's used for a therapeutic abortion, usually up to 12 weeks' gestation but occasionally as late as 16 weeks'.

Patient preparation

Prepare the patient for surgery:
• Make sure she has followed preoperative directions for fasting and has used an enema to empty her colon before admission.
• Remind her that she'll be groggy after the procedure and won't be able to drive. Make sure that she has arranged transportation home.
• Ask the patient to void before you administer preoperative medications, such as meperidine or diazepam.
• Start I.V. fluids (either dextrose 5% in water or normal saline solution) as ordered to facilitate administration of the anesthetic. The patient may receive a general anesthetic, a regional paracervical block, or a local anesthetic.

Tell the patient that she'll be groggy, so she should arrange transportation home.

Monitoring and aftercare

After surgery, take these measures:
• Administer an analgesic as ordered. Expect the patient to have moderate cramping and pelvic and lower back pain. Continuous, sharp abdominal pain that doesn't respond to the analgesic may indicate perforation of the uterus. Report it at once.
• Monitor the patient for hemorrhage and signs of infection such as purulent, foul-smelling vaginal drainage. Also monitor the color and volume of urine (hematuria indicates infection). Report any of these signs immediately.

• Administer fluids as tolerated, and allow food if the patient requests it. Keep the bed's side rails raised, and help the patient walk to the bathroom if she's unsteady on her feet.

Home care instructions

Include these home care instructions:

• Warn the patient to report signs of infection. Tell her not to use tampons or take tub baths until healing is complete because these activities increase the risk of infection.

• Tell her to expect moderate cramps and lower back pain, and to take analgesics as needed. Warn her that she should report unrelenting sharp pain immediately.

• Explain that spotting and discharge may last a week or longer (up to 4 weeks after an abortion procedure). She should report any bright red blood.

• Advise her to follow her doctor's instructions for scheduling an appointment for a routine checkup.

• Tell the patient to resume activity as tolerated but to follow her doctor's instructions concerning vigorous exercise and sexual intercourse. These are usually discouraged until 2 weeks after the follow-up visit.

• Advise the patient to seek birth control counseling if needed, and refer her to an appropriate center.

Hysterectomy

A hysterectomy involves removing the uterus. Although it can be performed using a vaginal or an abdominal approach, the abdominal approach allows better visualization of the pelvic organs and a larger operating field.

A different approach

The vaginal approach may be used to repair relaxed pelvic structures, such as cystocele or rectocele, at the same time as hysterectomy. (See *Types of hysterectomy*.)

Patient preparation

The patient will enter the hospital on the day of surgery or 1 day before. Prepare her for surgery:

• Take time to talk to her about what she expects from the surgery and about her menstrual and reproductive status after surgery.

• Review what the surgical approach involves and the extent of the excision.

• If the patient is having an abdominal hysterectomy, tell her that she'll need to:

Types of hysterectomy

Hysterectomy is classified three ways:

☝ A total hysterectomy (panhysterectomy) involves removal of the entire uterus.

✌ A subtotal hysterectomy removes only a portion of the uterus, leaving the cervical stump intact.

🤟 A radical hysterectomy involves removing all reproductive organs.

Total and subtotal hysterectomies are commonly performed for uterine myomas or endometrial disease. They may also be performed postpartum if the placenta fails to separate from the uterus after a cesarean delivery or if amnionitis is present.

A radical hysterectomy is the treatment of choice for cervical cancer.

– douche and have an enema the evening before surgery
– take a shower with an antibacterial soap shortly before surgery
– have her pubic area shaved
– have an indwelling urinary catheter inserted because surgery causes urine retention
– have a nasogastric (NG) tube or rectal tube inserted if she develops abdominal distention
– expect temporary abdominal cramping and pelvic and lower back pain after the procedure.
• If the patient is scheduled for a vaginal hysterectomy, tell her to expect abdominal cramping afterward. She'll also have a perineal pad in place because moderate amounts of drainage occur postoperatively.
• Inform the patient that after surgery she needs to lie in a supine position or in a low- to mid-Fowler's position.
• Demonstrate the exercises that she'll need to perform to prevent venous stasis.

Monitoring and aftercare
After surgery, take these measures:
• If the patient has had a vaginal hysterectomy, change her perineal pad frequently. Provide analgesics to relieve cramps.
• If she has had an abdominal hysterectomy, tell her to remain in a supine position or a low- to mid-Fowler's position. Encourage her to perform the prescribed exercises and to walk early and frequently to prevent venous stasis. Monitor her urine output because retention commonly occurs.
• If abdominal distention develops, relieve it by inserting an NG tube or rectal tube as ordered. Note bowel sounds during routine assessment.

Home care instructions
Include these home care instructions:
• If the patient had a vaginal hysterectomy, instruct her to report severe cramping, heavy bleeding, or hot flashes (common with oophorectomy) to her doctor immediately.
• If she had an abdominal hysterectomy, tell her to avoid heavy lifting, rapid walking, or dancing, which can cause pelvic congestion. Encourage her to walk a little more each day and to avoid sitting for a prolonged period. Tell her that swimming is permissible.
• Advise any posthysterectomy patient to eat a high-protein, high-residue diet to avoid constipation, which may increase abdominal pressure. The doctor may also order increased fluid intake (3 qt [2.8 L]/day).
• Mention that the doctor will inform her when she can resume sexual activity (usually 6 weeks after surgery).

• Explain to the patient and her family that abrupt hormonal fluctuations may cause the patient to feel depressed or irritable for a while. She may also have feelings of loss or depression for up to 1 year after the surgery. Encourage family members to respond calmly and with understanding.

• If her ovaries were removed, the patient may receive hormone replacement therapy, which requires monitoring.

Penile prosthesis implantation

A penile prosthesis is surgically implanted in the corpora cavernosa of the penis. Prostheses come in two types: those consisting of a pair of semirigid rods and those made of inflatable cylinders. They're used to treat both organic and psychogenic erectile dysfunction.

Look Ma, no hands

A semirigid penile prosthesis is especially helpful for the patient with limited hand or finger function because it doesn't require manual dexterity. However, the prosthesis keeps the penis semierect, which may embarrass the patient. Also, some couples complain that the semirigid prosthesis produces an erection that isn't sufficiently stiff to be sexually satisfying.

Closer to the real thing

An inflatable prosthesis provides a more natural erection. The patient controls the erection by squeezing a small pump in the scrotum that releases radiopaque fluid from a reservoir into the implanted cylinders. This device, however, is contraindicated in patients with iodine sensitivity.

Patient preparation

Prepare the patient for implant surgery:

• Reinforce the doctor's explanation of the surgery and answer any questions.

• Reassure the patient that the prosthesis won't affect ejaculation or orgasmic pleasure. If the patient experienced either before surgery, he can experience them afterward.

• Recognize that the patient and his partner are likely to be anxious before surgery, so provide emotional support.

• Instruct the patient to shower both the evening before and the morning of surgery, using an antimicrobial soap. Tell him that his pubic area will be shaved in the operating room to reduce the risk of infection.

• Begin antibiotic therapy if ordered.

Make sure the patient showers with antimicrobial soap the night before and the morning of surgery.

Monitoring and aftercare

After surgery, take these measures:
- Apply ice packs to the patient's penis for 24 hours after surgery.
- Empty the surgical drain when it's full, or as ordered, to reduce the risk of infection.
- If the patient has an inflatable prosthesis, tell him to pull the scrotal pump downward to ensure proper alignment.
- With the doctor's approval, encourage the patient to practice inflating and deflating the prosthesis when the pain subsides. Pumping promotes healing of the tissue sheath around the reservoir and pump.

Home care instructions

Include these home care instructions:
- Instruct the patient to wash the incision daily with an antimicrobial soap.
- Caution him to watch for signs of infection and to report them to the doctor immediately.
- Inform him that scrotal swelling and discoloration may last up to 3 weeks.

Nursing diagnoses

Two nursing diagnoses are commonly used when referring to patients with reproductive disorders. These diagnoses are discussed here, along with appropriate nursing interventions and rationales.

Sexual dysfunction

Related to altered body structure or psychological stress, *Sexual dysfunction* can be applied to such conditions as endometriosis, PID, arousal and orgasmic dysfunction, dyspareunia, vaginismus, impotence, or premature ejaculation.

Expected outcomes

- Patient states understanding of sexual dysfunction related to his current situation.
- Patient discusses concerns with spouse or significant other.
- Patient has resources for postdischarge support, including a sex counselor and other appropriate professional, if necessary.

Nursing interventions and rationales

• Provide a nonthreatening, nonjudgmental atmosphere. This enhances communication and understanding between patient and caregiver.

• Allow the patient to express his feelings openly. This encourages him to ask questions specifically related to his current situation.

• Suggest that the patient discuss concerns with his spouse or partner. Sharing concerns helps strengthen relationships.

• Provide support for the patient's spouse or partner. Supportive interventions (such as active listening) communicate concern, interest, and acceptance.

Encourage the patient to share his sexuality concerns with his partner.

• Educate the patient and his spouse or partner about limitations that the patient's physical condition imposes on sexual activity. Understanding these limitations helps the patient avoid complications or injury.

• Suggest referral to a sex counselor or other appropriate professional for future guidance and support.

Ineffective sexuality patterns

Related to illness or medical treatment, *Ineffective sexuality patterns* may be associated with genitourinary or gynecologic disorders or with STDs, such as AIDS, herpes, gonorrhea, and syphilis.

Expected outcomes

• Patient understands diagnosis and treatment.

• Patient communicates with spouse or partner concerns regarding change in sexual patterns.

Nursing interventions and rationales

• Plan for uninterrupted time to talk with the patient. This demonstrates your comfort with sexuality issues and reassures the patient that his concerns are acceptable for discussion.

• Provide a nonthreatening, nonjudgmental atmosphere to encourage the patient to express feelings about perceived changes in sexual identity and behaviors. This demonstrates unconditional positive regard for the patient and his concerns.

• Provide the patient and spouse or partner with information about the illness and its treatment. Answer questions and clarify

any misconceptions. This helps them focus on specific concerns, encourages questions, and avoids misunderstandings.
• Encourage social interaction and communication between the patient and spouse or partner. This fosters sharing of concerns and strengthens relationships.
• Offer referral to counselors or support persons, such as a mental health professional, a sex counselor, or an illness-related support group (such as I Can Cope, Reach for Recovery, and the Ostomy Association).

Disorders

This section discusses common female and male reproductive disorders, including STDs. For each disorder, you'll find information on causes, assessment findings, diagnostic tests, treatments, nursing interventions, patient teaching, and evaluation criteria.

Endometriosis

In endometriosis, endometrial tissue appears outside the lining of the uterine cavity. This ectopic tissue can appear anywhere in the body, but it usually remains in the pelvic area, around the ovaries, uterovesical peritoneum, uterosacral ligaments, and cul-de-sac.

The age of endometriosis

Active endometriosis usually occurs between ages 30 and 40, especially in women who postpone childbearing. It's uncommon before age 20. Severe symptoms of endometriosis may occur abruptly or develop slowly over many years.

Generally, endometriosis becomes progressively severe during the menstrual years, and then subsides after menopause. Infertility is the primary complication, although spontaneous abortion may also occur.

Going through stages

A scoring and staging system created by the American Fertility Society quantifies endometrial implants according to size, character, and location.
• Stage I is minimal disease.
• Stage II signifies mild disease.
• Stage III indicates moderate disease.
• Stage IV indicates severe disease.

Endometriosis may be in your future if you are between ages 30 and 40, and if you have postponed childbearing.

What causes it

The direct cause is unknown, but having a family member with the disease or having recent surgery that required opening the uterus (such as a cesarean birth) may predispose a woman to endometriosis. Other causes include immune system defects, inflammatory influence, spread through the lymphatic system, or environmental contaminants.

Pathophysiology

Ectopic endometrial tissue responds to estrogen and progesterone with proliferation and secretion. During menstruation, ectopic tissue bleeds and causes inflammation of the surrounding tissues. Inflammation leads to fibrosis, and fibrosis leads to adhesions that produce pain and infertility.

What to look for

Acquired dysmenorrhea is the classic symptom of endometriosis. Pain may be constant. It usually begins 5 to 7 days before menses and lasts for 2 to 3 days.

What a pain

The pain may be in the lower abdomen, vagina, posterior pelvis, and back. It commonly radiates down the legs. Multiple tender nodules occur on uterosacral ligaments or in the rectovaginal system. They enlarge and become more tender during menses. Ovarian enlargement may also be evident on palpation.

Location, location, location

Other signs and symptoms depend on the location of the ectopic tissue:
• appendix and small bowel: nausea and vomiting, which worsen before menses, and abdominal cramps
• bladder: suprapubic pain, dysuria, and hematuria
• cervix, perineum, and vagina: bleeding from endometrial deposits in these areas during menses
• colon and rectovaginal septum: painful bowel movements, rectal bleeding with menses, and pain in the coccyx or sacrum
• cul-de-sac or ovaries: deep-thrust dyspareunia
• ovaries and oviducts: infertility and profuse menses.

What tests tell you

Diagnosis of endometriosis is based on these characteristic tests and findings:

Contaminants like me can cause endometriosis.

• Laparoscopy may confirm the diagnosis and determine the stage of the disease.
• Barium enema rules out malignant or inflammatory bowel disease.

How it's treated

Treatment varies according to the stage of the disease, the patient's age, and her desire to have children. It includes:
• For young women who want to become pregnant: Conservative therapy includes androgens such as danazol, which produce a temporary remission in stages I and II. Progestins and hormonal contraceptives also relieve symptoms.
• With extensive disease (stages III and IV) or for women who don't want to become pregnant: When ovarian masses are present, they should be removed to rule out cancer. Although this may be accomplished with conservative surgery, the treatment of choice is a total abdominal hysterectomy performed with bilateral salpingo-oophorectomy.

What to do

During and after treatment, take these measures:
• Encourage the patient to contact a support group such as the Endometriosis Association for further information and counseling. Remind her to have an annual pelvic examination and Pap test.
• Note whether the patient is free from pain or can at least manage symptoms.
• Check for postoperative complications.
• Explain the possible consequences of delaying surgery if applicable.
• Make sure she understands the importance of frequent gynecologic examinations. (See *Endometriosis teaching tips*.)

Erectile dysfunction

Erectile dysfunction, also known as *impotence*, prevents a man from achieving or maintaining penile erection sufficient to complete intercourse. Two types of impotence exist:

Primary impotence means that the patient has never achieved a sufficient erection.

Secondary impotence (more common and less serious) means that the patient has achieved and maintained erections in the past, even though he can't do so now.

Education edge

Endometriosis teaching tips

If your patient has endometriosis:
• Advise her to use sanitary napkins instead of tampons if she's an adolescent. This helps prevent retrograde flow in a girl with a narrow vagina or small introitus.
• Warn her that infertility is a possible complication, so if she wants children, she shouldn't postpone childbearing.
• Stress the importance of treatment to prevent or postpone complications, which can include infertility.
• Teach her how to recognize endometrioma rupture and what to do if it occurs.
• Teach her how to relieve dyspareunia and how to recognize and prevent symptoms of anemia.

Erectile dysfunction affects men of all ages but is more common and frequent in older men. The prognosis depends on the severity and duration of impotence and on the underlying cause. Transient periods of impotence aren't considered dysfunctional and probably occur in 50% of adult males.

What causes it

Eighty percent of cases are believed to have an organic cause, such as vascular insufficiency or veno-occlusive dysfunction. Other organic causes include alcohol and drug abuse and medications such as amitriptyline, cimetidine, clonidine, desipramine, digoxin, hydralazine, methyldopa, nortriptyline, propranolol, thiazide diuretics, and tranylcypromine.

Twenty percent of cases are believed to be psychogenic in nature, resulting from sexual performance anxiety, low self-esteem, or past failures in sustaining an erection.

Pathophysiology

Inappropriate adrenergic stimulation can cause a lack of autonomic signal or impairment of perfusion. This may interfere with arteriolar dilation and cause premature collapse of the sacs of the corpus cavernosum.

Psychogenic causes may exacerbate emotional problems in a circular pattern; with anxiety causing fear of erectile dysfunction, which in turn causes further emotional problems.

Anticlimax

In addition, pelvic steal syndrome causes increased blood flow to the pelvic muscles, resulting in loss of erection before ejaculation.

What to look for

Because the patient's erectile dysfunction won't be obvious to you, you'll need to ask him questions to learn more about it. If he has secondary erectile dysfunction, base your questions on these categories:

 partial: patient can't achieve a full erection

 intermittent: patient is sometimes potent with the same partner

 selective: patient is potent only with certain partners.

Sorry, but I have to ask

Also ask the patient if he lost erectile function suddenly or gradually. If the cause of his erectile dysfunction is psychogenic, ask if he can still achieve erection through masturbation. Ask how he feels before trying to have intercourse — is he anxious, with sweating and palpitations? Is he totally disinterested in sexual activity?

Also ask the patient if he's depressed. Depression can cause psychogenic impotence and result from both psychogenic and organic impotence.

> Are you depressed? Depression can both cause and result from impotence.

What tests tell you

Diagnosis is confirmed when the patient meets either of two criteria of the *Diagnostic and Statistical Manual of Mental Disorders*, Fourth Edition, Text Revision:

☝ persistent or recurrent partial or complete failure to attain or maintain erection until completion of sexual activity

✌ marked distress or interpersonal difficulty as a result of erectile dysfunction.

Diagnosis must also rule out chronic disease, such as diabetes and other vascular, neurologic, or urogenital problems.

How it's treated

Treatment includes these measures:
• Sex therapy, largely directed at reducing performance anxiety, may cure psychogenic impotence. Such therapy should include both partners.
• If impotence is caused by drug or alcohol abuse, treatment of those specific problems may be the solution.
• Treatment of organic impotence focuses on reversing the cause if possible. If not, psychological counseling may help the couple deal realistically with their situation and explore alternatives for sexual expression.
• Certain patients suffering from organic impotence may benefit from surgically inserted penile implants; those with low testosterone levels, from testosterone injections.

What to do

During and after treatment, take these measures:
• Help the patient feel comfortable about discussing his sexuality. Assess his sexual health during your initial nursing history. When appropriate, refer him for further evaluation or treatment.

• Help prevent impotence by providing information about resuming sexual activity as part of your discharge instructions for any patient with a condition that requires modification of daily activities. Such patients include those with cardiac disease, diabetes, hypertension, or chronic obstructive pulmonary disease, and all postoperative patients.

• Evaluate the patient. He should report achieving and maintaining an erection and express satisfaction with his sexual relationships. (See *Erectile dysfunction teaching tips*.)

PID

PID refers to any acute, subacute, recurrent, or chronic infection of the oviducts and ovaries, with adjacent tissue involvement. It includes inflammation of the cervix (cervicitis), uterus (endometritis), fallopian tubes (salpingitis), and ovaries (oophoritis), which can extend to the connective tissue lying between the broad ligaments (parametritis). (See *Three types of PID*.)

No time to waste!

Early diagnosis and treatment prevent damage to the reproductive system. Complications of PID include infertility and potentially fatal septicemia, pulmonary emboli, and shock. Untreated PID may be fatal.

What causes it

PID can result from infection with aerobic or anaerobic organisms. About 60% of cases result from overgrowth of one or more of the common bacterial species found in cervical mucus, including staphylococci, streptococci, diphtheroids, chlamydiae, and coliforms such as *Pseudomonas* and *Escherichia coli*.

PID also results from infection with *Neisseria gonorrhoeae*. Finally, multiplication of typically nonpathogenic bacteria in an altered endometrial environment can cause PID. This occurs most commonly during parturition.

PID promoters

These factors increase the patient's chances of developing PID:
• history of STD
• more than one sexual partner

Three types of PID

Cause and signs and symptoms	Diagnostic findings
Cervicitis	
• *Acute:* purulent, foul-smelling vaginal discharge; vulvo-vaginitis, with itching or burning; red, edematous cervix; pelvic discomfort; sexual dysfunction; metrorrhagia; infertility; spontaneous abortion • *Chronic:* cervical dystocia, laceration or eversion of the cervix, ulcerative vesicular lesion (when cervicitis results from herpes simplex virus type 2)	• Cultures for *Neisseria gonorrhoeae* are positive. • With chronic cervicitis, causative organisms are usually staphylococcus or streptococcus. • Cytologic smears may reveal severe inflammation. • If cervicitis isn't complicated by salpingitis, white blood cell (WBC) count is normal or slightly elevated; erythrocyte sedimentation rate (ESR) is elevated. • With acute cervicitis, cervical palpation reveals tenderness.
Endometritis (usually postpartum or postabortion)	
• *Acute:* mucopurulent or purulent vaginal discharge oozing from cervix; edematous, hyperemic endometrium, possibly leading to ulceration and necrosis (with virulent organisms); lower abdominal pain and tenderness; fever; rebound pain; abdominal muscle spasm; thrombophlebitis of uterine and pelvic vessels • *Chronic:* recurring acute episodes (usually from having multiple sexual partners and sexually transmitted infections)	• With severe infection, palpation may reveal boggy uterus. • Uterine and blood samples are positive for causative organism, usually staphylococcus. • WBC count and ESR are elevated.
Salpingo-oophoritis	
• *Acute:* sudden onset of lower abdominal and pelvic pain, usually after menses; increased vaginal discharge; fever; malaise; lower abdominal pressure and tenderness; tachycardia; pelvic peritonitis • *Chronic:* recurring acute episodes	• Elevated or normal WBC count. • X-ray may show ileus. • Pelvic examination reveals extreme tenderness. • Smear of cervical or periurethral gland exudate shows gram-negative intracellular diplococci.

• conditions, such as uterine infection, or procedures, such as conization or cauterization of the cervix, that alter or destroy cervical mucus, allowing bacteria to ascend into the uterine cavity
• any procedure that risks transfer of contaminated cervical mucus into the endometrial cavity by instrumentation, such as use of a biopsy curet or an irrigation catheter, tubal insufflation, abortion, or pelvic surgery
• infection during or after pregnancy
• an infectious focus within the body, such as drainage from a chronically infected fallopian tube, a pelvic abscess, a ruptured appendix, or diverticulitis of the sigmoid colon.

Pathophysiology

Various conditions, procedures, or instruments can alter or destroy the cervical mucus, which usually serves as a protective barrier. As a result, bacteria enter the uterine cavity, causing inflammation of various structures.

What to look for

Signs and symptoms vary with the affected area and include:
• profuse, purulent vaginal discharge
• low-grade fever and malaise (especially if *N. gonorrhoeae* is the cause)
• lower abdominal pain
• extreme pain on movement of the cervix or palpation of the adnexa.

What tests tell you

PID is diagnosed based on these tests and findings:
• Gram stain of secretions from the endocervix or cul-de-sac to help identify the infecting organism.
• Culture and sensitivity testing to aid selection of the appropriate antibiotic. Urethral and rectal secretions may also be cultured.
• Ultrasonography to identify an adnexal or uterine mass.
• Culdocentesis to obtain peritoneal fluid or pus for culture and sensitivity testing.

How it's treated

Effective management eradicates the infection, relieves symptoms, and leaves the reproductive system intact. It includes:
• Aggressive therapy with multiple antibiotics beginning immediately after culture specimens are obtained. Therapy can be reevaluated as soon as laboratory results are available (usually after 24 to 48 hours). Infection may become chronic if treated inadequately.
• For PID resulting from gonorrhea: I.V. doxycycline and I.V. cefoxitin, followed by doxycycline by mouth (P.O.). Outpatient therapy may consist of I.M. cefoxitin, amoxicillin P.O., or ampicillin P.O. (each with probenecid), followed by doxycycline P.O. A patient with gonorrhea may also require therapy for syphilis.
• Supplemental treatment, including bed rest, analgesics, and I.V. therapy.
• Adequate drainage if a pelvic abscess develops.
• For a ruptured pelvic abscess (a life-threatening complication): Possible total abdominal hysterectomy with bilateral salpingo-oophorectomy.

• Nonsteroidal anti-inflammatory drugs for pain relief (preferred treatment); opioids if necessary.

What to do

During and after treatment, take these measures:
• After establishing that the patient has no drug allergies, administer antibiotics and analgesics, as ordered.
• Check for elevated temperature.
• Watch for abdominal rigidity and distention, possible signs of developing peritonitis.
• Provide frequent perineal care if vaginal drainage occurs.
• Evaluate the patient. She shouldn't have pain, discharge, fever, or recurring infection. However, many patients experience occasional pain, and up to 25% may become infertile after one episode of PID. (See *PID teaching tips*.)

STDs

STDs are the most common infections in the United States, and chlamydia is the most common STD. Morbidity and mortality depend on the type and stage of the disease. Many STDs are easy to treat when detected early.

What causes it

Transmission of the causative organism, which may include bacteria, viruses, protozoans, fungi, or ectoparasites, leads to infection. Patients at high risk include those:

 under age 25

 with multiple sexual partners

 with a history of STDs.

Four groups not to join

The incidence of STDs is higher among prostitutes, people having sexual contact with prostitutes, drug abusers, and prison inmates.

Pathophysiology

These contagious diseases are usually transmitted through intimate sexual contact with an infected person. Some are transmitted to an infant during pregnancy or childbirth.

Education edge

PID teaching tips

If your patient has pelvic inflammatory disease (PID), cover these important points:
• To prevent recurrence, encourage compliance with treatment, and explain the nature and seriousness of PID.
• Because PID may cause painful intercourse, advise the patient to consult with her doctor about sexual activity.
• Stress the need for the patient's sexual partner to be examined and treated for infection.
• To prevent infection after minor gynecologic procedures such as dilatation and curettage, tell the patient to immediately report fever, increased vaginal discharge, or pain. After such procedures, instruct her to avoid douching and intercourse for at least 7 days.

What to look for

The chief signs of STDs are vaginitis, recurrent vaginitis, vaginal or penile discharge, epididymitis, lower abdominal pain, pharyngitis, proctitis, and skin or mucous membrane lesions.

The stealthy STD

Many STDs produce no symptoms, especially in women. By the time the STD is detected, the woman may have severe complications, such as PID, infertility, ectopic pregnancy, or chronic pelvic pain.

What tests tell you

The diagnosis of a specific STD is made by physical examination, patient history, and laboratory tests to determine the causative organism.

How it's treated

Treatment is based on the specific causative organism. Treatment guidelines for each STD are available from the Centers for Disease Control and Prevention (CDC). (See *Sexually transmitted diseases.*)

Advice from on high

The CDC recommends that these resources be available for patients with STDs:
• medical evaluation and treatment facilities for patients with human immunodeficiency virus infection
• hospitalization facilities for patients with complicated STDs, such as PID and disseminated gonococcal infection
• referrals for medical, pediatric, infectious disease, dermatologic, and gynecologic-obstetric services
• family-planning services
• substance abuse treatment programs.

What to do

During and after treatment, take these measures:
• Ensure the patient's privacy and confidentiality. Avoid judging the patient's lifestyle and making assumptions about his sexual preference.
• Provide emotional support, and encourage the patient to discuss his feelings. He may be anxious and fearful and may experience altered self-esteem and self-image.
• Evaluate the patient. When assessing treatment outcome, note whether the patient remains asymptomatic without recurrent in-

Education edge

STD teaching tips

If your patient has a sexually transmitted disease (STD), include these points in your teaching:
• Discuss disease transmission, signs and symptoms, the length of the infectious period, infection prevention, and cure (if the STD can be cured).
• Explain the health consequences of improper treatment, and emphasize that the patient's partner is also at risk.
• Clarify common misconceptions, and promote understanding of healthful sexual practices.
• Tell the patient to seek immediate treatment if STD symptoms develop.
• Discuss modifications of sexual activity to prevent recurrence: reducing the number of sexual partners, avoiding partners who have multiple partners, and questioning partners about their STD history.

Sexually transmitted diseases

Name and organism	Possible signs and symptoms	Treatment	Special considerations
Chlamydia *Chlamydia trachomatis*	• Purulent discharge • *Males:* burning on urination and symptoms of epididymitis • *Females:* usually asymptomatic	Doxycycline or azithromycin	• All sexual contacts must be treated. • Potential complications in females are pelvic inflammatory disease (PID), infertility, and spontaneous abortion; in males, urethritis, epididymitis, and prostatitis. • Patient should take medication as prescribed, follow up in 7 to 10 days, and abstain from sexual activity until treatment is completed.
Genital herpes, herpes simplex Type 2	• *Females:* purulent vaginal discharge • Multiple vesicles on genital area, buttocks, or thighs • Painful dysuria • Fever • Headache • Malaise	Famciclovir; valacyclovir, acyclovir, topical anesthetic ointment	• Warm baths and mild analgesics may relieve pain. • Patient should avoid sexual activity during the prodromal stage and during outbreaks until all lesions have dried up. • Many patients have recurrences every 2 to 3 months; local hyperesthesias may occur 24 hours before outbreak of lesions.
Gonorrhea *Neisseria gonorrhoeae*	• Purulent discharge • Dysuria • Urinary frequency	Ceftriaxone plus azithromycin or doxycycline	• All sexual contacts must be treated. • Potential complications in females are PID, sterility, and ectopic pregnancy; in males, prostatitis, urethritis, epididymitis, and sterility. • Patient should take medication as prescribed, follow up in 7 to 10 days, and abstain from sexual activity until treatment is completed.
Human papillomavirus (HPV)	• Pink-gray soft lesions, singularly or in clusters	Podophyllin 10% to 25% to lesions, cryosurgery	• Patient should receive frequent Papanicolaou tests. • HPV has an 80% chance of recurrence. • HPV is the most common cause of cervical cancer.
Syphilis *Treponema pallidum*	• Chancre on genitalia, mouth, lips, or rectum • Fever • Lymphadenopathy • Positive results for Venereal Disease Research Laboratories test, fluorescent treponemal antibodies test, and rapid plasma reagin test	Penicillin	• Syphilis may be characterized as primary, secondary, or tertiary. • All sexual contacts must be treated. • Patient should take medication as prescribed, follow up in 7 to 10 days, and abstain from sexual activity until treatment is completed.

(continued)

Sexually transmitted diseases *(continued)*

Name and organism	Possible signs and symptoms	Treatment	Special considerations
Trichomoniasis *Trichomonas vaginalis*	• *Males:* urethritis or penile lesions; usually asymptomatic • *Females:* frothy vaginal discharge with erythema and pruritus; may be asymptomatic	Metronidazole	• All sexual contacts must be treated. • Complications in females include recurrent infections and salpingitis. • Patient should take medication as prescribed, follow up in 7 to 10 days, and abstain from sexual activity until treatment is completed.

fections. Make sure the patient understands how to prevent spreading the infection. (See *STD teaching tips*, page 642.)

Testicular torsion

Testicular torsion is the abnormal twisting of the spermatic cord that results from rotation of a testis or the mesorchium (a fold in the area between the testis and epididymis). It causes strangulation and, if untreated, eventual infarction of the testis.

This condition is almost always unilateral. Although it's most common between ages 12 and 18, it may occur at any age. The prognosis is good with early detection and prompt treatment.

What causes it

Testicular torsion is caused in part by abnormalities inside or outside the tunica vaginalis, the serous membrane covering the internal scrotal cavity.

Twist and shout

Intravaginal torsion is caused by:
• abnormality of the tunica vaginalis and the position of the testis
• incomplete attachment of the testis and spermatic fascia to the scrotal wall, leaving the testis free to rotate around its vascular pedicle.

Extravaginal torsion is caused by:
• loose attachment of the tunica vaginalis to the scrotal lining, causing spermatic cord rotation above the testis
• sudden forceful contraction of the cremaster muscle due to physical exertion or irritation of the muscle.

Help! I'm dying here!

Pathophysiology

In testicular torsion, the testis rotates on its vascular pedicle and twists the arteries and vein in the spermatic cord. This interrupts blood flow to the testis, resulting in vascular engorgement, ischemia, and scrotal swelling.

What to look for

Torsion produces excruciating pain in the affected testis or iliac fossa. Physical examination reveals tense, tender swelling in the scrotum or inguinal canal and hyperemia of the overlying skin. Scrotal swelling is unrelieved by rest or elevation of the scrotum.

What tests tell you

Doppler ultrasonography helps distinguish testicular torsion from strangulated hernia, undescended testes, or epididymitis.

How it's treated

If manual reduction is unsuccessful, torsion must be surgically corrected within 6 hours after the onset of symptoms to preserve testicular function (70% salvage rate). Treatment consists of immediate surgical repair by orchiopexy (fixation of a viable testis to the scrotum) or orchiectomy (excision of a nonviable testis).

Without treatment, the testis becomes dysfunctional and necrotic after 12 hours.

What to do

Before surgery, promote the patient's comfort as much as possible. After surgery, take these measures:
• Administer pain medication as ordered.
• Monitor voiding, and apply an ice bag with a cover to reduce edema.
• Protect the wound from contamination. Otherwise, allow the patient to perform as many normal daily activities as possible.
• Evaluate the patient. He shouldn't have pain or postoperative complications. (See *Testicular torsion teaching tips.*)

Education edge

Testicular torsion teaching tips

If your patient has testicular torsion:
• Explain the surgical procedure and postoperative care. Even if the testis must be removed, reassure him that his sexual function and fertility should be unaffected.
• Recommend that the patient routinely wear a scrotal support while exercising.

Uterine leiomyomas

Also known as *myomas, fibromyomas,* and *fibroids,* uterine leiomyomas are the most common benign tumors in women. They usually occur in the uterine corpus, although they may also appear on the cervix or on the round or broad ligament.

These neoplasms are usually multiple and occur in about 20% of women over age 35. They're three times more common in Blacks than in Whites. They become malignant (leiomyosarcoma) in only 0.1% of patients.

Where the leiomyomas are

Leiomyomas are classified three ways, according to location:

 intramural (in the uterine wall)

 submucosal (protruding into the endometrial cavity)

subserosal (protruding from the serosal surface of the uterus).

In all three cases, the uterine cavity may become larger, increasing the endometrial surface area and causing increased uterine bleeding.

What causes it

The cause of uterine leiomyomas is unknown, but steroid hormones, including estrogen and progesterone, and several growth factors, including epidermal growth factor, have been implicated as regulators of leiomyoma growth.

Pathophysiology

Excessive levels of estrogen and human growth hormone (hGH) probably contribute to uterine leiomyoma formation by stimulating susceptible fibromuscular elements. Large doses of estrogen and the later stages of pregnancy increase tumor size and hGH levels. Conversely, uterine leiomyomas usually shrink or disappear after menopause, when estrogen production decreases.

What to look for

Signs and symptoms of uterine leiomyomas include:
• submucosal hypermenorrhea (cardinal sign) and possibly other forms of abnormal endometrial bleeding, dysmenorrhea, and pain
• with large tumors, a feeling of heaviness in the abdomen, pain, intestinal obstruction, constipation, urinary frequency or urgency, and irregular uterine enlargement.

What tests tell you

Diagnosis of uterine leiomyomas is based on these tests and findings:
• Blood studies showing anemia support the diagnosis.
• D&C or submucosal hysterosalpingography detects submucosal leiomyomas.
• Laparoscopy shows subserous leiomyomas on the uterine surface.

The cause of leiomyomas remains elusive. Steroid hormones may, however, regulate leiomyoma growth.

How it's treated

Appropriate intervention depends on the severity of symptoms, the size and location of the tumors, and the patient's age, parity, pregnancy status, desire to have children, and general health. Treatment can include these measures.

• A surgeon may remove small leiomyomas that have caused problems in the past or that appear likely to threaten a future pregnancy. This is the treatment of choice for a young woman who wants to have children.

• Tumors that twist or grow large enough to cause intestinal obstruction require a hysterectomy, with preservation of the ovaries if possible.

• If a pregnant woman has a leiomyomatous uterus no larger than a 6-month normal uterus by the 16th week of pregnancy, surgery is usually unnecessary and the pregnancy outcome is favorable.

• If a pregnant woman has a leiomyomatous uterus the size of a 5-month to 6-month normal uterus by the 9th week of pregnancy, spontaneous abortion will probably occur, especially with a cervical leiomyoma. A hysterectomy may be performed 5 to 6 months after delivery (when involution is complete), with preservation of the ovaries if possible.

What to do

During and after treatment, take these measures:

• If your patient develops severe anemia from excessive bleeding, administer iron and blood transfusions as ordered.

• Evaluate the patient for abnormal bleeding or pain and postoperative complications. (See *Uterine leiomyoma teaching tips*.)

Education edge

Uterine leiomyoma teaching tips

If your patient has a uterine leiomyoma, include these points in your teaching:

• Tell the patient to report abnormal bleeding or pelvic pain immediately.

• If a hysterectomy or an oophorectomy is indicated, explain the effects of the operation on menstruation, menopause, and sexual activity. Reassure the patient that she won't experience premature menopause if her ovaries are left intact.

• If she must undergo a multiple myomectomy, make sure she understands that pregnancy is still possible.

• If the surgeon must enter the uterine cavity, explain that a cesarean delivery may be necessary.

Quick quiz

1. Spermatogenesis is:
   A. the growth and development of sperm into primary spermatocytes.
   B. the division of spermatocytes to form secondary spermatocytes.
   C. the entire process of sperm formation.
   D. the storage of newly developed sperm.

Answer: C. Spermatogenesis refers to the entire process of sperm formation, from the development of primary spermatocytes to the formation of fully functional spermatozoa.

2.   Which disorder is characterized by pain in the lower abdomen, vagina, posterior pelvis, and back that lasts for 2 to 3 days and occurs 5 to 7 days before menses?

    A.   Ovarian cyst

    B.   Endometriosis

    C.   PID

    D.   Uterine leiomyomas

Answer: B. The classic symptom of endometriosis, acquired dysmenorrhea, may produce the findings listed above.

3.   Which statement isn't true about PID?

    A.   Risk factors include more than one sexual partner and a history of STD.

    B.   Up to 25% of patients may become infertile after one episode of PID.

    C.   Untreated PID may be fatal.

    D.   The patient's sexual partners don't need to be examined and treated for infection.

Answer: D. It's necessary for the patient's sexual partners to be examined and treated for infection.

4.   Which STD is the most common in the United States?

    A.   Gonorrhea

    B.   Syphilis

    C.   Chlamydial infection

    D.   Genital herpes

Answer: C. Chlamydial infection is the most common STD in the United States. Transmission usually occurs unknowingly because chlamydia typically produces no symptoms until late in its development.

Scoring

✩✩✩   If you answered all four items correctly, bravo! You're the diva of reproductive disorders!

✩✩   If you answered three items correctly, encore! You win the Emmy for excellence in endoscopic tests!

✩   If you answered fewer than three items correctly, don't worry. A little review and you'll be performing like a star!

Musculoskeletal disorders

Just the facts

In this chapter, you'll learn:

♦ anatomy and physiology of the musculoskeletal system

♦ assessment techniques

♦ tests to diagnose musculoskeletal disorders

♦ typical nursing diagnoses

♦ common musculoskeletal disorders, including causes, pathophysiology, signs and symptoms, test results, treatments, nursing interventions, and patient teaching.

A look at musculoskeletal disorders

Be prepared to call on the full range of your nursing skills when providing musculoskeletal care. Why? Because some musculoskeletal problems are subtle and difficult to assess, whereas others are obvious, even traumatic, affecting the patient emotionally as well as physically.

Anatomy and physiology review

The three main parts of the musculoskeletal system are the bones, joints, and muscles.

Bones

The 206 bones of the skeleton support the organs and tissues and form the body's framework. The bones also serve as storage sites for minerals and produce blood cells. (See *A close look at the skeletal system*, page 650.)

A close look at the skeletal system

Of the 206 bones in the human skeletal system, 80 form the axial skeleton, or head and trunk, and 126 form the appendicular skeleton, or the extremities. Shown here are the body's major bones.

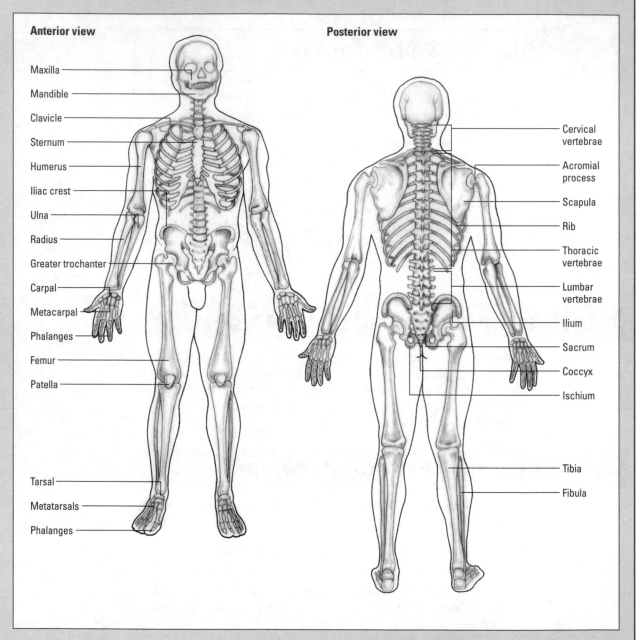

Anterior view

- Maxilla
- Mandible
- Clavicle
- Sternum
- Humerus
- Iliac crest
- Ulna
- Radius
- Greater trochanter
- Carpal
- Metacarpal
- Phalanges
- Femur
- Patella
- Tarsal
- Metatarsals
- Phalanges

Posterior view

- Cervical vertebrae
- Acromial process
- Scapula
- Rib
- Thoracic vertebrae
- Lumbar vertebrae
- Ilium
- Sacrum
- Coccyx
- Ischium
- Tibia
- Fibula

Bone function

Bones perform anatomic (mechanical) and physiologic functions, including:
- stabilizing and supporting the body
- providing a surface for muscle, ligament, and tendon attachment
- moving through "lever" action when contracted
- producing red blood cells (RBCs) in the bone marrow (hematopoiesis)
- storing mineral salts, including about 99% of the body's calcium
- protecting internal tissues and organs (For example, the 33 vertebrae surround and protect the spinal cord.).

Joints

The junction of two or more bones is called a *joint*. Joints stabilize the bones and allow a specific type of movement. There are two types of joints:

 nonsynovial

 synovial.

In nonsynovial joints, the bones are connected by fibrous tissue or cartilage. They may be immovable, like the sutures in the skull, or slightly movable, like the vertebrae.

Free to be...a synovial joint

Synovial joints move freely. The bones are separate from each other and meet in a cavity filled with synovial fluid, a lubricant. A layer of resilient cartilage covers the surfaces of opposing bones. This cartilage cushions the bones and allows full joint movement by making the surfaces of the bones smooth. (See *Synovial joint.*)

Some popular joints

Synovial joints come in several types, including ball-and-socket joints and hinge joints.

Ball-and-socket joints (found in the shoulders and hips) allow for:

 flexion (bending, which decreases the joint angle)

 extension (straightening, which increases the joint angle)

 adduction (moving toward midline)

 abduction (moving away from midline).

These joints also rotate in their sockets and are assessed by their degree of internal and external rotation.

Synovial joint

Typically, bones fit together. Cartilage—a smooth, fibrous tissue—cushions the end of each bone, and synovial fluid fills the joint space. This fluid lubricates the joint and eases movement, much as the brake fluid functions in a car.

Joint capsule

Cartilage

Bone

Joint space filled with synovial fluid

Hinge joints, such as the knee and elbow, usually move in flexion and extension only.

We've got you surrounded

Synovial joints are surrounded by a fibrous capsule that stabilizes the joint structures. The capsule also surrounds the joint's ligaments—the tough, fibrous bands that join one bone to another.

Muscles

Skeletal muscles are groups of contractile cells or fibers. These fibers contract and produce skeletal movement when they receive a stimulus from the central nervous system (CNS). The CNS is responsible for involuntary and voluntary muscle function. Skeletal muscles also maintain posture and generate body heat.

Tough guy, huh?

Tendons are tough, fibrous portions of muscle that attach the muscles to bone. Bursae—sacs filled with friction-reducing synovial fluid—are located in areas of high friction such as the knee.

Muscle movements

Skeletal muscle allows several types of movement. A muscle's functional name comes from the type of movement it permits. For example, a flexor muscle permits bending (flexion), an abductor muscle permits movement away from a body axis (abduction), and a circumductor muscle allows a circular movement (circumduction).

My muscles maintain posture and generate body heat.

Musculoskeletal assessment

Your sharp assessment skills will help you uncover musculoskeletal abnormalities and evaluate the patient's ability to perform activities of daily living (ADLs). However, because many musculoskeletal injuries are emergencies, you might not have time for a thorough patient history and physical examination.

Patient history

If possible, question the patient about his current illness, past illnesses, medications, and social history.

Current illness

Ask the patient about his chief complaint. Patients with joint injuries usually complain of pain, swelling, or stiffness; those with bone fractures have sharp pain when they move the affected area. Muscular injury is commonly accompanied by pain, swelling, and weakness.

Ask the patient if his ability to carry out ADLs is affected. Has he noticed grating sounds when he moves certain parts of his body? Does he use ice, heat, or other remedies to treat the problem?

Past health history

Inquire whether the patient has ever had gout, arthritis, tuberculosis (TB), or cancer, which may have bony metastases. Has he been diagnosed with osteoporosis?

Any ouchies?

Ask whether he has had a recent blunt or penetrating trauma. If so, how did it happen? For example, did he suffer knee and hip injuries after being hit by a car, or did he fall from a ladder and land on his coccyx? This information will help guide your assessment and predict hidden trauma.

Also ask the patient whether he uses an assistive device, such as a cane, walker, or brace. If so, watch him use the device to assess how he moves.

Medications

Question the patient about the medications he takes regularly. Many drugs can affect the musculoskeletal system. Corticosteroids, for example, can cause muscle weakness, myopathy, osteoporosis, pathologic fractures, and avascular necrosis of the heads of the femur and humerus.

Several drugs affect the musculoskeletal system.

Family history

Ask the patient if family member suffers from joint disease. Disorders with a hereditary component include:
• gout
• osteoarthritis of the interphalangeal joints
• spondyloarthropathies (such as ankylosing spondylitis, Reiter's syndrome, psoriatic arthritis, and enteropathic arthritis)
• rheumatoid arthritis.

Social history

Ask the patient about his job, hobbies, and personal habits. Knitting, playing football or tennis, working at a computer, or doing construction work can all cause repetitive stress injuries or injure the musculoskeletal system in other ways. Even carrying a heavy knapsack or purse can cause injury or increase muscle size.

> Working at a computer can cause repetitive stress injuries.

Physical examination

Perform a head-to-toe assessment, simultaneously evaluating the muscle and joint function of each body area. You'll need to observe the patient's posture, gait, and coordination, and inspect and palpate his muscles, joints, and bones.

Inspecting posture, gait, and coordination

Assessment begins the instant you see the patient. Good observation skills enable you to obtain a wealth of information about approximate muscle strength, facial muscle movement, body symmetry, and obvious physical or functional deformities or abnormalities.

Assess the patient's overall body symmetry as he assumes different postures and makes diverse movements. Note marked dissimilarities in side-to-side size, shape, and motion.

Posture

Posture is the attitude, or position, that body parts assume in relation to other body parts and to the external environment. Assessing posture includes inspecting spinal curvature and knee positioning.

Stand by your man (and woman)

To assess spinal curvature, instruct the patient to stand as straight as possible. Then stand at his side, behind his back, and in front of him, in that order, inspecting the spine for alignment and the shoulders, iliac crests, and scapulae for symmetry of position and height.

When the patient stands, his thoracic spine should have a convex curvature and his lumbar spine should have a concave curvature.

Next, have the patient bend forward from the waist with his arms relaxed and dangling. Stand behind him and inspect the straightness of his spine, noting flank and thorax position and symmetry.

Other normal findings include:

• a midline spine without lateral curvatures
• a concave lumbar curvature that changes to a convex curvature in the flexed position
• iliac crests, shoulders, and scapulae at the same horizontal level.

Gait

Direct the patient to walk away from you, turn around, and then walk back. Observe his posture, movement (such as pace and length of stride), foot position, coordination, and balance.

Smooth walker

Normal findings when walking include smooth, coordinated movements, the head leading the body when turning, and erect posture with approximately 2″ to 4″ (5 to 10 cm) of space between the feet. Be sure to remain close to an elderly or infirm patient and be ready to help if he should stumble or start to fall.

Coordination

Evaluate how well a patient's muscles produce movement. Coordination results from neuromuscular integrity; a lack of muscular or nervous system integrity, or both, impairs the ability to make voluntary and productive movements.

You're so fine and gross

Assess gross motor skills by having the patient perform body action involving the muscles and joints in natural directional movements, such as lifting the arm to the side and other range-of-motion (ROM) exercises. Assess fine motor coordination by asking the patient to pick up a small object from a desk or table.

Inspecting and palpating muscles

Expect to perform inspection and palpation simultaneously during the musculoskeletal assessment. You'll evaluate muscle tone, mass, and strength. Palpate the muscles gently, never forcing movement when the patient reports pain or when you feel resistance. Watch the patient's face and body language for signs of discomfort — he may suffer silently.

Tone and mass

Muscle tone is the consistency or tension in the resting muscle. Test it by palpating a muscle at rest and by performing passive ROM exercises. To palpate a muscle at rest, feel from the muscle attachment at the bone to the edge of the muscle. A relaxed muscle should feel soft, pliable, and nontender; a contracted muscle should feel firm.

Check out those muscles

Muscle mass is the size of a muscle. Assessment of muscle mass usually involves measuring the circumference of the thigh, calf, and upper arm. When measuring, mark landmarks with a pen to make sure you're measuring at the same location on each side of the body.

Check out my muscle mass!

Strength and joint ROM

Assessing joint ROM tests the joint's function. Assessing muscle strength against resistance tests the function of the muscles surrounding the joint. (See *Testing muscle strength*.)

Inspecting and palpating joints and bones

When evaluating joint and bone characteristics and joint ROM, never force joint movement if you feel resistance or if the patient complains of pain.

Departures from the norm

Deviations include pain, swelling, stiffness, deformities, altered ROM, crepitation (a grating sound or sensation accompanying joint movement), ankylosis (joint fusion or fixation), and contracture (muscle shortening).

Cervical spine

Have the patient sit or stand. Inspect the cervical spine from behind, from the side, and while facing the patient.

Drawing a line

Observe the alignment of the head with the body.

The nose should be in line with the midsternum and extend beyond the shoulders when viewed from the side. The head should align with the shoulders. Typically, the seventh cervical and first thoracic vertebrae appear more prominent than the others.

Clavicles

With the patient sitting or standing, inspect and palpate the length of the clavicles, including the sternoclavicular and acromioclavicular joints. Normal findings include firm, smooth, continuous bones.

Testing muscle strength

To test the muscle strength of your patient's arm and ankle muscles, use the techniques shown here.

Biceps strength

Ankle strength: Plantar flexion

Triceps strength

Ankle strength: Dorsiflexion

Scapulae

To inspect and palpate the scapulae, sit directly behind the patient as he sits with his shoulders thrust backward. Usually, the scapulae are located over thoracic ribs two through seven. Check for an equal distance from the medial scapular edges to the midspinal line.

Ribs

Have the patient remain sitting. After assessing the scapulae, inspect and palpate the anterior, posterior, and lateral surfaces of the ribs. Normal findings include firm, smooth, continuous bones.

Shoulders

With the patient still sitting, palpate the moving joints for crepitus. Inspect the skin overlying the shoulder joints for erythema, masses, or swelling.

Introducing the Ducts, Ad and Ab

Next, palpate the acromioclavicular joint and the area over the greater humeral tuberosity. Ask the patient to stand. Have him hold his arm at his side and then adduct his arm. Next, place your thumb on the anterior portion of the patient's shoulder joint and your fingers on the posterior portion of the shoulder joint. Ask the patient to abduct his arm. Palpate the shoulder joint as he does so.

Stand and rotate

Now stand behind the patient. With your fingertips placed over the greater humeral tuberosity, instruct him to rotate each shoulder internally by moving the corresponding arm behind his back. This allows you to palpate a portion of the musculotendinous rotator cuff as well as the bony structures of the shoulder joint.

Elbows

With the patient sitting or standing, inspect joint contour and skin over each elbow. Palpate the elbows at rest and during movement.

Wrists

With the patient sitting or standing, inspect the wrists for masses, erythema, skeletal deformities, and swelling. Palpate the wrist at rest and during movement by gently grasping it between your thumb and fingers.

Fingers and thumbs

With the patient sitting or standing, inspect the fingers and thumbs of each hand for nodules, erythema, spacing, length, and skeletal deformities. Palpate the fingers and thumbs at rest and during movement.

Thoracic and lumbar spine

In addition to evaluating the curvatures of the thoracic and lumbar spine during the postural assessment, you'll need to palpate the length of the spine for tenderness and vertebral alignment. With the patient standing, check for tenderness, percuss each spinous process (directly over the vertebral column) with the ulnar side of your fist.

Note whether the patient can move with a full ROM while maintaining balance, smoothness, and coordination.

We have all the right moves, along with balance, smoothness, and coordination!

Hips and pelvis

With the patient sitting or standing, inspect and palpate over the bony prominences of the hips and pelvis: iliac crests, symphysis pubis, anterior spine, ischial tuberosities, and greater trochanters. Palpate the hip at rest and during movement.

Knees

Inspect the knees with the patient seated. Palpate the knee at rest and during movement. Inspect and palpate the popliteal spaces behind the knee joint. Knee movements should be smooth.

Ankles and feet

With the patient sitting, inspect and palpate the ankles and feet at rest and during movement.

Toes

The patient may be sitting or lying supine for toe assessment. Inspect all toe surfaces. Palpate the toes at rest and during movement.

Diagnostic tests

Diagnostic tests help to confirm the diagnosis and identify the underlying cause of musculoskeletal problems. Common procedures include aspiration tests, endoscopic tests, and radiographic and imaging studies.

Aspiration tests

The doctor may aspirate a specimen from the joint capsule (arthrocentesis) or from the bone marrow to detect various disorders.

Arthrocentesis

Arthrocentesis is a joint puncture that's used to collect fluid for analysis to identify the cause of pain and swelling, to assess for infection, and to distinguish forms of arthritis, such as pseudogout and infectious arthritis. The doctor will probably choose the knee for this procedure, but he may tap synovial fluid from the wrist, ankle, elbow, or first metatarsophalangeal joint.

Telltale findings

In joint infection, for example, synovial fluid looks cloudy and contains more white blood cells (WBCs) and less glucose than

Hmmmmm...I see more WBCs and less glucose than normal. Could be a joint infection.

normal. When trauma causes bleeding into a joint, synovial fluid contains RBCs. In specific types of arthritis, crystals can confirm the diagnosis — for instance, urate crystals indicate gout.

Doing double duty

Arthrocentesis also has therapeutic value. For example, in symptomatic joint effusion, removing excess synovial fluid relieves pain.

Nursing considerations

Take these measures:
• Describe the procedure to the patient. Explain that he'll be asked to assume a certain position, depending on the joint being aspirated, and that he'll need to remain still.
• After the test, the doctor may ask you to apply ice or cold packs to the joint to reduce pain and swelling.
• If the doctor removed a large amount of fluid, tell the patient that he may need to wear an elastic bandage.
• Advise him not to use the joint excessively for 24 hours after the test to avoid joint pain, swelling, and stiffness.
• Instruct him to report these signs of infection: fever and increased pain, tenderness, swelling, warmth, or redness.

Bone marrow aspiration

Bone marrow aspiration can help diagnose many abnormalities, including rheumatoid arthritis, TB, amyloidosis, syphilis, bacterial or viral infection, parasitic infestation, tumors, and hematologic problems.

Aspiration usually involves the sternum or iliac crests.

Suck it up

The site is prepared as for any minor surgical procedure and then infiltrated with a local anesthetic such as lidocaine. The doctor inserts the marrow needle, with stylet in place, through the cortex into the marrow cavity. Marrow cavity penetration causes the patient to feel a collapsing sensation. Then the doctor removes the stylet, attaches a syringe to the needle hub, and aspirates 0.2 to 0.5 ml of fluid.

Nursing considerations

Take these measures:
• Tell the patient that he'll be sedated and that he'll receive a local anesthetic before needle insertion.
• Explain that the test takes about 10 minutes.

They're putting a needle in what?

- Warn the patient that he'll feel pressure as the doctor inserts the needle and that aspiration may hurt briefly.
- Watch for signs of infection after the procedure.
- Make sure bleeding stops, particularly if the patient has a clotting disorder.

Endoscopic tests

Endoscopic studies allow direct visualization of joint problems. Arthroscopy is a common endoscopic procedure.

Arthroscopy

Arthroscopy is usually used to evaluate the knee. It helps the doctor assess joint problems, plan surgical approaches, and document pathology.

Needling the knee

After inserting a large-bore needle into the suprapatellar pouch, the doctor injects sterile saline solution to distend the joint. Then he passes a fiber-optic scope through puncture sites lateral or medial to the tibial plateau, allowing direct visualization. With a large scope, he can remove articular debris and small, loose bodies or repair a torn meniscus.

Nursing considerations

Take these measures:
- Tell the patient that he can't eat or drink after midnight before the test.
- Explain that he'll receive a sedative immediately before the test, and that the area around the joint will be shaved. Determine if the patient requires skin preparation before the procedure.
- If the test will be performed under local anesthesia, check the patient history for hypersensitivity to local anesthetics. Warn the patient that he may feel transient discomfort during injection of the anesthetic.
- Explain that the doctor will make a small incision and insert the arthroscope into the joint cavity.
- Tell the patient that he'll be allowed to walk as soon as he's fully awake. He'll experience mild soreness and a slight grinding sensation in his knee for 1 to 2 days.
- Instruct him to notify the doctor if he feels severe or persistent pain or develops a fever with signs of local inflammation.

Take it easy for a few days after an arthroscopy.

• Advise against excessive use of the joint for a few days after the test. Tell the patient that he may resume his normal diet.
• Ask the doctor about specific leg exercises, ice application, and dressing changes that are necessary after the procedure and at home.
• Assess the patient for signs of complications, such as infection, hemarthrosis (blood accumulation in the joint), or a synovial cyst.

Radiographic and imaging studies

Radiographic and imaging studies include bone scans, computed tomography (CT) scans, dual energy X-ray absorptiometry (DEXA), magnetic resonance imaging (MRI), and X-rays.

Bone scan

A bone scan helps detect bony metastasis, benign disease, fractures, avascular necrosis, and infection.

Scintillating study

After I.V. introduction of a radioactive material, such as the radioisotope technetium polyphosphate, the isotope collects in areas of increased bone activity or active bone formation. A scintillation counter detects the gamma rays, indicating abnormal areas of increased uptake (positive findings). The radioisotope has a short half-life and soon passes from the patient's body.

A short half-life means that the radioisotope passes from the patient's body quickly.

Nursing considerations

Take these measures:
• Explain to the patient how this painless test commonly detects bone abnormalities earlier than conventional X-rays.
• Tell him that he can eat and drink as usual before the test.
• Describe how the doctor applies a tourniquet on the patient's arm and then injects a small dose of a radioactive isotope. Assure the patient that the isotope emits less radiation than a standard X-ray machine.
• Explain that after the isotope is injected, there's a 2- to 3-hour waiting period before the scan is done. During this time, the patient must drink four to six glasses of fluid.
• Explain that when it's time for the scan, he'll lie supine on a table within the scanner. The scanner moves back and forth slowly, recording images for about 1 hour. Instruct the patient to lie as still as possible and to expect to assume various positions.

CT scan

A CT scan aids diagnosis of bone tumors and other abnormalities. It helps assess questionable cervical or spinal fractures, fracture fragments, bone lesions, and intra-articular loose bodies.

Beam me up, Scotty

Multiple X-ray beams from a computerized body scanner are directed at the body from different angles. The beams pass through the body and strike radiation detectors, producing electrical impulses. A computer then converts these impulses into digital information, which is displayed as a three-dimensional image on a video monitor.

Nursing considerations

Take these measures:
- If the patient is scheduled to receive a contrast medium, inform him that he must not eat for 4 hours before the test. Check his records to make sure he isn't hypersensitive to any contrast media.
- Tell the patient that he needs to put on a hospital gown, remove all jewelry, and empty his bladder before the test.
- Instruct him to remain still during the test. Although he'll be alone in the room, assure him that he can communicate with the technician through an intercom system.
- If the patient received a contrast medium by mouth, encourage him to drink plenty of fluids after the test to help flush the contrast medium from his body.

DEXA

DEXA can assess the bone density of the entire body, or just the hip or spine. It's used to help diagnose osteoporosis, especially before a fracture occurs. This noninvasive technique uses a radiography tube to measure bone mineral density and exposes the patient to only minimal radiation.

The test uses low-dose radiation to measure bone density and is usually given to women considered at high risk for osteoporosis.

Several other machines are also used to measure bone density. (See *A bevy of bone density tests*, page 664.)

Nursing considerations

Take these measures:
- Reassure the patient that this test is painless and noninvasive and usually takes less than 15 minutes.

• Have the patient remove jewelry from the area that will be examined.

MRI

MRI can show irregularities of the spinal cord and is especially useful for diagnosing disk herniation.

Must be your animal magnetism

The MRI scanner uses a powerful magnetic field and radiofrequency energy to produce images based on the hydrogen content of body tissues. The computer processes signals and displays the resulting high-resolution image on a video monitor. The patient can't feel the magnetic fields, and no harmful effects have been observed.

Nursing considerations

Take these measures:
• Explain to the patient that he'll be positioned on a narrow bed that slides into a large cylinder housing the MRI magnets.
• Tell him that he'll be asked to put on a hospital gown and to remove all metal objects, including bobby pins, jewelry, watches, eyeglasses, hearing aids, and dental appliances. He should also remove clothes with metal zippers, buckles, or buttons as well as credit, bank, and parking cards, because the scan could erase the magnetic codes.
• Tell the patient he'll hear soft thumping noises during the test. Ask if claustrophobia has ever been a problem for him. If so, sedation may help him tolerate the scan.
• Instruct him to remain still during the test. Although he'll be alone in the room, assure him that he can communicate with the technician through an intercom system.

X-rays

Anteroposterior, posteroanterior, and lateral X-rays allow three-dimensional visualization. They help diagnose:
• traumatic disorders, such as fractures and dislocations
• bone disease, including solitary lesions, multiple focal lesions in one bone, or generalized lesions involving all bones
• joint disease, such as arthritis, infection, degenerative changes, synoviosarcoma, osteochondromatosis, avascular necrosis, slipped femoral epiphysis, and inflamed tendons and bursae around a joint
• masses and calcifications.
    If the doctor needs further clarification of standard X-rays, he may order a CT scan or MRI.

A bevy of bone density tests

These tests measure bone density or mass and are helpful in diagnosing osteoporosis.
• Single energy X-ray absorptiometry measures the wrist or heel.
• Peripheral dual energy X-ray absorptiometry measures the wrist, heel, or finger.
• Single photon absorptiometry measures the wrist.
• Dual photon absorptiometry measures the hip, spine, or total body.
• Radiographic absorptiometry calculates bone density using an X-ray of the hand.

Nursing considerations

Take these measures:

• Make sure the patient removes all jewelry from the area to be X-rayed.

• Verify that the X-ray order includes pertinent recent history, such as trauma, and identifies the point tenderness site. It should also include past fractures, dislocations, or surgery involving the affected area.

> X-rays can help diagnose trauma, bone and joint disease, and masses and calcifications — but oh boy, is this table cold and hard!

Treatments

Pain and impaired mobility provide good motivation for obtaining medical care. Consequently, most patients with musculoskeletal problems eagerly seek treatment.

Get up and go again

To restore a patient's mobility, several treatments are used alone or in combination:

• a balanced program of exercise and rest

• a splint, brace, or other device to support a weakened or injured limb or joint

• drug therapy to control pain, inflammation, or muscle spasticity.

• nonsurgical treatments, including closed reduction or immobilization

• surgery with subsequent immobilization with a cast, brace, or other device.

Drug therapy

Salicylates are the first line of defense against arthropathies. Other drug therapy includes analgesics, nonsteroidal anti-inflammatory drugs (NSAIDS), corticosteroids, and skeletal muscle relaxants.

Nonsurgical treatments

Some patients with musculoskeletal disorders require nonsurgical treatment. Such treatment may include closed reduction of a fracture or immobilization.

> I'm tuned up and ready to mobilize!

Closed reduction

Closed reduction involves external manipulation of fracture fragments or dislocated joints to restore their normal position and alignment. It may be done under local, regional, or general anesthesia.

Patient preparation

Prepare the patient for reduction:
• If he'll be receiving a general anesthetic, instruct him not to eat after midnight. Tell him he'll receive a sedative before the procedure.
• If appropriate, explain how traction can reduce pain, relieve muscle spasms, and maintain alignment while he awaits the procedure.

Monitoring and aftercare

Take these measures:
• Assess for pain and provide pain management, as needed.
• Be prepared to care for a bandage, sling, splint, or cast after the procedure. These devices immobilize the fracture or dislocation.
• Tell the patient that he'll have an X-ray to evaluate the closed reduction.

Home care instructions

Give the patient these instructions:
• Before discharge, teach the patient how to apply (if appropriate) and care for the immobilization device. Tell him to regularly check his skin under and around the device for irritation and breakdown.
• Stress the importance of following prescribed exercises.

Immobilization

Immobilization devices are commonly used to maintain proper alignment and limit movement. They also relieve pressure and pain.

Don't move a muscle!

Immobilization devices include:
• plaster and synthetic casts applied after closed or open reduction of fractures or after other severe injuries
• splints to immobilize fractures, dislocations, or subluxations
• slings to support and immobilize an injured arm, wrist, or hand, or to support the weight of a splint or hold dressings in place

• skin or skeletal traction, using a system of weights and pulleys to reduce fractures, treat dislocations, correct deformities, or decrease muscle spasms
• braces to support weakened or deformed joints
• cervical collars to immobilize the cervical spine, decrease muscle spasms, and possibly relieve pain.

Traction uses pulleys and weights to reduce fractures.

Patient preparation

Prepare the patient for immobilization:
• Explain the purpose of the immobilization device the doctor has ordered. If possible, show the patient the device before application and demonstrate how it works. Tell him approximately how long the device will remain in place.
• Explain that he'll have discomfort initially, but reassure him that this will resolve as he becomes accustomed to the device. (See *Comparing traction techniques*, page 668.)
• If the patient is in pain, give analgesics and muscle relaxants as ordered.

Monitoring and aftercare

Take these measures:
• Take steps to prevent complications of immobility, especially if the patient is in traction or requires long-term bed rest. For example, reposition him frequently to enhance comfort and prevent pressure ulcers.
• As ordered, assist with active or passive ROM exercises to maintain muscle tone and prevent contractures.
• Encourage regular coughing and deep breathing to prevent pulmonary complications.
• Stress adequate fluid intake to prevent urinary stasis and constipation.
• Encourage the bedridden patient to engage in hobbies or other activities to relieve boredom. This also helps maintain the positive mental outlook that's important to recovery.
• Encourage ambulation, if appropriate, and provide assistance as necessary.
• Provide analgesics as ordered. If you're administering opioid analgesics, watch for signs of toxicity or oversedation.

Home care instructions

Give the patient these instructions:

Comparing traction techniques

Traction restricts movement of a patient's affected limb or body part and may confine the patient to bed rest for an extended period. The limb is immobilized by pulling with equal force on each end of the injured area — an equal mix of traction and countertraction. Weights provide the pulling force. Countertraction is produced by using other weights or by positioning the patient's body weight against the traction pull.

Although traction commonly requires confinement to a hospital bed, it does allow the patient limited motion of his affected extremity and permits exercise of his unaffected body parts.

Skin traction

Skin traction immobilizes a body part intermittently over an extended period through direct application of a pulling force on the patient's skin. The force may be applied using adhesive or nonadhesive traction tape or other skin traction devices, such as a boot, belt, or halter. Adhesive attachment allows more continuous traction, whereas nonadhesive attachment allows easier removal for daily care.

Skeletal traction

Skeletal traction immobilizes a body part for prolonged periods by attaching weighted equipment directly to the patient's bones. This may be accomplished with pins, screws, wires, or tongs.

• Tell him to promptly report signs of complications, including increased pain, drainage, or swelling in the involved area.
• Stress the need for strict compliance with activity restrictions while the immobilization device is in place.
• If the patient has been given crutches to use with a leg or ankle cast, splint, or knee immobilizer, make sure he understands how to use them. If the patient has a removable device, such as a knee immobilizer, make sure he knows how to apply it correctly.
• Advise the patient to keep scheduled medical appointments to evaluate healing.

Walking with crutches takes practice!

Surgery

For some patients with musculoskeletal disorders, surgery can offer a bright alternative to a life of chronic pain and disability. Surgical procedures include amputation, joint replacement, laminectomy and spinal fusion, and open reduction and internal fixation.

Amputation

Perhaps more than any other surgery, amputation can dramatically change a patient's life. Your role includes providing support and detailed instruction in postoperative care.

Patient preparation

Prepare the patient for amputation:
• Before surgery, reinforce the doctor's explanation of the procedure and clear up any misconceptions the patient may have.
• Support the patient as he comes to grips with the emotions surrounding loss of a limb.

Monitoring and aftercare

Take these measures:
• After surgery, be prepared to care for the cast or elastic wrap that the doctor applies around the stump. This helps control swelling, minimize pain, and mold the stump so that it fits comfortably into a prosthesis.
• As appropriate, instruct the patient to report drainage through the cast, warmth, tenderness, or a foul smell.
• Warn the patient that the cast may slip off as swelling subsides. If so, he should immediately wrap the stump or slip on a custom-fitted elastic stump shrinker.

Home care instructions

Give the patient these instructions:
• Emphasize that proper home care of the stump can speed healing. Tell the patient to inspect the stump carefully each day, using a mirror. He should call the doctor if the incision is open, red or swollen, warm, painful to touch, or seeping drainage. Teach him to clean the stump daily with mild soap and water; then rinse and dry it thoroughly.
• Instruct the patient to rub the stump with alcohol daily to toughen the skin. Because alcohol may cause irritation in some patients, warn him to watch for and report this. Tell him not to apply powder or lotion because this may soften or irritate the skin.
• Tell him to massage the stump toward the suture line to mobilize the scar and prevent its adherence to bone.
• Advise him to avoid exposing the skin around the stump to excessive perspiration, which can be irritating. He may need to change his elastic bandages or stump socks during the day to avoid this.

• As stump muscles adjust to amputation, tell the patient he may have twitching, spasms, or phantom limb pain. Heat (for example, a hot bath, heating pad, or warm compress), massage, or gentle pressure will decrease these symptoms. If his stump is sensitive to touch, tell him to rub it with a dry washcloth for 4 minutes three times per day.

• Stress the importance of performing prescribed exercises to help minimize complications, maintain muscle strength and tone, prevent contractures, and promote independence.

• Stress the importance of positioning to prevent contractures.

• To prepare the stump for a prosthesis, teach progressive resistance maneuvers. First, the patient should push his stump gently against a soft pillow. Have him progress to pushing it against a firm pillow, a padded chair, and finally, a hard chair.

Joint replacement

Total or partial replacement of a joint with a synthetic prosthesis restores mobility and stability, relieves pain, and increases the patient's sense of independence and self-worth.

A pretty hip joint

Recent improvements in surgical techniques and prosthetic devices have made joint replacement a common treatment of severe chronic arthritis, degenerative joint disorders, and extensive joint trauma. All joints except the spine can be replaced with prostheses, with hip and knee replacements being the most common.

Patient preparation

Prepare the patient for joint replacement:

• Tell the patient that because of the complexity of joint replacement, he'll start having extensive tests and studies long before the day of surgery.

• Discuss postoperative recovery with the patient and his family. Explain that he'll probably remain in bed for 2 days after surgery. While confined to bed, he'll begin an exercise program to maintain joint mobility.

• As appropriate, show him ROM exercises. If he's having a total knee replacement, demonstrate the continuous passive motion (CPM) device he'll use during recovery.

• Point out that surgery may not relieve his pain immediately. In fact, the pain may worsen for several weeks. Reassure him that pain will diminish dramatically after edema subsides, and that analgesics will be available as needed.

Every joint in the body can be replaced, except for the spine. Groovy!

Monitoring and aftercare

Take these measures:

• After surgery, keep the patient on bed rest for the prescribed period. Turn him no more than 45 degrees every 2 hours. Maintain the affected joint in proper alignment. If traction is used, periodically check the weights and other equipment.

• Assess the patient's level of pain and provide analgesics, as ordered. If you're administering opioid analgesics, be alert for signs of toxicity or oversedation.

Dangerous globules

• During recovery, monitor for complications of joint replacement, particularly hypovolemic shock from blood loss during surgery. Also watch for signs of fat embolism. This potentially fatal complication is caused by release of fat molecules in response to increased intermedullary canal pressure from the prosthesis. The fat globules then combine with platelets to form emboli, which may occlude vessels that supply the brain, lungs, kidneys, or other organs. Symptoms typically occur within 24 to 72 hours but may occur up to a week after injury.

• Inspect the incision frequently for signs of infection. Change the dressing as necessary, maintaining strict sterile technique. Periodically assess neurovascular and motor status distal to the joint replacement site.

• Immediately report abnormalities or complications, such as a dislocated total hip replacement. Signs and symptoms of this are sudden, severe pain, shortening, or internal or external rotation of the involved leg.

• Reposition the patient often to enhance comfort and prevent pressure ulcers.

• Encourage coughing and deep breathing to prevent pulmonary complications.

• Stress adequate fluid intake to avert urinary stasis and constipation.

• Have the patient begin exercising the affected joint, as ordered, perhaps even on the day of surgery. The doctor may prescribe CPM (using a machine or a system of suspended ropes and pulleys) or a series of active or passive ROM exercises.

• Before the patient with a knee or hip replacement is discharged, make sure that he has a walker and knows how to use it.

Home care instructions

Give the patient these instructions:

• Reinforce the doctor's and physical therapist's instructions for an exercise regimen. Remind the patient to closely adhere to the

Sudden, severe pain is a symptom of a dislocated total hip replacement. Report it immediately!

prescribed schedule and not to rush rehabilitation, no matter how good he feels.

• Review prescribed activity limitations.

• If the patient has undergone hip replacement, instruct him to keep his hips abducted and not to cross his legs when sitting. This helps reduce the risk of dislocating the prosthesis. Also tell him to avoid flexing his hips more than 90 degrees when rising from a bed or chair. Encourage him to sit in chairs with high arms and a firm seat and to sleep only on a firm mattress.

• Caution the patient to promptly report signs of infection, such as persistent fever and increased pain, tenderness, and stiffness in the joint and surrounding area. Remind him that infection may still develop several months after joint replacement.

• Tell the patient to report a sudden increase of pain, which may indicate dislodgment of the prosthesis.

Laminectomy and spinal fusion

In laminectomy, the surgeon removes one or more of the bony laminae that cover the vertebrae. This procedure has two main uses:

To relieve pressure on the spinal cord or spinal nerve roots resulting from a herniated disk (most common)

To treat compression fracture or dislocation of vertebrae or a spinal cord tumor.

Nothin' confusin' about fusion

After removing the lamina, the surgeon may stabilize the spine by performing spinal fusion using bone chip grafts between vertebral spaces.

Spinal fusion may also be done without a laminectomy in patients whose vertebrae are seriously weakened by trauma or disease. Usually, spinal fusion is done only when more conservative treatments — such as prolonged bed rest, traction, or a back brace — prove ineffective. (See *Alternatives to laminectomy.*)

Patient preparation

Prepare the patient for laminectomy and spinal fusion:

• Discuss postoperative recovery and rehabilitation. Point out that surgery won't relieve back pain immediately and that pain may even worsen after the operation. Explain that relief will come only after chronic nerve irritation and swelling subside, which may take several weeks. Reassure him that analgesics and muscle relaxants will be available during recovery.

Alternatives to laminectomy

Percutaneous automated diskectomy and chemonucleolysis represent alternatives to laminectomy, the traditional surgical treatment of a herniated disk.

Percutaneous automated diskectomy

In percutaneous automated diskectomy, the surgeon uses a suction technique and X-ray visualization to remove only the disk portion that is causing pain. Depending on the patient's and surgeon's preference, this procedure can be done under local or general anesthesia and on an inpatient or outpatient basis.

Because the procedure causes little muscle trauma, it produces minimal pain. The patient should be on bed rest for the first few days and then gradually resume activities over the next 2 months. A mild analgesic or anti-inflammatory is usually sufficient for pain control.

Chemonucleolysis

Chemonucleolysis involves injection of the drug chymopapain or collagenase to destroy the disk. Usually performed with radiographic visualization, it eliminates the need for surgery.

Chemonucleolysis isn't without risks, however. Studies indicate disk space narrowing after chemonucleolysis, leading to irreversible osteoarthritis-like changes.

Nursing care after chemonucleolysis involves monitoring the patient for changes in neurologic status, such as worsened back pain and decreased sensation below the injection site. This may suggest bleeding into the disk space (most common) or an antigenic reaction to the drug.

• Tell the patient that he'll return from surgery with a dressing over the incision and that he'll be kept on bed rest for the duration prescribed by the surgeon.
• Explain that he'll be turned often to prevent pressure ulcers and pulmonary complications. Show him the logrolling method of turning, and explain that he'll use this method later to get in and out of bed by himself.
• Just before surgery, perform a baseline assessment of motor function and sensation in the patient's lower trunk, legs, and feet. Carefully document the results for comparison with postoperative findings.

Monitoring and aftercare

Take these measures:
• After surgery, keep the head of the patient's bed flat for at least 24 hours. Urge him to remain in the supine position for the prescribed period to prevent strain on the involved vertebrae.
• When he can assume a side-lying position, make sure he keeps his spine straight with his knees flexed and drawn up toward his chest. Insert a pillow between his knees to relieve pressure on the spine from hip adduction.

• Inspect the dressing frequently for bleeding or cerebrospinal fluid (CSF) leakage, and report either immediately. The surgeon will probably perform the initial dressing change, and you may be asked to perform subsequent changes.
• Assess motor and neurologic function in the patient's trunk and lower extremities, and compare the results with baseline findings. Also evaluate circulation in the patient's legs and feet and report any abnormalities. Give analgesics and muscle relaxants as ordered.
• Every 2 to 4 hours, assess urine output and auscultate for the return of bowel sounds. If the patient doesn't void within 8 to 12 hours after surgery, notify the doctor and prepare to insert a catheter to relieve retention. If the patient can void normally, assist him in getting on and off a bedpan while maintaining proper alignment.

Home care instructions
Give the patient these instructions:
• Teach the patient and his caregiver proper incision care measures. Tell them to check the incision site often for signs of infection — such as increased pain and tenderness, redness, swelling, and changes in the amount and character of drainage — and to report any signs immediately.
• Make sure the patient understands the importance of resuming activity gradually after surgery. As ordered, instruct him to start with short walks and to slowly progress to longer distances.
• Review any prescribed exercises, such as pelvic tilts, leg raises, and toe pointing. Advise him to rest frequently and avoid overexertion.

Get up, stand up

• Review any prescribed activity restrictions. Usually, the doctor will prohibit sitting for prolonged periods, lifting heavy objects, bending over, and climbing long flights of stairs. He may also impose other restrictions, depending on the patient's condition.
• Teach the patient proper body mechanics to lessen strain and pressure on his spine.
• Instruct the patient to sleep only on a firm mattress. If necessary, advise him to purchase a new one or to insert a bed board between his mattress and box spring.

> Sleeping on a firm mattress is recommended after laminectomy or spinal fusion.

Open reduction and internal fixation
During open reduction, the surgeon restores the normal position and alignment of fracture fragments or dislocated joints. He then

inserts internal fixation devices—such as pins, screws, wires, nails, rods, or plates—to maintain alignment until healing can occur.

Patient preparation

Prepare the patient for open reduction and internal fixation:
• Because this procedure requires general or regional anesthesia, instruct the patient not to eat after midnight the night before.
• Tell the patient that he'll receive a sedative and antibiotics before going to the operating room.

Monitoring and aftercare

Take these measures:
• Describe to the patient the bulk dressing and surgical drain that he'll have in place for several days postoperatively.
• Tell him that he may need a cast or splint for support when the drain is removed and swelling subsides.

Home care instructions

Give the patient these instructions:
• Teach him how to apply and care for the device, if appropriate. Tell him to check his skin regularly under and around the device, if possible, for irritation and breakdown. Also instruct him to watch for signs of incisional infection (redness, swelling, drainage, and foul odor from the site).
• Advise him to follow the doctor's orders about exercising and placing weight on the affected joint. (See *Reviewing internal fixation devices*, page 676.)

Nursing diagnoses

Several nursing diagnoses are used for patients with musculo-skeletal disorders. Common ones appear in this section, along with appropriate nursing interventions and rationales.

Activity intolerance

Related to impaired physical mobility, *Activity intolerance* may be associated with pain or edema. Alternatively, the patient's activity may be severely restricted by such conditions as fractures requiring skeletal traction, rheumatoid arthritis, vertebral fractures, neurogenic arthropathy, Paget's disease, muscular dystrophy, and other disorders.

Reviewing internal fixation devices

Fractures can be stabilized with various internal devices: pins, nails, rods, or screwplates. Choice of a specific device depends on the location, type, and configuration of the fracture.

For instance, in trochanteric or subtrochanteric fractures, the surgeon may use a hip pin or nail (with or without plate) or a screwplate. Because weight bearing imposes great stresses on this area, the patient requires strong control of both proximal and distal bone fragments. A pin or plate with extra nails stabi-lizes the fracture by impacting the bone ends at the fracture site.

In an uncomplicated fracture of the femoral shaft, the surgeon may use an intramedullary rod. This device permits early ambulation with partial weight bearing.

In an upper extremity fracture, the surgeon may use a plate, rod, or nail. Most radius and ulna fractures may be fixed with plates, whereas humerus fractures may be fixed with rods.

Hip pin with screwplate

Pelvis

Femur

Intramedullary rod

Femur

Pins in humerus

Humerus

Radius

Ulna

Screwplate in tibia

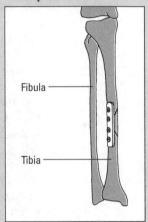

Fibula

Tibia

Expected outcomes

- Patient reports factors that decrease his activity tolerance.
- Patient progresses to his highest level of possible activity.

Nursing interventions and rationales

- Perform active or passive ROM exercises to all extremities every 2 to 4 hours to foster muscle strength and tone, maintain joint mobility, and prevent contractures.
- Turn and reposition the patient every 2 hours to prevent skin breakdown and improve breathing. Establish a turning schedule for the dependent patient. Post a schedule at the patient's bedside and monitor frequency.
- Maintain proper body alignment at all times to avoid contractures and maintain optimal musculoskeletal balance and physiologic function.

• Encourage active exercise. Provide a trapeze or other assistive device whenever possible. Such devices simplify moving and turning for many patients and allow them to strengthen some upper-body muscles.
• Teach isometric exercises to allow the patient to maintain or increase muscle tone and joint mobility.
• Have the patient perform self-care activities. Begin slowly and increase daily, as tolerated. These activities help the patient regain his health.

You can do it!

• Provide emotional support and encouragement to help improve patient self-concept and provide the motivation to perform ADLs.
• Involve the patient in care-related planning and decision making to improve compliance.
• Monitor physiologic responses to increased activity level, including respirations, heart rate and rhythm, and blood pressure to ensure that they return to normal within a few minutes after exercising.
• Teach caregivers to assist the patient with self-care activities in a way that maximizes the patient's potential. This encourages caregivers to participate in patient care and to support patient independence. Place needed objects within reach to encourage independence.
• Explain the importance of following the prescribed medical and physical therapy regimens. As the patient's understanding of his condition improves, his compliance increases.

Deficient knowledge

Deficient knowledge is related to a lack of information about management and control of disease. Your patient's understanding of his condition will directly affect his ability to cope and his recovery.

Expected outcomes

• Patient reports an increase in knowledge regarding disease.
• Patient demonstrates ability to perform new skill related to his lifestyle.

Nursing interventions and rationales

• Assess the patient's level of understanding of the disease, its course, and its management. This helps you formulate an appropriate teaching plan. Provide a quiet environment, conducive to teaching and learning.

• Provide information at a pace and in a form appropriate for the patient to enhance his understanding and retention of information.

• Identify the patient's learning style. Then select teaching strategies — such as discussion, demonstration, role-playing, and visual materials — that are appropriate to his style. This makes your teaching more effective.

• Identify and teach the skills the patient must incorporate into his daily lifestyle. Ask for a return demonstration of each new skill to help him gain confidence.

• Have the patient incorporate learned skills into his daily routine during hospitalization. This allows him to practice them and receive feedback.

• Provide the patient with the names and telephone numbers of resource people or organizations to provide continuity of care and follow-up after discharge.

Impaired physical mobility

Impaired physical mobility is related to many musculoskeletal disorders involving joint inflammation as well as to fractures, bone disorders, and other disorders that cause decreased mobility.

Expected outcomes

• Patient demonstrates safety measures while increasing mobility.
• Patient reports an increase or optimum mobility.
• Patient describes ways to increase physical mobility.

Nursing interventions and rationales

• Instruct the patient in ROM exercises (active and passive) to increase strength.
• Teach him how to use adaptive aids for mobility so that he can do as much as possible for himself.
• Encourage increased mobility for short durations several times per day to increase strength and confidence.
• Provide emotional support and encouragement to help improve the patient's self-concept and provide motivation.
• Teach the patient how to walk and transfer from a wheelchair safely to prevent falls or accidents.

Teaching the patient how to use adaptive aids will help her become more independent.

Disorders

This section discusses musculoskeletal disorders. For each disorder you'll find information on causes, assessment findings, diagnostic tests, treatments, nursing interventions, and patient teaching.

Carpal tunnel syndrome

Carpal tunnel syndrome is the most common nerve entrapment syndrome. It results from compression of the median nerve at the wrist, within the carpal tunnel (formed by the carpal bones and the transverse carpal ligament). The median nerve, along with blood vessels and flexor tendons, passes through this tunnel to the fingers and thumb.

Definitely a hands-on disorder

Carpal tunnel syndrome usually occurs in women between ages 30 and 60 and poses a serious occupational health problem. Assembly-line workers, packers, and people who repeatedly use poorly designed tools are most likely to develop this disorder. Any strenuous use of the hands aggravates this condition.

Make sure you have the proper support when using me! Strenuous use of the hands can aggravate carpal tunnel syndrome.

What causes it

The cause of carpal tunnel syndrome is unknown, but damage to the median nerve may result from:

 repetitive wrist motions involving excessive flexion or extension

 dislocation

🖐 acute sprain.

Pathophysiology

The median nerve controls motions in the forearm, wrist, and hand and supplies sensation to the index, middle, and ring fingers. Compression of the median nerve results in sensory and motor changes in the median distribution of the hand.

What to look for

Signs and symptoms of carpal tunnel syndrome include weakness, pain, burning, numbness, or tingling in one or both hands. This paresthesia affects the thumb, forefinger, middle finger, and one-half of the fourth finger.

A surplus of signs and symptoms

Other indications include decreased sensation to light touch or pinpricks in the affected fingers; an inability to clench the hand into a fist; nail atrophy; dry, shiny skin; and pain, possibly spreading to the forearm and, in severe cases, as far as the shoulder.

What tests tell you

Diagnosis of carpal tunnel syndrome is based on these characteristic tests and findings:
• Tinel's sign: Tingling occurs over the median nerve on light percussion.
• Phalen's maneuver: Carpal tunnel syndrome symptoms occur when the patient holds his forearms vertically and allows both hands to drop into complete flexion at the wrists for 1 minute.
• compression test: Blood pressure cuff inflated above systolic pressure on the forearm for 1 to 2 minutes provokes pain and paresthesia along the distribution of the median nerve.
• electromyography: A median nerve motor conduction delay of more than 5 milliseconds suggests carpal tunnel syndrome.

How it's treated

Conservative treatment includes resting the hands by splinting the wrists in neutral extension for 1 to 2 weeks. If a definite link has been established between the patient's occupation and carpal tunnel syndrome, he may have to seek other work.

Effective treatment may also require correction of an underlying disorder.

Free at last!

When conservative treatment fails, the only alternative is surgical decompression of the nerve by sectioning the entire transverse carpal tunnel ligament. Neurolysis (freeing of the nerve fibers) may also be necessary.

What to do

During and after treatment, take these measures:
• Administer mild analgesics as needed. Encourage the patient to use his hands as much as possible; however, if the dominant hand is impaired, you may have to help with eating and bathing.
• After surgery, monitor vital signs, and regularly check the color, sensation, and motion of the affected hand. Suggest occupational

counseling for the patient who has to change jobs because of carpal tunnel syndrome.

• Evaluate the patient. Following successful interventions (such as splinting and surgery), muscle strength and normal ROM in the affected hand and wrist should progressively return. The patient should be free from pain or paresthesia in the affected hand. (See *Carpal tunnel syndrome teaching tips.*)

Herniated intervertebral disk

A herniated disk occurs when all or part of the nucleus pulposus (the soft, gelatinous, central portion of an intervertebral disk) forces through the weakened or torn anulus fibrosus (outer ring).

Impingement is irritating

The extruded disk may impinge on spinal nerve roots as they exit from the spinal canal or on the spinal cord itself, resulting in back pain and other signs of nerve root irritation. Most herniation occurs in the lumbar and lumbosacral regions.

What causes it

Herniated intervertebral disk has two causes:

 Trauma or strain

 Degenerative disk disease.

Pathophysiology

The ligament and posterior capsule of the disk are usually torn, allowing the nucleus pulposus to extrude, compressing the nerve root. Occasionally, the injury tears the entire disk loose, causing protrusion onto the nerve root or compression of the spinal cord. Large amounts of extruded nucleus pulposus or complete disk herniation of the capsule and nucleus pulposus may compress the spinal cord. (See *What happens when a disk herniates?* page 682.)

What to look for

The overriding symptom of lumbar herniated disk is severe lower back pain that radiates to the buttocks, legs, and feet (usually unilaterally). The pain intensifies with Valsalva's maneuver, coughing, sneezing, or bending.

Education edge

Carpal tunnel syndrome teaching tips

Include these points in your patient teaching:

• Teach the patient how to apply a splint. Warn him not to make it too tight.

• Show him how to remove the splint and how to perform gentle range-of-motion exercises. Advise him to do these exercises daily.

• Recommend that, after discharge, the patient exercise his hands occasionally in warm water. If his arm is in a sling, tell him to remove the sling several times per day to exercise his elbow and shoulder.

What happens when a disk herniates?

The spinal column is made of verte-brae that are separated by cartilage called *disks.* Within each disk is a soft, gelatinous center that acts as a cushion during vertebral movement. When severe trauma or strain or in-tervertebral joint degeneration oc-cur, the outer fibrous ring can weak-en or tear, the pulpy nucleus can be forced through, and the extruded disk can impinge on the spinal nerve root or the spinal column itself.

The patient may also experience motor and sensory loss in the area innervated by the compressed spinal nerve root and, in later stages, weakness and atrophy of leg muscles.

What tests tell you

Although the straight-leg-raising test and Lasègue's test are per-haps the best tests to determine herniated disk, other tests are used as well.

• Straight-leg-raising test: The patient lies supine while the exam-iner places one hand on the ilium (to stabilize the pelvis) and the other hand under the ankle. Then the examiner slowly raises the patient's leg. This test is positive only if the patient complains of sciatic (posterior leg) pain and not lower back pain.

• Lasègue's test: The patient lies supine while the examiner flexes his thigh and knee to a 90-degree angle. Resistance and pain as well as absent or decreased ankle or knee deep tendon reflexes in-dicate spinal root compression.

• Myelography, CT scan, and MRI: These tests provide the most specific diagnostic information, showing spinal compression caused by the herniated disk. CT scan and MRI have, for the most part, replaced myelography.

X out the X-rays

Although X-ray is essential to rule out other abnormalities, it isn't a good diagnostic tool for herniated intervertebral disk. Marked disk herniation can be present despite a normal X-ray.

How it's treated

Initially, conservative treatment consists of several days of bed rest (possibly with pelvic traction), heat applications, and an exercise program.

Medications that mend

Drug therapy includes aspirin to reduce inflammation and edema at the injury site and (rarely) corticosteroids for the same purpose. The patient may also benefit from muscle relaxants, especially diazepam, methocarbamol, or the analgesic hydrocodone with acetaminophen.

Calling the disk doctor

If neurologic impairment progresses rapidly, or a herniated disk fails to respond to conservative treatment, surgery may be necessary.
• Laminectomy, the most common procedure, involves excision of a portion of the lamina and removal of the protruding disk.
• Spinal fusion may be necessary to overcome segmental instability if laminectomy doesn't alleviate pain and disability. Laminectomy and spinal fusion may be performed concurrently to stabilize the spine.
• Chemonucleolysis — injection of the enzyme chymopapain into the herniated disk to dissolve the nucleus pulposus — is a possible alternative to laminectomy. However, this procedure isn't as popular as it once was because it has been found to be less effective than other treatments and may cause severe allergic reaction or nerve damage.
• Microdiskectomy can be used to remove fragments of nucleus pulposus. This form of microsurgery is becoming more popular.

What to do

To help the patient cope with the discomfort and frustration of chronic lower back pain, take these measures:
• During conservative treatment, watch for a deterioration in neurologic status (especially during the first 24 hours after admission). This may indicate an urgent need for surgery.
• Use antiembolism stockings or a sequential pressure device (stockings) as prescribed, and encourage the patient to move his

Microdiskectomy is being used more and more for herniated disks.

legs as allowed. Provide high-topped sneakers to prevent foot-drop.
• Work closely with the physical therapy department to ensure a consistent regimen of leg- and back-strengthening exercises.
• Give plenty of fluids to prevent renal stasis and constipation and remind the patient to cough, deep-breathe, and use an incentive spirometer to help prevent pulmonary complications.
• Provide good skin care.

Rollin', rollin', rollin'

• After laminectomy, diskectomy, or spinal fusion, enforce bed rest as ordered. Monitor vital signs and check for bowel sounds and abdominal distention. Use a logrolling technique to turn the patient.
• If a closed drainage system is in use, check the tubing frequently for kinks and a secure vacuum. Empty the Hemovac at the end of each shift as ordered, and record the amount and color of drainage. Report colorless moisture on dressings (possible CSF leakage) or excessive drainage immediately. Observe the neurovascular status of the legs, including color, motion, temperature, and sensation.
• Administer analgesics as ordered, especially 30 minutes before initial attempts at sitting or walking. Assist the patient during his first attempt to walk. Provide a straight-backed chair for limited sitting.
• Before chemonucleolysis, make sure the patient isn't allergic to meat tenderizers (chymopapain is a similar substance). Such an allergy contraindicates the use of this enzyme, which can produce severe anaphylaxis in a sensitive patient.
• After chemonucleolysis, enforce bed rest as ordered. Administer analgesics and apply heat as needed. Urge the patient to cough and breathe deeply. Assist with special exercises, and tell the patient to continue these exercises after discharge.
• Provide emotional support. Try to raise the patient's spirits during periods of frustration and depression. Assure him of his progress and offer encouragement.
• Evaluate the patient's response to treatment: Look for absence of pain, ability to maintain adequate mobility, and ability to perform ADLs. The patient should also express an understanding of his treatments and any adjustments he must make in his lifestyle. (See *Herniated intervertebral disk teaching tips.*)

Gout

In gout, urate deposits lead to painfully arthritic joints. It can strike any joint but occurs most commonly in the feet and legs.

Education edge

Herniated intervertebral disk teaching tips

Include these points in your patient teaching:
• Teach the patient who has undergone spinal fusion how to wear a brace if ordered.
• Teach proper body mechanics when lifting: bending at the knees and hips (never at the waist), and standing straight.
• Advise the patient to lie down when tired. He should sleep on his side (never on his abdomen) or in a semi-Fowler's position, using an extra-firm mattress or a bed board to reduce tension on his spine.
• Advise the patient to maintain proper weight to avoid lordosis caused by obesity.
• Warn the patient who must take a muscle relaxant of possible adverse effects. Advise him to avoid activities that require alertness until he has built up a tolerance to the drug's sedative effects.

Primary gout usually occurs in men age 30 and older and in post-menopausal women. Secondary gout occurs in the elderly.

All about gout

Gout follows an intermittent course and commonly leaves patients symptom-free for years between attacks. It can lead to chronic disability or incapacitation and, rarely, severe hypertension and progressive renal disease. Prognosis is good with treatment.

What causes it

Although the cause of primary gout remains unknown, it appears to be linked to a genetic defect in purine metabolism, which causes hyperuricemia (overproduction of uric acid), retention of uric acid, or both.

Secondary gout develops during the course of other diseases, such as obesity, diabetes mellitus, hypertension, polycythemia, leukemia, myeloma, sickle cell anemia, and renal disease. It can also follow drug therapy, especially after hydrochlorothiazide or pyrazinamide.

Pathophysiology

In gout, increased concentration of uric acid leads to tophi (urate deposits) in joints or tissues. These crystals trigger an immune response, causing local necrosis or fibrosis.

What to look for

Gout develops in four stages:

 asymptomatic

 acute

 intercritical

 chronic.

In asymptomatic gout, serum urate levels rise but produce no symptoms. As the disease progresses, it may cause hypertension or nephrolithiasis with severe back pain.

You can't flout gout

The first acute attack strikes suddenly and peaks quickly. Although it usually involves only one joint or a few joints, it's extremely painful. Affected joints appear hot, tender, inflamed, dusky red, or cyanotic.

Even though only one or a few joints are affected, the first acute attack of gout is extremely painful!

The metatarsophalangeal joint of the great toe usually becomes inflamed first (podagra), and then the instep, ankle, heel, knee, or wrist joints. Sometimes a low-grade fever is present. Mild acute attacks typically subside quickly but tend to recur at irregular intervals. Severe attacks may persist for days or weeks.

A gap between attacks

Intercritical periods are the symptom-free intervals between gout attacks. Most patients have a second attack within 6 months to 2 years, but in some people, the second attack is delayed for 5 to 10 years.

Delayed attacks are more common in those who are untreated and tend to be longer and more severe than initial attacks. Such attacks are also polyarticular, invariably affecting joints in the feet and legs, and are sometimes accompanied by fever.

Persistent and painful

Eventually, chronic polyarticular gout sets in. This final, unremitting stage of the disease — also called chronic or tophaceous gout — is marked by persistent painful polyarthritis, with large, subcutaneous tophi in cartilage, synovial membranes, tendons, and soft tissue.

Tophi form in the fingers, hands, knees, feet, ulnar sides of the forearms, helix of the ear, Achilles tendons, and, rarely, in internal organs, such as the kidneys and myocardium. The skin over the tophus may ulcerate and release a chalky, white exudate or pus. Chronic inflammation and tophaceous deposits precipitate secondary joint degeneration, with eventual erosions, deformity, and disability.

Kidney involvement, with associated tubular damage, leads to chronic renal dysfunction. Hypertension and albuminuria occur in some patients and urolithiasis is common.

Nothing fake about the symptoms

Pseudogout also causes abrupt joint pain and swelling but results from an accumulation of calcium pyrophosphate in periarticular joint structures.

What tests tell you

Diagnosis of gout is based on these characteristic tests and findings:
• Urate monohydrate crystals in synovial fluid taken from an inflamed joint or tophus establish the diagnosis. Arthrocentesis (aspiration of synovial fluid) or aspiration of tophaceous material reveals needlelike intracellular crystals of sodium urate.

• Although hyperuricemia isn't specifically diagnostic of gout, tests reveal above-normal serum uric acid levels. Uric acid levels are usually higher in secondary gout than in primary gout.

• Initially, X-ray examinations are normal. However, in chronic gout, X-rays show a punched-out look when urate acids replace bony structures. As the disorder destroys cartilage, the joint space narrows and degenerative changes become evident. Outward displacement of the overhanging margin from the bone contour characterizes gout.

How it's treated

Management goals are to terminate an acute attack, reduce hyperuricemia, and prevent recurrence, complications, and calculi formation. Treatment of the patient with acute gout consists of bed rest; immobilization and protection of inflamed, painful joints; and local application of heat or cold.

In chronic gout, X-rays show a punched-out look when urate acids replace bony structures.

A medley of meds

Analgesics, such as acetaminophen or ibuprofen, relieve the pain associated with mild attacks. Acute inflammation requires concomitant treatment with I.V. or oral colchicine every hour for 8 hours, until the pain subsides or until signs of overdose develop, such as nausea, vomiting, cramping, or diarrhea.

Phenylbutazone or indomethacin in therapeutic doses may be used instead but are less specific. Resistant inflammation may require corticosteroids or I.V. drip or I. M. corticotropin or joint aspiration and an intra-articular corticosteroid injection.

Down with serum uric acid!

Treatment of chronic gout aims to decrease serum uric acid levels. The doctor may order a continuing maintenance dosage of allopurinol to suppress uric acid formation or control uric acid levels and prevent further attacks. However, use this powerful drug cautiously in a patient with renal failure. Colchicine prevents recurrent acute attacks until uric acid returns to its normal level, but the drug doesn't affect the acid level.

Uricosuric agents — such as probenecid and sulfinpyrazone — promote uric acid excretion and inhibit accumulation of uric acid, but their value is limited in a patient with renal impairment. Don't administer these drugs to patients with calculi.

Adjunctive therapy emphasizes a few dietary restrictions, primarily avoiding alcohol and high-purine foods. Obese patients should try to lose weight because obesity puts additional stress on painful joints.

Say good-bye to tophi

In some cases, surgery may be necessary to improve joint function or correct deformities. Tophi must be excised and drained if they become infected or ulcerated. They can also be excised to prevent ulceration, improve the patient's appearance, or make it easier for him to wear shoes or gloves.

What to do

To help the patient with gout, take these measures:
• Encourage bed rest, but use a bed cradle to keep covers off extremely sensitive, inflamed joints.
• Give pain medication as needed, especially during acute attacks. Administer anti-inflammatory medication and other drugs as ordered. Watch for adverse effects. Be alert for GI disturbances with colchicine.
• Apply hot or cold packs to inflamed joints.
• Urge the patient to drink plenty of fluids (up to 2 qt [2 L] per day) to prevent calculi formation. When forcing fluids, record intake and output accurately. Be sure to monitor serum uric acid levels regularly. Alkalinize urine with sodium bicarbonate or another agent if ordered.
• Watch for acute gout attacks that may occur 24 to 96 hours after surgery. Even minor surgery can precipitate an attack. Before and after surgery, administer colchicine as ordered to help prevent gout attacks.
• Evaluate the patient. When assessing response to treatment, note whether the patient's pain is relieved or controlled. Also note whether he's complying with drug therapy and dietary restrictions to maintain normal serum urate levels and avoid recurrence of acute episodes. (See *Gout teaching tips.*)

Osteoarthritis

Osteoarthritis is the most common form of arthritis. Symptoms usually begin in middle age and may progress with age. A thorough physical examination confirms typical symptoms, and lack of systemic symptoms rules out an inflammatory joint disorder such as rheumatoid arthritis.

Disability depends on the site and severity of involvement and can range from minor limitation of the fingers to severe disability in people with hip or knee involvement. The rate of progression varies, and joints may remain stable for years in an early stage of deterioration.

Education edge

Gout teaching tips

Include these points in your patient teaching:
• Make sure the patient understands the importance of checking serum uric acid levels.
• Warn him to avoid high-purine foods, such as anchovies, liver, sardines, lentils, and alcoholic beverages, which raise the urate level.
• Explain the principles of a gradual weight reduction diet to obese patients. Such a diet features foods containing moderate amounts of protein and little fat.
• Advise the patient receiving allopurinol, probenecid, and other drugs to report adverse effects. Warn the patient taking probenecid or sulfinpyrazone to avoid aspirin or any other salicylate. Their combined effect causes urate retention.
• Inform the patient that long-term colchicine therapy is essential for the first 3 to 6 months of treatment with uricosuric drugs or allopurinol.

What causes it

The cause of osteoarthritis is unknown. Primary osteoarthritis, a normal part of aging, results from many things, including metabolic, genetic, chemical, and mechanical factors.

Fateful event

Secondary osteoarthritis usually follows an identifiable predisposing event, most commonly trauma, congenital deformity, or another disease such as Paget's disease. It leads to degenerative changes.

Pathophysiology

This chronic condition causes deterioration of the joint cartilage and reactive new bone formation at the margins and subchondral areas. Degeneration results from a breakdown of chondrocytes, most commonly in the hips and knees. Cartilage flakes irritate the synovial lining, and the cartilage lining becomes fibrotic, causing limited joint movement. Synovial fluid leaks in to bone defects, causing cysts.

What to look for

The severity of these signs and symptoms increases with poor posture, obesity, and occupational stress:
• joint pain (the most common symptom) that occurs particularly after exercise or weight bearing and is usually relieved by rest
• stiffness in the morning and after exercise that's usually relieved by rest
• achiness during changes in weather
• "grating" of the joint during motion
• limited movement.

Irreparable damage

In addition, osteoarthritis of the interphalangeal joints causes irreversible changes in the distal joints (Heberden's nodes) and proximal joints (Bouchard's nodes). Nodes may be painless at first but eventually become red, swollen, and tender, causing numbness and loss of dexterity. (See *Signs of osteoarthritis*, page 690.)

What tests tell you

Diagnosis of osteoarthritis is based on these characteristic tests and findings:
• X-rays of the affected joint may show narrowing of the joint space or margins, cystlike bony deposits in the joint

Well, your posture's good and you certainly aren't obese. Could occupational stress be causing your joint pain?

Signs of osteoarthritis

Heberden's nodes appear on the dorsolateral aspect of the distal interphalangeal joints. These bony and cartilaginous enlargements are usually hard and painless. They typically occur in middle-aged and elderly patients with osteoarthritis. Bouchard's nodes are similar to Heberden's nodes but are less common and appear on the proximal interphalangeal joints.

Heberden's nodes

Bouchard's nodes

space and margins, joint deformity from degeneration or articular damage, and bony growths at weight-bearing areas (such as the hips and knees).
• MRI shows the affected joint, adjacent bones, and disease progression.
• Synovial fluid analysis rules out inflammatory arthritis.

How it's treated

Most measures are palliative. Medications for relief of pain and joint inflammation include aspirin (or other nonopioid analgesics), phenylbutazone, indomethacin, ketorolac, ibuprofen, propoxyphene, rofecoxib and, in some cases, intra-articular injections of corticosteroids. Such injections may delay the development of nodes in the hands.

Stabilizing influences

Effective treatment also reduces joint stress by supporting or stabilizing the joint with crutches, braces, a cane, a walker, a cervical collar, or traction. Other supportive measures include massage, moist heat, paraffin dips for hands, protective techniques for preventing undue stress on the joints, adequate rest (particularly after activity), and, occasionally, exercise when the knees are affected.

Surgery for severe cases

Patients who have severe osteoarthritis with disability or uncontrollable pain may undergo one or more of these surgical procedures:
• arthroplasty (partial or total): replacement of a deteriorated joint with a prosthetic appliance
• arthrodesis: surgical fusion of bones, which is used primarily in the spine (laminectomy)
• osteoplasty: scraping of deteriorated bone from a joint
• osteotomy: excision of bone to change alignment and relieve stress.

What to do

To help the patient with osteoarthritis, take these measures:
• Promote adequate rest, particularly after activity. Plan rest periods during the day, and provide for adequate sleep at night. Moderation is the key; so teach the patient to pace daily activities.
• Assist with physical therapy and encourage the patient to perform gentle ROM exercises. Provide emotional support and reassurance to help the patient cope with limited mobility. Explain that osteoarthritis isn't a systemic disease.
• Other specific nursing measures depend on the affected joint.
  – Hand. Apply hot soaks and paraffin dips as ordered to relieve pain.
  – Spine (lumbar and sacral). Recommend a firm mattress or bed board to decrease morning pain.
  – Spine (cervical). Check the cervical collar for constriction; watch for redness with prolonged use.
  – Hip. Use moist heat pads to relieve pain, and administer antispasmodic drugs, as ordered. Assist with ROM and strengthening exercises, making sure that the patient gets the proper rest afterward.

  Check crutches, braces, cane, or walker for proper fit, and teach the patient how to use them correctly. For example, the patient with unilateral joint involvement should use an orthopedic appliance (such as a cane or walker) on the unaffected side. Advise the use of cushions when sitting and suggest an elevated toilet seat.
  – Knee. Twice daily, assist with prescribed ROM exercises, exercises to maintain muscle tone, and progressive resistance exer-

cises to increase muscle strength. Provide elastic supports or braces if needed.

• Evaluate the patient. Assess whether compliance with the exercise regimen slows down the debilitating effects of osteoarthritis. The patient should maintain or improve his ability to perform ADLs. He should also be able to obtain and use appropriate assistive devices. Note whether he understands and makes use of pain control interventions for involved joints. (See *Osteoarthritis teaching tips*.)

Osteomyelitis

A pyogenic bone infection, osteomyelitis may be chronic or acute. The infection causes tissue necrosis, breakdown of bone structure, and decalcification. Although it commonly remains localized, osteomyelitis can spread through the bone to the marrow, cortex, and periosteum.

Blood-borne bone breakdown

Usually a blood-borne disease, acute osteomyelitis most commonly affects rapidly growing children, especially boys.

In children, the most common sites of infection are the lower end of the femur and the upper ends of the tibia, humerus, and radius. In adults, the most common sites are the pelvis and vertebrae, usually the result of contamination associated with surgery or trauma. With prompt treatment, the prognosis is good.

Chronic osteomyelitis, which is rare, is characterized by multiple draining sinus tracts and metastatic lesions. More prevalent in adults, it carries a poor prognosis.

What causes it

Causes of osteomyelitis include:
• minor traumatic injury
• acute infection originating elsewhere in the body
• organisms, such as *Staphylococcus aureus* (most common), *Streptococcus pyogenes*, *Pneumococcus*, *Pseudomonas aeruginosa*, *Escherichia coli*, and *Proteus vulgaris*
• fungi or viruses.

Pathophysiology

Organisms settle in a hematoma or weakened area and spread directly to the bone. Pus is produced and pressure builds within the rigid medullary cavity. Then pus is forced through the haversian canals. A subperiosteal abscess forms, depriving the bone of its

Education edge

Osteoarthritis teaching tips

To minimize the long-term effects of osteoarthritis, include these points in your patient teaching:

• Tell the patient to plan for adequate rest during the day, after exertion, and at night.

• Warn him to avoid overexertion. He should also stand and walk correctly and be especially careful when stooping or picking up objects.

• Caution him to take his medication exactly as prescribed and to report adverse effects.

• Advise him to wear well-fitting, supportive shoes.

• Tell him to install safety devices at home such as bathroom handrails.

• Remind him to perform ROM exercises as gently as possible.

• Urge him to maintain proper body weight to lessen joint stress.

• Tell him to discuss any alternative therapy with the doctor before starting it.

blood supply. Necrosis results and new bone formation is stimulated. Dead bone detaches and exits through an abscess or the sinuses.

What to look for

Usually, the clinical signs for chronic and acute osteomyelitis are similar. However, chronic infection can persist intermittently for years, flaring up spontaneously after minor trauma. Sometimes the only sign of chronic infection is persistent drainage of pus from an old pocket in a sinus tract. Acute osteomyelitis usually has a rapid onset.

Three sure signals

Local signs and symptoms include:
- sudden pain in the affected bone
- tenderness, heat, and swelling over the affected area
- restricted movement.

What tests tell you

Diagnosis of osteomyelitis is based on these characteristic tests and findings:
- WBC shows leukocytosis, and the patient has an elevated erythrocyte sedimentation rate (ESR).
- Blood culture results enable the doctor to identify the causative organisms.
- X-rays may not show bone involvement until the disease has been active for some time, usually 2 to 3 weeks. Bone scans may enable the doctor to detect infection early.

How it's treated

To prevent further bone damage, interventions against acute osteomyelitis may begin before definitive diagnosis. Measures include:
- administration of large doses of I.V. antibiotics after blood cultures are taken (usually a penicillinase-resistant penicillin, such as nafcillin or oxacillin)
- early surgical drainage to relieve pressure buildup and formation of sequestrum (dead bone fragments that separate from sound bone during necrosis)
- immobilization of the affected bone by plaster cast, traction, or bed rest
- supportive treatment, such as analgesics and I.V. fluids.

Attacking an abscess

If an abscess forms, treatment includes incision and drainage, followed by a culture of the drainage matter. Antibiotic therapy to control infection includes administration of systemic antibiotics, intracavitary instillation of antibiotics through closed-system continuous irrigation with low intermittent suction, limited irrigation with a closed drainage system with suction, and local application of packed, wet, antibiotic-soaked dressings.

If an infected artificial joint is the cause, it's usually removed. Antibiotic therapy is given for 2 to 3 weeks before surgery.

Bad to the bone

Besides antibiotic and immobilization therapy, patients with chronic osteomyelitis usually need surgery to remove dead bone and promote drainage. Even after surgery, the prognosis remains poor. The patient usually feels great pain and requires prolonged hospitalization. Therapy-resistant chronic osteomyelitis in an arm or leg may necessitate amputation.

What to do

Your major concerns are to control infection, protect the bone from injury, and offer meticulous supportive care. To help meet these needs, follow these guidelines:
• Use strict sterile technique when changing dressings and irrigating wounds. If the patient is in skeletal traction for compound fractures, cover insertion points of pin tracks with small, dry dressings, and tell him not to touch the skin around the pins and wires.
• Administer I.V. fluids to maintain adequate hydration as needed. Provide a diet high in protein and vitamin C.
• Assess vital signs every 4 hours. Assess wound appearance and new pain sites, which may indicate secondary infection, daily.
• Carefully monitor suctioning equipment. Don't let containers of instilled solution become empty—this allows air into the system. Monitor the amount of solution instilled and suctioned.
• Support the affected limb with firm pillows. Keep the limb level with the body, and don't let it sag. Provide good skin care. Turn the patient gently every 2 hours, and watch for signs of developing pressure ulcers.
• Provide good cast care. Support the cast with firm pillows, and "petal" the edges with pieces of adhesive tape or moleskin to smooth roughness. Check circulation and drainage every 4 hours for the first 24 hours postoperatively. Promptly report excessive drainage or signs of neurovascular deficits.

Stand guard against infection. Protect the bone from injury at all costs!

• Protect the patient from mishaps, such as jerky movements and falls that may threaten bone integrity. Report sudden pain, crepitus, or deformity immediately. Watch for sudden malposition of the limb, which may indicate fracture.

• Evaluate the patient. Note whether he sustained any neurovascular deficit secondary to treatment. He should achieve pain relief or pain control. New areas of pain, possibly indicating secondary infection, shouldn't appear.

• Also assess whether the patient pursues meaningful, satisfying activities that avoid the risk of fracture. Is he following therapeutic interventions? If so, look for normal body temperature, absence of pain and edema, and full ROM. (See *Osteomyelitis teaching tips.*)

Osteoporosis

In osteoporosis, bones lose calcium and phosphate salts and become abnormally vulnerable to fracture. Osteoporosis may be primary or secondary to an underlying disease.

Primarily postmenopausal

Primary osteoporosis most commonly develops in postmenopausal women. It's called *postmenopausal osteoporosis* if it occurs in women ages 50 to 75 and senile osteoporosis if it occurs between ages 70 and 85. Risk factors include inadequate intake or absorption of calcium, estrogen deficiency, and sedentary lifestyle.

Osteoporosis primarily affects the weight-bearing vertebrae, ribs, femurs, and wrist bones. Vertebral and wrist fractures are common.

What causes it

The cause of primary osteoporosis remains unknown. Secondary osteoporosis may result from:

• prolonged therapy with steroids, aluminum-containing antacids, heparin, anticonvulsants, or thyroid preparations

• total immobility or disuse of a bone (as with hemiplegia).

Osteoporosis is also linked to alcoholism, malnutrition, malabsorption, scurvy, lactose intolerance, hyperthyroidism, osteogenesis imperfecta, and Sudeck's atrophy (localized to hands and feet, with recurring attacks).

Pathophysiology

In osteoporosis, the rate of bone resorption accelerates as the rate of bone formation decelerates. Decreased bone mass results, and bones become porous and brittle.

Education edge

Osteomyelitis teaching tips

Include these points in your patient teaching:

• Before discharge, counsel him on how to protect and clean his wound.

• Teach him how to recognize signs of recurring infection, such as increased body temperature, redness, localized heat, and swelling.

• Stress the need for follow-up examinations.

• Urge the patient to seek prompt treatment for possible sources of recurrence, such as blisters, boils, sties, and impetigo.

What to look for

Although osteoporosis develops insidiously, the disease is usually discovered suddenly. An elderly person typically becomes aware of the disorder when he bends to lift something, hears a snapping sound, and then feels a sudden pain in the lower back. Any movement or jarring aggravates the backache.

Other ominous signs

Other signs and symptoms include:
- pain in the lower back that radiates around the trunk
- deformity
- kyphosis (humpback)
- loss of height
- a markedly aged appearance.

What tests tell you

Diagnosis of osteoporosis is based on these characteristic tests and findings:
- X-rays show typical degeneration in the lower thoracic and lumbar vertebrae. The vertebral bodies may appear flattened, with varying degrees of collapse and wedging, and may look denser than normal. Loss of bone mineral becomes evident in later stages.
- CT scan accurately assesses spinal bone loss.
- Bone scans show injured or diseased areas.
- Serum calcium, phosphorus, and alkaline phosphatase levels are within normal limits, but parathyroid hormone levels may be elevated.

X-ray is one way to diagnose osteoporosis.

How it's treated

The patient receives symptomatic treatment aimed at preventing additional fractures and controlling pain. Measures may include:
- a physical therapy program emphasizing gentle exercise and activity
- estrogen to decrease the rate of bone resorption and calcium and vitamin D to support normal bone metabolism (However, drug therapy merely arrests osteoporosis; it doesn't cure it.)
- a back brace to support weakened vertebrae
- surgery to correct pathologic fractures of the femur by open reduction and internal fixation. Colles' fracture, a fracture of the radius where it joins the wrist, requires reduction followed by plaster-cast immobilization for 4 to 10 weeks.

An *ounce of prevention*

Adequate intake of dietary calcium and regular weight-bearing exercise may reduce a person's chances of developing senile osteoporosis. Although hormone therapy may offer some preventive benefit, it also has risks and adverse effects.

Secondary osteoporosis can be prevented through effective treatment of the underlying disease and by judicious use of steroid therapy, early mobilization after surgery or trauma, decreased alcohol consumption, careful observation for signs of malabsorption, and prompt treatment of hyperthyroidism.

What to do

Your care plan should focus on the patient's fragility, stressing careful positioning, ambulation, prescribed exercises, and injury prevention strategies. Take these steps:
• Check the patient's skin daily for redness, warmth, and new sites of pain, which may indicate new fractures.
• Encourage activity by helping the patient walk several times daily. As appropriate, perform passive ROM exercises, or encourage the patient to perform active exercises. Make sure the patient regularly attends scheduled physical therapy sessions.
• Provide a balanced diet high in nutrients that support skeletal metabolism, such as vitamin D, calcium, and protein.
• Administer analgesics as needed. Apply heat to relieve pain.
• Evaluate the patient. Assess whether adherence to the prescribed regimen of medication, exercise, and dietary intake of calcium, vitamin D, and protein is preventing progression of the disease. Note whether the patient demonstrates good body mechanics and if she can identify and subsequently avoid activities that increase the risk of fracture. (See *Osteoporosis teaching tips*.)

Paget's disease

Paget's disease is a slowly progressive metabolic bone disease. It usually localizes in one or several areas of the skeleton (most commonly the lower torso), although occasionally, widely distributed skeletal deformity occurs. Paget's disease can be fatal, particularly if associated with heart failure (widespread disease creates a continuous need for high cardiac output), bone sarcoma, or giant cell tumors.

What causes it

The cause remains unknown, but one theory holds that early viral infection (possibly with mumps virus) causes a dormant skeletal

Education edge

Osteoporosis teaching tips

Include these points in your patient teaching:
• Thoroughly explain osteoporosis to the patient and her family. They may feel the fractures could have been prevented if they were more careful.
• Before discharge, make sure the patient and her family understand the drug regimen.
• Tell the patient to report new pain sites immediately, no matter how slight the pain.
• Advise her to sleep on a firm mattress and to avoid excessive bed rest.
• If she has a back brace, make sure she knows how to wear it. Teach her good body mechanics.
• If a female patient is taking estrogen, emphasize the need for routine gynecologic checkups, including Papinocolaou tests and mammographys. Tell her to report abnormal vaginal bleeding. Instruct her in the proper technique for breast self-examination and instruct her to perform one monthly.

infection that erupts many years later as Paget's disease. The disease also tends to run in families.

Pathophysiology

In the initial phase of Paget's disease (osteoclastic phase), excessive bone resorption occurs. The second phase (osteoblastic phase) involves excessive abnormal bone formation. Affected bones enlarge and soften, and the new bone structure is chaotic, fragile, and weak.

What to look for

Although Paget's disease produces no symptoms in the early stages, it eventually produces severe, persistent pain that intensifies with weight bearing and may impair movement. Characteristic cranial enlargement occurs over frontal and occipital areas (hat size may increase). Headaches also occur with skull involvement. Bony infringement on cranial nerves may impair hearing and visual acuity.

Other signs may include kyphosis, barrel-shaped chest, and asymmetrical bowing of the tibia and femur. The pagetic sites may be warm and tender, with slow and incomplete healing of fractures. The patient may walk with a waddling gait and have increased susceptibility to pathologic fractures.

What tests tell you

Diagnosis of Paget's disease is based on these characteristic tests and findings:
• X-rays may show increased bone expansion and density before overt symptoms develop.
• A bone scan (more sensitive than an X-ray) clearly shows early pagetic lesions. Radioisotope concentrates in areas of active disease.
• A bone biopsy reveals the characteristic mosaic pattern.
• Blood tests reveal anemia and elevated serum alkaline phosphatase levels. Routine biochemical screens, which include serum alkaline phosphatase, make early diagnosis more common.
• A 24-hour urine test shows an elevated hydroxyproline level. (Hydroxyproline is an amino acid excreted by the kidneys and is an index of osteoclastic hyperactivity.)

Drug therapy is the main treatment in Paget's disease.

How it's treated

Drug therapy is the primary intervention. It includes the hormone calcitonin, given subcutaneously or I. M.; etidronate, taken by mouth; and plicamycin, a cytotoxic antibiotic.

Retarding resorption and reducing levels

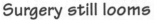

Calcitonin and etidronate retard bone resorption and reduce serum alkaline phosphatase levels and urinary hydroxyproline secretion. Although calcitonin requires long-term maintenance therapy, improvement is noticeable after the first few weeks of treatment. Etidronate produces improvement in 1 to 3 months.

Plicamycin decreases calcium, urinary hydroxyproline, and serum alkaline phosphatase levels. This medication produces remission of symptoms within 2 weeks and biochemical improvement in 1 to 2 months. However, it may destroy platelets or compromise renal function.

Surgery still looms

Self-administration of calcitonin and etidronate helps patients with Paget's disease lead near-normal lives. Nevertheless, these patients may need surgery to reduce or prevent pathologic fractures, correct secondary deformities, and relieve neurologic impairment.

To decrease the risk of excessive bleeding from hypervascular bone, drug therapy with calcitonin and etidronate or plicamycin must precede surgery. Joint replacement is difficult if bonding material (methyl methacrylate) is used because it doesn't set properly on pagetic bone.

Other treatment is supportive and varies according to symptoms. Aspirin, indomethacin, or ibuprofen usually controls pain.

What to do

To help the patient with Paget's disease, take these measures:
• To evaluate the effectiveness of analgesics, assess the patient's level of pain daily. Watch for new areas of pain or restricted movement, which may indicate new fracture sites. Also watch for sensory or motor disturbances, such as difficulty hearing, seeing, or walking.
• Monitor serum calcium and alkaline phosphatase levels.
• Monitor intake and output. Encourage adequate fluid intake to minimize renal calculi formation.
• If the patient is on prolonged bed rest, prevent pressure ulcers by providing good skin care. Reposition the patient frequently and

use a flotation mattress. Provide high-topped sneakers to prevent footdrop.

• Evaluate the patient and assess the success of therapy by asking yourself these questions:

– Does the patient avoid activities that increase the risk of fracture, while at the same time maintaining ROM?

– Does the patient have neurologic deficits, such as footdrop, because of progression of the disease or interventions?

– Does the patient demonstrate effective coping skills for dealing with his illness?

– Has adherence to the prescribed medication and dietary regimens prevented progression of the disease? (See *Paget's disease teaching tips.*)

Rheumatoid arthritis

Rheumatoid arthritis (RA) is a chronic, systemic inflammatory disease that primarily attacks peripheral joints and surrounding muscles, tendons, ligaments, and blood vessels. Spontaneous remissions and unpredictable exacerbations mark the course of the disease. Potentially crippling, RA usually requires lifelong treatment and sometimes surgery.

From intermittent to incessant

In most patients, the disease follows an intermittent course and allows normal activity. However, 10% of patients suffer total disability from severe articular deformity and associated extra-articular symptoms, or both. Prognosis worsens with the development of nodules, vasculitis, and high titers of rheumatoid factor (RF).

What causes it

RA is currently believed to have an autoimmune basis, although the cause remains unknown.

Pathophysiology

Cartilage damage resulting from inflammation triggers further immune responses, including complement activation. Complement, in turn, attracts polymorphonuclear leukocytes and stimulates the release of inflammatory mediators, which exacerbates joint destruction.

Education edge

Paget's disease teaching tips

Include these points in your patient teaching:

• Demonstrate how to inject calcitonin and rotate injection sites. Advise that adverse effects may occur, although they are usually mild.

• Warn him to use analgesics as prescribed.

• Tell the patient receiving etidronate to take the medication with fruit juice 2 hours before or 2 hours after meals, as milk and high-calcium fluids impair absorption, and to divide dosage to minimize adverse effects.

• Tell the patient receiving plicamycin to watch for signs of infection, easy bruising, bleeding, and temperature elevation and to report for regular follow-up tests.

• Teach him how to pace activities, use assistive devices, and follow a recommended exercise program. Suggest a firm mattress or a bed board to minimize spinal deformities. Advise him to remove small obstacles at home.

What to look for

Initial symptoms may include fatigue, malaise, anorexia, persistent low-grade fever, weight loss, and lymphadenopathy. The patient may also experience vague articular symptoms.

Sooner and later

Later, the patient may develop joint pain, tenderness, warmth, and swelling. Usually, joint symptoms occur bilaterally and symmetrically. Other symptoms may include morning stiffness; paresthesia in the hands and feet; and stiff, weak, or painful muscles. The patient may also develop rheumatoid nodules — subcutaneous, round or oval, nontender masses, usually on pressure areas such as the elbow.

Advanced signs include joint deformities and diminished joint function. (See *Joint deformities.*)

What tests tell you

In early stages, X-rays show bone demineralization and soft-tissue swelling. Later, they help determine the extent of cartilage and bone destruction, erosion, subluxations, and deformities and show the characteristic pattern of these abnormalities. Other tests and findings include:
• Positive RF test occurs in 75% to 80% of patients (as indicated by a titer of 1:160 or higher).
• Synovial fluid analysis usually shows increased volume and turbidity but decreased viscosity and complement (C3 and C4) levels, with WBC count possibly exceeding 10,000/μl.
• Serum globulins are elevated.
• ESR is elevated.
• Complete blood count shows moderate anemia and slight leukocytosis.

How it's treated

Salicylates, particularly aspirin, provide the mainstay of RA therapy because they decrease inflammation and relieve joint pain. Other useful medications include:
• NSAIDS, such as indomethacin, ketorolac, and ibuprofen
• antimalarials, such as chloroquine and hydroxychloroquine
• gold sodium thiomalate
• penicillamine
• corticosteroids, such as prednisone
• immunosuppressives, such as methotrexate, cyclophosphamide, and azathioprine.

Joint deformities

In advanced rheumatoid arthritis, marked edema and congestion cause spindle-shaped interphalangeal joints and severe flexion deformities.

Sleep well, eat right, and rest often

Supportive measures include 8 to 10 hours of sleep every night, adequate nutrition, frequent rest periods between daily activities, and splinting to rest inflamed joints. A physical therapy program, including ROM exercises and carefully individualized therapeutic exercises, forestalls loss of joint function.

Application of heat relaxes muscles and relieves pain. Moist heat, such as hot soaks, paraffin baths, and whirlpools, usually works best for patients with chronic disease. Ice packs are effective during acute episodes.

Advanced disease may require synovectomy, joint reconstruction, or total joint arthroplasty.

What to do

Here are some important interventions for caring for a patient with RA:

• Assess all joints carefully. Look for deformities, contractures, immobility, and inability to perform ADLs.

• Monitor vital signs and note weight changes, sensory disturbances, and level of pain. Administer analgesics as ordered and watch for adverse effects.

• Give meticulous skin care. Use lotion or cleansing oil, not soap, for dry skin.

• Explain all diagnostic tests and procedures. Tell the patient to expect multiple blood samples to allow firm diagnosis and accurate monitoring of therapy.

The benefits of bubble baths

• Monitor the duration, not the intensity, of morning stiffness because duration more accurately reflects the severity of the disease. Encourage the patient to take hot showers or baths at bedtime or in the morning to reduce the need for pain medication.

• Apply splints carefully. Observe for pressure ulcers if the patient is in traction or wearing splints.

• Explain the nature of RA. Make sure the patient and his family understand that RA is a chronic disease that requires major lifestyle changes.

• Encourage a balanced diet, but make sure the patient understands that special diets won't cure RA. Stress the need for weight control because obesity adds further stress to joints.

• Urge the patient to perform ADLs, such as dressing and feeding himself. Supply easy-to-open cartons, lightweight cups, and unpackaged silverware.

Monitor weight changes. Obesity can put more stress on joints.

Can we talk?

• Provide emotional support. Encourage the patient to discuss his fears about dependency, sexuality, body image, and self-esteem. Refer the patient to an appropriate social service agency as needed.
• Discuss sexual aids, such as alternative positions, pain medication, and moist heat to increase mobility.
• Before discharge, make sure the patient knows how and when to take his prescribed medication and how to recognize adverse effects such as GI bleeding from salicylate therapy.
• Evaluate the patient. When assessing his response to therapy, note whether compliance with exercise and dietary regimen slows progression of debilitating effects. Has he maintained or improved his ability to perform ADLs? Does he use effective pain control measures? Does he use appropriate assistive devices? (See *RA teaching tips*.)

Scoliosis

Scoliosis—a lateral curvature of the spine—may occur in the thoracic, lumbar, or thoracolumbar spinal segment. The curve may be convex to the right (more common in thoracic curves) or to the left (more common in lumbar curves). Rotation of the vertebral column around its axis occurs and may cause rib cage deformity.

There are two types of scoliosis: functional (postural) and structural. Both types are commonly associated with kyphosis and lordosis.

What causes it

Functional scoliosis isn't a fixed deformity of the vertebral column. It results from poor posture or a discrepancy in leg lengths.

Three sorts of structural scoliosis

Structural scoliosis involves deformity of the vertebral bodies. It may be:

 congenital,

 paralytic (musculoskeletal)

 idiopathic.

Congenital scoliosis is usually related to a congenital defect, such as wedge vertebrae, fused ribs or vertebrae, or hemivertebrae.

Paralytic or musculoskeletal scoliosis develops several months after asymmetrical paralysis of the trunk muscles from polio, cerebral palsy, or muscular dystrophy.

Idiopathic scoliosis, the most common form, may be transmitted as an autosomal dominant or multifactorial trait. It appears in a previously straight spine during the growing years.

Pathophysiology

In scoliosis, the vertebrae rotate, forming the convex part of the curve. The rotation causes rib prominence along the thoracic spine and waistline asymmetry in the lumbar spine.

What to look for

The most common curve in functional or structural scoliosis arises in the thoracic segment, with convexity to the right. This curve results in compensatory curves (S curves) in the cervical segment above and the lumbar segment below, both with convexity to the left. These curves develop to maintain body balance and mark the deformity.

When the disease becomes well established, backache, fatigue, and dyspnea may occur.

Unequal and asymmetrical

Physical examination reveals unequal shoulder heights, elbow levels, and heights of the iliac crests. Muscles on the convex side of the curve may be rounded, whereas those on the concave side are flattened, producing asymmetry of paraspinal muscles. (See *Testing for scoliosis*.)

What tests tell you

Diagnosis of scoliosis is based on these characteristic tests and findings:
• Anterior, posterior, and lateral spinal X-rays, taken with the patient standing upright and bending, confirm scoliosis and determine the degree of curvature and flexibility of the spine.
• Bone growth studies may help determine skeletal maturity.

How it's treated

The severity of the deformity and potential spine growth determine appropriate treatment. Interventions include close observation, exercise, a brace (for example, a Milwaukee brace), surgery, or a combination of these. To be most effective, treatment should begin early, when spinal deformity is still subtle.

Testing for scoliosis

When assessing the patient for an abnormal spinal curve, use this screening test for scoliosis.

Have the patient remove her shirt and stand as straight as she can with her back to you. Instruct her to distribute her weight evenly on each foot. While the patient does this, observe both sides of her back from neck to buttocks. Look for these signs:

• uneven shoulder height and shoulder blade prominence
• unequal distance between the arms and the body
• asymmetrical waistline
• uneven hip height
• a sideways lean.

With the patient's back still facing you, ask the patient to do the "forward-bend" test. In this test, she places her palms together and slowly bends forward, keeping her head down. Look for these signs:

Rib hump

Asymmetrical thoracic spine

Asymmetrical waistline

• asymmetrical thoracic spine or prominent rib cage (rib hump) on either side
• asymmetrical waistline.

Mild curve

A mild curve (less than 25 degrees) can be monitored by X-rays and an examination every 3 months. An exercise program may strengthen torso muscles and prevent curve progression. A heel lift may help.

Moderate curve

A curve of 25 degrees to 40 degrees requires spinal exercises and a brace. Alternatively, the patient may undergo transcutaneous electrical nerve stimulation. A brace halts progression in most patients but doesn't reverse established curvature.

Dangerous curve

A curve of 40 degrees or more requires surgery (spinal fusion, usually with instrumentation) because a lateral curve progresses at the rate of 1 degree per year even after skeletal maturity. Preoperative preparation may include Cotrel-Dubousset segmental instrumentation for 7 to 10 days.

Education edge

Scoliosis teaching tips

If the patient needs a brace, include these points in your patient teaching:
• Tell her to wear the brace 23 hours per day, and to remove it only for bathing and exercise. While she's adjusting to the brace, tell her to lie down and rest several times per day.
• To prevent skin breakdown, advise the patient not to use lotions, ointments, or powders on areas where the brace contacts the skin. Instead, she should use rubbing alcohol or compound benzoin tincture to toughen the skin. Tell her to keep the skin dry and clean and to wear a snug T-shirt under the brace.
• Instruct the patient to turn her whole body, not just her head, when looking to the side.

Casts and traction
If the patient needs traction or a cast before surgery, explain these procedures to her and her family. Remember that application of a body cast can be traumatic because it's done on a special frame and the patient's head and face are covered throughout the procedure.

Postoperative care commonly requires immobilization in a localizer cast (Risser jacket) for 3 to 6 months. Periodic checkups follow for several months to monitor stability of the correction.

What to do

The patient with scoliosis needs emotional support, meticulous skin and cast care, and thorough teaching.
• If the patient needs traction or a cast before surgery, check the skin around the cast edge daily. Keep the cast clean and dry and the edges of the cast "petaled" (padded).

Under your skin

• Warn the patient not to insert anything or let anything get under the cast and to immediately report cracks in the cast, pain, burning, skin breakdown, numbness, or odor. Watch for skin breakdown and signs of cast syndrome (such as nausea, abdominal pressure, and vague abdominal pain).
• Evaluate the patient. Make sure that she doesn't develop a neurovascular deficit or loss of skin integrity because of bracing, traction, or surgery. Can she maintain an activity level normal for her age and developmental level?
• Evaluate the results of surgery, if appropriate. Is pain absent or controlled? Are breath sounds, skin color and turgor, elimination patterns, and arterial blood gas levels normal? Are shoulders and hips aligned horizontally? (See *Scoliosis teaching tips*.)

Quick quiz

1. If your patient can't move his right arm away from his side, you document this as impaired:

    A.   supination.

    B.   abduction.

    C.   eversion.

    D   adduction.

Answer: B. Abduction is the ability to move a limb away from the midline.

2. What's a positive sign of carpal tunnel syndrome?

    A.   Trousseau's sign

    B.   Phalen's sign

    C.   Tzanck test

    D.   Tinel's sign

Answer: D. Tinel's sign, a complaint of tingling over the median nerve on light percussion, is a positive sign of carpal tunnel syndrome.

3. Irreversible changes in the distal joints of the fingers caused by osteoarthritis are known as:

    A.   Bouchard's nodes.

    B.   lymph nodes.

    C.   Heberden's nodes

    D.   supraclavicular nodes.

Answer: C. Heberden's nodes are the result of changes in the distal joints of the fingers.

4. Osteoporosis is characterized by:

    A.   crystal deposition and brittleness.

    B.   brittleness and swelling of the joints.

    C.   porosity and brittleness.

    D.   joint stiffness and deformity.

Answer: C. Osteoporosis is a metabolic bone disorder in which bone loses calcium and phosphate and becomes porous, brittle, and abnormally vulnerable to fractures.

5. Which medication is used to treat RA?

    A.   Aspirin

    B.   Acetominophen

    C.   Calcitonin

    D.   Etidronate

Answer: A. Salicylates, particularly aspirin, provide the mainstay of RA therapy because they decrease inflammation and relieve joint pain.

Scoring

☆☆☆ If you answered all five items correctly, way to go! You're a bred in the bone musculoskeletal maven!

☆☆   If you answered three or four items correctly, impressive! Make no bones about it, you have a mastery of musculoskeletal matters!

☆   If you answered fewer than three items correctly, don't become unhinged! Just bone up a bit, and you'll be playing ball and socket with the big boys soon.

Hematologic and lymphatic disorders

Just the facts

In this chapter, you'll learn:

♦ about the anatomy and physiology of the hematologic system

♦ how to assess the hematologic system

♦ causes, pathophysiology, and diagnostic tests for common hematologic and lymphatic disorders

♦ nursing interventions appropriate for patients with these disorders.

Because the hematologic system affects every body system, caring for a patient with a hematologic disorder can be especially challenging. For example, a patient's dyspnea may lead you to suspect a respiratory or cardiovascular condition — when his primary problem is anemia.

To help ensure accurate diagnosis and effective care, you'll need to obtain an especially thorough history and physical assessment. With astute, sensitive care founded on a firm understanding of hematologic basics, you can help patients survive these disorders. Even when the prognosis is poor, you can help patients make the necessary adjustments to maintain an optimal quality of life.

Anatomy and physiology

The hematologic system consists of blood — the major body fluid tissue — and the bone marrow, which manufactures new blood cells in a process called *hematopoiesis*. Blood delivers oxygen and nutrients to all tissues, removes wastes, and performs many other tasks. (See *Mapping out blood cell formation*, pages 710 and 711.)

(Text continues on page 712.)

A closer look

Mapping out blood cell formation

Blood cells form and develop in the bone marrow by a process called *hematopoiesis*. This chart breaks down the process from the time the five unipotential stem cells are "born" from the multipotential stem cell until they each reach "adulthood" as fully formed cells — erythrocytes, granulocytes, agranulocytes, or platelets.

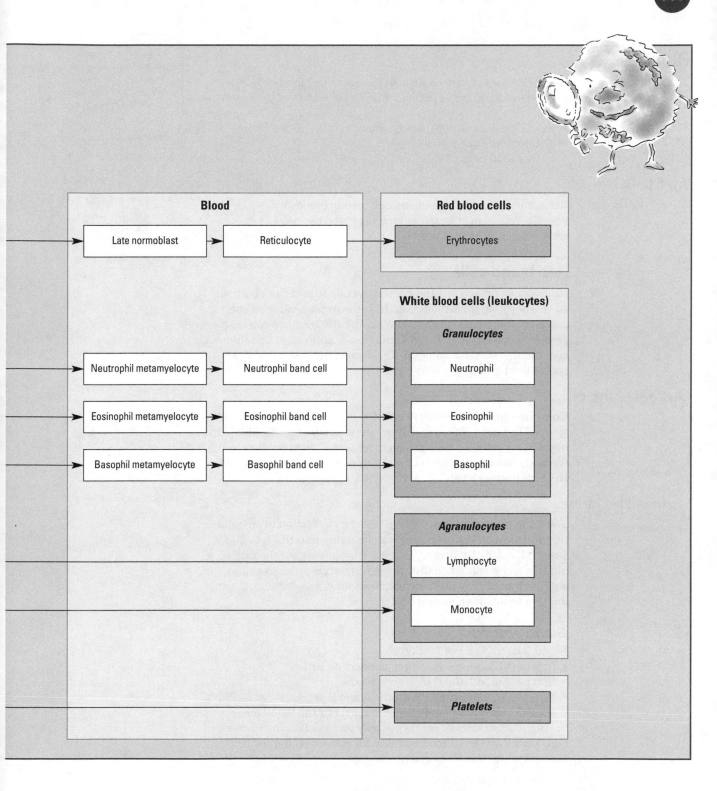

Blood

Late normoblast → Reticulocyte

Red blood cells

Erythrocytes

Neutrophil metamyelocyte → Neutrophil band cell

Eosinophil metamyelocyte → Eosinophil band cell

Basophil metamyelocyte → Basophil band cell

White blood cells (leukocytes)

Granulocytes

Neutrophil

Eosinophil

Basophil

Agranulocytes

Lymphocyte

Monocyte

Platelets

Blood

Blood consists of various formed elements, or blood cells, suspended in a fluid called *plasma*. Formed elements of the blood include:
- red blood cells (RBCs), or erythrocytes
- platelets (thrombocytes)
- white blood cells (WBCs), or leukocytes.

Turf talk

RBCs and platelets function entirely within blood vessels. WBCs, in contrast, act mainly in the tissues outside the blood vessels.

> RBCs like me never leave blood vessels. But my friend here is a WBC, and she likes to roam around in the tissues.

Red blood cells

RBCs transport oxygen and carbon dioxide to and from body tissues. They contain hemoglobin (Hb), the oxygen-carrying substance that gives blood its red color. The RBC surface carries antigens (substances that trigger formation of antibodies that interact specifically with that antigen). These antigens determine a person's blood group, or blood type.

Out with the old...

Constant circulation wears out RBCs, which have an average life span of 120 days. The spleen sequesters, or isolates, the old, worn-out RBCs, removing them from circulation. This process requires the body to manufacture billions of new cells daily to maintain RBCs at normal levels.

... In with the new

The bone marrow releases RBCs into the circulation in an immature form called *reticulocytes*, which mature into RBCs in about 1 day. The rate of reticulocyte release usually equals the rate of old RBC removal. When RBC depletion occurs—for example, with hemorrhage—the bone marrow increases reticulocyte production to maintain normal RBC levels.

Blood groups

Blood falls into one of four types:
- In type A blood, the A antigen appears on RBCs.
- In type B blood, the B antigen appears.
- Type AB blood contains both the A and B antigens.
- Type O blood has neither the A antigen nor the B antigen.

Blood from any of these types may also contain the Rhesus (Rh) factor antigen. Blood with the Rh antigen is Rh-positive; blood without it is Rh-negative.

Antagonistic actions

Plasma may contain antibodies (immunoglobulins) that interact with these antigens, causing the cells to agglutinate (clump together). However, plasma can't contain antibodies to its own cell antigen, or it would destroy itself. Thus, type A blood has A antigen but no anti-A antibodies, although it does have anti-B antibodies.

This principle is important for blood transfusions: The donor's blood type must be compatible with the recipient's. Otherwise, the transfusion may be fatal. That's why precise blood typing and crossmatching (mixing and observing for agglutination of donor cells) are essential.

I knew it would come to this! I'm type A, and I'm just not compatible with type B.

Compatible couplings

These blood groups are compatible:
- Type A with type A or O
- Type B with type B or O
- Type AB with type A, B, AB, or O
- Type O with type O.

Platelets

Platelets are small, colorless, disk-shaped, cytoplasmic fragments split from very large bone marrow cells called *megakaryocytes*. Their life span is approximately 10 days.

Platelets perform three vital functions:
- They initiate contraction of damaged blood vessels to minimize blood loss.
- They form hemostatic plugs in injured blood vessels to help stop bleeding.
- Along with plasma, they provide materials that accelerate blood clot formulation, or coagulation.

White blood cells

Five types of WBCs participate in the body's defense and immune systems. WBCs are classified as granulocytes or agranulocytes based on:
- shape of the nucleus (the sphere that contains the genetic codes for maintaining and reproducing that cell)
- presence or absence of granules (small particles) in the cytoplasm (all of the cell's contents excluding the nucleus)
- affinity for laboratory stains or dyes.

Granulocytes

Granulocytes contain a single multilobed nucleus and prominent cytoplasmic granules. Types of granulocytes include neutrophils, eosinophils, and basophils.

Polly wants a shorter name

Collectively, these cells are called *polymorphonuclear leukocytes*. However, each cell type exhibits different properties, and each is activated by different stimuli.

Neutrophils

Neutrophils, the most abundant type of granulocyte, account for 48% to 77% of circulating WBCs. Like granulocytes, neutrophils are phagocytic.

Neutrophils leave the bloodstream by passing through intact capillary walls into surrounding tissues — a process called *diapedesis*. Then they migrate to and accumulate at infection sites.

Eating the enemy

Neutrophils are phagocytes — cells that engulf, ingest, and digest waste material, harmful microorganisms, and other foreign bodies. Consequently, they serve as the body's first line of cellular defense against foreign organisms.

Strike up the bands

Worn-out neutrophils form the main component of pus. Bone marrow produces their replacements — immature neutrophils called *bands*. In response to infection, the bone marrow must produce many immature cells and release them into the circulation, which elevates the band count.

Hey, cootie — prepare to be engulfed by Sgt. Bug Eater, First Phagocyte Division!

Eosinophils

Eosinophils account for only 0.3% to 7% of circulating WBCs. These granulocytes also migrate from the bloodstream by diapedesis, but do so in response to an allergic reaction. Eosinophils accumulate in loose connective tissue, where they take part in ingesting antigen-antibody complexes.

Basophils

Basophils usually account for less than 2% of circulating WBCs. These cells have little or no phagocytic ability. However, their cytoplasmic granules secrete histamine (a vasodilator) in response to certain inflammatory and immune stimuli. This action causes an increase in vascular permeability and eases fluid passage from capillaries into body tissues.

Agranulocytes

WBCs in this category—monocytes and lymphocytes—lack specific cytoplasmic granules and have nuclei without lobes.

Monocytes

Monocytes, the largest of the WBCs, constitute only 0.6% to 10% of WBCs in circulation. Like neutrophils, monocytes are phagocytic and diapedetic. Outside the bloodstream, they enlarge and mature, becoming tissue macrophages (also called *histiocytes*).

Protection from infection

As macrophages, monocytes may roam freely through the body when stimulated by inflammation. Usually, however, they remain immobile, populating most organs and tissues.

Collectively, monocytes are components of the mononuclear phagocyte system (MPS), formerly called the reticuloendothelial system. The MPS defends against infection and disposes of cell breakdown products.

Fluid finders

Macrophages concentrate in structures that filter large amounts of body fluid—such as the liver, spleen, and lymph nodes—where they defend against invading organisms.

Macrophages are efficient phagocytes of bacteria, cellular debris (including worn-out neutrophils), and necrotic (dead) tissue. When mobilized at an infection site, they engulf and destroy cellular remnants and promote wound healing.

Lymphocytes

Lymphocytes, the smallest of the WBCs and the second most numerous (16% to 43%), derive from stem cells in the bone marrow. They exist in two types:
- T lymphocytes, which directly attack an infected cell
- B lymphocytes, which produce antibodies against specific antigens.

> We T cells attack infections directly. B cells, like my buddy here, produce antibodies that do the dirty work for them.

Assessment

Many signs and symptoms of hematologic disorders are nonspecific. However, certain ones are more specific and can help you focus on possible disorders. These include:
- abnormal bleeding
- bone and joint pain
- exertional dyspnea

- shortness of breath
- ecchymoses (bruising)
- fatigue and weakness
- fever
- lymphadenopathy (enlarged lymph nodes
- petechiae (tiny purplish spots caused by minute hemorrhages).

If your patient has one of these more specific signs or symptoms, turn your attention to assessing his hematologic system.

History

Start your assessment by taking a thorough patient history. To increase the patient's cooperation, develop a trusting relationship with him.

Current health status

Ask the patient why he's seeking medical help. Document his response in his own words. Keep in mind that signs and symptoms of hematologic problems can appear in any body system, so patient complaints may be nonspecific — such as lack of energy, light-headedness, or nosebleeds.

Picking out patterns

Nonspecific complaints aren't diagnostic in themselves. However, when considered in the context of a complete patient history, they may establish a pattern that suggests a hematologic disorder.

Previous health status

Ask about the patient's medical history, which may provide clues to his present condition. Stay alert for disorders (such as acute leukemia, Hodgkin's disease, or sarcoma) that necessitated aggressive immunosuppressant or radiation therapies.

If your patient was hospitalized, ask why. Could a previous surgical intervention, such as a splenectomy, be causing a medical problem?

Has the patient received blood products? If so, note when and how many he received to help assess his risk of harboring an infection transmitted by transfusion.

Finally, document all the medications he's taking — prescription and over-the-counter.

Family history

Ask about deceased family members, recording the cause of death and their ages at death. Note heredi-

Document all the medications your patient takes, including over-the-counter preparations.

tary hematologic disorders, such as hemophilia, von Willebrand's disease, and sickle cell anemia. Plot these disorders on a family genogram to determine the inheritance risk.

Social history

Ask your patient about:
• alcohol intake, diet, sexual habits, and possible drug abuse, which can impair hematologic function
• exposure to such hazardous substances as benzene or Agent Orange, which can cause bone marrow dysfunction (especially leukemia).

Physical examination

Because a hematologic disorder can involve almost every body system, be sure to conduct a complete physical examination.

A seemly sequence

When assessing the abdomen, be sure to inspect first, then auscultate, percuss, and palpate. Palpating or percussing the abdomen before you auscultate it can change the character of bowel sounds and lead to an inaccurate assessment.

Inspection

Focus your inspection on the areas most relevant to a hematologic disorder—the skin, mucous membranes, fingernails, eyes, lymph nodes, liver, and spleen.

Skin and mucous membranes

Skin color directly reflects body fluid composition. Observe for pallor, cyanosis, and jaundice. Because normal skin color can vary widely among individuals, ask the patient if his present skin tone is normal.

Inspect the patient's face, conjunctivae, hands, and feet for plethora (a ruddy color)—a symptom of polycythemia (a disorder marked by excess RBCs). Also look for erythema (redness) of the skin, which may indicate local inflammation or fever.

Not-so-mellow yellow

Next, assess the skin and mucous membranes for jaundice. Be sure to observe the patient in natural light rather than incandescent light, which can mask a yellowish tinge. With a dark-skinned patient, inspect the buccal mucosa, palms, and soles for a yellowish tinge. In a patient with edema, examine the inner forearm for jaundice.

Purplish purpuric patches

If you suspect a blood-clotting abnormality, check the skin for purpuric lesions — purplish spots or patches that vary in size and usually result from thrombocytopenia. With dark-skinned patients, check the oral mucosa or conjunctivae for petechiae or ecchymoses (bruising).

Anemic indicators

Check the skin for dryness and coarseness, which may indicate iron deficiency anemia.

Mucous membrane appraisal

Finally, inspect the patient's mucous membranes, especially the gingivae (gums). Look for bleeding, redness, swelling, and ulcers.

Fingernails

Inspect the patient's fingernails for longitudinal striations, koilonychia (spoon nail), platyonychia (abnormally broad or flat nails), and nail clubbing (enlargement).

Eyes

Examine the patient's eyes for yellowish sclerae and for retinal hemorrhages and exudates.

Lymph nodes, liver, and spleen

Inspect the abdominal area for enlargement, distention, and asymmetry. Liver and spleen enlargement may result from congestion caused by blood cell overproduction (as in polycythemia or leukemia) or excessive blood cell destruction (as in hemolytic anemia).

Abdominal auscultation

With the patient lying down, auscultate the abdomen before palpation and percussion to avoid altering bowel sounds. Listen for loud, high-pitched tinkling sounds, which herald the early stages of intestinal obstruction.

Finding friction

Next, auscultate the liver and spleen. Listen carefully over both organs for friction rubs — grating sounds that fluctuate with respiration. These sounds usually indicate inflammation of the organ's peritoneal covering.

Check your patient's skin for jaundice. If he's dark-skinned, look for a yellowish tinge to the palms, soles, and buccal mucosa.

Percussion of the liver and spleen

To determine liver and spleen size (and possibly detect tumors), percuss all four abdominal quadrants and compare your findings. The normal liver sounds dull.

Establish the organ's approximate size by percussing for its upper and lower borders at the midclavicular line. To determine medial extension, percuss to the midsternal landmark.

How dull can it get?

Like the liver, the normal spleen sounds dull. Percuss it from the midaxillary toward the midline. The average-sized spleen lies near the eighth, ninth, or tenth intercostal space. You might want to mark liver and spleen borders with a pen for later reference during palpation of these organs.

Palpation of the lymph nodes, liver, and spleen

Palpate the patient's neck, axillary, epitrochlear, and inguinal lymph nodes. Using your finger pads, move the skin over each area.

As you palpate each node, note its location, size, tenderness, texture (hard, soft, or firm), and fixation (whether it's movable or fixed). For each node group, note the symmetry.

Liver look-over

Accurate liver palpation is difficult and can depend on the patient's size, present comfort level, and whether fluid is present. If necessary, repeat the procedure, checking your hand position and the pressure you exert.

Quadruple scrutiny

Lightly palpate all four abdominal quadrants to distinguish tender sites and muscle guarding. Deeper palpation helps delineate abdominal organs and masses.

Be sure to palpate tender areas last. Avoid continued palpation if a tumor is suspected.

Man, that spleen sounds dull! And, dig this — that's what passes for normal!

Diagnostic tests

Diagnostic tests allow direct analysis of the blood, its formed elements, and the bone marrow. Such tests include agglutination tests, coagulation screening tests, and bone marrow aspiration and biopsy.

Agglutination tests

Agglutination tests evaluate the ability of the blood's formed elements to react to foreign substances by clumping together. They include ABO blood typing, crossmatching, and Rh blood typing.

ABO blood typing

ABO blood typing classifies blood into A, B, AB, or O groups according to the presence of major antigens A and B on RBC surfaces, and according to serum antibodies anti-A and anti-B.

Go forward, then reverse

To prevent a lethal transfusion reaction, both forward and reverse blood typing are required. In *forward* typing, a blood sample is mixed with serum containing anti-A antibodies; another sample is then mixed with serum that contains anti-B antibodies. Clotting patterns are observed and recorded.

In *reverse* typing, the blood sample is mixed with type A and type B blood, and clotting patterns are observed and recorded.

Nursing considerations

• Before the patient receives a transfusion, compare current and past ABO typing and crossmatching to detect mistaken identification and help prevent transfusion reactions. Remember — if the recipient's blood type is A, he may receive type A or O blood. If his blood type is B, he may receive type B or O blood. If his blood type is AB, he may receive type A, B, AB, or O blood. If his blood type is O, he may receive *only* type O blood.
• Note that recent administration of dextran or I.V. contrast media causes cells to aggregate similarly to agglutination. If the patient received blood during the past 3 months, antibodies to the donor blood may have developed and lingered, interfering with compatibility testing.

Crossmatching

Crossmatching establishes whether donor and recipient blood are compatible and serves as the final check for such compatibility. Lack of agglutination indicates compatibility between donor and recipient blood, which means the blood transfusion can proceed.

Crossmatching in a crisis

Blood is always crossmatched before transfusion, except in extreme emergencies. A complete crossmatch may take 45

Memory jogger

To remember which blood types are compatible, visualize the letter "O" as an orb representing the universe, because type O blood is the universal donor blood. Patients with any blood type can receive it.

But O also means "odd man out": Patients with type O blood can receive only type O blood.

Don't even think about giving a transfusion until ABO typing and crossmatching have been done!

minutes to 2 hours, so an incomplete (10-minute) crossmatch may be acceptable in an emergency. Meanwhile, transfusion can begin with limited amounts of group O packed RBCs.

An emergency transfusion must proceed with special awareness of the complications that may result from incomplete typing and crossmatching. After crossmatching, compatible units of blood are labeled and a compatibility record is completed.

If more than 48 hours have elapsed since the previous transfusion, donor blood must be crossmatched with a new recipient blood sample.

Nursing considerations
• If more than 48 hours have elapsed since the previous transfusion, previously crossmatched donor blood must be crossmatched with a new recipient blood sample to detect newly acquired incompatibilities before transfusion.

Verifying protocols
• If the recipient hasn't received the transfusion, donor blood need not be crossmatched again for 72 hours. Check facility transfusion protocols.
• If the patient is scheduled for surgery and has received blood during the previous 3 months, his blood must be crossmatched again to detect recently acquired incompatibilities.

Rh blood typing
The Rh system classifies blood by the presence or absence of the Rh°(D) antigen on the surface of RBCs. This test is used to establish blood type according to the Rh system to determine if the donor and recipient are compatible before transfusion and determine if the patient needs a RhoGAM injection.

Get right with Rh
Classified as Rh-positive, Rh-negative, or Rh-positive D^u, donor blood may be transfused only if it's compatible with the recipient's blood. (D^u is an Rho[D] variant.)

Nursing considerations
Encourage the patient to carry a blood group identification card in his wallet to protect him in an emergency. Most laboratories will provide such a card on request.

Coagulation screening tests
Coagulation screening tests help detect bleeding disorders and specific coagulation defects. Commonly ordered coagulation tests include partial thromboplastin time (PTT), bleeding time, plasma

thrombin time, and prothrombin time (PT). (See *Common coagulation tests.*)

Nursing considerations

- Perform a clean venipuncture. Blood contaminated with tissue thromboplastin causes misleading test results.
- Place the blood sample on ice immediately after obtaining it to preserve its labile factors.
- Allow no more than 4 hours between blood sampling and coagulation testing. Allow only 2 hours between blood centrifugation and coagulation testing; after being centrifuged, RBCs lose their buffering effect on the plasma.

Common coagulation tests

Commonly ordered coagulation tests include partial thromboplastin time (PTT), bleeding time, plasma thrombin time, and prothrombin time (PT).

Partial thromboplastin time

The PTT test evaluates all intrinsic pathway clotting factors (except factors VII and XIII) by measuring the time needed for a fibrin clot to form after calcium and phospholipid emulsion is added to a plasma sample. PTT relies on the activator kaolin to shorten clotting time.

Bleeding time

The bleeding time test measures bleeding duration after a standard skin incision. Bleeding time depends on blood vessel wall elasticity, platelet count, and ability to form a hemostatic plug. The test should involve two separate punctures, and the results should be averaged.

Plasma thrombin time

Also known as the *thrombin clotting time test,* the plasma thrombin time test measures how quickly a clot forms after a standard amount of bovine thrombin is added to a platelet-poor plasma sample from the patient and to a normal plasma control sample.

Quick but questionable

Because thrombin rapidly converts fibrinogen to a fibrin clot, this test provides a rapid but imprecise estimate of plasma fibrinogen levels.

Prothrombin time

The PT test determines the time needed for a fibrin clot to form in a citrated plasma sample after calcium ion and tissue thromboplastin (factor III) are added. It then compares this time with the fibrin clotting time in a control plasma sample.

Profiting from prothrombin time

This test indirectly measures prothrombin (factor II) and serves as an excellent screening method in evaluating prothrombin, fibrinogen, and extrinsic coagulation factors V, VII, and X. It's the test of choice for monitoring oral anticoagulant therapy.

Biopsy

Biopsy procedures involve removing a small tissue sample for further testing. Bone marrow aspiration is an important test for evaluating the blood's formed elements.

Bone marrow aspiration and needle biopsy

Because most hematopoiesis occurs in the bone marrow, histologic and hematologic bone marrow examination yields valuable diagnostic information about blood disorders. Bone marrow aspiration and needle biopsy provide the material for this examination.

Doubling the diagnostic odds

Aspiration biopsy removes a fluid specimen containing bone marrow cells in suspension. Needle biopsy removes a marrow core containing cells but no fluid. Using both methods provides the best possible marrow specimens.

Bone marrow biopsy helps:
• diagnose aplastic, hypoplastic, and vitamin B_{12} deficiency anemias; granulomas; leukemias; lymphomas; myelofibrosis; and thrombocytopenia
• evaluate primary and metastatic tumors
• determine infection causes
• stage such diseases as Hodgkin's disease
• evaluate chemotherapy effectiveness
• monitor myelosuppression.

Hematologic analysis, including the WBC differential and myeloid-erythroid ratio, can suggest various disorders.

Nursing considerations

• When preparing your patient, explain that the test provides a bone marrow specimen for microscopic examination. Inform him that he need not restrict food or fluids beforehand. Explain who will perform the biopsy, that it usually takes only 5 to 10 minutes, and that results usually are available in 1 day. Inform him that more than one bone marrow specimen may be necessary and that before the biopsy, he'll need to give a blood sample for laboratory testing.
• Check the patient's history for hypersensitivity to the local anesthetic.
• After checking with the person who will perform the procedure, tell the patient which bone will serve as the biopsy site (usually the posterior iliac crest). Inform him that he'll receive a local anesthetic but will feel pressure with biopsy needle insertion and a brief pulling pain with

Before bone marrow aspiration, tell the patient that more than one bone marrow specimen may be needed.

Bone marrow aspiration and biopsy sites

These drawings show the most common sites for bone marrow aspiration and biopsy. These sites are used because the involved bone structures are relatively accessible and rich in marrow cavities.

Posterior superior iliac crest
The posterior superior iliac crest is the preferred site because no vital organs or vessels are nearby. With the patient lying in a prone or lateral position with one leg flexed, the doctor or nurse anesthetizes the bone and inserts the needle several centimeters lateral to the iliosacral junction. Directed downward, the needle enters the bone plane crest and is advanced toward the anterior interior spine. In some cases, the needle enters a few centimeters below the crest at a right angle to the bone surface.

Spinous process
The spinous process is preferred if multiple punctures are necessary or if marrow is absent at other sites. The patient sits on the edge of the bed, leaning over the bedside stand. (If he's uncooperative, he may be placed in the prone position with restraints.) The doctor selects the spinous process of the third or fourth lumbar vertebrae and inserts the needle at the crest or slightly to one side, advancing it in the direction of the bone plane.

Sternum
The sternum involves the greatest risk but provides the best access. The patient is placed in a supine position on a firm bed or an examination table, with a small pillow beneath his shoulders to raise his chest and lower his head. The doctor secures the needle guard 3 to 4 mm from the tip of the needle to avoid accidentally puncturing the heart or a major vessel. Then he inserts the needle at the midline of the sternum at the second intercostal space.

marrow removal. (See *Bone marrow aspiration and biopsy sites.*)
- As ordered, administer a mild sedative 1 hour before the test.
- After the procedure, check the biopsy site for bleeding and inflammation. Observe the patient for signs of hemorrhage and infection—rapid pulse rate, low blood pressure, and fever. Change the dressing over the biopsy site every 24 hours to reduce the risk of infection.

Treatments

Treatments for hematologic and lymphatic disorders include drug therapy, transfusions, and surgery.

Drug therapy

Drugs used to treat hematologic and lymphatic disorders include:
• hematinics, which fight anemia by increasing the amount of Hb in the blood
• anticoagulants and heparin antagonists, which impede blood clotting
• hemostatics, which arrest blood flow or reduce capillary bleeding
• blood derivatives, which replace blood loss caused by diseases or surgical procedures
• thrombolytic enzymes, which treat thrombotic disorders
• vitamins, which correct deficiencies of vitamins (such as vitamin B_{12}).

Transfusions

Transfusion procedures allow administration of a wide range of blood products. Here are some examples:
• RBC transfusions revive oxygen-starved tissues.
• Leukocyte transfusions combat infections beyond the reach of antibiotics.
• Transfusions of clotting factors, plasma, and platelets help patients with hemophilia live virtually normal lives.

Factor replacement

I.V. infusion of deficient clotting factors is a major part of treatment of coagulation disorders. Factor replacement typically corrects clotting factor deficiencies, thereby stopping or preventing hemorrhage. The blood product used depends on the specific disorder being treated.

Cold comfort

Fresh frozen plasma, for instance, helps treat clotting disorders whose causes aren't known, clotting factor deficiencies resulting from hepatic disease or blood dilution, consumed clotting factors secondary to disseminated intravascular coagulation (DIC), and deficiencies of clotting factors (such as factor V) for which no specific replacement product exists.

For cryin' out loud

Administration of cryoprecipitate, which forms when fresh frozen plasma thaws slowly, helps treat von Willebrand's disease, fibrinogen deficiencies, and factor XIII deficiencies. It's also used for hemophilia patients who are young or whose disease is mild.

Fresh frozen plasma may be given to treat clotting factor deficiencies caused by liver disease, blood dilution, DIC, and certain other conditions.

Eight is really great

Factor VIII (antihemophilic factor) concentrate is the long-term treatment of choice for hemophilia A because it contains a less variable amount of factor VIII than cryoprecipitate. It's given I.V. to hemophiliac patients who have sustained injuries.

Pooled assets

Prothrombin complex—which contains factors II, VII, IX, and X—is used to treat hemophilia B, severe liver disease, and acquired deficiencies of the factors it contains. However, it carries a high risk of transmitting hepatitis because it's collected from large pools of donors.

Patient preparation
• Explain the procedure to the patient.
• Assemble the necessary equipment: a standard blood administration set for giving fresh frozen plasma or prothrombin complex, a component syringe or drip set for giving cryoprecipitate, a plastic syringe for I.V. injection of factor VIII, or a plastic syringe and infusion set for I.V. infusion.
• Obtain the plasma fraction from the blood bank or pharmacy. Check the expiration date, and carefully inspect the plasma fraction for cloudiness and turbidity. If you'll be transfusing fresh frozen plasma, administer it within 4 hours because it doesn't contain preservatives.
• Take the patient's vital signs. If an I.V. line isn't in place, perform venipuncture and infuse normal saline solution at a keep-vein-open rate.

Inspect the plasma fraction closely for cloudiness and turbidity. Also check the expiration date.

Monitoring and aftercare
• During and after administration of clotting factors, monitor the patient for signs and symptoms of anaphylaxis, other allergic reactions, and fluid overload.
• Monitor for fever, bleeding, and increased pain or swelling at the transfusion site.
• Closely monitor the patient's PTT.
• Alert the doctor if adverse reactions occur or if you suspect bleeding.
• Follow your facility's protocol for monitoring vital signs.

Home care instructions
The patient or his family can administer factor replacement therapy at home. If home therapy is ordered, cover these topics:
• Demonstrate correct venipuncture and infusion techniques to the patient and his family.

• Tell them to keep factor replacement and infusion equipment readily available and to start treatment immediately if the patient experiences bleeding.
• Teach them to watch for signs and symptoms of anaphylaxis, allergic reactions, and fluid overload. Instruct them to call the doctor immediately if such reactions occur. Also tell them to watch for signs of hepatitis, which may appear 3 weeks to 6 months after treatment with blood components.
• Caution the patient and his family to never reuse needles or syringes.

Surgery

Surgical removal of the spleen is sometimes done to treat various hematologic disorders.

Splenectomy

The spleen may be removed to reduce the rate of RBC and platelet destruction, to remove a ruptured spleen, or to stage Hodgkin's disease. It's also done as an emergency procedure to stop hemorrhage after traumatic splenic rupture.

Look Ma, no spleen

Splenectomy is the treatment of choice for such diseases as hereditary spherocytosis and chronic idiopathic thrombocytopenic purpura in patients who don't respond to steroids or danazol therapy. Besides bleeding and infection, splenectomy can cause other complications, such as pneumonia and atelectasis.

Infection alert

Keep in mind that the spleen's location close to the diaphragm and the need for a high abdominal incision restrict lung expansion after surgery. Also, splenectomy patients—especially children—are vulnerable to infection because of the spleen's role in the immune response.

Patient preparation
• Explain to the patient that splenectomy involves removal of the spleen under general anesthesia. Inform him that he can lead a normal life without the spleen, although he'll be more prone to infection.

You can lead a normal life without your spleen, but you'll need to take extra precautions against infection.

• Obtain the results of blood studies, including coagulation tests and complete blood count (CBC), and report them to the doctor.
• If ordered, transfuse blood to correct anemia or hemorrhagic loss. Similarly, give vitamin K to correct clotting factor deficiencies. Give pneumonia vaccine as ordered.
• Take the patient's vital signs and perform a baseline respiratory assessment. Note signs and symptoms of respiratory tract infection, such as fever, chills, crackles, rhonchi, and cough. Notify the doctor if you suspect such infection; he may delay surgery.
• Teach the patient coughing and deep-breathing techniques to help prevent postoperative pulmonary complications.

Monitoring and aftercare

• During the early postoperative period, check closely (especially if the patient has a bleeding disorder) for bleeding from the wound or drain and for signs of internal bleeding, such as hematuria (bloody urine) or hematochezia (bloody feces).
• Know that leukocytosis (an increased WBC count) and thrombocytosis (an increased platelet count) follow splenectomy and may persist for years. Because thrombocytosis may predispose the patient to thromboembolism, help him exercise and walk as soon as possible after surgery. Encourage him to perform coughing and deep-breathing exercises to reduce the risk of pulmonary complications.
• Watch for signs and symptoms of infection, such as fever and sore throat, and monitor the results of hematologic studies. If infection develops, give an antibiotic as prescribed.

Home care instructions

• Inform the patient that he's at increased risk for infection, and urge him to report signs and symptoms of infection promptly.
• Teach him measures to help prevent infection, such as getting the pneumococcal pneumonia vaccine.

Nursing diagnoses

When caring for patients with hematologic disorders, you'll typically use several nursing diagnoses. These diagnoses appear here, along with appropriate nursing interventions and rationales.

Fatigue

Related to anemia caused by decreased hematocrit (HCT) and Hb, *Fatigue* may be associated with sickle cell anemia, pernicious anemia, folic acid and iron deficiency anemias, aplastic or hypoplastic anemias, thalassemias, leukemia, and sideroblastic anemias.

Expected outcomes

- Patient demonstrates that he's adequately rested by being able to participate in routine daily activities.
- Patient identifies measures to prevent or modify fatigue.
- Patient states that he has increased energy.

Nursing interventions and rationales

- Help the patient avoid unnecessary activity—for example, avoid scheduling two energy-draining procedures on the same day. Consult an occupational therapist for practical suggestions in modifying the home and work environments. Using energy-conserving techniques avoids overexertion and potential for exhaustion.
- Help the patient conserve energy through rest, planning, and setting priorities, to prevent or alleviate fatigue.
- Alternate activities with periods of rest. Encourage the patient to engage in activities that he can complete in short periods or divide into several segments—for example, reading one chapter of a book at a time. Regular rest periods help decrease fatigue and increase stamina.
- Discuss the effects of fatigue on daily living and personal goals. Explore with the patient the relationship between fatigue and his disorder, to enhance his ability to cope.

Be less demanding

- Minimize demands on the patient—for example, ask one family member to call at specified times and relay messages to others. This reduces stress.
- Structure the patient's environment to encourage compliance with the treatment regimen. For example, devise a daily schedule based on his needs and desires.
- Encourage the patient to eat foods rich in iron and minerals, unless contraindicated, to help prevent anemia and demineralization.
- Provide small, frequent feedings to conserve the patient's energy and encourage increased dietary intake.
- Establish a regular sleeping pattern. Getting 8 to 10 hours of sleep nightly helps reduce fatigue.
- Avoid highly emotional situations, which worsen fatigue. Encourage the patient to explore feelings and emotions with a sup-

portive counselor, clergy, or other professional to help cope with illness.

Ineffective tissue perfusion: Cardiopulmonary

Related to inadequate blood volume or HCT, *Ineffective tissue perfusion: Cardiopulmonary* may be associated with hemophilia, thrombocytopenia, various purpuras, DIC, and von Willebrand's disease.

Expected outcomes

- Patient's vital signs are within baseline values.
- Patient's pulse oximetry value is within normal limits.

Nursing interventions and rationales

- Monitor the patient's vital signs every 4 hours. Assess for signs and symptoms of both *minor* bleeding (such as bleeding gums, ecchymoses, epistaxis [nosebleed], and petechiae) and *serious* bleeding (such as changed mental status, headache, hematemesis [vomiting of blood], hemoptysis [coughing up of blood], hypotension, melena [black, tarry stools], orthostatic changes, and tachycardia). Detecting bleeding early helps control complications.
- Take steps to prevent bleeding. Avoid invasive measures, such as injections, rectal enemas or suppositories, and urinary catheterization. Avoid giving aspirin or aspirin-containing products if possible. Shave the patient with an electric razor only. Give oral care with a soft toothbrush. These measures prevent complications by maintaining skin integrity.

Memory jogger

Think BEEP to remember the signs of minor bleeding:

B: Bleeding gums

E: Ecchymoses (bruises)

E: Epistaxis (nosebleed)

P: Petechiae (tiny purplish spots)

If your patient has ineffective cardiopulmonary tissue perfusion, don't perform invasive measures, such as giving injections, enemas, or suppositories.

Common hematologic disorders

This section discusses common hematologic disorders, from anemias (such as aplastic anemia and sickle cell anemia) to hemorrhagic disorders (such as hemophilia and thrombocytopenia).

Aplastic anemia

Aplastic, or hypoplastic, anemia results from injury to or destruction of stem cells in the bone marrow or the bone marrow matrix, causing pancytopenia (deficiency of RBCs, WBCs, and platelets) and bone marrow hypoplasia (underdevelopment).

(Text continues on page 731.)

Diabetes mellitus

What's diabetes?

Diabetes is the name for a group of chronic or life-long diseases that affect the way the body uses food to make the energy necessary for life. Primarily, diabetes is a disruption of carbohydrate (sugar and starch) metabolism that also affects fats and proteins. There are two main forms of diabetes (type 1 and type 2), as well as conditions of glucose intolerance, gestational diabetes, and diabetes caused by pancreatic disorders. Regardless of the form of diabetes, metabolic control under the care of a doctor is essential for good health.

What's insulin?

Insulin is an essential hormone produced in the pancreas and released into the bloodstream. Insulin attaches itself to cells at places called *insulin receptors*. Once attached, insulin allows sugar or glucose from the food we eat to enter the liver, fat, and muscle cells, where it's used for energy.

Type 1 diabetes mellitus

In type 1 diabetes, the pancreas makes little or no insulin. Without insulin, sugar can't enter cells to be used for energy. The body's tissues are starved and blood glucose levels grow dangerously high. The disorder begins most often in youth, but it may also occur in older adults. Type 1 diabetes occurs in 5% to 10% of patients with diabetes, who require insulin therapy for treatment.

Type 2 diabetes mellitus

In type 2 diabetes, the pancreas produces some insulin, but it's either too little or isn't effective. In addition, insulin receptors that control the transport of sugar into cells may not work properly or are reduced in number. Type 2 diabetes most often develops in people over age 40. The majority of newly diagnosed type 2 patients are overweight but can control their diabetes through diet and weight loss. Some patients may require oral medications or insulin injections to achieve glucose control.

Diabetes can be a chronic or lifelong illness that affects the way the body uses food to make energy.

Type 1 diabetes

Pancreas with no insulin production

Cell
Glucose
Closed glucose channel
Open glucose channel

Type 2 diabetes

Pancreas producing little or ineffective insulin

Insulin receptor
Insulin

Osteoporosis

Osteoporosis is a metabolic bone disorder in which the rate of bone resorption accelerates while the rate of bone formation slows, causing a loss of bone mass. Bones affected by this disease lose calcium and phosphate salts and become porous, brittle, and abnormally vulnerable to fractures.

Calcium

Normal absorption of calcium by intestines

Increased calcium resorption from bone

Lining of intestine

Calcium stored in bone

Normal bone

Ineffective absorption of calcium by intestines

Osteoporotic bone

Bones affected by osteoporosis lose calcium and become brittle. Not to brag or anything, but I have lots of calcium!

Sickle cell anemia

Sickle cell crisis is triggered by infection, cold exposure, high altitudes, overexertion, and other conditions that cause cellular oxygen deprivation. Here's what happens:

• Deoxygenated, sickle-shaped erythrocytes adhere to the capillary wall and to each other, blocking blood flow and causing cellular hypoxia.

• The crisis worsens as tissue hypoxia and acidic waste products cause more sickling and cell damage.

• With each new crisis, organs and tissues are destroyed and areas of tissue die slowly—especially in the spleen and kidneys.

Peripheral blood smear in sickle cell anemia

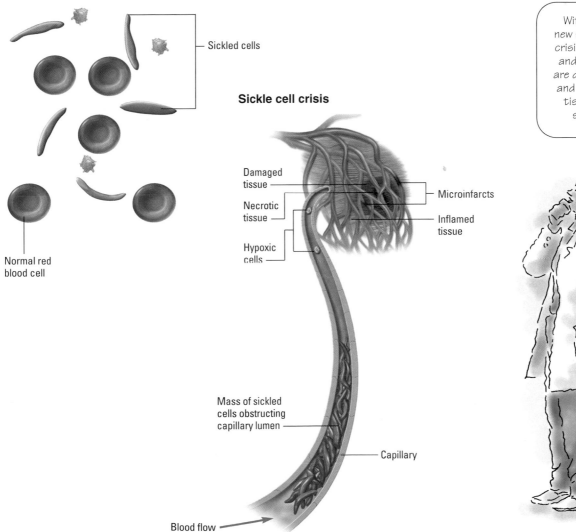

Sickled cells

Normal red blood cell

Sickle cell crisis

Damaged tissue

Necrotic tissue

Hypoxic cells

Microinfarcts

Inflamed tissue

Mass of sickled cells obstructing capillary lumen

Capillary

Blood flow

With each new sickle cell crisis, organs and tissues are destroyed and areas of tissue die slowly.

With early detection, most skin cancers can be removed in a simple outpatient surgical procedure.

Skin cancer

Types of skin cancer

Changes in an existing growth on the skin or new growth that doesn't heal or ulcerates could indicate skin cancer or precancer, a collection of abnormal cells that may become cancerous without intervention. The key to successful treatment of skin cancer is early detection. Most early skin cancers can be removed in a simple outpatient surgical procedure. If left untreated, skin cancers can spread, leading to disability or even death.

Less severe

Cancer

Basal cell carcinoma, the most common skin cancer, begins as a papule, enlarges, and develops a central crater. This cancer usually only spreads locally.

Squamous cell carcinoma begins as a firm, red nodule or scaly, crusted flat lesion. If not treated, this cancer can spread.

Malignant melanoma can arise on normal skin or from an existing mole. If not treated promptly, it can spread downward into other areas of the skin, lymph nodes, or internal organs.

Precancer

Actinic keratosis exhibits abnormal changes in keratinocytes that could someday become squamous cell carcinoma.

Dysplastic nevus exhibits abnormal growth of cells in a mole (melanocytes) that may someday become melanoma.

The ABCDs of malignant melanoma

Asymmetry	Borders	Color	Diameter

6 mm

More severe

C8

Alarming mortality

Although commonly used interchangeably with other terms for bone marrow failure, aplastic anemia properly refers to pancytopenia resulting from decreased functional capacity of a hypoplastic, fatty bone marrow. Aplastic anemia with severe pancytopenia carries a mortality of 80% to 90%. Death may result from bleeding or infection.

What causes it

Aplastic anemia may result from:
• adverse drug reactions
• exposure to toxic agents, such as benzene and chloramphenicol
• radiation
• immunologic factors
• severe disease, especially hepatitis
• preleukemia and neoplastic infiltration of bone marrow
• congenital abnormalities
• induced changes in fetal development (suspected as a cause when no consistent genetic history of aplastic anemia exists).

Pathophysiology

Aplastic anemia usually develops when damaged or destroyed stem cells inhibit RBC production. Less commonly, it arises when damaged bone marrow microvasculature creates an unfavorable environment for cell growth and maturation.

What to look for

Clinical features of aplastic anemia vary with the severity of pancytopenia. They commonly develop gradually, and may include:
• pallor, ecchymoses, and petechiae
• retinal hemorrhages
• weakness and fatigue
• alterations in level of consciousness
• bibasilar crackles
• tachycardia
• gallop murmur
• fever
• oral and rectal ulcers
• sore throat
• nausea.

Memory jogger

Having difficulty distinguishing hypoplasia from hyperplasia? When you see plasia in any word, think of plastic. Plastic, in turn, means forming or developing.

As for hypo and hyper, that's the easy part. Hypo means under, or below normal. Hyper means excessive, or above normal.

Thus, hypoplasia means underdevelopment, and hyperplasia means overdevelopment.

Adverse drug reactions are among the many possible causes of aplastic anemia.

What tests tell you

Confirmation of aplastic anemia requires a series of laboratory tests:

• RBC tests usually show RBCs of normal size, shape, and color, although larger-than-normal RBCs and RBCs of varying size may be present. Total RBC count is 1 million/µl or less.

• Absolute reticulocyte count is very low.

• Serum iron level is elevated (unless bleeding occurs), but total iron-binding capacity is normal or slightly reduced. Hemosiderin (a blood protein) is present, and tissue iron storage is visible microscopically.

• Platelet and WBC counts fall. A lower platelet count is reflected in abnormal coagulation tests (bleeding time).

• Bone marrow biopsies taken from several sites may yield a "dry tap" or show severely hypocellular or aplastic marrow, with a varying amount of fat, fibrous tissue, or gelatinous replacement; absence of tagged iron and megakaryocytes; and depression of RBC elements.

In aplastic anemia, the absolute reticulocyte count, platelet count, and WBC count fall below normal.

How it's treated

Effective treatment must eliminate identifiable causes of anemia and provide vigorous supportive measures, such as packed RBC, platelet, and experimental human leukocyte antigen (HLA)-matched leukocyte transfusions. Even then, recovery may take months.

Bone marrow transplantation is the preferred treatment of anemia stemming from severe aplasia and for patients needing constant RBC transfusions.

Going the reversal route

Patients with low WBC counts may need reverse isolation to avoid infection. They may receive antibiotics, but prophylactic use encourages resistant strains of organisms. Patients with low Hb levels may need oxygen therapy and blood transfusion.

Stimulate, suppress, or complement

Other treatments for aplastic anemia include:

• bone marrow-stimulating agents, such as androgens (controversial)

• immunosuppressants (if the patient doesn't respond to other therapies)

• colony-stimulating factors, which encourage growth of specific cellular components in patients who have had chemotherapy or radiation therapy; agents include granulocyte colony-stimulating factor, granulocyte-macrophage colony-stimulating factor, and erythropoietic stimulating factor

• alternative and complementary therapies to treat associated fatigue. Osteopaths may use manipulation techniques, either alone or with conventional allopathic treatments, to treat chronic fatigue.

What to do

• If the patient's platelet count is below 20,000/µl, take steps to prevent hemorrhage. For instance, avoid I.M. injections; suggest that the patient use an electric razor and a soft toothbrush; give humidifying oxygen, if ordered, to prevent drying of mucous membranes (dry mucosa may bleed); and promote regular bowel movements through stool softeners and a proper diet. Also, apply pressure to venipuncture sites until bleeding stops. Detect bleeding early by checking for blood in the urine and stools and assessing the skin for petechiae.

• Help prevent infection by washing your hands thoroughly before entering the patient's room, making sure the patient eats a nutritious diet high in vitamins and proteins to boost his resistance, and encouraging meticulous mouth and perianal care. Make sure routine throat, urine, and blood cultures are done regularly to check for infection.

Keep an eye on it

• Watch for life-threatening hemorrhage, infection, adverse drug reactions, and transfusion reaction.

• Schedule frequent rest periods for a patient with a low Hb level.

• Administer oxygen therapy as needed and ordered.

• If blood transfusions are given, assess for transfusion reaction by checking the patient's temperature and monitoring him for rash, hives, itching, back pain, restlessness, and shaking chills.

• To prevent aplastic anemia, monitor blood drug levels carefully if the patient is receiving a drug that could cause anemia.

• Evaluate the patient. He should experience fewer infections, his blood cell counts should return to normal, he should breathe easily, and he should no longer experience trauma-induced hemorrhagic episodes. He and his family should demonstrate knowledge of energy-saving strategies. (See *Aplastic anemia teaching tips*.)

Education edge

Aplastic anemia teaching tips

• Reassure and support the patient and his family by teaching them about aplastic anemia and its treatment, particularly if the patient has recurring acute episodes.

• Teach the patient how to recognize signs and symptoms of infection, and tell him to report these immediately.

• If the patient doesn't require hospitalization, encourage him to continue his normal lifestyle with appropriate restrictions (such as regular rest periods) until remission occurs.

Disseminated intravascular coagulation

DIC is a grave blood coagulation disorder that occurs as a complication of conditions that accelerate clotting. It causes small blood vessel occlusion, organ necrosis, depletion of circulating clotting factors and platelets, and activation of the fibrinolytic (blood-clot promoting) system.

The case of the consumed clotting factors

These processes, in turn, can provoke severe hemorrhage as clotting factors are consumed. Clotting in the microcirculation usually affects the kidneys and extremities, but also may occur in the brain, lungs, pituitary and adrenal glands, and GI mucosa.

Although usually acute, DIC may be chronic in cancer patients. Prognosis depends on early detection and treatment, hemorrhage severity, and treatment of the underlying disease.

What causes it

DIC can result from:
• infection, such as gram-negative or gram-positive septicemia; viral, fungal, or rickettsial infection; or protozoal infection (falciparum malaria)
• obstetric complications, such as abruptio placentae, amniotic fluid embolism, or retained dead fetus
• neoplastic disease, such as acute leukemia or metastatic carcinoma
• tissue necrosis from extensive burns or trauma, brain tissue destruction, transplant rejection, or hepatic necrosis.

Other possible causes of DIC include cardiac arrest, heatstroke, shock, poisonous snakebite, cirrhosis, fat embolism, incompatible blood transfusions, intraoperative cardiopulmonary bypass, giant hemangioma (a benign vascular tumor), severe venous thrombosis, and purpura fulminans (a severe, rapidly fatal form of nonthrombocytopenic purpura).

In DIC, small blood vessel occlusion is one in a series of events leading to severe hemorrhaging.

Pathophysiology

DIC arises when one of the predisposing conditions listed above activates the coagulation system. Excess fibrin forms (triggered by the action of thrombin, an enzyme) and becomes trapped in the microvasculature along with platelets, causing clots.

Horrific hemorrhaging

Blood flow to the tissues then decreases, resulting in acidemia, blood stasis, and tissue hypoxia. These conditions may lead to organ failure. Both fibrinolysis (fibrin dissolution) and antithrombotic mechanisms induce anticoagulation. Platelets and clotting factors are consumed, and massive hemorrhage may ensue. (See *Deciphering DIC.*)

What to look for

Abnormal bleeding, without a history of a serious hemorrhagic disorder, can signal DIC. Signs of such bleeding include:
• cutaneous oozing

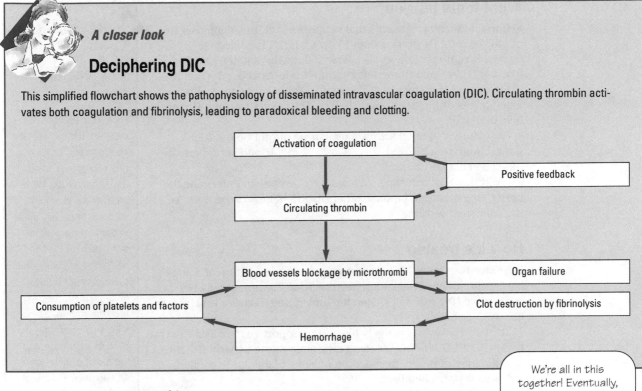

A closer look

Deciphering DIC

This simplified flowchart shows the pathophysiology of disseminated intravascular coagulation (DIC). Circulating thrombin activates both coagulation and fibrinolysis, leading to paradoxical bleeding and clotting.

- petechiae
- ecchymoses
- hematomas
- bleeding from sites of surgical or invasive procedures (such as incisions and I.V. sites)
- GI tract bleeding.

Assessment add-ons

Also, assess the patient for acrocyanosis (symmetrical cyanosis) and acute tubular necrosis (damage to renal tubule cells, leading to renal failure).

Related symptoms and other possible effects of DIC include:
- nausea and vomiting
- dyspnea
- oliguria (reduced urine output)
- seizures
- coma
- shock
- severe muscle, back, and abdominal pain
- failure of major organ systems.

We're all in this together! Eventually, major organ systems may fail in DIC.

What tests tell you

• Initial laboratory findings that support a tentative diagnosis of DIC include PT greater than 15 seconds, PTT exceeding 60 seconds, fibrinogen levels below 150 mg/dl, platelet count below 100,000/µl, and fibrin degradation products above 100 µg/ml.
• Supportive data may include positive fibrin monomers, diminished levels of factors V and VIII, RBC fragmentation, and Hb level below 10 g/dl.
• Assessment of renal status shows urine output below 30 ml/hour, blood urea nitrogen level above 25 mg/dl, and serum creatinine level above 1.3 mg/dl.

Additional diagnostic measures may be done to determine the underlying disorder, because other disorders may cause many of the same test results.

How it's treated

Effective treatment of DIC requires prompt recognition and adequate treatment of the underlying disorder. Treatment may be supportive (for example, when the underlying disorder is self-limiting) or highly specific.

If the patient isn't actively bleeding, supportive care alone may reverse DIC. But active bleeding may necessitate heparin I.V. and transfusions of blood, fresh frozen plasma, platelets, or packed RBCs to support hemostasis.

Dissension over heparin

Heparin therapy is controversial. It may be used early in DIC to prevent microclotting or as a last resort in an actively bleeding patient. In thrombosis, heparin therapy is usually mandatory. In most cases, it's given with transfusion therapy.

What to do

Focus patient care on early recognition of the primary signs and symptoms of abnormal bleeding, prompt treatment of the underlying disorder, and prevention of further bleeding. Implement these measures:
• To prevent clots from dislodging, don't scrub bleeding areas.
• Use pressure, cold compresses, and topical hemostatic agents to control bleeding.
• Protect the patient from injury. Enforce complete bed rest during bleeding episodes. If the patient is agitated, pad the side rails.
• Check all I.V. and venipuncture sites frequently.
• Apply pressure to injection sites for at least 10 minutes.

Education edge

DIC teaching tips

• If your patient has disseminated intravascular coagulation (DIC), explain diagnostic tests and procedures. Allow time for questions.
• Inform the family of the patient's progress. Prepare them for his appearance, including the possibility of I.V. lines, nasogastric tubes, bruises, and dried blood.
• Provide emotional support. As needed, enlist the aid of a social worker, chaplain, and other health care team members in providing such support.

• Monitor fluid intake and output hourly in patients with acute DIC, especially when giving blood products. Watch for transfusion reactions and indications of fluid overload.
• To measure the amount of blood lost, weigh dressings and linens and record drainage.
• Weigh the patient daily, particularly if there's renal involvement.
• Check the patient for headache, and assess neurologic status periodically.
• Watch for GI and genitourinary tract bleeding. To detect intra-abdominal bleeding, measure the patient's abdomen at least every 4 hours and monitor closely for signs and symptoms of shock. Monitor the results of serial blood studies (especially HCT, Hb levels, and coagulation times).
• Evaluate the patient. With successful treatment, he should be free from bleeding, and tests should show his coagulation parameters and renal status within normal limits. (See *DIC teaching tips*.)

If your patient has acute DIC, monitor his fluid intake and output every hour — especially when giving blood products.

Hemophilia

Hemophilia is a hereditary bleeding disorder that results from lack of specific clotting factors. It occurs in two main forms:
• Hemophilia A (classic hemophilia), seen in more than 80% of hemophilia cases, results from deficiency of factor VIII.
• Hemophilia B (Christmas disease), which accounts for roughly 15% of hemophilia cases, results from deficiency of factor IX.

A prettier picture

Treatment advances have greatly improved prognosis, and many hemophiliacs have normal life spans. Surgery can be done safely under a hematologist's guidance at special hemophilia treatment centers.

What causes it

Hemophilia A and B are inherited as X-linked recessive traits. This means female carriers have a 50% chance of transmitting the gene to each son or daughter. Daughters who receive the gene are carriers; sons who receive it are born with hemophilia.

Nonfunctional factors?

Although traditionally seen as a deficiency of clotting factors, recent evidence suggests that hemophilia may result from nonfunctioning factors VIII and IX.

Some experts think hemophilia reflects nonfunctioning of certain clotting factors, not a deficiency of these factors.

Pathophysiology

Hemophilia produces abnormal bleeding. Depending on the degree of factor deficiency, the bleeding may be mild, moderate, or severe. Overall prognosis is best in patients with mild hemophilia, which doesn't cause spontaneous bleeding or joint deformities.

Plugs that preclude clots

After a platelet plug forms at a bleeding site, lack of clotting factors impairs formation of a stable fibrin clot. Delayed bleeding is more common than immediate hemorrhage.

What to look for

Signs and symptoms vary with the severity of hemophilia.
• With *mild* hemophilia, bleeding doesn't occur spontaneously or after minor trauma. However, major trauma or surgery typically causes prolonged bleeding.
• With *moderate* hemophilia, spontaneous bleeding occurs occasionally. Surgery or trauma causes excessive bleeding.
• With *severe* hemophilia, bleeding occurs spontaneously and may be severe even with minor trauma, leading to large subcutaneous and deep I.M. hematomas.

Bleeding and deformity

Bleeding into joints and muscles also may occur and causes pain, swelling, extreme tenderness and, possibly, permanent deformity.

What tests tell you

Characteristic findings in patients with hemophilia A include:
• factor VIII assay 0% to 30% of normal
• prolonged PTT
• normal platelet count and function, bleeding time, and PT.
  Characteristic findings in patients with hemophilia B include:
• deficient factor IX assay
• baseline coagulation results similar to those in hemophilia A, except with normal factor VIII levels.

Three degrees of deficiency

With either hemophilia A or B, the degree of factor deficiency determines the severity of the illness:
• mild hemophilia: factor levels 5% to 40% of normal
• moderate hemophilia: factor levels 1% to 5% of normal
• severe hemophilia: factor levels less than 1% of normal.

These test results show that my patient's factor levels are 4% of normal. That means he has moderate hemophilia.

How it's treated

Although hemophilia isn't curable, treatment can prevent crippling deformities and prolong life expectancy. Correct treatment quickly stops bleeding by increasing plasma levels of deficient clotting factors. This helps prevent disabling deformities that result from repeated bleeding into muscles and joints.

Treatment includes:
• For hemophilia A, cryoprecipitated antihemophilic factor (AHF), lyophilized AHF, or both are given in doses large enough to raise clotting factor levels above 25% of normal to support normal hemostasis. Before surgery, AHF is given to raise clotting factors to hemostatic levels. Levels are then kept within a normal range until the wound has healed. Fresh frozen plasma also can be given.

Multiple risks

• Inhibitors to factor VIII develop after multiple transfusions in 10% to 20% of patients with severe hemophilia, causing resistance to factor VIII infusions. Desmopressin may be given to stimulate release of stored factor VIII, raising the blood level of this factor. In hemophilia B, administering factor IX concentrate during bleeding episodes increases factor IX levels.
• A patient who undergoes surgery needs careful management by a hematologist experienced in caring for hemophiliacs. The deficient factor must be replaced before and after surgery (possibly even minor surgery such as dental extractions). Aminocaproic acid is commonly used for oral bleeding, to inhibit the active fibrinolytic system in the oral mucosa. Human immunodeficiency virus screening reduces the risk of acquired immunodeficiency syndrome from transfusion.

What to do

Implement these measures:
• During bleeding episodes, administer the deficient clotting factor or plasma as ordered. The body uses up AHF in 48 to 72 hours, so repeat the infusion, as ordered, until bleeding stops.
• Apply cold compresses or ice bags, and raise the injured part.
• To prevent recurrent bleeding, restrict the patient's activity for 48 hours after bleeding is under control.
• If bleeding into a joint occurs, immediately elevate the affected joint.
• Control pain with an analgesic, such as acetaminophen, propoxyphene, codeine, or meperidine, as ordered.
• Know that aspirin and aspirin-containing medications are contraindicated because they decrease platelet adherence and may worsen bleeding.

• Avoid I.M. injections because of possible hematoma formation at the injection site.
• After bleeding episodes and surgery, watch closely for signs and symptoms of further bleeding, such as increased pain and swelling, fever, or indications of shock. Closely monitor PTT.
• To restore mobility in an affected joint, begin range-of-motion exercises, if ordered, at least 48 hours after bleeding is controlled. Tell the patient to avoid bearing weight on the joint until bleeding stops and swelling subsides.
• Evaluate the patient. He should be free from bleeding; he should understand how to minimize bleeding risks and know what to do if bleeding occurs. (See *Hemophilia teaching tips.*)

Sickle cell anemia

A type of congenital hemolytic anemia (shortened RBC survival and inability of bone marrow to compensate for decreased RBC life span), sickle cell anemia occurs mainly in African-Americans. It results from a defective Hb molecule (HbS), which causes RBCs to roughen and become sickle shaped and more fragile.

Renegade RBCs

The abnormal RBCs impair circulation, resulting in chronic ill health, periodic crises, long-term complications, and premature death.

What causes it

Sickle cell anemia may stem from homozygous inheritance of the HbS–producing gene, which causes the amino acid valine to replace glutamic acid in the HBB chain. (See *Understanding sickle cell trait.*)

Pathophysiology

Blood vessel obstruction by rigid, tangled RBCs causes tissue oxygen starvation and possible necrosis. These conditions, in turn, lead to painful vaso-occlusive crisis, a hallmark of the disease. Bone marrow depression results in aplastic (megaloblastic) crisis.

Crises and their causes

Factors that predispose a patient to sickle cell crisis include deoxygenation (as from pneumonia, hypoxia, or scuba diving), cold exposure, acidosis, and infection.

Education edge

Hemophilia teaching tips

• Teach the parents of a child with hemophilia which precautions they must take to prevent bleeding episodes as well as proper procedures for managing these episodes when they occur.
• Refer new patients to a hemophilia treatment center for evaluation. The center can develop a treatment and management plan for the patient's primary care doctor and serve as a resource for medical personnel, dentists, or others involved in the patient's care.

What to look for

Signs and symptoms of sickle cell anemia include:
- aching bones
- cardiomegaly (heart enlargement)
- chest pain
- chronic fatigue
- diastolic and systolic murmurs
- exertional or unexplained dyspnea
- hepatomegaly (liver enlargement)
- increased susceptibility to infection
- ischemic leg ulcers (especially on the ankles)
- jaundice
- joint swelling
- pallor
- tachycardia.

Crisis components

During a painful vaso-occlusive crisis, the patient may experience:
- severe abdominal, thoracic, muscular, or bone pain
- low-grade fever
- possible increased jaundice and dark urine
- in chronic disease, spleen shrinkage. (See *Caring for a patient in sickle cell crisis*, page 742.)

What tests tell you

- Stained blood smear showing sickle-shaped RBCs and Hb electrophoresis showing HbS confirm the diagnosis.
- CBC shows low RBC and elevated WBC and platelet counts. Hb levels may be low or normal.
- Erythrocyte sedimentation rate and RBC survival time are decreased; serum iron levels and reticulocyte counts are increased.

How it's treated

Although sickle cell anemia can't be cured, treatment can ease symptoms and prevent painful crises. Treatment includes:
- Polyvalent pneumococcal and *Haemophilus influenzae* B vaccinations; anti-infectives, such as low-dose oral penicillin; and chelating agents, such as deferoxamine, help minimize complications.
- Analgesics can relieve the pain of vaso-occlusive crisis.
- An iron supplement may be given if folic acid levels are low.
- An antisickling agent may be given. However, the most commonly used agent, sodium cyanate, has many adverse effects.

Understanding sickle cell trait

Sickle cell trait is a relatively benign condition that results from heterozygous inheritance of a sickle hemoglobin S (HbS) gene. Like sickle cell anemia, sickle cell trait is most common in African-Americans. However, sickle cell trait *never* progresses to sickle cell anemia.

The woes of low O_2

In people with sickle cell trait (called *sickle cell carriers*), 20% to 40% of the total Hb is HbS; the rest of the Hb is normal. These people rarely experience symptoms, have normal Hb levels and hematocrit, and can have a normal life span.

But, they must avoid situations that provoke oxygen deficiency (hypoxia), because these sometimes cause a sickling crisis similar to that in sickle cell anemia.

Genetic risks

Genetic counseling is essential for sickle cell carriers. If two sickle cell carriers marry, each of their children has a 25% chance of inheriting sickle cell anemia.

What do I do?

Caring for a patient in sickle cell crisis

Suspect a sickle cell crisis if your patient has these signs and symptoms:
• severe pain
• a temperature over 104.7° F (40.4° C) or a fever of 100.7° F (38.2° C) lasting at least 2 days
• pale lips, tongue, palms, or nailbeds
• lethargy or listlessness
• difficulty awakening
• irritability.

Taking action
Implement these measures:
• Provide effective pain management, including use of opioid analgesics if needed. Assess the patient's pain frequently. Have him rate the pain on a scale of 0 to 10 (or according to your facility's policy). Give opioid analgesics as prescribed.

• Apply warm compresses to painful areas. Never use cold compresses because they may aggravate the condition.
• Cover the patient with a blanket.
• Give an analgesic-antipyretic, such as aspirin or acetaminophen as ordered.
• Encourage bed rest, and place the patient in a sitting position.
• If dehydration or severe pain occurs, hospitalization may be necessary.

• During an acute sequestration crisis, treatment may include sedation, analgesia, blood transfusions, oxygen therapy, and large amounts of oral or I.V. fluids.

What to do
• Advise the patient to avoid tight clothing that restricts circulation.
• Emphasize the need for prompt treatment of infection.
• Evaluate the patient. He should be free from pain and infection. He and his family should understand what steps to take to avoid exacerbating the disease. (See *Sickle cell anemia teaching tips*.)

Thrombocytopenia

The most common hemorrhagic disorder, thrombocytopenia is characterized by a deficiency of circulating platelets. Because platelets play a vital role in blood clotting, this disorder seriously threatens hemostasis.

Predicting recovery

Drug-induced thrombocytopenia carries an excellent prognosis if the causative drug is withdrawn; recovery may be immediate. Otherwise, prognosis depends on the patient's response to treatment of the underlying cause.

What causes it

Thrombocytopenia may be congenital or acquired (more common). In either case, it usually results from:
• decreased or defective platelet production in the bone marrow
• increased platelet destruction outside the marrow, caused by an underlying disorder (such as cirrhosis of the liver, DIC, or severe infection)
• sequestration (as in hypothermia or increased RBC destruction in the spleen) or platelet loss.

An acquired affliction

Acquired thrombocytopenia may result from such drugs as non-steroidal anti-inflammatory agents, sulfonamides, histamine blockers, alkylating agents, or antibiotic chemotherapeutic agents.

Fleeting forms

In children, thrombocytopenia of unknown cause (idiopathic thrombocytopenia) is common. Transient thrombocytopenia may follow a viral infection, such as Epstein-Barr or infectious mononucleosis.

Pathophysiology

In thrombocytopenia, lack of platelets may cause inadequate hemostasis. The four responsible mechanisms include:
• decreased platelet production
• decreased platelet survival
• pooling of blood in the spleen
• intravascular dilution of circulating platelets.

Minding megakaryocytes

Platelet production falls when the number of megakaryocytes decreases or when platelet production becomes dysfunctional.

What to look for

Watch for these signs and symptoms:
• abnormal bleeding (typically of a sudden onset, with skin petechiae or ecchymoses, or bleeding into mucous membranes)
• malaise and fatigue
• general weakness and lethargy
• large, blood-filled bullae (elevations) in the mouth.

What tests tell you

• Coagulation tests show diminished platelet count with prolonged bleeding time.

Education edge

Sickle cell anemia teaching tips

• Instruct the patient to avoid strenuous exercise, vasoconstricting medications, cold temperatures, unpressurized aircraft, high altitudes, and conditions that provoke hypoxia.
• Stress meticulous wound care, good oral hygiene, regular dental and eye checkups, and a balanced diet as safeguards against infection.
• Advise to maintain a high fluid intake to prevent dehydration.
• Recommend that family members be screened to determine if they're heterozygous carriers of the sickle cell trait.
• Warn a female patient that both pregnancy and oral contraceptives can pose risks for her. Refer her to a gynecologist for birth control counseling.
• Inform a male patient that he may experience sudden, painful episodes of priapism (abnormal errection of the penis. Frequent or severe episodes may lead to impotence.

• Bone marrow studies may reveal increased megakaryocytes and shortened platelet survival.

How it's treated

The underlying cause must be treated. In drug-induced thrombocytopenia, the offending drug is withdrawn.

Outlining the options

Treatment may include:
• splenectomy for hypersplenism
• chemotherapy for acute or chronic leukemia
• corticosteroids to enhance vascular integrity
• steroids, danazol, or I.V. immune globulin for idiopathic thrombocytopenia
• platelet transfusions (to reduce the risk of spontaneous bleeding) if the platelet count falls below 20,000/µl.

What to do

• Take every possible precaution against bleeding, including guarding the patient from trauma. Keep the bed side rails up and pad them, if possible. Instruct him to use an electric razor and a soft toothbrush. Avoid all invasive procedures, such as venipuncture or urinary catheterization, if possible. When venipuncture is unavoidable, exert pressure on the puncture site for at least 20 minutes or until bleeding stops.
• Monitor platelet counts daily. Test stools for occult blood, and test urine and vomitus for blood. Watch for signs of bleeding (including petechiae, ecchymoses, surgical or GI bleeding, and menorrhagia).
• When the patient is bleeding, enforce strict bed rest if necessary.
• When giving platelet concentrate, remember that platelets are extremely fragile. Infuse them quickly, using the administration set recommended by the blood bank. During platelet transfusion, monitor the patient for febrile reaction (flushing, chills, fever, headache, tachycardia, and hypertension).
• Be aware that HLA–typed platelets may be ordered when the patient no longer responds to pooled platelets (because of antibody development). WBC–depleted platelets may be ordered to reduce the risk of febrile reactions. A patient with a history of minor reactions may benefit from acetaminophen and diphenhydramine before the transfusion.
• During steroid therapy, monitor the patient's fluid and electrolyte balance and blood glucose level. Watch for infection, pathologic fractures, and mood changes.

Don't roll the dice when giving platelet concentrates. We're fragile, so be sure to infuse us quickly.

• Evaluate the patient. He should lack signs and symptoms of gross and microscopic bleeding. He and his family should know how to reduce bleeding risks. (See *Thrombocytopenia teaching tips*.)

Quick quiz

1. The blood cells that transport oxygen and carbon dioxide to and from body tissues are:
- A. RBCs.
- B. WBCs.
- C. platelets.
- D. granulocytes.

Answer: A. RBCs transport oxygen and carbon dioxide. Because of their biconcave shape, they have the flexibility to travel through blood vessels of different sizes.

2. A patient with blood type B can receive a transfusion of:
- A. type A or type O blood.
- B. type B or type O blood.
- C. type AB or type O blood.
- D. type A or type B.

Answer: B. Type B blood contains B antigens and anti-A antibodies, but no anti-B antibodies. Therefore, a patient with type B blood can receive type B or type O blood (which contains neither anti-A nor anti-B antibodies).

3. Which type of anemia results from deficiency of all the blood's formed elements, caused by failure of the bone marrow to generate enough new cells?
- A. Sickle cell anemia
- B. Folic acid deficiency anemia
- C. Aplastic anemia
- D. Iron deficiency anemia

Answer: C. Aplastic anemia usually develops when damaged or destroyed stem cells inhibit RBC production.

4. Which disorder results from a deficiency of circulating platelets?
- A. Hemophilia
- B. Sickle cell anemia
- C. Von Willebrand's disease
- D. Thrombocytopenia

Education edge

Thrombocyto-penia teaching tips

• Caution the patient to avoid aspirin in any form as well as other drugs that impair coagulation. Teach him how to recognize aspirin compounds listed on labels of over-the-counter preparations.

• Advise the patient to avoid coughing and straining at stool. Both can lead to increased intracranial pressure, possibly causing cerebral hemorrhage in someone with thrombocytopenia. Provide a stool softener if necessary.

• If thrombocytopenia is drug-induced, stress the importance of avoiding the offending drug.

• If the patient must receive long-term steroid therapy, teach him to watch for and report cushingoid signs (such as acne, moon face, hirsutism, and edema). Emphasize that steroids must never be stopped suddenly; they must be discontinued gradually.

Answer: D. Thrombocytopenia, the most common hemorrhagic disorder, results from a deficiency of circulating platelets.

Scoring

☆☆☆ If you answered all four items correctly, you're certainly brainy about blood! Whatever your blood type, on this test you're clearly an A+!

☆☆ If you answered three items correctly, nice phagocytic footwork! You've obviously ingested and absorbed the bulk of this chapter!

☆ If you answered fewer than three items correctly, your hematologic expertise is a bit anemic. We recommend rereading this chapter for a quick knowledge transfusion.

Immunologic disorders

Just the facts

In this chapter, you'll learn:

♦ about the anatomy and physiology of the immune system

♦ effects of the immune system on other body systems

♦ how to assess the immune system

♦ causes, pathophysiology, and diagnostic tests for common immune disorders

♦ treatments and nursing interventions for patients with these disorders.

A normally functioning immune system guards against the effects of invasion by microorganisms and maintains equilibrium within the body by governing degradation and removal of damaged cells. When the immune system functions abnormally, physiologic effects can be devastating.

Immunologic disorders can result from — or cause — problems in other systems. This makes accurate assessment and intervention both crucial and challenging.

Besides endangering the patient's health — or even his life — some immunologic disorders pose a serious health risk to caregivers. This is yet another of the many challenges you'll face when caring for a patient with an immunologic disorder.

Anatomy and physiology

The immune system consists of specialized blood cells (lymphocytes and macrophages) and specialized structures, including the lymph nodes, spleen, thymus, bone marrow, tonsils, adenoids, and appendix.

The blood is an important part of this protective system. Although the blood and immune system are distinct entities, they're closely related. Their cells share a common origin in the bone marrow, and the immune system uses the bloodstream to transport its components to the site of an invasion.

The immune system and blood are closely related. Immune system cells and blood cells both originate in the bone marrow.

Immunity

Immunity refers to the body's capacity to resist invading organisms and toxins, thus preventing tissue and organ damage. The cells and organs of the immune system perform that function. (See *Unraveling the immune system*, pages 750 and 751.)

Scavengers on surveillance

The immune system recognizes, responds to, and eliminates foreign substances (antigens), such as bacteria, fungi, viruses, and parasites. It also preserves the internal environment by scavenging dead or damaged cells and by performing surveillance.

Triple tactics

To perform these functions efficiently, the immune system uses three basic defense strategies:

 physical and chemical barriers to infection

 inflammatory response

 immune response.

   Physical barriers, such as the skin and mucous membranes, prevent most organisms from invading the body. Organisms that penetrate this first barrier simultaneously trigger the inflammatory and immune responses. Both responses involve stem cells — primitive cells in the bone marrow from which all types of blood cells derive.

Types of immunity

In general host defenses, all foreign substances elicit the same response. In contrast, particular microorganisms or molecules activate *specific* immune responses, and initially can involve specialized sets of immune cells. These specific responses are classified as either *humoral* or *cell-mediated* immunity. Lymphocytes (B cells and T cells) produce the responses.

T and B cells like us play crucial roles in humoral and cell-mediated immunity. If we don't function well, the body has trouble fighting off infection.

Humoral immunity

In the humoral response, an invading antigen causes B cells to divide and differentiate into plasma cells. Each plasma cell, in turn, produces and secretes large amounts of antigen-specific immunoglobulins (Ig) into the bloodstream.

Mind your Igs

Immunoglobulins exist in five types — IgA, IgD, IgE, IgG, and IgM. Each type serves a particular function:

- IgA, IgG, and IgM guard against viral and bacterial invasion.
- IgD acts as an antigen receptor of B cells.
- IgE causes an allergic response.

Thanks for the complement

Indispensable to humoral immunity, the complement system consists of about 25 enzymes that "complement" the work of antibodies by aiding phagocytosis or destroying bacterial cells (through puncture of their cell membranes).

Cell-mediated immunity

Cell-mediated immunity protects the body against bacterial, viral, and fungal infections. It also resists transplanted cells and tumor cells. In the cell-mediated immune response, a type of scavenger cell called a *macrophage* processes the antigen, which is then presented to T cells.

> **Memory jogger**
>
> A stand-up comedian who gets no laughs might say his audience has humoral immunity. But humor is the Latin word for "liquid," and humoral immunity comes from elements in the blood — specifically, antibodies.
>
> Contrast this with cellular immunity, which comes about through the actions of T cells.

Assessment

Accurately assessing the immune system can challenge your skills because immune disorders commonly cause vague symptoms, such as fatigue or dyspnea. Initially, these symptoms may seem to be related to other body systems.

History

Begin your assessment with a thorough history. Because the immune system affects all body functions, be sure to investigate the patient's overall health.

Current health status

Among patients with immunologic disorders, common complaints include fatigue or lack of energy, lightheadedness, frequent bruising, and slow wound healing.

> The wound you got when you charged that lion last month isn't healing well. I'll need to assess you for an immune problem.

(Text continues on page 752.)

Unraveling the immune system

The immune system includes organs and tissues in which *lymphocytes* (a type of white blood cell) predominate as well as cells that circulate in peripheral blood. The central lymphoid organs are the bone marrow and thymus. Peripheral lymphoid organs include the lymph nodes and vessels, spleen, tonsils, adenoids, appendix, and intestinal lymphoid tissue (Peyer's patches).

Bringing up baby cells

The bone marrow and thymus play a role in developing the primary immune system cells—B lymphocytes (B cells) and T lymphocytes (T cells). Both cell types probably originate in the bone marrow.

B cells may also mature and differentiate from pluripotential stem cells in the bone marrow. T cells mature and differentiate in the thymus, a two-lobed endocrine gland in the upper mediastinum. B and T cells are distributed throughout the tissue of peripheral lymphoid organs, especially the lymph nodes and spleen.

Lymph nodes

Most abundant in the head, neck, axillae, abdomen, pelvis, and groin, lymph nodes are small, oval-shaped structures located along a network of lymph channels. They help remove and destroy antigens (such as toxins, bacteria, and other foreign matter) that circulate in the blood and lymph. Lymph nodes are also a primary source of circulating lymphocytes, which provide specific immune responses.

Surrounding each lymph node is a fibrous capsule. Bands of connective tissue (trabeculae) from the capsule extend into the node, dividing it into three compartments: superficial cortex, deep cortex, and medulla.
• The *superficial cortex* contains follicles consisting mainly of B cells. During an immune response, the follicles enlarge and develop a germinal area with large proliferating cells.
• The *deep cortex* consists mostly of T cells, as do the areas between follicles.
• The *medulla* contains numerous plasma cells that secrete immunoglobulins (antibodies) during an immune response.

Lymphatic vessels

Afferent lymphatic vessels carry lymph (a colorless fluid consisting mainly of water with dissolved salts and protein) into the node's subcapsular sinus. From here, lymph flows through cortical sinuses and smaller radial medullary sinuses. In the deep cortex and medullary sinuses, phagocytes (cells that engulf, ingest,

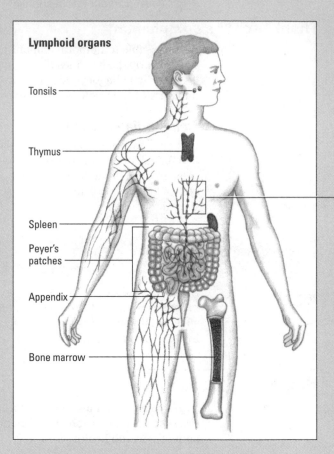

Lymphoid organs

Tonsils

Thymus

Spleen

Peyer's patches

Appendix

Bone marrow

and digest foreign material) attack the antigen. The antigen may also be trapped in the follicles of the superficial cortex.

Wayfaring lymph

Clean lymph leaves the node through efferent lymphatic vessels at the hilum. These vessels drain into specific lymph node chains that, in turn, drain into large lymph vessels known as trunks, which empty into the subclavian vein of the vascular system. In most parts of the body, lymphatic vessels and lymphatic capillar-

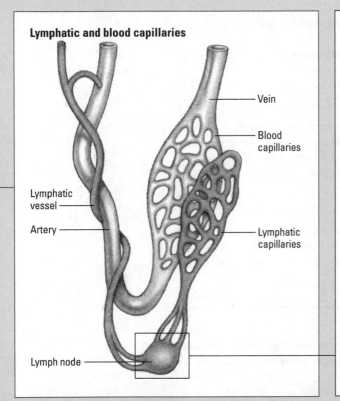

Lymphatic and blood capillaries

- Vein
- Blood capillaries
- Lymphatic vessel
- Artery
- Lymphatic capillaries
- Lymph node

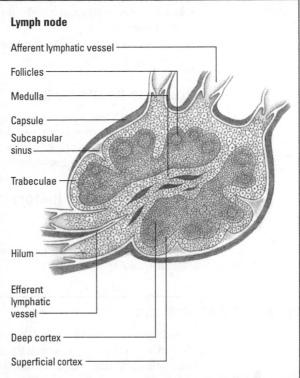

Lymph node

- Afferent lymphatic vessel
- Follicles
- Medulla
- Capsule
- Subcapsular sinus
- Trabeculae
- Hilum
- Efferent lymphatic vessel
- Deep cortex
- Superficial cortex

ies help veins and blood capillaries function by draining body tissues and increasing the return of blood to the heart.

Protecting the center

Lymph usually travels through more than one lymph node because numerous nodes line the lymphatic channels that drain a particular region. For example, axillary nodes filter drainage from the arms, whereas femoral nodes (located in the inguinal region) filter drainage from the legs. This arrangement prevents organisms that enter peripheral body areas from migrating unchallenged to central areas.

Spleen

The spleen is located in the left upper quadrant of the abdomen beneath the diaphragm. It gathers and isolates worn-out red blood cells, foreign materials, and cellular debris. It also stores blood and about 20% to 30% of the body's platelets.

Accessory organs

Other lymphoid tissues—tonsils, adenoids, appendix, thymus, and Peyer's patches—also remove foreign debris in much the same way as lymph nodes do. They're positioned in food and air passages—likely areas of microbial access.

Key queries

Ask these questions to elicit details about your patient's current illness:
• Have you noticed enlarged lymph nodes?
• Have you experienced weakness or joint pain? If so, when did you first notice the problem? Does it affect one side of your body or both sides?
• Have you recently had a rash, abnormal bleeding, or a slow-healing sore?
• Have you experienced vision disturbances, fever, or changes in elimination patterns?

Previous health status

Explore the patient's previous major illnesses, recurrent minor illnesses, accidents or injuries, surgical procedures, and allergies. Ask if he has had a procedure that could affect the immune system, such as a blood transfusion or an organ transplant.

Family and social history

Find out if the patient has a family history of cancer or hematologic or immune disorders. Ask about his home and work environments to help determine if he's being exposed to hazardous chemicals or other agents.

Physical examination

The effects of immune disorders are far-reaching and may materialize in several body systems. Pay special attention to the skin, hair, nails, and mucous membranes.

Inspection

• Observe for pallor, cyanosis (blue-tinged skin), and jaundice. Also check for erythema (redness), indicating a local inflammation, and plethora (a red, florid complexion).
• Evaluate skin integrity. Note signs or symptoms of inflammation or infection, such as redness, swelling, heat, tenderness, poor wound healing, wound drainage, induration (tissue hardening), and lesions.
• Check for rash, and note its distribution.
• Observe hair texture and distribution, noting alopecia (hair loss) on the arms, legs, or head.

- Inspect nails for color, texture, longitudinal striations, onycholysis (separation from the nail bed), and clubbing (enlargement of the fingertips).
- Inspect the oral mucous membranes for fluffy white patches, white plaques, lesions, swollen gums, redness, and bleeding.
- Inspect areas where the patient reports "swollen glands" or "lumps" for color abnormalities and visible lymph node enlargement.
- Observe respiratory rate, rhythm, and energy expenditure related to respiratory effort. Note the position the patient assumes to ease breathing.
- Assess peripheral circulation. Inspect for Raynaud's phenomenon (intermittent arteriolar vasospasm of the fingers or toes and, sometimes, the ears and nose).
- Inspect the anus for inflammation or breaks in the mucosal surface.

Your gums are swollen. Unless you've gone back to flossing with wildebeest horns, the swelling could mean your immune system is weak.

Palpation

Palpate the peripheral pulses, which should be symmetrical and regular. Next, palpate the abdomen, noting enlarged organs and tenderness; and the joints, checking for swelling, tenderness, and pain.

Taking notes on nodes

Then palpate superficial lymph nodes in the head and neck and in the axillary, epitrochlear, inguinal, and popliteal areas. If palpation reveals an enlarged node or other abnormalities, note the node's location, size, shape, surface, consistency, symmetry, mobility, color, tenderness, temperature, pulsations, and vascularity. (See *Locating lymph nodes in the head and neck*, page 754.)

Percussion

Percuss the anterior, lateral, and posterior thorax, comparing one side with the other. A dull sound indicates consolidation, which may occur with pneumonia. Hyperresonance (increased percussion sounds) may result from trapped air, as from bronchial asthma.

Auscultation

Auscultate over the lungs to check for adventitious (abnormal) sounds. Wheezing suggests asthma or an allergic response. Crackles may signal a respiratory tract infection such as pneumonia.

Locating lymph nodes in the head and neck

This illustration shows the location of the lymph nodes in the head and neck.

Occipital

Postauricular

Superficial cervical

Anterior cervical

Posterior cervical

Supraclavicular

Preauricular

Tonsillar

Submandibular

Submental

Auscultate the patient's lungs for adventitious sounds, over the precordium for abnormal heart sounds, and the abdomen for bowel sounds.

Auscultation agenda

Auscultate for heart sounds over the precordium. Normal auscultation reveals only the first and second heart sounds (lub-dub).

Next, auscultate the abdomen for bowel sounds. With autoimmune disorders that cause diarrhea, bowel sounds increase. With scleroderma (skin hardening and thickening, with degeneration of connective tissue) and other autoimmune disorders that cause constipation, bowel sounds decrease.

Diagnostic tests

Commonly ordered studies to evaluate the immune response include general cellular tests (which help diagnose immunodeficiency disorders), general humoral tests (which help detect immunomediated disease), and delayed hypersensitivity skin tests (which evaluate the cell-mediated immune response).

General cellular tests

General cellular tests, such as T- and B-lymphocyte assays, aid the diagnosis of primary and secondary immunodeficiency disorders.

T- and B-lymphocyte surface marker assays

Surface marker assays identify specific cells involved in the immune response and examine the balance between the regulatory activities of several interacting cell types — notably, T-helper and T-suppressor cells. These tests use highly specific monoclonal antibodies to define levels of lymphocyte differentiation and to analyze both normal and malignant cells.

Plethora of purposes

The results of T- and B-lymphocyte surface marker assays help to:
- assess immunocompetence in chronic infections
- evaluate immunodeficiencies
- classify lymphocytic leukemia, lymphoma, and immunodeficiency diseases such as acquired immunodeficiency syndrome (AIDS)
- identify immunoregulation associated with autoimmune disorders
- diagnose disorders marked by abnormal numbers and percentages of T-helper cells, T-suppressor cells, and B lymphocytes.

Nursing considerations
- Inform the patient that the test requires a blood sample.
- As ordered, perform a venipuncture. Send the blood sample to the laboratory immediately to ensure viable lymphocytes. The sample must not be refrigerated or frozen.
- Many patients with T- and B-cell changes have a compromised immune system, so be sure to keep the venipuncture site clean and dry. If a hematoma develops, apply warm soaks.

Be sure to send the blood sample to the laboratory immediately. Lymphocytes don't stay viable too long.

Delayed hypersensitivity skin tests

Delayed hypersensitivity skin tests evaluate the cell-mediated immune response. They include intradermal skin tests and scratch and puncture allergy tests.

Intradermal skin tests

For intradermal skin tests, recall antigens (antigens to which the patient may have been previously sensitized) are injected into the superficial skin layer with a needle and syringe or a sterile four-pronged lancet.

TB or not TB?

Tuberculin skin tests (such as the tine, Aplitest, or Mantoux) produce a delayed hypersensitivity reaction in patients with active or dormant tuberculosis (TB).

Recalling past antigens

Recall antigen tests for blastomycosis, coccidioidomycosis, and histoplasmosis induce depressed or negative delayed hypersensitivity reactions in patients with these diseases.

Recall antigen tests induce positive delayed hypersensitivity reactions in patients who can maintain a nonspecific inflammatory response to the antigen.

Nursing considerations

• Tell the patient when he can expect a reaction to appear. Check his history for hypersensitivity to the test antigens and for previous reactions to a skin test.
• Using alcohol, clean the volar surface (palm side) of the arm, about 2 or 3 fingerbreadths distal to the antecubital space (triangle of the elbow) to protect the wheal from potential infection. You may also clean the area with acetone to remove skin oils that may interfere with test results.
• Make sure the test site you've chosen has adequate subcutaneous tissue and is free from hair and blemishes. Let the skin dry completely before administering the injection to avoid inactivating the antigen.
• Instruct an outpatient to return at the prescribed time to have test results read.

Scratch and puncture allergy tests

Skin scratch and puncture allergy tests evaluate the immune system's ability to respond to known allergens. A tiny amount of allergen is scratched across or lightly pricked into the skin of a hairless area, such as the scapula, volar surface of the forearm, or anterior surface of the thigh. If the patient has an allergy, the specific allergens he's allergic to will cause redness and swelling.

Teensy weensy doses

These tests provoke delayed hypersensitivity reactions mediated by T cells. Although minute amounts of test allergens usually can demonstrate an intact immune response, test results may indicate an anergic (diminished or absent) reaction in elderly patients as well as in patients with acute leukemia, Hodgkin's disease, congenital immunodeficiencies, or overwhelming infections.

Scratch and puncture tests are contraindicated in patients with inflammation, skin diseases, or significant immunologic impairment.

This scratch and puncture test may tell us which substances you're allergic to.

Nursing considerations

• Use the volar surface of the arm to perform the test in an adult; use the upper back in a child.
• After 20 minutes, check for a pale, raised, urticarial area around the puncture or scratch site (wheal), surrounded by a reddened area that's generally round (flare). This indicates a positive response, meaning a patient is allergic to the specific allergen tested.
• Record the greatest diameter of the wheal and flare for each allergen.

Treatments

Treatments for immune disorders include drug therapy and bone marrow transplantation. Both may cause additional immunosuppression, so you'll need to take special precautions to maintain strict asepsis and prevent infection and injury.

Drug therapy

Many immune disorders are treated with drugs, so you'll need to be familiar with the indications, dosages, and nursing considerations for such drugs as:
• antihistamines, which prevent or relieve allergic reactions

- immunosuppressants, used to combat tissue rejection and help control autoimmune disorders
- corticosteroids, which prevent or suppress the cell-mediated immune response and reduce inflammation
- cytotoxic drugs, which kill immunocompetent cells
- adrenergics, which stimulate the sympathetic nervous system.

Epinephrine should be given immediately to a patient who's suffering an acute anaphylactic reaction.

Epi vs. anny

Drugs are the primary treatment for certain immune disorders. For instance, epinephrine is the drug of choice for treating acute anaphylactic reaction. For other immune disorders, drugs are prescribed to treat associated symptoms.

Medication roster

Besides epinephrine, other drugs used to treat immune disorders include:
- azathioprine
- cyclosporine
- cytomegalovirus immune globulin (human)
- didanosine
- hepatitis B immune globulin, human
- immune globulin
- lamivudine
- levamisole
- $Rh_o(D)$ immune globulin
- stavudine
- zalcitabine
- zidovudine (AZT).

Immunosuppressant therapy

Iatrogenic (treatment-induced) immunodeficiency may be a complicating adverse effect of chemotherapy or other treatment.

Oh no! It's immunosuppressant therapy! I wonder how many of us lymphocytes will survive.

In some cases, however, it's the goal of therapy—for instance, to suppress immune-mediated tissue damage from an autoimmune disorder or to prevent rejection of an organ transplant. To induce immunodeficiency, a patient may receive various types of immunosuppressant drugs.

Antilymphocyte serum

Antilymphocyte serum is a powerful nonspecific immunosuppressant that destroys circulating lymphocytes. It reduces T-cell number and function, thus suppressing cell-mediated immunity. It has been used effectively to prevent cell-mediated rejection of tissue grafts or transplants.

Antithymocyte globulin

Antithymocyte globulin (ATG) causes specific destruction of T lymphocytes. Usually, it's given immediately before transplantation and continued for some time afterward.

Sickening the serum

Adverse effects of ATG include anaphylaxis and serum sickness. Arising 1 to 2 weeks after ATG injection, serum sickness is marked by fever, malaise, rash, arthralgias and, sometimes, glomerulonephritis or vasculitis.

Corticosteroids

Corticosteroids are adrenocortical hormones used widely to treat immune-mediated disorders because of their potent anti-inflammatory and immunosuppressant effects. They stabilize the vascular membrane, blocking tissue infiltration by neutrophils and monocytes and thus inhibiting inflammation. They also "kidnap" T cells in the bone marrow, causing lymphopenia.

Lymphocyte bounce-back

However, because these drugs aren't toxic to cells, lymphocyte concentration can quickly return to normal within 24 hours after the corticosteroid is withdrawn. Also, corticosteroids seem to inhibit immunoglobulin synthesis and interfere with binding of immunoglobulin to antigen.

Cyclosporine

Cyclosporine selectively suppresses the proliferation and development of T-helper cells, resulting in depressed cell-mediated immunity.

Cytotoxic drugs

Cytotoxic drugs kill immunocompetent cells while they're replicating. Unfortunately, most of these agents aren't selective, which means they interfere with all rapidly proliferating cells. As a result, they cause depletion of lymphocytes and phagocytes and interfere with lymphocyte synthesis and release of immunoglobulins and lymphokines.

Dicey drug therapy

Cyclophosphamide, a potent cytotoxic drug commonly used as an immunosuppressant, initially depletes B cells, suppressing humoral immunity. Long-term therapy also depletes T cells, suppressing cell-mediated immunity, too. Cyclophosphamide may be

Memory jogger

Searching for a "hook" to use when assessing patients for serum sickness? Just think of the word FARM. Each letter stands for a key sign or symptom of serum sickness.

F: Fever

A: Arthralgias

R: Rash

M: Malaise

given to patients with systemic lupus erythematosus (SLE), Wegener's granulomatosis, or certain autoimmune disorders.

Because it nonselectively destroys rapidly dividing cells, the drug can cause severe bone marrow suppression with abnormally low levels of red blood cells, or RBCs (anemia), neutrophils (neutropenia), or platelets (thrombocytopenia). It also may lead to gonadal suppression, resulting in sterility, alopecia, hemorrhagic cystitis, nausea and vomiting, stomatitis, and an increased risk of lymphoproliferative neoplasm.

Other immune busters

Other cytotoxic drugs used to suppress the immune system include:
• azathioprine, commonly used in kidney transplant
• methotrexate, occasionally used in rheumatoid arthritis and other autoimmune disorders.

Nonsurgical intervention

Patients with certain immune disorders may be candidates for bone marrow transplant. This procedure also is being explored as a treatment of certain hematologic disorders and cancers, such as multiple myeloma and some solid tumors.

Bone marrow transplantation

In bone marrow transplantation, bone marrow cells are collected from the patient or another donor and then administered to the patient after his diseased bone marrow is destroyed by chemotherapy or total body radiation. The goal is to allow the patient to resume normal blood cell production.

The preferred treatment of aplastic anemia and severe combined immunodeficiency syndrome (SCID), bone marrow transplantation also is used to treat leukemia patients who are at high risk for relapse or who have undergone high-dose chemotherapy and total body radiation therapy.

Patient preparation

• Inform the patient that bone marrow transplant will deplete his white blood cells (WBCs), putting him at high risk for infection immediately after the procedure. As a safeguard, he'll be placed in reverse isolation for several weeks.
• Prepare him for the pretransplant regimen, which may include cytotoxic chemotherapy and total body radiation. During this regimen, he should expect adverse reactions, such as parotitis (inflammation or infection of the parotid salivary glands), diarrhea,

Patients with certain immunologic diseases may receive a bone marrow transplant so their bone marrow can resume normal blood cell production.

fever, nausea, vomiting, and symptoms of bone marrow depression (such as fever, fatigue, chills, bruising, and bleeding).

Monitoring and aftercare
• During the transfusion, monitor the patient's vital signs closely to allow prompt detection of such reactions as fever, dyspnea, and hypotension.
• Assess the patient every 4 hours for infection symptoms, such as fever and chills.
• Maintain strict asepsis when caring for the patient. Take measures to protect him from injury.
• Watch for signs of graft-versus-host (GVH) disease, such as dermatitis, hepatitis, hemolytic anemia, and thrombocytopenia. GVH disease usually occurs during the first 90 days after the transplant and may become chronic — or it may cause transplant failure, lymphatic depletion, infection, or death.

Home care instructions
• Tell the patient to guard against infection. Warn him that he may remain unusually vulnerable to infection for up to 1 year after bone marrow transplantation.
• Urge him to keep regular medical appointments so the doctor can monitor his progress and detect late complications.

If your patient is in reverse isolation, apply a clean mask every time you enter his room, and make sure visitors do the same.

Nursing diagnoses

When caring for patients with immunologic disorders, you'll find that several nursing diagnoses can be used over and over. Commonly used diagnoses appear here, along with appropriate nursing interventions and rationales.

Risk for infection

Related to external or internal factors, *Risk for infection* may be associated with AIDS, SCID, pernicious anemia, and other immune disorders.

Expected outcomes
• Patient remains free from signs and symptoms of infection.
• Patient maintains adequate respiratory function.
• Patient states ways to prevent infection, including proper hand washing and good personal hygiene.

Nursing interventions and rationales

• Practice strict hand washing before and after patient contact to avoid spreading pathogens.
• Monitor the patient closely for signs and symptoms of infection, such as fever and chills. Check vital signs every 4 hours. Close monitoring allows for timely intervention.
• Maintain skin and mucous membrane integrity to help prevent infection. Encourage ambulation, and help turn the patient every 2 hours. Don't give an enema or a suppository or take the patient's rectal temperature. Encourage mouth care with sodium bicarbonate and natural saline rinse (1 teaspoonful per 8 oz) to inhibit microbial growth. Perform daily hygiene and oral assessment.
• Assist the patient in performing coughing and deep-breathing exercises to prevent pulmonary stasis. Removal of secretions helps prevent respiratory tract infections.
• Make sure visitors and staff members with upper respiratory tract infections wear masks when with the patient to protect him from pathogens.
• Teach the patient measures to minimize the risk of infection. Participating in his care encourages his compliance with therapy and lifestyle modifications.

Ineffective coping

Related to perceived or impending personal loss, *Ineffective coping* may be associated with life-threatening immunodeficiency disorders.

Expected outcomes

• Patient identifies mechanisms for coping effectively.
• Patient demonstrates an active role in self-care activities.
• Patient identifies appropriate resources to maximize his status.

Nursing interventions and rationales

• Encourage the patient and his family to discuss past coping mechanisms and their effectiveness. Doing this reinforces successful coping behaviors and fosters a sense of control.
• Urge the patient and his family to participate in care and ongoing decision making, to increase their sense of self-worth and mastery over the current situation and allow the patient to progress at his own pace.
• Refer the patient and his family to appropriate community resources as needed for continued support to restore and maintain psychological equilibrium and prevent future crisis.

Common immunologic disorders

Immunologic disorders range from mild ailments (such as hypersensitivity vasculitis) to life-threatening ones (such as anaphylaxis). Some are congenital, whereas others are acquired.

Immunologic disorders may result from:
- hyperreactivity, as in allergic rhinitis
- autoimmunity, as in SLE
- immunodeficiency, as in AIDS.

Acquired immunodeficiency syndrome

Marked by progressive weakening of cell-mediated immunity, AIDS increases susceptibility to opportunistic infections and unusual cancers. (See *Opportunistic infections in AIDS*, page 764.)

Diagnosis comes from careful correlation of the patient's history and clinical features with counts of certain types of T cells.

Time and mortality

The time between probable exposure to the human immunodeficiency virus (HIV, the agent that causes AIDS) and diagnosis averages 1 to 3 years. Children seem to have a shorter incubation time, with a mean of 8 months.

More than 75% of AIDS patients die within 2 years of diagnosis. Patients may be HIV-positive and asymptomatic for varying periods.

What causes it

AIDS is caused by infection with HIV, a retrovirus present in body fluids, such as blood and semen. Modes of HIV transmission include:
- sexual contact, especially associated with trauma to the rectal or vaginal mucosa
- transfusion of contaminated blood or blood products
- use of contaminated needles
- placental transmission from an infected mother to a fetus through cervical or blood contact at delivery
- breast milk from an infected woman.

Compromising circumstances

Risk factors for AIDS include:
- multiple sexual contacts with homosexual or bisexual men
- heterosexual contact with someone who has AIDS or is at risk for it

Opportunistic infections in AIDS

This chart shows the complicating infections that may occur in patients with acquired immunode-ficiency syndrome (AIDS). Other opportunistic conditions seen in AIDS patients include Kaposi's sarcoma, wasting disease, and AIDS dementia complex.

Microbiological agent	Organism	Condition
Protozoa	*Pneumocystis carinii* *Cryptosporidium* *Toxoplasma gondii* *Histoplasma*	*Pneumocystis carinii* pneumonia Cryptosporidiosis Toxoplasmosis Histoplasmosis
Fungi	*Candida albicans* *Cryptococcus neoformans*	Candidiasis Cryptococcosis
Viruses	Herpes Cytomegalovirus	Herpes simplex 1 and 2 Cytomegalovirus retinitis
Bacteria	*Mycobacterium tuberculosis* *M. avium-intracellulare*	Tuberculosis Mycobacteriosis

- present or past abuse of I.V. drugs
- transfusion of blood or blood products.

Prenatal and perinatal exposure to AIDS increases the risk of AIDS in infants, as does breast-feeding if the mother has AIDS or is at risk for it.

Pathophysiology

HIV attaches to helper T-cells having an antigen called *CD4+* on their surface. CD4+ serves as a receptor for the virus, allowing it to enter the cell. After invading the cell, HIV replicates, leading to cell death; or the virus becomes latent.

By hook or by crook

HIV infection results in profound pathology — either directly or indirectly. Direct pathologic effects come about through destruction of CD4+ cells, other immune cells, and neuroglial cells. Indirect pathologic consequences occur through the secondary effects of CD4+ T-cell dysfunction and the resulting immunosuppression.

A patient with a history of injectable drug use is at risk for AIDS, which can be transmitted through contaminated needles.

What to look for

After initial exposure, an infected person may have no signs or symptoms—or may have a flulike illness (seroconversion illness) and then remain asymptomatic for years.

Cunning contagion

However, as the syndrome progresses, he may have neurologic symptoms caused by HIV encephalopathy or symptoms of an opportunistic infection or disease, such as *Pneumocystis carinii* pneumonia, cytomegalovirus, or cancer. Eventually, repeated opportunistic infections overwhelm his weakened immune defenses, invading every body system.

What tests tell you

The Centers for Disease Control and Prevention defines AIDS as a CD4+ cell count below 200 cells/µl or when a patient has an opportunistic infection in the setting of HIV infection.

Enzyme-linked immunosorbent assay and a confirmatory Western blot assay detect HIV antibodies to diagnose HIV infection. Levels of circulating HIV ("viral load") are measured regularly to assess the risk of disease progression and the patient's response to therapy.

CD4+ cells like me must be monitored closely. If our count falls below 200/µl, the patient officially has AIDS.

How it's treated

Although no cure exists for AIDS, signs and symptoms can be managed with treatment. Primary therapy for HIV infection includes three different types of antiretroviral drugs:
• protease inhibitors, such as ritonavir, indinavir, nelfinavir, and saquinavir
• nucleoside reverse transcriptase inhibitors, such as zidovudine (AZT), didanosine, zalcitabine, lamivudine, and stavudine
• nonnucleoside reverse transcriptase inhibitors, such as nevirapine and delaviridine.

Used in various combinations, these drugs are designed to inhibit HIV viral replication.

Ambivalence over AZT

Treatment with AZT effectively slows the progression of HIV infection, decreasing the number of opportunistic infections, prolonging survival, and slowing the progress of associated dementia. However, the drug can cause severe adverse and toxic reactions.

Tweaking the immune system

Other drug therapies used in AIDS include immunomodulatory drugs, designed to boost the weakened immune system, and anti-infective and antineoplastic agents, used to combat opportunistic infections and associated cancers.

What to do

- Monitor the patient for fever, noting its pattern.
- Assess for tender, swollen lymph nodes, and check laboratory values regularly.
- Watch for signs and symptoms of infection, such as skin breakdown, cough, sore throat, and diarrhea.
- Encourage daily oral rinsing with normal saline or bicarbonate solution.
- Follow standard precautions as directed by your facility, depending on the patient's disease stage and condition.
- Offer support in coping with the social impact and discouraging prognosis of AIDS
- Evaluate the patient. After counseling and treatment, he should be able to state the early signs and symptoms of infection, explain how HIV is transmitted, and describe the limitations AIDS may impose on his lifestyle. He also should be able to maintain an optimal nutritional status. (See *AIDS teaching tips*.)

Anaphylaxis

Anaphylaxis is an exaggerated hypersensitivity reaction to a previously encountered antigen. A severe anaphylactic reaction may induce vascular collapse leading to systemic shock and, in some cases, death.

What causes it

An anaphylactic reaction results from systemic exposure to a sensitizing drug or other antigen, such as:
- penicillin (the most common cause) or other antibiotics
- serums
- vaccines
- allergen extracts
- enzymes
- hormones
- sulfonamides
- local anesthetics
- salicylates
- polysaccharides.

Education edge

AIDS teaching tips

- Explain how acquired immunodeficiency syndrome (AIDS) affects the immune response and makes him susceptible to opportunistic infection. Discuss ways to prevent infection.
- Discuss measures to prevent the spread of AIDS, such as wearing a condom during vaginal or anal intercourse; not sharing needles or syringes; and not donating blood, body organs or tissue, or sperm.
- Discuss contraceptive measures with a female patient. Explain that a mother can transmit AIDS to her fetus during pregnancy and to an infant through her breast milk.
- Teach the patient about your facility's infection-control policies and how they're implemented.

Sulfites, cysts, and venom

Anaphylaxis may also result from diagnostic chemicals (including radiographic contrast media containing iodine), foods, sulfites, insect venom (such as from a bee sting) and, rarely, a ruptured hydatid cyst (a liver cyst containing tapeworm larvae).

Pathophysiology

Here's how an anaphylactic reaction occurs:
• On initial exposure to an antigen, the immune system responds by producing IgE antibodies in the lymph nodes. Helper T cells enhance this process.
• Antibodies bind to membrane receptors located on mast cells in connective tissues and on basophils.
• The next time the person encounters this antigen, the IgE antibodies, or cross-linked IgE receptors, recognize it as foreign and activate the release of powerful chemical mediators.

As an antibody, it's my job to fight antigens. The Vegas bookies have even money on this match.

What to look for

An anaphylactic reaction usually produces sudden distress within seconds or minutes after exposure to an allergen. (A delayed or persistent reaction may occur up to 24 hours later.) Symptom severity depends on the original sensitizing dose of antigen, amount and distribution of antibodies, and the antigen's entry route and dose.

Right out of the gate...

Initial signs and symptoms of anaphylaxis include:
• a feeling of impending doom or fright
• weakness
• sweating
• sneezing
• pruritus (itching)
• urticaria (an itchy skin eruption causing wheals) and angioedema (acute swelling of the face, neck, lips, larynx, hands, feet, genitalia, or internal organs)
• cardiovascular changes, such as hypotension, shock, and arrhythmias
• respiratory signs and symptoms, including swelling of the nasal mucosa, profuse runny nose, nasal congestion, sudden sneezing attacks, and hoarseness, stridor, and dyspnea (early signs of acute respiratory failure)

• GI and genitourinary signs and symptoms (severe stomach cramps, nausea, diarrhea, and urinary urgency and incontinence).

How it's treated

Anaphylaxis is always an emergency. It requires an immediate injection of epinephrine 1:1,000 aqueous solution, repeated every 5 to 20 minutes, as necessary.

Epi to the rescue

In the early stages of anaphylaxis, when the patient still has normal blood pressure and is conscious, give epinephrine I.M. or subcutaneously (S.C.) Massage the injection site to help the drug move into circulation faster.

With severe reactions, when the patient has lost consciousness and is hypotensive, give epinephrine I.V.

What to do

• Maintain a patent airway. Observe the patient for early signs of laryngeal edema (stridor, hoarseness, and dyspnea), which typically necessitate endotracheal intubation or a tracheotomy and oxygen therapy. If he's in cardiac arrest, begin cardiopulmonary resuscitation (CPR) at once.
• Watch for hypotension and shock, and maintain circulatory volume with volume expanders (plasma, saline solution, and albumin), as needed and ordered.
• After the initial emergency, give other medications as ordered: epinephrine solution or suspension S.C., corticosteroids and diphenhydramine I.V. for long-term management, and aminophylline I.V. over 10 to 20 minutes for bronchospasm. Keep in mind that rapid aminophylline infusion may cause or aggravate severe hypotension.
• If a patient must receive a drug to which he's allergic, help prevent a severe reaction by making sure he's carefully desensitized beforehand with gradually increasing doses of the antigen or advance steroid administration.
• Evaluate the patient. On recovery, his blood pressure should be within normal limits and his respirations should be regular and unlabored. (See *Anaphylaxis teaching tips.*)

Education edge

Anaphylaxis teaching tips

• To prevent anaphylaxis, teach the patient to avoid exposure to known allergens. If he has a food or drug allergy, tell him to avoid the offending food or drug in all its forms. If he's allergic to insect bites or stings, tell him to avoid open fields and wooded areas during the insect season and to carry an anaphylaxis kit (containing epinephrine, antihistamine, tourniquet) when outdoors.
• Advise the patient to wear medical identification jewelry identifying his allergy or allergies.

If your anaphylactic patient goes into cardiac arrest, start CPR immediately.

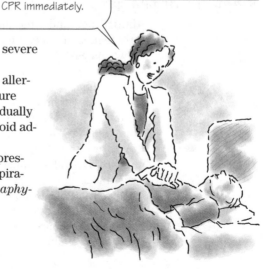

Asthma

A chronic reactive airway disorder, asthma causes episodic, reversible airway obstruction with bronchospasm, increased mucus secretion, and mucosal edema. Although this common condition can strike at any age, children under age 10 account for 50% of the cases.

From within or without

Asthma can be intrinsic or extrinsic. Intrinsic asthma results from sensitivity to specific external allergens. In intrinsic asthma, the allergen isn't obvious.

All in the family?

About one-third of all asthmatics share the condition with at least one member of their immediate family, and roughly three-fourths of children with two asthmatic parents also have asthma.

What causes it

• Extrinsic asthma follows exposure to pollen, animal dander, house dust or mold, pillows containing feathers or a silky material called kapok, food additives containing sulfites, or other sensitizing substances.
• Intrinsic asthma may result from irritants, emotional stress, fatigue, endocrine changes, temperature and humidity changes, or exposure to noxious fumes.

Aspirin and asthma

Other causes of asthma include aspirin, various nonsteroidal anti-inflammatory drugs (NSAIDs, such as indomethacin and mefenamic acid), tartrazine (a yellow food dye), exercise, and occupational exposure to an allergenic factor (such as platinum).

Pathophysiology

In asthma, tracheal and bronchial linings overreact to various stimuli, causing episodic smooth-muscle spasms that severely narrow the airways. Mucosal edema and thickened secretions further block the airways.

Collapse and resistance

During an asthma attack, expiratory airflow decreases, trapping gas in the airways and causing alveoli to hyperinflate. Atelectasis (lung tissue collapse) may occur in some lung regions. Increased airway resistance leads to labored breathing.

Noxious fumes, emotional stress, temperature changes, and certain other conditions may trigger intrinsic asthma.

What to look for

Usually, extrinsic asthma is accompanied by signs and symptoms of atopy (IgE–mediated allergy), such as eczema and allergic rhinitis. It commonly follows a severe respiratory tract infection, especially in adults.

Drama and distress

An acute asthma attack may begin dramatically, with simultaneous onset of severe multiple symptoms. Sometimes, however, onset is slow, with gradually increasing respiratory distress. Asthma that causes cyanosis, confusion, and lethargy indicates the onset of life-threatening status asthmaticus and respiratory failure.

Signs and symptoms of asthma include:
• sudden dyspnea, wheezing, and tightness in the chest
• coughing that produces thick, clear, or yellow sputum
• tachypnea and use of accessory respiratory muscles.

Other findings may include a rapid pulse, profuse perspiration, hyperresonant lung fields, and diminished breath sounds.

What tests tell you

• Pulmonary function studies reveal signs of obstructive airway disease (decreased flow rates and forced expiratory volume in 1 second), low-normal or diminished vital capacity, and increased total lung and residual capacity.
• Arterial blood gas analysis reveals reduced partial pressure of oxygen and partial pressure of arterial carbon dioxide ($Paco_2$). With severe asthma, $Paco_2$ may be normal or elevated, indicating severe bronchial obstruction.
• Chest X-ray may show lung hyperinflation, with areas of local atelectasis.
• Skin testing for specific allergens may be necessary if the patient lacks a history of allergy.
• Inhalation bronchial challenge testing evaluates the significance of allergens identified by skin testing.

If your patient has asthma, a chest X-ray may show hyperinflated lungs with areas of atelectasis.

How it's treated

Treatment usually is tailored to each patient and focuses on identifying and avoiding precipitating factors, such as allergens or irritants. Usually, such stimuli can't be removed entirely. Although desensitization to specific antigens may be helpful, it's rarely totally effective or persistent.

Drug therapy usually includes a bronchodilator and proves more effective when begun soon after symptom onset. Other drugs used to treat asthma may include:

- rapid-acting epinephrine
- epinephrine in oil (not recommended for infants)
- terbutaline
- aminophylline
- theophylline and oral preparations containing theophylline
- oral sympathomimetics
- corticosteroids
- aerosolized sympathomimetics, such as isoproterenol and albuterol
- cromolyn and nedocromil to help prevent release of the chemical mediators (histamine and leukotrienes) that cause bronchoconstriction.

What to do

- During an acute asthma attack, take appropriate measures to maintain respiratory function and relieve bronchoconstriction, while allowing mucus plug expulsion.
- If the attack was caused by exertion, have the patient sit down, rest, and sip warm water.
- Severe breathing difficulty is terrifying. Reassure the patient that you'll help him. Place him in semi-Fowler's position, encourage diaphragmatic breathing, and urge him to relax as much as possible.
- Know that status asthmaticus unrelieved by epinephrine is a medical emergency. Give humidified oxygen by nasal cannula at 2 L/minute, as ordered, to ease breathing difficulty and increase arterial oxygen saturation.
- Administer drugs and I.V. fluids as ordered.
- Evaluate the patient. With successful treatment, his respirations should be regular and unlabored; he should exhibit signs of adequate gas exchange, such as absence of cyanosis and confusion. Also, the patient and his family should be able to identify predisposing factors and state measures to eliminate them. (See *Asthma teaching tips*.)

Systemic lupus erythematosus

A chronic inflammatory disorder of the connective tissue, SLE affects multiple organ systems (as well as the skin) and can be fatal. It's marked by recurring remissions and exacerbations, which are especially common during the spring and summer.

SLE strikes eight times as many women as men, increasing to 15 times as many during childbearing years. SLE occurs worldwide, and is most prevalent among Asians and blacks.

Education edge

Asthma teaching tips

- Help the patient identify asthma triggers. Explain how these triggers cause bronchospasm, airway edema, and mucus production.
- Explain how to recognize and prevent respiratory tract infection.
- Teach him how to control an asthma attack.
- Discuss prescribed drugs and how to use them. Teach the patient how to use an oral inhaler. Explain that he should keep his nebulizer handy at all times. Caution him to take no more than two or three inhalations every 4 hours. If he needs the nebulizer more frequently, advise him to call the doctor. Explain that nebulizer overuse can weaken his response and diminish the drug's therapeutic effect. Warn him that extended overuse can lead to cardiac arrest and death.
- Tell the patient about asthma support groups such as the American Lung Association.

Mixed prognosis

The prognosis improves with early detection and treatment, but is poor for patients who develop cardiovascular, renal, or neurologic complications or severe bacterial infections.

About 1 out of 20 patients with discoid lupus erythematosus, another form of lupus erythematosus, later develops SLE.

During the childbearing years, SLE strikes 15 times more women than men.

What causes it

The cause of SLE remains a mystery, but evidence points to interrelated immunologic, environmental, hormonal, and genetic factors as possible causes.

Grab bag of causes

Factors that may increase the risk of SLE include:
• genetic predisposition
• stress
• streptococcal or viral infections
• exposure to sunlight or ultraviolet light
• immunization
• pregnancy
• abnormal estrogen metabolism.

Medications that increase the risk of SLE include procainamide, hydralazine, anticonvulsants and, less commonly, penicillins, sulfa drugs, and hormonal contraceptives.

Pathophysiology

Autoimmunity is thought to be the prime mechanism associated with SLE. The body produces antibodies against components of its own cells, resulting in immune complex disease. Patients with SLE may produce antibodies against various tissue components (such as RBCs, neutrophils, platelets, lymphocytes) or virtually any organ or tissue in the body.

What to look for

Characteristic findings in SLE include facial erythema (butterfly rash), nonerosive arthritis, and photosensitivity. (See *Recognizing butterfly rash.*)

Sun-induced rash

The patient may also experience discoid rash (an itchy, scaly, or flaky round or oval rash most common on the face, scalp, neck and chest after sun exposure), oral or nasopharyngeal ulcers, pleuritis, pericarditis, seizures, patchy alopecia, and even psychoses.

Recognizing butterfly rash

In the classic butterfly rash of systemic lupus erythematosus, lesions appear on the cheeks and the bridge of the nose, creating a characteristic butterfly pattern. The rash may vary in severity from malar erythema (redness of the cheeks) to discoid lesions (plaques).

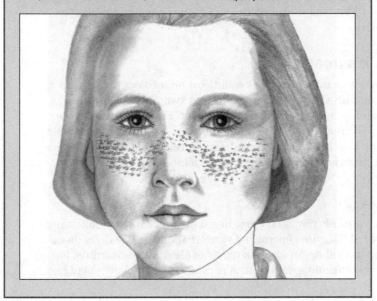

Systemic tip-offs

Also, she may have some combination of these systemic signs and symptoms: aching, malaise, fatigue, low-grade or spiking fever, chills, anorexia, weight loss, lymph node enlargement, abdominal pain, nausea and vomiting, diarrhea or constipation, and irregular menses or amenorrhea.

What tests tell you

- For most patients with active disease, antinuclear antibody, anti–deoxyribonucleic acid, and lupus erythematosus cell tests are the most specific SLE tests.
- Complete blood count with differential may show anemia and decreased WBC counts. Platelet count also may be decreased.
- Erythrocyte sedimentation rate may be elevated.

Sun exposure may trigger an itchy discoid rash on the face of a patient with SLE.

• Serum electrophoresis may show hypergammaglobulinemia (an excess of gamma globulins in the blood).
• Urine studies may show urinary RBCs and WBCs, urine casts and sediment, and significant urine protein loss (more than 3.5 g/24 hours).
• Blood studies showing decreased serum complement (C3 and C4) levels indicate active disease.
• Chest X-ray may show pleurisy or lupus pneumonitis (lung inflammation).

How it's treated

Patients with mild disease need little or no medication. Aspirin and other NSAIDs may control arthritis symptoms.

Skin lesions require topical treatment. For acute lesions, corticosteroid creams, such as flurandrenolide, are recommended. Refractory skin lesions are treated with intralesional corticosteroids or antimalarial drugs, such as hydroxychloroquine and chloroquine.

Singling out steroids

Corticosteroids remain the treatment of choice for systemic symptoms of SLE, acute generalized exacerbations, and serious disease related to vital organ systems (such as pleuritis, pericarditis, lupus nephritis, vasculitis, and central nervous system involvement).

What to do

• Watch for signs and symptoms, such as joint pain or stiffness, weakness, fever, fatigue, and chills.
• Observe the patient for dyspnea, chest pain, and edema of the arms and legs.
• Note the size, type, and location of skin lesions.
• Check the urine for blood.
• Inspect the scalp for hair loss, and check skin and mucous membranes for petechiae (tiny purplish spots indicating minute hemorrhages), bleeding, ulcers, pallor, and bruising.
• Provide a balanced diet. A patient with renal involvement may require a low-sodium, low-protein diet.
• Apply heat packs to relieve joint pain and stiffness. Encourage regular exercise to maintain full range of motion and prevent contractures.
• Monitor vital signs, fluid intake and output, weight, and laboratory findings.

A patient with SLE should eat a balanced diet. If she has renal involvement, instruct her to limit sodium and protein intake.

• Evaluate the patient. With successful therapy, she should be free from pain and stiffness and her vital signs should be within normal limits.

Quick quiz

1. If a patient who's allergic to peanut butter eats five peanut butter cookies, which antigen-specific immunoglobulin will his body produce?

    A.   IgA
    B.   IgD
    C.   IgE
    D.   IgG

Answer: C. IgE is responsible for allergic reactions.

2. The most common anaphylaxis-causing agent is:

    A.   shellfish.
    B.   contrast dye.
    C.   bee venom.
    D.   penicillin.

Answer: D. Penicillin is the most common anaphylaxis-causing antigen because of its systemic effects on the body.

3. Asthma is most strongly associated with:

    A.   a family history of asthma.
    B.   a history of anaphylactic reactions.
    C.   high blood pressure.
    D.   a history of frequent upper respiratory infections.

Answer: A. About one-third of asthmatics share the condition with at least one member of their immediate family, and three-fourths of children with two asthmatic parents also have asthma.

4. In most cases, the treatment of choice for SLE is:

    A.   antibiotics.
    B.   antifungals.
    C.   corticosteroids.
    D.   cyclosporine.

Answer: C. Corticosteroids are the treatment of choice for systemic symptoms of SLE.

Scoring

☆☆☆ If you answered all four items correctly, we're impressed! Your top score has earned you immunity from having to reread this chapter!

☆☆ If you answered three items correctly, well done! Your knowledge of the immune system is a far cry from deficient!

☆ If you answered fewer than three items correctly, don't break out in hives! Just read this chapter again to improve your anergic performance!

Skin disorders

Just the facts

In this chapter, you'll learn:

♦ about the anatomy and physiology of the skin and its appendages

♦ how to assess the skin and its appendages

♦ causes, pathophysiology, and diagnostic tests for common skin disorders

♦ treatments and nursing interventions for patients with these disorders.

Anatomy and physiology

The skin (integument) covers the body's internal structures and protects them from the external world. The skin has two distinct layers.
• The *epidermis*, or outer layer, is made up of squamous epithelial tissue, which itself contains several layers—the stratum corneum, stratum lucidum, stratum spinosum, and stratum basale.
• The *dermis*, the deeper second layer, consists of connective tissue and an extracellular material called *matrix*, which contributes to the skin's strength and pliability. The dermis contains and supports the blood vessels, lymphatic vessels, nerves, and sweat and sebaceous glands and serves as the site of wound healing and infection control. Beneath the dermis lies the subcutaneous tissue. (See *Skin: The inside story*, page 778.)

Value-added appendages

Numerous epidermal appendages occur throughout the skin. They include the hair, nails, sebaceous glands, and sweat glands. The two types of sweat glands are the *apocrine* glands (found in the axillae and groin near hair follicles) and the *eccrine* glands (located over most of the body except the lips).

Skin: The inside story

This cross section of the skin illustrates major skin structures.

Back off, bacteria! The skin serves as armor against injury and invasion by harmful microorganisms.

Skin functions

The skin performs many functions. It:
- protects the tissues from trauma and bacteria
- prevents loss of water and electrolytes from the body
- allows temperature, pain, touch, and pressure sensation
- regulates body temperature through sweat production and evaporation
- synthesizes vitamin D
- promotes wound repair by intensifying normal cell replacement mechanisms.

Assessment

Skin disorders may involve or stem from disorders that originate in other body systems. During your assessment, be sure to investigate even minor symptoms and systemic complaints.

History

Begin the assessment by taking a thorough history. With a skin disorder, expect the patient to complain of such problems as changes in the skin's appearance, pruritus (itching), pain, or drainage from lesions.

Current health status

Ask these questions to elicit information about the patient's chief complaint:
• How long have you had this problem? When did it begin? Have you had it before?
• What does the problem area look like, including its shape, size, color, location, character, and distribution?
• Is the area painful? Tender? Numb? Warm?
• Does anything seem to trigger the problem (such as stress, menstruation, or sunlight exposure)? Does anything make it worse? Does anything relieve it?
• Have you had recent contact with detergents, chemicals, or plants?
• Did you recently change soaps?
• Have you tried using anything to make the condition feel better, such as compresses, lotions, or over-the-counter preparations?

Previous health status

Ask whether the patient has ever had a similar skin condition. (Some skin disorders, such as psoriasis, can recur.) Find out if he has ever had an allergic reaction to medication, food, or other substances (such as cosmetics). Past and present allergies — including those caused by cutaneous, ingested, or inhaled allergens — may predispose a patient to other skin disorders.

Also find out if the patient has a history of diabetes mellitus, venous insufficiency, or immunodeficiency.

I think of myself as a good guy. But in some people, foods can trigger allergic skin conditions.

Family history

Some skin disorders, such as atopic dermatitis, acne, and psoriasis, tend to run in families. Contagious skin problems, such as scabies, may be transmitted by family members. Ask the patient if anyone in his family has had a skin problem. If so, what was it and when did it occur?

Allergies also may run in families. Find out if any family members have allergies. If so, what are they and how have they been treated?

Social history

Obtain relevant information about the patient's lifestyle, including occupation, travel, diet, smoking, alcohol and drug use, sun exposure, stress, casual social contact, and sexual contact.

Physical examination

Start by observing the overall appearance of the patient's skin to identify areas that need further assessment. Then inspect and palpate the skin one area at a time, focusing on color, texture, turgor, moisture, and temperature. Be sure to check for and note skin lesions.

Color

Look for localized areas of ecchymosis (bruising), cyanosis, pallor, and erythema (redness). Check for color uniformity and for areas with darker or lighter pigmentation than the rest of the patient's body. Remember that color changes may vary depending on skin pigmentation.

Texture and turgor

Inspect and palpate the skin's texture, noting its thickness and mobility. It should look smooth and be intact.

Turgor on trial

Assess turgor by gently grasping and pulling up a fold of skin, releasing it, and observing how quickly it returns to normal shape. Skin usually resumes its flat shape immediately.

Moisture

Observe the skin's moisture content. The skin should be relatively dry, with a minimal amount of perspiration. Skin-fold areas also should be fairly dry.

Temperature

Palpate for skin temperature by using the back (dorsal surface) of your fingers or hands, which are most sensitive to temperature perception. The skin should feel warm to cool, and areas should feel the same bilaterally.

Lesions

Whenever you see a skin lesion, evaluate it to determine its origin. Start by classifying it as primary or secondary. A *primary* lesion is new. (See *Identifying primary skin lesions*.)

Collateral damage

Changes in a primary lesion constitute a *secondary* lesion. Examples of secondary lesions include fissures, scales, crusts, scars, and excoriations.

- Measure and record the lesion's size, shape or configuration, color, degree of elevation or depression, pedunculation (connection to the skin by a stem or stalk), and texture.
- Evaluate the lesion's odor, color, consistency, and amount of exudate.
- Assess the lesion's distribution pattern, including the extent and pattern of involvement. Note the location of the lesion or lesions, such as on a specific dermatome (cutaneous

Use the backs of your fingers or hands when palpating skin temperature. They're more sensitive to temperature perception.

Identifying primary skin lesions

Are you having trouble identifying your patient's skin lesion? Here's a quick look at three common lesions. Remember to keep a centimeter ruler handy so you can measure lesion size accurately.

Macule
Flat circumscribed area of altered skin color, generally less than 1 cm. Examples: freckle, flat nevus

Papule
Raised, circumscribed, solid area; generally less than 1 cm. Examples: elevated nevus, wart

Vesicle
Circumscribed, elevated lesion; contains serous fluid; less than 1 cm. Example: early chickenpox

nerve ending), on flexor or extensor surfaces, in skin folds, on clothing or jewelry lines, or on palms or soles — or whether lesions appear randomly.

• Accurately describe the arrangement of lesions to help determine their cause. Is each lesion discrete? Are the lesions grouped? Do they merge together? Are they diffuse? Linear? Annular (ring shaped)? Arciform (curved or arced)? Do the lesions revolve around a fixed point (gyrate)?

Diagnostic tests

Several studies can help differentiate among integumentary disorders. They include the patch test, potassium hydroxide (KOH) preparation, skin biopsy, and Tzanck test.

Patch test

The patch test identifies the cause of allergic contact sensitization. Indicated in patients with suspected allergies or allergies from an unknown cause, this test uses a sample of common allergens, or antigens, to determine if one or more will produce a positive reaction. If the doctor suspects a particular causative agent, he may test it for a positive reaction.

Nursing considerations
• If the patient has an acute inflammation, postpone the patch test until the inflammation subsides, because a patch test may worsen it.
• Apply the patch to normal, hairless skin on the back or on the inner surface of the forearm.
• Instruct the patient to leave the patch in place for 48 hours — but to remove it immediately if pain, itching, or irritation develops.
• Check findings after removing the patch, and then recheck 48 hours later for a delayed reaction.

Set the alarm for 48 hours. That's when your patient's patch test results should be read.

Potassium hydroxide preparation

KOH preparation helps identify fungal skin infections. It involves scraping scales from the skin, mixing them with a few drops of 10% to 25% KOH on a glass slide, and then lightly heating the slide. Skin cells dissolve, leaving fungal elements (hyphae and spores) visible on microscopic examination.

Nursing considerations

• Gently scrape the border of a rash or skin lesion with a sterile scalpel blade to obtain a specimen. After scraping, inspect the area for bleeding and apply light pressure, if necessary.
• Tell the patient that the KOH preparation may identify a fungal infection—but because the test may be inconclusive, he should comply with treatment until fungal culture results are known.

Skin biopsy

During a skin biopsy, a small piece of tissue from a suspected malignancy or other skin lesion is excised. One of three techniques—excision, shave, or punch—may be used to secure the specimen.
• An *excision* biopsy removes a small lesion in its entirety. This technique is indicated for rapidly expanding lesions; sclerotic, bullous, or atrophic lesions; and examination of the border of a lesion and surrounding normal skin.
• A *shave* biopsy cuts the lesion above the skin line, leaving the lower dermal layers intact.
• A *punch* biopsy removes an oval core from the center of a lesion.

Nursing considerations

• Explain to the patient that he'll first receive a local anesthetic.
• After the procedure, apply pressure to the biopsy site to stop bleeding, if necessary, and apply a dressing.
• After the biopsy specimen is obtained, place it in a container with 10% formaldehyde solution.
• If the patient has sutures, instruct him to keep the area clean and as dry as possible. Tell him when the sutures will be removed.
• If the patient has adhesive strips, instruct him to leave them in place for 14 to 21 days.

Tzanck test

In the Tzanck test, vesicular fluid or exudate from an ulcer is smeared on a glass slide and stained with Papanicolaou's, Wright's, Giemsa, or methylene blue stain. Herpesvirus is confirmed if microscopic examination of the slide reveals multinucleated giant cells, intranuclear inclusions, and ballooning degeneration.

Nursing considerations

• To obtain a specimen for staining, unroof an intact vesicle and, using a sterile scalpel blade, scrape the base of the lesion to ob-

> **Memory jogger**
> Did you know that the doctor uses ESP to perform a skin biopsy? No, that doesn't mean he uses extrasensory perception. ESP simply refers to the three different techniques — Excision, Shave, or Punch — used to secure a skin biopsy specimen.

OK, so I'm exaggerating a little. But after a skin biopsy, you may need to apply a pressure dressing to the site.

tain fluid and skin cells. Apply the specimen to a glass slide and stain.

• Wear gloves while obtaining the specimen because herpesvirus is transmissible.

Treatments

Usually, treatment for skin disorders involves hands-on care. Most medications are applied topically. Surgery is usually performed with only a local anesthetic, and monitoring depends less on laboratory tests than on simple observation.

Drug therapy

Categories of drugs used to treat skin disorders include:
• anti-infectives, such as acyclovir, bacitracin, clotrimazole, lindane, and mupirocin
• astringents, such as aluminum acetate and aluminum acetate and calcium acetate
• corticosteroids (topical), such as hydrocortisone, hydrocortisone acetate, and triamcinolone
• demulcents, emollients, and protectants, such as calamine, oatmeal, and para-aminobenzoic acid
• keratolytics, such as podophyllum and salicylic acid
• miscellaneous agents, such as acitretin, anthralin, isotretinoin, minoxidil (topical), selenium sulfide, and tretinoin.

Surgery

Surgical techniques used to treat skin disorders include cryosurgery, laser surgery, Mohs' micrographic surgery, and skin grafting.

Cryosurgery

Cryosurgery is a common procedure in which extreme cold is applied to the skin to induce tissue destruction. Cryosurgery causes epidermal-dermal separation above the basement membranes, helping to prevent scarring after reepithelialization.

Simple or sophisticated

The procedure can be performed quite simply, using nothing more than a cotton-tipped applicator dipped in liquid nitrogen

Brrrr! With cryosurgery, extreme cold is applied to the skin to cause tissue destruction.

and applied to the skin, or it may involve a complex cryosurgical unit.

Patient preparation
• Ask the patient if he has any allergies or hypersensitivities, especially to iodine or cold.
• Tell him he'll initially feel cold, followed by a burning sensation, during the procedure.

Monitoring and aftercare
• After cryosurgery, clean the area gently with a cotton-tipped applicator soaked in hydrogen peroxide.
• If necessary, apply an ice bag to relieve swelling and give the patient an analgesic, as ordered, to relieve pain.

Home care instructions
• Tell the patient that he should expect pain, redness, and swelling, and that a blister will form within 24 hours of treatment. The blister may be large, and it may bleed. Usually, it flattens within a few days and sloughs off in 2 to 3 weeks. Serous exudation may follow during the first week, and a crust or a dry scab may develop.
• To promote healing and prevent infection, warn the patient not to touch the blister. Tell him that if the blister becomes uncomfortable or interferes with daily activities, he should call the doctor, who can decompress it with a sterile blade or pin.
• Tell the patient to clean the area gently with soap and water, alcohol, or a cotton-tipped applicator soaked in hydrogen peroxide, as ordered.
• To prevent hypopigmentation, instruct him to cover the wound with a loose dressing when he's outdoors. After the wound heals, he should apply a sunblock over the area.

Laser surgery

Laser surgery uses the intense, highly focused light of a laser beam to treat dermatologic lesions. Performed on an outpatient basis, laser surgery spares normal tissue, promotes faster healing, and helps prevent postsurgical infection.

Patient preparation
• If the surgical suite has windows, keep shades or blinds closed. Cover reflective surfaces and remove flammable materials.
• Make sure everyone in the room, including the patient, is wearing safety goggles, because reflection of the laser beam may damage the eyes.

During laser surgery, everyone in the room — patient included — must wear goggles to protect their eyes.

Monitoring and aftercare
• After the procedure, apply direct pressure over any bleeding wound for 20 minutes.
• Initial wound care varies with the procedure.

Home care instructions
• Tell the patient to dress the wound daily. Permit him to take showers but advise him not to immerse the wound site in water.
• If bleeding occurs, instruct the patient to apply direct pressure on the site with clean gauze or a washcloth for 20 minutes. If pressure doesn't control the bleeding, he should call the doctor immediately.
• To avoid pigmentation changes, caution the patient to protect the wound from sun exposure.

Mohs' micrographic surgery

Mohs' micrographic surgery involves serial excision and histologic analysis of cancerous or suspected cancerous tissues. By allowing step-by-step tumor excision, Mohs' surgery minimizes the size of the scar (important if the treatment is done on the face) and helps prevent recurrence by removing all malignant tissue. This surgery is especially effective in basal cell carcinomas.

With Mohs' surgery, excised tissue is examined after each stage of the procedure.

Scar sequelae

Mohs' surgery has two common complications: bleeding and facial scarring. Bleeding is easily controlled with direct pressure. The potentially devastating psychological effects of a large facial scar or defect are harder to treat and require considerable emotional support.

Patient preparation
• Make sure the patient understands that the procedure takes many hours, most of which will be spent waiting for histologic results. Reassure him that a long wait doesn't mean his cancer is grave.
• Explain that the doctor will use electrocauterization to control bleeding and that a grounding plate will be affixed to the patient's leg or arm to complete the circuit between the cautery pencil and generator. Warn him to expect a burning odor.

Monitoring and aftercare
• Assess the patient's level of pain, and provide an analgesic, as ordered.
• Periodically check for excessive bleeding. If it occurs, remove the dressing and apply pressure over the site for 20 minutes.

Memory jogger

The word MOHS can help you remember a chief benefit of Mohs' surgery:

M: Minimizing

O: Of

H: His (or Her)

S: Scar

Home care instructions

• Tell the patient to leave the dressing in place for 24 hours and to change the dressing daily afterward.
• If he experiences frank bleeding, advise him to reinforce the bandage and apply direct pressure to the wound for 20 minutes, using clean gauze or a clean washcloth. If this measure doesn't control bleeding, he should call the doctor.
• Instruct the patient to report signs or symptoms of infection.
• Advise him to refrain from alcohol, aspirin, and excessive exercise for 48 hours to prevent bleeding and promote healing.
• Recommend acetaminophen for discomfort.

Skin grafting

Skin grafting covers defects caused by burns, trauma, and surgery. This procedure is indicated when:
• primary closure isn't possible or cosmetically acceptable
• primary closure would interfere with functioning
• the defect is on a weight-bearing surface
• a skin tumor is excised and the site needs to be monitored for recurrence.

Grafting may be done using a general or local anesthetic. It can be performed on an outpatient basis for small facial or neck defects.

Getting graphic about grafts

Types of skin grafts include:
• split-thickness grafts, which consist of the epidermis and a small portion of dermis
• full-thickness grafts, which include all of the dermis as well as the epidermis
• composite grafts, which also include underlying tissues, such as muscle, cartilage, or bone.

Patient preparation

• Because successful skin grafting begins with a good graft, take steps to preserve potential donor sites by providing meticulous skin care.
• Assess the recipient site. The graft's survival depends on close contact with the underlying tissue. Ideally, the recipient site should consist of healthy granulation tissue free from eschar (a dry crust or thick scab appearing after a burn), debris, or the products of infection.

Be sure to provide meticulous skin care at potential donor graft sites.

Monitoring and aftercare

After the procedure, your primary role is to ensure graft survival.
• Position the patient so he isn't lying on the graft. If possible, keep the graft area elevated and immobilized.
• Modify your nursing care to protect the graft. For example, never use a blood pressure cuff over a graft site.
• Use sterile technique when changing the dressing, and work gently to avoid dislodging the graft.
• Provide care to the donor site.

Home care instructions

• Advise the patient not to disturb the dressings on the graft or donor sites for any reason. If they need to be changed, instruct him to call the doctor.
• If grafting was done as an outpatient procedure, stress that the graft site must be immobilized to promote proper healing.
• After the graft has healed, instruct the patient to apply cream to the site several times daily to keep the skin pliable and aid scar maturation.
• Because sun exposure can affect graft pigmentation, advise the patient to limit his time in the sun and to use a sunblock on all grafted areas.
• Explain that when scar maturation is complete, the doctor may use other plastic surgery techniques to improve graft appearance.

Debridement

Debridement may involve mechanical, chemical, or surgical techniques to remove necrotic tissue from a wound. Although debridement can be extremely painful, it's necessary to prevent infection and promote healing of burns and skin ulcers.

Mechanical debridement

Mechanical debridement consists of wet-to-dry dressings, irrigation, hydrotherapy, and bedside debridement.
• Wet-to-dry dressings are appropriate for partially healed wounds with only slight amounts of necrotic tissue and minimal drainage.
• Irrigation of a wound with an antiseptic solution cleans tissues and removes cell debris and excess drainage.
• Hydrotherapy (commonly called "tubbing" or "tanking") involves immersing the patient in a tank of warm water, which is agitated intermittently. Hydrotherapy is often performed on burn patients.

Irrigation provides mechanical debridement. The antiseptic solution cleans tissues and removes cell debris.

• Bedside debridement of a burn wound involves careful prying and cutting of loosened eschar with forceps and scissors to separate it from viable tissue beneath. One of the most painful types of debridement, it may be the only practical way to remove necrotic tissue from a severely burned patient.

Chemical debridement

In chemical debridement, topical debriders are used to absorb exudate and particulate debris. These agents also absorb bacteria, thus reducing the risk of infection.

Surgical debridement

Surgical debridement is done under general or regional anesthesia. It provides the fastest and most complete debridement, but it's usually reserved for burn patients or those with extremely deep or large ulcers. It's commonly performed with skin grafting.

Patient preparation
• Explain the type of debridement the patient will undergo. Reassure him that he'll receive an analgesic if needed.
• If ordered, give analgesics 20 minutes before the procedure.

Monitoring and aftercare
• Assess the patient's pain and provide analgesics, as ordered.
• During dressing changes, note the amount of granulation tissue, necrotic debris, and drainage. Watch for signs of wound infection.
• If the patient's arm or leg was debrided, keep it elevated to promote venous return — especially if the patient has a stasis ulcer.

Home care instructions
• Teach the patient how to perform dressing changes if appropriate.
• Instruct him to watch for and report signs or symptoms of infection or poor healing.

Nursing diagnoses

When caring for patients with skin disorders, you'll find that several nursing diagnoses are applicable to many situations. These nursing diagnoses appear here, along with appropriate nursing interventions and rationales.

Impaired skin integrity

Related to illness, *Impaired skin integrity* can be associated with bacterial and fungal infections, parasitic infestations, follicular and glandular disorders, inflammatory reactions, and other skin disorders.

Expected outcomes

• Patient verbalizes and demonstrates an understanding of all procedures and skin care regimens, to prevent further tissue breakdown.
• Patient verbalizes feelings about his skin condition.

Nursing interventions and rationales

• Inspect the patient's skin daily and document findings, particularly noting any change in status. Early detection prevents or minimizes skin breakdown.
• Perform the prescribed treatment regimen for the patient's skin condition; monitor progress. Report favorable and adverse responses to treatment so the current regimen can be maintained or modified as needed.
• Assist the patient with general hygiene and comfort measures as needed to promote comfort and a general sense of well-being.
• Apply a bed cradle to protect lesions from bed covers.
• Encourage the patient to express his feelings about his skin condition. This helps allay anxiety and aids him in developing coping skills.
• Discuss precipitating factors if known. If the patient has a skin allergy to food, explain dietary restrictions to help reduce the occurrence and severity of skin reactions.
• Teach the patient about his skin care regimen to ensure compliance.
• Refer the patient to a psychiatric liaison nurse, social service, or support group, as appropriate.

Risk for infection

Related to impaired skin integrity, *Risk for infection* may also apply to any condition that impairs the skin's ability to guard against invasion by microorganisms.

Expected outcomes

• Patient remains free from additional infections.

• Patient maintains normal temperature and laboratory values.

Nursing interventions and rationales

• Minimize the patient's risk of infection through proper hand washing and by using standard precautions when providing direct care.

• Take the patient's temperature at least every 4 hours. Report elevations immediately. Sustained postoperative fever may signal the onset of pulmonary complications, wound infection or dehiscence (premature splitting open of the wound layers), urinary tract infection, or thrombophlebitis.

• Monitor white blood cell (WBC) count as ordered. Report elevations or depressions. An elevated WBC count indicates infection.

• Inspect skin lesions for erythema, warmth, or purulent drainage to detect secondary infection.

• Culture urine, respiratory secretions, wound drainage, or blood according to facility policy and doctor's orders. This procedure identifies pathogens and guides antibiotic therapy.

• Instruct the patient to wash his hands before and after meals and after using the bathroom, bedpan, or urinal.

• Ensure adequate nutritional intake. Offer high-protein supplements, unless contraindicated, to aid healing, stabilize weight, and improve muscle tone and mass.

• Teach the patient about good hand-washing technique, factors that increase his infection risk, and signs and symptoms of infection. Doing this helps him participate in care and modify his lifestyle to maintain optimal health.

If your patient is at risk for infection, report an elevated or depressed WBC count to the doctor.

Common skin disorders

This section covers common skin disorders and includes information on their causes, assessment findings, diagnostic tests, treatment, nursing interventions, patient teaching, and evaluation criteria.

Cellulitis

A diffuse inflammation of the dermis and subcutaneous tissue, cellulitis commonly appears around a skin break—usually a fresh wound or small puncture site. With timely treatment, prognosis is usually good.

What causes it

Cellulitis usually results from infection by group A beta-hemolytic streptococci. It may also stem from infection by other streptococci, *Staphylococcus aureus*, *Haemophilus influenzae*, or various fungi.

Pathophysiology

A break in skin integrity almost always precedes infection. As the offending organism invades the compromised area, it overwhelms the defensive cells (such as neutrophils, eosinophils, basophils, and mast cells) that usually contain and localize the inflammation. As cellulitis progresses, the organism invades tissue around the initial wound site.

We're the A-team, short for group A beta-hemolytic streptococci. I don't mean to brag, but we're usually responsible for cellulitis.

What to look for

Signs and symptoms of cellulitis include:
- a tender, warm, erythematous, swollen area, which is usually well demarcated
- a warm, red, tender streak following the course of a lymphatic vessel
- fever or chills.

What tests tell you

Although diagnosis usually can be made from the clinical presentation, the doctor may order a Gram stain and culture of skin tissue. If the patient is acutely ill, blood cultures may be taken.

I just love a break in the skin! That's when I get to invade!

How it's treated

Preventing widespread skin destruction requires antibiotic therapy. The doctor may prescribe oral penicillin to treat small, localized areas of cellulitis on the legs or trunk.

Planning on penicillin

Cellulitis of the face or hands or with lymphatic involvement calls for parenteral penicillin or a penicillinase-resistant antibiotic.

If gangrene occurs, the patient must undergo surgical debridement and incision and drainage of surrounding tissue.

What to do

- Monitor the patient's vital signs (especially temperature) every 4 hours.
- Assess the patient every 4 hours for an increase in the size of the affected area or worsening of pain.
- Administer an antibiotic, an analgesic, and warm soaks, as ordered.
- Evaluate the patient. He should show signs of resolution of erythema, pain, and warmth and improved skin integrity. (See *Cellulitis teaching tips*.)

Education edge

Cellulitis teaching tips

- If your patient has cellulitis, emphasize the importance of complying with treatment to prevent relapse.
- Teach the patient how to apply compresses.
- Advise him to elevate the affected limb to reduce swelling.
- Tell him to limit activity until his condition improves.

Cutaneous ulcers

Cutaneous ulcers are localized areas of cellular necrosis, usually arising in areas of inadequate circulation. The ulcers may be superficial (caused by local skin irritation with subsequent surface maceration) or deep (originating in underlying tissue). Deep lesions typically go undetected until they penetrate the skin, but by then they've usually caused subcutaneous damage.

The two types of cutaneous ulcers are pressure ulcers (bedsores) and stasis ulcers.

What causes them

Cutaneous ulcers can result from pressure and chronic venous stasis.

Provocation for pressure ulcers

Conditions that increase the risk of developing pressure ulcers include:
- altered mobility
- inadequate nutrition (leading to weight loss with reduction of subcutaneous tissue and muscle bulk)
- breakdown in skin or subcutaneous tissue (from edema or incontinence).

Other predisposing factors for pressure ulcers are fever, pathologic conditions, and obesity.

Standing and stasis ulcers

Predisposing factors for stasis ulcers include obesity and prolonged standing in one position.

While I'm in traction, I'm at increased risk for developing pressure ulcers.

Pathophysiology

Pressure ulcers are caused by pressure that interrupts normal circulatory function. Intensity and duration of the pressure determine ulcer severity. Pressure exerted over an area for a moderate length of time (1 to 2 hours) produces tissue ischemia and increased capillary pressure, leading to edema and multiple small-vessel thromboses.

From inflamed to infected

An inflammatory reaction gives way to ulceration and necrosis of ischemic cells. In turn, necrotic tissue predisposes to bacterial invasion and subsequent infection.

Stasis ulcers result from chronic venous stasis caused by varicose veins or venous thrombosis.

What to look for

Pressure ulcers commonly develop over bony prominences. Early features of superficial lesions are:
• shiny, erythematous changes over the compressed area, caused by localized vasodilation when pressure is relieved
• superficial erythema progressing to small blisters or erosions and, ultimately, to necrosis and ulceration.

Other signs of pressure ulcers include:
• inflamed area on the skin surface
• foul-smelling, purulent discharge
• black eschar developing around and over the lesion.

Gauging the stage

Staging of pressure ulcers is recommended in the Clinical Practice Guidelines of the U.S. Department of Health and Human Services. Staging should be documented in the patient record on the first notice of redness and at least weekly thereafter. (See *Staging pressure ulcers.*)

Stasis ulcers sites

Stasis ulcers appear on the skin of the lower legs (usually over the medial malleolus). Before they develop, the skin may appear patchy brown from chronic venous stasis. It then becomes erythematous and pruritic.

What tests tell you

Wound culture and sensitivity testing of ulcer exudate identify infecting organisms and help determine whether an antibiotic is needed.

Memory jogger

RIDES is your clue to the key signs of pressure ulcers.

R: Red

I: Inflamed

D: Discharge

E: Eschar

S: Shiny

Experts recommend staging pressure ulcers at their onset and at least every week thereafter.

Staging pressure ulcers

To help your patient prevent pressure ulcer complications, learn to recognize the four stages of ulcer formation.

Stage I
The skin stays red for 5 minutes after removal of pressure and may develop an epidermal abrasion. (A black person's skin may look purple.) The skin feels warm and firm. Usually, the sore reverses after pressure is removed.

Stage II
Skin breaks appear and discoloration may occur. The sore penetrates to the subcutaneous fat layer; it's painful and visibly swollen. If pressure is removed, the sore may heal within 1 to 2 weeks.

Stage III
A hole develops, and oozes foul-smelling yellow or green fluid. The ulcer extends into the muscle and may develop eschar (a black leathery crust) at its edges and eventually at its center. The ulcer isn't painful, but healing may take months.

Stage IV
The ulcer destroys tissue from the skin to the bone and becomes necrotic. Findings include foul drainage and deep tunnels that extend from the ulcer. The ulcer may take months or even a year to heal.

How they're treated

Treatment is similar for both types of cutaneous ulcers. Open lesions are cleaned with normal saline solution. Dressings, if needed, should be porous and taped lightly to healthy skin. Composite dressings (such as Coverderm and Tegaderm) are appropriate for wounds with minimal to heavy drainage, necrotic tissue, or healthy granulation tissue.

Excise and debride

Debridement of necrotic tissue may be necessary to allow healing.

What to do

• Clean the skin with warm water and a mild cleaning agent; then apply moisturizer.
• Turn and reposition the patient every 1 to 2 hours, unless contraindicated. For patients who can't turn themselves or who are turned on a schedule, use a pressure-relieving mattress.
• Ensure adequate dietary intake of protein and calories.
• Use pressure reduction devices.

• Evaluate the patient: With successful treatment, the ulcer should reepithelialize. The patient and caregivers should take adequate measures to prevent recurrence of cutaneous ulcers. (See *Cutaneous ulcer teaching tips*.)

Herpes zoster

Also called *shingles*, herpes zoster is an acute unilateral and segmental inflammation of certain nerve roots. Usually appearing in adults over age 40, herpes zoster causes localized vesicular skin lesions confined to a dermatome (an area of the skin innervated by sensory fibers from a single spinal nerve).

No gain from this pain

Severe neuralgic pain occurs in peripheral areas fed by the nerves arising in the inflamed ganglia.

What causes it

Herpes zoster results from the varicella-zoster virus, a herpesvirus that also causes chickenpox. Roughly 20% of people who have had chickenpox eventually get herpes zoster.

It isn't known what causes the virus to reactivate in healthy people. Perhaps a temporary weakness in immunity, as from illness, trauma, or stress, allows it to multiply and travel along nerve fibers toward the skin.

Pathophysiology

Herpes zoster erupts when the varicella-zoster virus reactivates after dormancy in the cerebral ganglia (extramedullary ganglia of the cranial nerves) or the ganglia of posterior nerve roots. The virus may multiply as it reactivates, and antibodies remaining from the initial infection may neutralize it.

An attack of nerves

Without opposition from the effective antibodies, the virus continues to multiply in the ganglia, destroys neurons, and spreads down the sensory nerves to the skin.

What to look for

• Onset of herpes zoster is characterized by fever and malaise. Within 2 to 4 days, severe deep pain, pruritus, and paresthesia (burning, itching, prickling, or tingling sensations) or hyperesthesia (increased sensitivity to touch) develop — usually on the trunk

Education edge

Cutaneous ulcer teaching tips

• Advise the patient to eat a diet with adequate calories, protein, and vitamins.

• Teach a patient with venous stasis ulcers to avoid prolonged standing, to elevate the legs often to promote venous return, and to wear antiembolism stockings during the day.

• Emphasize the importance of changing positions regularly. Teach the patient and his family how to change the patient's position correctly.

• Tell the patient to avoid heat lamps and harsh soaps because they dry the skin. Advise him to treat dry skin with moisturizers after bathing.

• Caution the patient to avoid vigorous massage, which can damage capillaries.

• If he's confined to a chair or uses a wheelchair, advise him to shift his weight every 30 minutes to promote blood flow to compressed tissues.

and occasionally on the arms and legs. Pain may be continuous or intermittent.

• Small, red, nodular skin lesions then usually erupt over the painful areas and spread unilaterally around the thorax or vertically over the arms or legs. They quickly become vesicles, or blisters, filled with clear fluid or pus. About 10 days after they appear, the vesicles dry and form scabs. (See *Zooming in on herpes zoster.*)

What tests tell you

The dermatomic distribution of lesions is usually sufficient to confirm the diagnosis. A Tzanck test of vesicular fluid and infected tissue shows eosinophilic intranuclear inclusions and varicella virus. In unusual cases, confirmation may require a Tzanck smear, biopsy, and viral culture.

How it's treated

Relief of itching and neuralgic pain may require calamine lotion or another topical antipruritic, or aspirin (possibly with codeine or another analgesic). If bacteria have infected ruptured vesicles, treatment includes a systemic antibiotic.

Zooming in on herpes zoster

The classic vesicles of herpes zoster, shown here, have erupted along a peripheral nerve in the torso.

This illustration shows the lesions about 10 days later—that is, after they've begun to dry and form scabs.

Potent potions

Trigeminal zoster with corneal involvement calls for instillation of idoxuridine ointment or another antiviral agent. To help the patient cope with the intractable pain of postherpetic neuralgia, the doctor may order analgesics, a systemic corticosteroid to reduce inflammation, or a tranquilizer, sedative, or tricyclic antidepressant with a phenothiazine.

Acyclovir is used to stop progression of the skin rash and prevent visceral complications.

What to do

• Promote patient comfort.
• Administer medications as ordered.
• If lesions are severe and widespread, apply a wet dressing. If vesicles rupture, apply a cold compress as ordered.
• Watch an immunosuppressed patient closely for signs and symptoms of dissemination (such as generalized lesions) and central nervous system infection (such as headache, weakness, fever, and stiff neck).
• Evaluate the patient. With successful treatment, he should show resolution of all skin lesions. Determine whether he has postherpetic neuralgia. (See *Herpes zoster teaching tips.*)

Psoriasis

A chronic disorder, psoriasis is a noncontagious inflammatory skin disease marked by reddish papules (solid elevations) and plaques covered with silvery scales. The condition takes a recurrent course, with remissions and exacerbations. Psoriatic lesions vary widely in severity and distribution.

Psoriasis occurs in about 1% of the North American population, with usual onset between ages 25 and 30.

What causes it

The tendency to develop psoriasis is genetically determined. Researchers have found a significantly higher-than-normal incidence of human leukocyte antigen (HLA) in patients with psoriasis, suggesting a possible autoimmune deficiency.

Pathophysiology

Psoriatic skin cells have a shortened maturation time as they migrate from the basal membrane to the surface or stratum corneum.

Education edge

Herpes zoster teaching tips

• Focus on helping the patient with herpes zoster minimize pain and prevent infection spread.
• Instruct him to avoid scratching the lesions.
• To decrease the pain of oral lesions, advise him to use a soft toothbrush, eat a soft diet, and use saline solution mouthwash. Reassure him that herpetic pain will subside eventually.
• Provide diversionary activities to take his mind off the pain and pruritus.
• Caution the patient to avoid close contact with people who haven't had chickenpox until his eruption has resolved.

Plaque attack

As a result, the stratum corneum develops thick, scaly plaques (the chief sign of psoriasis).

Some people have a genetic predisposition for psoriasis. Interventions vary because no permanent cure exists.

What to look for

Small, erythematous papules usually are the initial sign of psoriasis. These lesions enlarge or merge to form red, elevated plaques with silver scales. Most commonly, they're seen on the scalp, face, chest, elbows, knees, back, buttocks, and genitalia.

Other features of psoriasis include pruritus, nail pitting, and joint stiffness.

What tests tell you

- Skin biopsy helps rule out other disorders.
- The serum uric acid level is usually elevated.
- In early-onset familial psoriasis, tests typically show presence of the known as Cw6, B13, and Bw57.

How it's treated

Interventions for psoriasis vary because no permanent cure exists. All treatments are merely palliative.

Lukewarm baths and application of occlusive ointment bases (petroleum jelly or preparations containing urea) or salicylic acid preparations may soften and remove psoriatic scales. Steroid creams are also useful.

A sunny suggestion

To slow rapid cell proliferation, the doctor may recommend exposure to ultraviolet light (wavelength B [UVB] or natural sunlight) to the point of minimal redness.

Advice on anthralin

Anthralin, combined with a paste mixture, may be used for well-defined plaques. However, this drug must not be applied to unaffected areas because it may cause inflammation. Anthralin irritates and stains the skin. It also stains clothing and household items such as the bathtub.

Tar? Sounds bizarre

For a patient with severe chronic psoriasis, the Goeckerman treatment—which combines tar application and UVB treatments—may help achieve remission and clear the skin.

The Ingram technique, a variation of the Goeckerman treatment, uses anthralin instead of tar. Psoralen plus ultraviolet A (PUVA) therapy combines methoxsalen (a psoralen derivative) with exposure to ultraviolet A light. Methotrexate may help severe, refractory psoriasis.

Oatmeal, emollients, and aspirin

Low-dosage antihistamines, oatmeal baths, emollients (perhaps with phenol and menthol), and open wet dressings may relieve pruritus.

Aspirin and local heat alleviate the pain of psoriatic arthritis; severe cases may require nonsteroidal anti-inflammatory drugs, such as indomethacin.

For scalp psoriasis, therapy usually consists of a tar shampoo, followed by application of a steroid lotion while the hair is still wet.

Not much for nails

No effective treatment exists for psoriasis of the nails. However, the nails usually improve as skin lesions improve.

What to do

• Monitor for adverse reactions to therapy. The patient may develop allergic reactions to anthralin; atrophy and acne from steroids; and burning, itching, nausea, and skin cancer from PUVA. Methotrexate may cause liver or bone marrow toxicity.
• Evaluate the patient. With successful treatment, skin eruptions should be under control; he should be able to demonstrate proper skin care. Note whether he keeps follow-up appointments required to monitor for adverse reactions to therapy. (See *Psoriasis teaching tips*.)

Quick quiz

1. Functions of the skin include:
    A. protection, regulation of temperature and blood pressure, and excretion.
    B. sensory perception, immunity, and blood pressure regulation.
    C. regulation of temperature, blood pressure, and respirations; protection; and immunity.
    D. cell formation, sensory perception, and immunity.

Education edge

Psoriasis teaching tips

• Teach the patient how to apply prescribed creams and lotions.
• Tell the patient using the Goeckerman treatment to apply tar with a downward motion to avoid rubbing it into the follicles.
• Instruct him to apply anthralin to psoriatic plaques only. Advise him to wear gloves because anthralin stains the skin. After application, he may dust himself with powder to prevent anthralin from rubbing off on his clothes. Warn him never to put an occlusive dressing over anthralin. Suggest using mineral oil, then soap and water, to remove anthralin. Caution to avoid scrubbing his skin vigorously.
• Tell him that flare-ups are commonly related to specific environmental and systemic factors.
• Inform the patient undergoing psoralen plus ultraviolet A therapy that treatment may cause burning, itching, nausea, and skin cancer.

Answer: A. The skin's many functions include protection, sensory perception, temperature and blood pressure regulation, vitamin synthesis, and excretion.

2. Which nursing diagnosis is most likely to be applicable to a patient with a skin disorder?
- A. Risk for imbalanced nutrition: More than body requirements
- B. Ineffective tissue perfusion
- C. Risk for infection
- D. Impaired physical mobility

Answer: C. *Risk for infection* may apply to any condition that impairs the skin's ability to guard against invasion by microorganisms.

3. Wet-to-dry dressings, irrigation, hydrotherapy, and bedside debridement are components of which type of debridement?
- A. Surgical
- B. Chemical
- C. Prophylactic
- D. Mechanical

Answer: D. Mechanical debridement uses wet-to-dry dressings, irrigation, hydrotherapy, and bedside debridement.

4. Conditions that increase the risk of pressure ulcers include:
- A. altered mobility and inadequate nutrition.
- B. obesity and high blood pressure.
- C. high blood pressure and altered mobility.
- D. skin breaks and increased metabolism.

Answer: A. Conditions that increase the risk of pressure ulcers include altered mobility, inadequate nutrition (leading to weight loss and subsequent reduction of subcutaneous tissue and muscle bulk), and breakdown of skin or subcutaneous tissue (from edema or incontinence). Other predisposing factors include fever, pathologic conditions, and obesity.

5. Your patient complains of an itchy rash. On inspection, you note red, scaly, silvery patches on her back. Which disorder can cause these findings?
- A. Scabies
- B. Cellulitis
- C. Psoriasis
- D. Herpes zoster

Answer: C. Psoriasis is characterized by red, elevated plaques with silvery scales.

Scoring

☆☆☆ If you answered all five items correctly, excellent! Your integumentary intelligence quotient has hit the uppermost stratum!

☆☆ If you answered four items correctly, kudos! You've added several
layers to your comprehension of cutaneous matters!

☆ If you answered fewer than three items correctly, don't overwork
your sweat glands! Just settle into a nice therapeutic bath
and review this chapter until it really gets under your skin!

Cancer care

Just the facts

In this chapter, you'll learn:

♦ epidemiology and pathophysiology of cancer

♦ risk factors for cancer

♦ how cancer is staged and graded

♦ assessment, diagnosis, and treatment of specific cancers

♦ nursing interventions for patients with cancer.

Cancer is an umbrella term for a group of disorders in which certain cells grow and multiply uncontrollably, eventually forming tissue masses called *tumors*. About 200 different types of cancer are known.

Cancer causes more than 550,000 deaths in the United States annually, making it the second leading killer after cardiovascular disease. The American Cancer Society (ACS) estimates that roughly 83 million Americans now living will eventually have some form of cancer.

Pathophysiology

In many cases, the exact cause of cancer remains unknown. However, specific factors have been implicated in some types of cancer. They include:
• chemical carcinogens
• ultraviolet (UV) light exposure
• hereditary predisposition.

Where there's smoke...

Smoking can cause lung cancer and has been strongly implicated in cancers of the mouth, throat, bladder, kidney, and several other organs. Although not everyone who smokes will get cancer, smoking increases the cancer risk. Similarly, high alcohol intake increases the risk of oral cancers.

Genetic mutation

Smoking and other risk factors can affect the cell's genetic material, interfering with normal gene replication before cell division (mitosis) takes place. Such interference can increase the likelihood of a mutation — an abnormal change in some portion of the cell's gene complement. (See *Reviewing cancer risk factors*.)

Genetic mutation may result from aging; exposure to chemicals, radiation, or hormones; and other factors. Over time, numerous gene mutations may occur in a cell, permitting it to divide and grow in a way that eventually leads to cancer.

> I can feel a nasty change coming on. Oh no — it's the dreaded genetic mutation!

Uncontrolled growth

Cancer cells first develop from a genetic mutation in a single cell. (See *Cancer cell characteristics*.) This cell grows without the control that characterizes normal cell growth. Also, it fails to mature into the type of normal cell from which it originated.

Uncontrolled localized growth follows. Unlike normal cells, cancer cells keep growing and multiplying even after lost cells have been replaced.

Metastasis

In addition to this uncontrolled localized growth, cancer cells may spread from their origin site in a process called *metastasis*. Cancer cells metastasize in three ways:
- by circulation through the bloodstream and lymphatic system
- by accidental transplantation during surgery or other invasive procedures
- by spreading to adjacent organs and tissues.

Cancer classifications

Cancer is classified by the tissues or blood cells in which it originates. Most cancers derive from epithelial tissues and are called *carcinomas*.

Other cancers arise from these tissues and cells:
- glandular tissues (adenocarcinomas)
- connective, muscle, and bone tissues (sarcomas)

Cancer cell characteristics

Cancer cells are characterized by uncontrolled cellular growth and development. Typically, these cells:
- vary in size and shape
- aren't encapsulated
- undergo abnormal mitosis
- function abnormally
- don't resemble their cells of origin
- produce substances rarely associated with the original cell or tissue
- can spread to other sites.

Reviewing cancer risk factors

Although cancer can strike anyone, adults and children alike, its incidence rises with age. Many other factors, internal and external, contribute to an individual's predisposition to cancer. Here are some examples.

Internal risk factors

Internal risk factors include age, gender, race, and genetic, immunologic and psychological factors.

Age

Age of exposure to carcinogens may increase the cancer risk. Fetuses, infants, and children are at greater risk because they're still developing. Blistering sunburns in children under age 12 may predispose them to skin cancer.

Researchers are examining the effects of low electromagnetic fields, as in electric blankets or high-voltage power lines, on children.

Gender

Overall, women have a lower cancer incidence than men and higher survival rates. In females, breast, colon, lung, and uterine cancers are the most common. In males, prostate, lung, GI tract, and bladder cancers predominate.

Race

Cancer incidence and mortality are higher in blacks due to economic, social, and environmental factors that may delay prompt detection and increase exposure risk to industrial carcinogens.

Genetic factors

Certain cancers tend to run in families. For example, women who have first-degree relatives (mothers or sisters) with breast cancer are at greater risk than the general population.

Immunologic factors

According to the immune surveillance theory, antigenic differences between normal and cancerous cells may help the body eliminate malignant cells. Thus, immunosuppression may increase susceptibility to cancer.

Psychological factors

Emotional stress may increase a person's cancer risk by leading to poor health habits (such as frequent smoking), by depressing the immune system, or by leading him to ignore early warning signs.

External risk factors

External risk factors include exposure to chemical carcinogens or radiation, viruses, diet, tobacco and alcohol use, and chemotherapeutic drugs.

Chemical carcinogens

The most important external risk factor for cancer is exposure to chemical carcinogens, such as those used in nickel refining or in the asbestos industry.

Chemical carcinogens typically cause cancer in a two-step process—initiation and promotion.
• *Initiation* involves exposure to the carcinogen. This irreversible step converts normal cells into latent tumor cells.
• In *promotion*, repeated exposure to the same or some other substance stimulates the latent cells to become actively neoplastic.

Radiation

Ionizing radiation of all kinds (from X-rays to nuclear radiation) are carcinogenic, although their potencies vary.

Fair-skinned people have a higher risk for skin cancer from ultraviolet radiation. Skin cancer develops on exposed extremities, and its incidence correlates with the amount of exposure.

Viruses

Some human viruses have carcinogenic potential. The Epstein-Barr virus, for example, has been linked to lymphoma and nasopharyngeal carcinoma.

Deoxyribonucleic acid viruses (such as herpes simplex virus type 2) have been associated with uterine cervical cancer. Ribonucleic acid viruses are linked to breast cancer in mice.

Diet

Certain foods may supply carcinogens (or precarcinogens), affect carcinogen formation, or modify other carcinogens' effect. Diet has been implicated in colon cancer, which may result from low fiber intake and excessive fat consumption.

(continued)

Reviewing cancer risk factors *(continued)*

Liver tumors are linked to food additives, such as nitrates (commonly used in smoked and processed meat) and alfatoxin (a fungus that grows on stored grains, nuts, and other food-stuffs).

Tobacco use

Lung cancer is the leading cause of cancer deaths in both men and women. Cigarette smoking accounts for about 30% of all cancers and is implicated in cancers of the mouth, pharynx, larynx, esophagus, pancreas, cervix, and bladder. Pipe smoking and chewing tobacco are linked to oral cancer.

Studies show increased cancer risks associated with inhalation of secondhand smoke by nonsmokers (particularly children).

Alcohol use

Alcohol may act synergistically with tobacco. Smokers who drink heavily run an increased risk of head, neck, and esophageal cancers. Heavy beer consumption may increase the risk of colorectal cancer through an unknown mechanism.

Chemotherapeutic drugs

Some chemotherapeutic drugs may be directly carcinogenic or may enhance neoplastic development by suppressing the immune system.

By altering the body's normal endocrine balance, hormones may contribute to (rather than directly stimulate) neoplastic development—especially in endocrine-sensitive organs, such as the breast or prostate. The risk of secondary cancers from these agents must be weighed carefully against their benefits.

- brain and spinal cord tissues (gliomas)
- pigmented cells (melanomas)
- plasma cells (myelomas)
- lymphatic tissue (lymphomas)
- leukocytes (leukemia)
- erythrocytes (erythroleukemia).

Cancers

This section discusses the most prevalent cancers of each body system. For each disorder, you'll find information on causes, assessment findings, diagnostic tests, treatment, nursing interventions, patient teaching, and evaluation criteria.

Acute leukemia

In acute leukemia, cancerous white blood cell (WBC) precursors called *blasts* proliferate in the bone marrow or lymph tissue and then accumulate in peripheral blood, bone marrow, and body tissues. Untreated, acute leukemia invariably leads to death, usually from complications of leukemic cell infiltration of bone marrow or vital organs.

Acute leukemia ranks 20th as a cause of cancer-related deaths among people of all ages. With treatment, prognosis varies. Among children, acute leukemia is the most common cancer.

How many lymphoblasts can you cram into the bone marrow? This is no joke — it's acute lymphoblastic leukemia.

Classifying acute leukemia

The most common forms of acute leukemia are:
• acute lymphoblastic leukemia (ALL), marked by abnormal growth of lymphocyte precursors (lymphoblasts)
• acute myelogenous leukemia (AML), characterized by rapid accumulation of myeloid precursors (myeloblasts)
• acute monocytic leukemia, or Schilling's type, which involves a marked increase in monocyte precursors (monoblasts).

Other leukemia variants include acute myelomonocytic leukemia and acute erythroleukemia.

Survival stats

In ALL, treatment induces remission in 90% of children; average survival time is 5 years. In adults, treatment induces remission in 65%, with an average survival time of 1 to 2 years. Children between ages 2 and 8 have the best survival rate — about 50% — with intensive therapy.

In AML, average survival is only 1 year after diagnosis, even with aggressive treatment.

In acute monocytic leukemia, treatment induces remissions lasting 2 to 10 months in 40% of children. Adults survive only about 1 year after diagnosis, even with treatment.

What causes it

The cause of acute leukemia is unknown. According to some experts, risk factors include:
• a combination of viruses
• genetic and immunologic factors
• exposure to radiation and certain chemicals.

Pathophysiology

The pathogenesis of acute leukemia isn't clearly understood. Immature, nonfunctioning WBCs appear to accumulate first in the tissue where they originate (lymphocytes in lymph tissue, granulocytes in bone marrow). These immature WBCs then spill into the bloodstream and infiltrate other tissues. Eventually, they cause organ malfunction from encroachment or hemorrhage.

What to look for

Typical clinical features of acute leukemia include:
- high fever of sudden onset
- abnormal bleeding
- easy bruising with even minor trauma
- prolonged menses.

Nonspecific signs and symptoms include low-grade fever, pallor, and weakness and lassitude that may persist for days or months before other symptoms arise.

Possible signs and symptoms of ALL, AML, and acute monocytic leukemia include dyspnea, fatigue, malaise, tachycardia, palpitations, systolic ejection murmur, and abdominal or bone pain. In meningeal leukemia, early symptoms typically include confusion, lethargy, and headache.

What tests tell you

- Bone marrow biopsy is performed in a patient with typical clinical findings but whose aspirate is dry or free from leukemic cells. Bone marrow aspiration typically shows proliferation of immature WBCs and confirms the diagnosis.
- WBC differential determines cell type.
- Complete blood count (CBC) shows decreased levels of hemoglobin (anemia), platelets (thrombocytopenia) and neutrophils (neutropenia).
- Lumbar puncture detects meningeal involvement.
- Uric acid measurement may be done to detect hyperuricemia.

> A slew of immature white blood cells, plus anemia, thrombocytopenia, and neutropenia. These test results definitely suggest leukemia.

How it's treated

Systemic chemotherapy aims to eradicate leukemic cells and induce remission, restoring normal bone marrow function. Chemotherapy varies with the specific leukemia:
- for meningeal leukemia — intrathecal instillation of methotrexate or cytarabine, along with cranial radiation
- for ALL — vincristine and prednisone with intrathecal methotrexate or cytarabine; I.V. asparaginase, daunorubicin, and doxorubicin; maintenance with mercaptopurine and methotrexate
- for AML — a combination of I.V. daunorubicin or doxorubicin, cytarabine, and oral thioguanine. If these agents fail to induce remission, the patient may receive a combination of cyclophosphamide, vincristine, prednisone, or methotrexate; high-dose cytarabine alone or with other drugs; amsacrine; mitoxantrone; or maintenance with additional chemotherapy.

Other treatments

Treatment may also include antibiotics, antifungals, and antivirals (given along with granulocyte injections to control infection and platelet transfusions to prevent bleeding). Red blood cell (RBC) transfusions may be given to prevent anemia. For some patients, bone marrow transplantation is an option.

What to do

• Control infection by placing the patient in a private room and imposing reverse isolation, if necessary. (Benefits of reverse isolation are controversial.) Coordinate care so the patient doesn't come in contact with staff who also care for patients with infections or infectious diseases. Avoid using indwelling catheters and giving intramuscular injections, which can pave the way for infection. Screen staff and visitors for contagious diseases. Watch for and report signs and symptoms of infection.

• Monitor the patient's vital signs every 2 to 4 hours. A temperature over 101° F (38.3° C) accompanied by a decreased WBC count calls for prompt antibiotic therapy.

• Watch for bleeding. If it occurs, apply ice compresses and pressure, and elevate the affected extremity. Avoid giving aspirin and aspirin-containing drugs. Also avoid taking rectal temperatures, giving rectal suppositories, and performing digital rectal examinations (DRE).

Safe in supine

• Watch for signs and symptoms of meningeal leukemia. If these occur, provide care after intrathecal chemotherapy. After instillation, place the patient in the Trendelenburg position for 30 minutes. Give plenty of fluids, and keep him supine for 4 to 6 hours. Check the lumbar puncture site often for bleeding.

• If the patient has received cranial radiation, teach him about potential adverse effects, and try to minimize them.

• Take steps to prevent hyperuricemia — a possible result of rapid chemotherapy-induced leukemic cell lysis. Give the patient about 2 qt (2 L) of fluids daily, and administer acetazolamide, sodium bicarbonate tablets, and allopurinol, as ordered. Check urine pH often — it should be above 7.5. Watch for rash and other hypersensitivity reactions to allopurinol.

• Control mouth ulcers by checking often for obvious ulcers and gum swelling and by providing frequent mouth care and saline solution rinses.

• Check the rectal area daily for induration, swelling, erythema, skin discoloration, and drainage.

If your patient is being treated for leukemia, don't give aspirin, take rectal temperatures, or perform digital rectal exams.

• Minimize stress by providing a calm, quiet atmosphere that promotes rest and relaxation.

• Provide psychological support by establishing a trusting relationship with the patient. Allow him and his family to express their anger, anxiety, and depression. Encourage them to participate in patient care as much as possible. Refer them to a local chapter of the Leukemia Society of America.

• For a patient with terminal disease that resists chemotherapy, provide supportive care directed at promoting comfort; managing pain, fever, and bleeding; and offering emotional support. Provide the opportunity for religious counseling, if appropriate. Discuss the option of home or hospice care.

• Evaluate the patient. He and his family should understand the rationale for treatment and potential complications of chemotherapy. They should also know how to recognize signs and symptoms of infection and understand that they must notify the doctor if these occur. They should be able to discuss treatment options and verbalize concerns about a poor prognosis. (See *Acute leukemia teaching tips*.)

Breast cancer

Breast cancer is the most common cancer among females in the United States and the second leading cause of cancer deaths in women ages 35 to 54. Breast cancer also occurs in men, although it's rare.

Thanks to earlier diagnosis and expanded treatment options, the 5-year survival rate for patients with localized breast cancer has improved from 78% in 1940 to 92% today.

Surviving in situ

For noninvasive cancer in situ (confined to the origin site without invading neighboring tissue), the survival rate is near 100%. If the cancer has spread regionally, the survival rate is 71%. With distant metastasis, it falls to 18%.

What causes it

Although the exact cause of breast cancer is unknown, certain risk factors exist. Primary risk factors include:
• gender (more than 90% of breast cancers occur in women)
• age (risk increases after age 50)
• personal history of the disease (15% of women develop breast cancer in the opposite breast)

Education edge

Acute leukemia teaching tips

• If your patient has leukemia, teach him and his family the signs and symptoms of infection (such as fever, chills, cough, and sore throat) and abnormal bleeding (such as bruising and small purplish spots, or petechiae, caused by tiny hemorrhages). Also teach them how to stop bleeding, such as by applying pressure or ice.
• Instruct the patient to use a soft-bristle toothbrush and to avoid hot, spicy foods and the overuse of commercial mouthwashes.

• family history of the disease (women who have a first-degree relative with breast cancer have a twofold to threefold increased risk).

Secondary risk factors

Secondary risk factors for breast cancer include:
• never having given birth
• giving birth to a first child after age 30
• prolonged hormonal stimulation (menarche before age 12 and menopause after age 50)
• atypical hyperplasia (abnormal cell multiplication) on a previous breast biopsy
• exposure to excessive ionizing radiation (as in Hodgkin's disease treatment)
• history of endometrial, ovarian, or colon cancer.

Breast cancer genes

The discovery of specific genes linked to breast cancer, called *BRCA1* and *BRCA2*, indicates that the disease can be inherited. Someone who inherits either gene has roughly an 80% chance of developing breast cancer.

Pathophysiology

Breast cancer is more commonly found in the left breast than the right. It's also more common in the upper outer quadrant. (See *Breast tumor sites*, page 812.)

Growth rates vary. Theoretically, slow-growing breast cancer may take up to 8 years to become palpable at 1 cm in size.

Spread pattern

Breast cancer spreads via the lymphatic system and bloodstream, through the right side of the heart to the lungs, and eventually to the other breast, chest wall, liver, bone, and brain.

What to look for

Signs and symptoms of breast cancer include:
• painless lump or mass in the breast
• changes in breast symmetry or size
• changes in breast skin, such as dimpling (called *peau d'orange*), edema, or ulcers
• changes in nipples; for instance, itching, burning, erosion, or retraction
• skin temperature changes (a warm, hot, or pink area).

If you detect any of these changes, suspect cancer in a nonlactating woman past childbearing age until proven

Memory jogger

ASH is an easy way to remember the primary risk factors for breast cancer.

A Age: The risk increases after age 50.

S Sex: About 90% of breast cancers are found in women.

H History: A personal or family history of breast cancer increases the risk for the disease.

Breast cancer more commonly affects the left breast than the right, and is more common in the upper outer quadrant.

Breast tumor sites

This illustration shows the location and frequency of breast cancer. The upper outer quadrant is the most common breast cancer site.

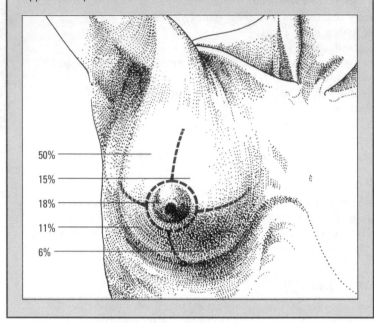

- 50%
- 15%
- 18%
- 11%
- 6%

otherwise. Investigate spontaneous discharge of any kind in a non–breast-feeding, nonlactating woman.

Signs and symptoms of metastasis

Metastatic disease may cause shoulder, hip, or pelvic pain; cough; anorexia; persistent dizziness; or enlarged axillary or supraclavicular lymph nodes.

What tests tell you

- Detection of a breast lump or tumor on breast self-examination, clinical breast examination, or mammography, suggests breast cancer. (See *Breast cancer screening recommendations.*)
- Diagnosis hinges on biopsy and pathologic evaluation of the suspicious tissue. The staging workup may include chest X-rays as well as liver and bone scans.
- A hormonal receptor assay of tumor tissue obtained by biopsy can determine whether the tumor's growth requires estrogen

Breast cancer staging may warrant chest X-rays and liver and bone scans.

(estrogen-dependent) or progesterone (progesterone-dependent). Such determination guides therapeutic decisions.

How it's treated

Treatment may include one or any combination of the following options.

Chemotherapy

Chemotherapy for breast cancer may involve various cytotoxic drug combinations. In patients with axillary lymph node involvement but no evidence of distant metastasis, chemotherapy may be adjuvant (used after the primary tumor has been removed), or neoadjuvant (used as a preliminary therapy preceding a necessary second treatment modality).

If metastasis has occurred, chemotherapy may be done as primary therapy based on such factors as the patient's premenopausal or postmenopausal status.

Chemo combos

Commonly used drug combinations include:
- cyclophosphamide, methotrexate, and fluorouracil
- doxorubicin and cyclophosphamide
- cyclophosphamide, doxorubicin, and fluorouracil.

Other drug treatments

Paclitaxel and docetaxel are used to treat recurrent or metastatic breast cancer. Herceptin is a monoclonal antibody used to treat metastatic breast cancer in patients with an overexpression of Hcr-2/ncu, a protein associated with a more aggressive tumor. About 30% of breast cancer patients are candidates for herceptin therapy.

Radiation therapy

Primary radiation therapy typically begins 2 to 4 weeks after surgery, when incisions have healed. It may be given before, during, or after chemotherapy.

Radiation therapy may also be used as adjunctive therapy for tumors that are located near the chest wall or are locally advanced or recurrent as well as for inflammatory breast cancer. If cancer has spread to the bone, radiation therapy may be targeted to specific bone sites to reduce pain.

Surgery

Lumpectomy, or tumor excision, usually is the initial surgery. It also provides biopsy material to determine tumor cell type.

Typically, lumpectomy is performed on an outpatient basis. For some patients — especially those with small tumors and no evidence of axillary node involvement — it's the only surgery required. However, lumpectomy is commonly combined with radiation therapy.

Lumpectomy is performed in two stages. First, the surgeon removes the lump and confirms malignancy. Then he discusses treatment options with the patient.

Other surgical options

Other surgical procedures for breast cancer include:
• lumpectomy with axillary lymph node dissection, which removes the tumor and axillary lymph nodes while leaving the breast intact
• simple mastectomy, which removes the breast but not axillary lymph nodes or pectoral muscles
• modified radical mastectomy, which removes the breast and axillary nodes
• radical mastectomy, which removes the breast, pectoralis major and minor muscles, and axillary nodes.

Rebuilding the breast

Postmastectomy reconstructive surgery can create a breast mound if the patient desires it and doesn't show evidence of advanced disease.

Other methods

Other breast cancer treatments may include:
• estrogen, progesterone, or androgen therapy
• antiandrogen therapy with aminoglutethimide
• antiestrogen therapy.

Antiestrogen therapy involves administration of tamoxifen, a drug with few adverse effects that inhibits deoxyribonucleic acid synthesis. Used in postmenopausal women, tamoxifen most effectively combats estrogen-dependent tumors.

Surgical slack-off

The success of drug therapies — along with growing evidence that breast cancer is a systemic rather than local disease — has led to a decline in types of surgery that remove the breast.

What to do

• Obtain a patient history. Assess the patient's feelings and knowledge about her diagnosis, and determine her expectations.

In a lumpectomy with axillary lymph node dissection, the doctor removes only the tumor and the lymph nodes under the arm — not the breast itself.

• Explain treatment options at the patient's level of understanding.
• Evaluate the patient. With effective treatment, she should recover uneventfully from surgery, radiation, chemotherapy, or other treatments. She should perform appropriate exercises and understand postoperative safety precautions for the affected arm. Also, she should correctly demonstrate breast self-examination. (See *Breast cancer teaching tips*.)

Cervical cancer

The third most common cancer of the female reproductive system (after uterine and ovarian cancer), cervical cancer may be preinvasive or invasive. With early detection and proper treatment, the preinvasive form is curable in 75% to 90% of cases.

Unwelcome invasion

If untreated (and depending on the exact cancer form), the disease may progress to become invasive. Invasive cervical cancer causes 6,000 deaths annually in the United States. Rare before age 20, it usually occurs between ages 30 and 50.

What causes it

The cause of cervical cancer is unknown. Risk factors include:
• presence of certain viruses (human papillomavirus and herpes)
• initiation of sexual intercourse during adolescence
• multiple sex partners
• cigarette smoking.

Pathophysiology

Preinvasive cervical cancer ranges from minimal cervical dysplasia, in which the lower third of the epithelium contains abnormal cells, to carcinoma in situ, which involves the full thickness of epithelium.

No basement bargains

In invasive cancer, cancer cells penetrate the basement membrane and may spread directly to adjacent pelvic structures or to distant sites via the lymph system.

What to look for

Preinvasive cervical cancer is asymptomatic. Abnormal vaginal bleeding, persistent vaginal dis-

Education edge

Breast cancer teaching tips

• To promote early diagnosis and treatment of breast cancer, teach female patients the importance of monthly breast self-examination, mammography, and appropriate follow-up care.
• Postoperatively, instruct the patient to continue these practices to detect new breast lesions.

The survival odds for a patient with preinvasive cervical cancer are pretty good. About 75% to 90% of cases are curable.

charge, and postcoital pain and bleeding may signal early invasive disease.

Advanced disease may cause pelvic pain or vaginal leakage of urine and feces from a fistula, along with anorexia, weight loss, and fatigue.

What tests tell you

• A Papanicolaou (Pap) test can detect cervical cancer before symptoms arise. The ACS recommends annual Pap tests starting no later than age 21. Women ages 30 to 70 with three or more consecutive satisfactory examinations with normal findings should have a Pap test every 2 to 3 years. For women age 70 and older with three or more consecutive satisfactory examinations and no abnormal Pap tests in the last 10 years, screening may stop.
• Colposcopy (examination of the vaginal and cervical epithelium using a colposcope) can reveal the presence and extent of preclinical lesions.
• Biopsy and histologic examination confirm the diagnosis.
• Additional studies, such as lymphangiography, cystography, and scans, can detect metastasis.

How it's treated

Effective treatment is tailored to the cancer stage. Preinvasive lesions may warrant total excisional biopsy, cryosurgery, laser destruction of the tumor, conization (removal of a cone-shaped section of the cervix) with frequent Pap test follow-up or, rarely, hysterectomy. Invasive squamous cancer may require radical hysterectomy and radiation therapy (internal, external, or both).

What to do

• Provide comprehensive patient teaching and emotional and psychological support.
• If the patient will receive internal radiation, determine if the radioactive source will be inserted while she's in the operating room (preloaded) or at the bedside (afterloaded). Remember that safety precautions—time, distance, and shielding—must start as soon as the radioactive source is in place. Tell the patient she'll require a private room.
• Check the patient's vital signs every 4 hours. Watch for skin reactions, vaginal bleeding, abdominal discomfort, and evidence of dehydration.
• Make sure she can reach everything she needs without stretching or straining. Assist her in range-of-motion arm exercises; be aware that leg exercises and other body movements could dis-

Invasive cervical cancer requires more aggressive treatment, such as radical hysterectomy or radiation therapy.

lodge the radiation source. If ordered, give a tranquilizer to help her relax and stay still.

• Organize the time you spend with the patient to minimize your radiation exposure. Inform visitors of safety precautions, and hang a sign listing these precautions on the patient's door.

• Evaluate the patient. When assessing her response to treatment, note how well she tolerates the therapy. She should understand that it won't impair her ability to have sex. Also she should understand the importance of complying with the treatment regimen. (See *Cervical cancer teaching tips*.)

Colorectal cancer

Colorectal cancer is the second most common visceral cancer in the United States and Europe. It affects men and women equally.

Nearly all colorectal cancers are adenocarcinomas. About 50% are rectosigmoid lesions that adhere closely to the mucosal surface (called *sessile*). The rest are polyps.

Slow to spread, easier to cure

Because colorectal cancer spreads slowly, it's potentially curable with early diagnosis. The 5-year survival rate is 91% for colon cancer and 83% for rectal cancer. After the cancer spreads regionally, survival drops to 60% for colon cancer and 50% for rectal cancer.

What causes it

The cause of colorectal cancer remains unknown. Studies show, however, that it's prevalent in areas of higher economic development. This suggests it's linked to a high-fat diet.

Other factors that increase the risk for this disease include:
• age over 40
• other GI tract diseases
• history of ulcerative colitis (average interval before cancer onset is 11 to 17 years)
• inherited tendency toward colon polyps (cancer almost always develops by age 50)
• breast and gynecologic cancers.

Pathophysiology

Most lesions of the large bowel are moderately differentiated adenocarcinomas. Tumors tend to grow slowly and remain asymptomatic for long periods.

Stretching the circumference

Tumors in the sigmoid and descending colon grow circumferentially and constrict the intestinal lumen. At diagnosis, tumors in the ascending colon are usually large and palpable on physical examination.

What to look for

Signs and symptoms of colorectal cancer include malaise and fatigue. Other findings result from local obstruction and, in later stages, from direct extension to adjacent organs (such as the bladder, prostate, ureters, vagina, and sacrum) or from distant metastasis (usually to the liver).

Later signs and symptoms include:
• weight loss
• pain
• pallor
• cachexia (malnutrition, weakness, and emaciation)
• ascites (buildup of serous fluid in the abdominal cavity)
• hepatomegaly (liver enlargement)
• lymphangiectasis (widening of the lymphatic vessels).

What tests tell you

• Only a tumor biopsy can verify colorectal cancer, but other tests help detect it. For women and men age 50 and older, the ACS recommends one of the following tests: fecal occult blood test (FOBT) every year, flexible sigmoidoscopy every 5 years, FOBT every year plus flexible sigmoidoscopy every 5 years, colonoscopy every 10 years, or double-contrast barium enema every 5 years.)
• DRE detects nearly 15% of colorectal cancers. It can be used to detect suspicious rectal and perianal lesions.
• FOBT detects blood in stools, a warning sign of rectal cancer.
• Proctoscopy or sigmoidoscopy permits visualization of the lower GI tract and can detect up to two-thirds of colorectal cancers.
• Colonoscopy allows visual inspection (and photographs) of the colon up to the ileocecal valve. It also provides access for polypectomy and biopsy of suspected lesions.
• Barium X-ray, using dual contrast with air, can locate lesions that are manually or visu-

People age 50 and older should have fecal occult blood tests every year, flexible sigmoidoscopy every 5 years, or colonoscopy every 10 years.

ally undetectable. This test should follow endoscopy because barium sulfate interferes with endoscopy.
• Carcinoembryonic antigen testing, although not specific or sensitive enough for early diagnosis, helps monitor the patient before and after treatment to detect metastasis or recurrence.

How it's treated

Surgery seeks to remove the cancerous tumor and adjacent tissues as well as lymph nodes that may contain cancer cells. The type of surgery depends on tumor location. (See *Treating colorectal cancer.*)

Treating colorectal cancer

The most effective treatment for colorectal cancer is surgery to remove the malignant tumor, adjacent tissues, and cancerous lymph nodes. The surgical site depends on tumor location.

This illustration shows the different locations in the colon that may be resected for tumor removal.

Postoperative treatment

After surgery, treatment typically includes chemotherapy or radiation therapy. If the cancer has spread to other sites or the patient has residual disease or a recurrent inoperable tumor, chemotherapy is essential.

- Transverse colon
- Ascending colon
- Descending colon
- Rectum

Surgical options

• For tumors of the cecum or ascending colon, right hemicolectomy for advanced disease may include resection of the terminal segment of the ileum, cecum, ascending colon, and right half of the transverse colon with corresponding mesentery.

• For tumors of the proximal and middle transverse colon, right colectomy includes transverse colon and mesentery corresponding to midcolonic vessels. Alternatively, the surgeon may perform segmental resection of the transverse colon and associated midcolonic vessels.

• For sigmoid colon tumors, surgery is usually limited to the sigmoid colon and mesentery.

• Upper rectum tumors usually call for anterior or low anterior resection. A newer method, using a stapler, allows resections much lower than were previously possible.

• For tumors in the lower rectum, abdominoperineal resection and permanent sigmoid colostomy are usually performed.

Better living through chemotherapy

Chemotherapy may be used as adjuvant therapy or for patients with metastasis, residual disease, or recurrent inoperable tumors. Commonly used drugs include:

• 5-fluorouracil, with or without leucovorin
• lomustine
• mitomycin
• methotrexate
• vincristine
• cisplatin
• levamisole.

Other treatments

Radiation therapy may induce tumor regression and may be used before and after surgery. Biotherapy (alone or with chemotherapy) is still experimental.

What to do

• If the patient will have colorectal surgery, monitor his diet and give laxatives, enemas, and antibiotics, as ordered (to clean the bowel and minimize abdominal and perineal cavity contamination during surgery).

• Evaluate the patient. He should verbalize an understanding of the treatment regimen, including ostomy care, and the need for long-term follow-up. (See *Colorectal cancer teaching tips.*)

Education edge

Colorectal cancer teaching tips

• If your patient with colorectal cancer will have a colostomy, teach him and his family about the procedure. Consider referring the patient to an enterostomal therapist before surgery.

• Because a history of colorectal cancer increases the risk for other primary cancers, instruct the patient to have close follow-up and screening and to increase his dietary fiber intake. Instruct his family about the familial risks of colorectal cancer, and teach them about dietary modifications to reduce their risk. Also teach them how to recognize early signs and symptoms of colorectal cancer.

Hodgkin's disease

Hodgkin's disease is a lymphatic cancer marked by painless, progressive enlargement of the lymph nodes, spleen, and other lymphoid tissue. Left untreated, it follows a variable but progressive and ultimately fatal course.

Promising odds

However, recent advances in therapy make Hodgkin's disease potentially curable, even in advanced stages. Appropriate treatment yields long-term survival in about 90% of patients.

What causes it

The exact cause of Hodgkin's disease is unknown, although indirect evidence suggests it may involve a virus. The disease is most common in young adults.

Pathophysiology

Enlargement of the lymph nodes, spleen, and other lymphoid tissues results from proliferation of lymphocytes, histiocytes, eosinophils, and Reed-Sternberg cells. The latter cells are hallmarks of the disease.

What to look for

Usually, the first sign is painless swelling in a cervical lymph node (or, occasionally, in a lymph node in another area). Other signs and symptoms include pruritus (itching), persistent fever, night sweats, fatigue, weight loss, and malaise.

Late-stage signs and symptoms include facial and neck edema, jaundice, nerve pain, enlarged retroperitoneal lymph nodes, and nodular infiltration of the spleen, liver, and bones.

What tests tell you

• Lymph node biopsy reveals abnormal histologic proliferation, nodular fibrosis, necrosis, and Reed-Sternberg cells. (See *Looking at Reed-Sternberg cells*, page 822.) Lymph node biopsy is also used to determine lymph node and organ involvement.
• Blood tests show mild to severe normocytic anemia (anemia with RBCs of normal size); normochromic anemia (marked by normal hemoglobin amounts) in 50% of cases; an elevated, normal, or reduced WBC count; and WBC differential showing any combination of neutrophilia (excessive neutrophil levels), lymphocytopenia (deficient lymphocyte levels), monocytosis (exces-

In Hodgkin's disease, lymphocytes, histiocytes, eosinophils, and Reed-Sternberg cells proliferate.

Looking at Reed-Sternberg cells

This enlarged, abnormal histiocyte, or Reed-Sternberg cell, from an excised lymph node suggests Hodgkin's disease. Note the large, distinct nucleoli. Reed-Sternberg cells must be present in a patient's blood and lymph tissue to confirm the diagnosis of Hodgkin's disease.

sive monophil levels), and eosinophilia (excessive eosinophil levels).
• Serum alkaline phosphatase levels may be elevated, indicating liver or bone involvement.
• A staging laparotomy is necessary for patients under age 55 and for those without obvious advanced disease (stages III or IV), lymphocyte predominance histology, or medical contraindications.

How it's treated

Depending on the disease stage, treatment may include chemotherapy, radiation, or both. Choice of therapy depends on careful physical examination, accurate histologic interpretation, and proper clinical staging. Correct treatment prolongs survival and induces an apparent cure in many patients.

Alleviation through radiation

Radiation therapy is used alone for patients with:
• stage I disease, which involves a single lymph node region or a single extralymphatic organ

> Radiation therapy is used alone in patients with early-stage Hodgkin's disease.

• stage II disease, which involves two or more nodes on the same side of the diaphragm, plus an extralymphatic organ and one or more node regions on the same side of the diaphragm.

Radiation is used in conjunction with combination chemotherapy for patients with unfavorable prognostic factors. Therapy for patients with stage III disease usually combines radiation and chemotherapy. For patients with stage IV disease, chemotherapy is used; it sometimes induces complete remission.

What to do

• Monitor the patient closely for indications of toxicity caused by chemotherapy or radiation. As appropriate, manage symptoms to help prevent the need for a treatment hiatus or reduction.
• Provide emotional support and offer appropriate counseling and reassurance. Ease the patient's anxiety by sharing your optimism about his prognosis.
• Evaluate the patient. He should understand and comply with the self-care regimen for radiation and chemotherapy. He should know how to recognize adverse effects of treatment and know when to notify the doctor. He should also be able to control weight loss and remain free from infection. (See *Hodgkin's disease teaching tips*.)

Education edge

Hodgkin's disease teaching tips

• If your patient has Hodgkin's disease, teach him and his family what they can do to relieve the adverse effects of treatment. Also teach them when to contact the doctor to help manage symptoms.
• Inform the patient and his family that local chapters of the American Cancer Society and Leukemia Society of America are available for information, financial assistance, and supportive counseling.

Lung cancer

Although largely preventable, lung cancer is the most common cause of cancer deaths in men and women. It usually develops within the wall or epithelium of the bronchial tree.

Histologic headings

The most common histologic (tissue) types of lung cancer are:
• epidermoid (squamous cell) carcinoma
• adenocarcinoma (which involves cells that line the lungs' walls)
• small cell (oat cell) carcinoma (cancer of the wall of a major bronchus, having round or elongated cells)
• large cell (anaplastic) carcinoma (a bronchogenic tumor with undifferentiated large cells).

Frail forecast

Prognosis is generally poor, but varies with cell type and extent of spread at the time of diagnosis. Only 13% of patients with lung cancer survive 5 years after diagnosis.

What causes it

Tobacco smoking accounts for approximately 90% of lung cancers and is closely associated with all histologic types. Other risk factors include genetic predisposition and exposure to carcinogenic industrial or air pollutants (such as asbestos, uranium, arsenic, nickel, iron oxides, chromium, radioactive dust, and coal dust).

Pathophysiology

Lung tumors show bronchial epithelial changes progressing from squamous cell changes or metaplasia (abnormal changes in adult cells) to carcinoma in situ. Tumors originating in the bronchi produce more mucus.

Tumor growth causes partial or complete airway blockage, resulting in collapse of lung lobes distal to the tumor.

Thoracic sprawl

Early metastasis occurs to other thoracic structures, such as the hilar lymph nodes and mediastinum. Distant metastasis may involve the brain, liver, bone, and adrenal glands.

Tobacco smoking (cough) accounts for about 90% (cough) of lung cancers (cough).

What to look for

Because early-stage lung cancer tends to have a gradual onset, the disease is usually well developed by the time it's diagnosed.

With small cell cancer and squamous cancers, late-stage respiratory findings include smoker's cough, hoarseness, wheezing, dyspnea, hemoptysis (expectoration of blood), and chest pain. With large cell cancer and adenocarcinoma, findings include fever, weakness, weight loss, anorexia, and shoulder pain.

Hormonal disharmony

Sometimes, lung cancer causes hormone-related changes, including:
• gynecomastia, or breast enlargement in males (with large cell cancer)
• bone and joint pain (with large cell cancer and adenocarcinoma)
• signs or symptoms of Cushing's syndrome, such as central obesity, round face, supraclavicular fat pads, muscle atrophy, edema, and emotional changes (with small cell cancer)
• signs or symptoms of carcinoid syndrome, such as flushing, diarrhea, cramps, skin lesions, labored breathing, and palpitations (with small cell cancer)

• signs or symptoms of hypercalcemia, such as muscle pain and weakness (with squamous cancer).

Findings in metastatic disease

If lung cancer spreads, signs and symptoms vary. With bronchial obstruction, metastatic signs and symptoms include hemoptysis, atelectasis (lung tissue collapse), pneumonitis (lung inflammation), and dyspnea.

With recurrent nerve invasion, findings may include vocal cord paralysis. With chest wall invasion, the patient may have piercing chest pain, increasing dyspnea, and severe shoulder pain radiating down the arm. With local lymphatic spread, expect cough, hemoptysis, stridor (a harsh sound on expiration), and pleural effusion.

What tests tell you

• Chest X-ray usually shows an advanced lesion, but can detect a lesion up to 2 years before symptoms appear. It also defines tumor size and location.
• Bronchoscopy can locate the tumor site. Bronchoscopic washings provide material for cytologic and histologic examination. Using a flexible fiber-optic bronchoscope increases test effectiveness.
• Needle biopsy uses biplane fluoroscopic visual control to detect peripheral tumors, allowing firm diagnosis in 80% of patients.
• Tissue biopsy of accessible metastatic sites includes supraclavicular and mediastinal node and pleural biopsy.
• Thoracentesis (removal of fluid from the chest cavity) allows chemical and cytologic examination of pleural fluid.
• Tests to detect metastasis include bone scan (a positive scan may lead to bone marrow biopsy; bone marrow biopsy is also recommended for patients with small cell cancer); computed tomography scan of the brain; liver function studies; and gallium scan (noninvasive nuclear scan) of the liver, spleen, and bone.

A chest X-ray can detect a lung tumor up to 2 years before symptoms appear.

How it's treated

Treatment involves combinations of surgery, radiation, and chemotherapy. Although treatment may improve prognosis and prolong survival, it's largely palliative because it generally doesn't start until an advanced disease stage.

Surgery

Surgery is the main treatment for squamous cancer, adenocarcinoma, and large cell cancer — unless the tumor is nonresectable or other conditions (such as cardiac disease) rule out surgery. Surgery may involve partial removal of a lung (as in wedge resection and lobectomy) or total lung removal (as in pneumonectomy and radical pneumonectomy).

Radiation therapy

Preoperative radiation therapy may reduce tumor bulk to allow surgical resection, but its value is questionable. Radiation therapy is generally recommended for early stage (stage I and stage II) lesions if surgery is contraindicated, and as an adjunct to surgery (either preoperatively or postoperatively).

Prophylactic cranial irradiation may be used to prevent or slow brain metastasis in small cell lung cancer. Some patients undergo radiation to control cancer-related symptoms or to prolong their functional lives.

Chemotherapy

Several new chemotherapy combinations show promise. The combination of fluorouracil, vincristine, and mitomycin induces remission in 40% of patients with adenocarcinomas.

Chemotherapy is the primary treatment for small cell cancer. Promising combinations include:
- cyclophosphamide, doxorubicin, and vincristine
- carboplatin, paclitaxel, and etoposide
- vincristine, ifosfamide, cisplatin, carboplatin, and etoposide.

Other treatments

Research continues on the use of biotherapy and laser therapy in treating lung cancer.

What to do

- Provide comprehensive supportive care and patient teaching to minimize complications and promote recovery from surgery, radiation, or chemotherapy.
- Evaluate the patient. He should experience an uneventful recovery from surgery, radiation, or chemotherapy. He and his family should verbalize an understanding of risk factors and alter their smoking behavior as appropriate. The patient should follow the treatment regimen and understand the need for good pulmonary hygiene and follow-up. He should also recognize signs and symptoms of respiratory tract infection and understand the need to report these immediately. (See *Lung cancer teaching tips*.)

Education edge

Lung cancer teaching tips

- Before discharge, teach the patient with lung cancer how to use home oxygen therapy. Make sure the patient and his family know the signs and symptoms of respiratory tract infection, and the need to report them to the doctor.
- To help prevent lung cancer, teach high-risk patients to stop smoking. Refer smokers who want to quit to the local branch of the American Cancer Society or American Lung Association. Inform patients that nicotine gum or a nicotine patch and an antidepressant may be prescribed in combination with educational and support groups.
- Encourage patients with recurring or chronic respiratory tract infections and those with chronic lung disease to see the doctor promptly for evaluation if they detect changes in the character of a cough.

Malignant melanoma

The most lethal form of skin cancer, malignant melanoma remains uncommon but is increasing at a rate of about 4% per year. An estimated 47,700 new cases develop each year, with about 7,700 deaths. Peak incidence occurs from ages 45 to 55.

The four types of melanoma are:
- superficial spreading melanoma
- nodular melanoma
- acral-lentiginous melanoma
- lentigo maligna melanoma.

I know I'm setting a bad example! Even though I've slathered on the sunscreen, that won't necessarily stop me from getting melanoma.

What causes it

The cause of malignant melanoma is unknown. Risk factors include a family tendency, a history of melanoma or dysplastic nevi, excessive sun exposure, a history of severe sunburns, and fair skin.

Ancestral affliction

Most people who develop melanoma have blond or red hair, fair skin, and blue eyes; are prone to sunburn; and are of Celtic or Scandinavian ancestry. Other risk factors are immunosuppressant therapy and psoralen UVA treatment for psoriasis.

Pathophysiology

Melanoma arises from melanocytes (cells that synthesize the pigment melanin. In addition to the skin, melanocytes are found in the meninges (membranes of the brain and spinal cord), alimentary canal, respiratory tract, and lymph nodes.

Metastatic itinerary

Melanoma spreads through the lymphatic and vascular systems to the regional lymph nodes, skin, liver, lungs, and central nervous system. Prognosis varies with tumor thickness. Typically, superficial lesions are curable, whereas deeper lesions tend to metastasize.

Crystal gazing

Prognosis is better for a tumor on an extremity (which is drained by one lymphatic network) than for one on the head, neck, or trunk (drained by several networks).

Memory jogger

Use the ABCD rule to assess a mole's malignant potential.

A Asymmetry: Is the mole irregular in shape?

B Border: Is its border irregular, notched, or poorly defined?

C Color: Does the color vary — for example, between shades of brown, red, white, or black?

D Diameter: Is the diameter more than 6 mm?

Recognizing potentially malignant nevi

Skin lesions called *nevi* (moles) commonly are pigmented and may be hereditary. They begin to grow in childhood and become more numerous during young adulthood.

Up to 70% of patients with melanoma have a history of a preexisting nevus at the tumor site. Of these, about one-third are congenital; the remainder develop later in life.

Changes in nevi (for example, in color, size, shape, or texture or onset of ulceration, bleeding, or itching) suggest possible malignant transformation. Presence or absence of hair within a nevus has no significance.

Types of nevi include blue nevi, compound nevi, dermal nevi, dysplastic nevi, junctional nevi, and lentigo maligna.

Blue nevi

Blue nevi are flat or slightly elevated lesions from 0.5 to 1 cm in diameter. Twice as common in women as in men, they appear on the head, neck, arms, and back of the hands. Their blue color results from dermal pigment and collagen, which reflect blue light but absorb other wavelengths. They must be excised to rule out pigmented basal cell epithelioma or melanoma, or for cosmetic reasons.

Compound nevi

Compound nevi usually are tan to dark brown and slightly raised, although size and color vary. They contain melanocytes in the dermis and epidermis, and rarely undergo malignant transformation. Excision may be needed to rule out malignant transformation or for cosmetic reasons.

Dermal nevi

Dermal nevi are elevated lesions from 2 to 10 mm in diameter that vary in color from tan to brown. Typically, they develop in older adults on the upper part of the body. They're generally removed only to rule out malignant transformation.

Dysplastic nevi

Dysplastic nevi usually are more than 5 mm in diameter, with irregularly notched or indistinct borders. Most often, they're tan or brown but sometimes have red, pink, or black pigmentation. No two of these lesions are exactly alike. They occur in great numbers (typically over 100 at a time), rarely singly—most commonly on the back, scalp, chest, and buttocks.

Dysplastic nevi are potentially malignant, especially in patients with a personal or family history of melanoma. Skin biopsy confirms diagnosis; treatment is by surgical excision, followed by regular physical examinations (every 6 months) to detect new lesions or changes in existing lesions.

Junctional nevi

Junctional nevi are flat or slightly raised and light to dark brown, with melanocytes confined to the epidermis. Usually, they appear before age 40. They may change into compound nevi if junctional nevus cells proliferate and penetrate the dermis.

Lentigo maligna

Also called *melanotic freckle or Hutchinson's melanotic freckle,* lentigo maligna is a precursor to malignant melanoma. About one-third of them eventually give rise to malignant melanoma.

Typically, they occur in persons over age 40, especially on exposed skin areas such as the face. At first, these lesions are flat tan spots, but they gradually enlarge and darken, developing black speckled areas against their tan or brown background. Removal by simple excision (not electrodessication and curettage) is recommended.

What to look for

Suspect melanoma when any skin lesion or nevus enlarges, changes color, becomes inflamed or sore, itches, ulcerates, bleeds, changes texture, or shows signs of surrounding pigment regression (halo nevus or vitiligo). (See *Recognizing potentially malignant nevi.*)

Superficial spreading melanoma

Features of superficial spreading melanoma, the most common type, include:

- a red, white, and bluish tinge over a brown or black background
- irregular, notched margins
- an irregular surface
- a small, elevated nodule that may ulcerate and bleed
- horizontal growth pattern.

Nodular malignant melanoma

Nodular malignant melanoma usually grows vertically, invades the dermis, and metastasizes early. It commonly appears as a polyp and has uniformly dark discoloration; sometimes, it's grayish, resembling a blackberry. Occasionally, it matches the patient's skin color. Pigment flecks may appear around the lesion's base, which may be inflamed.

Nodular malignant melanoma appears uniformly dark and may resemble a blackberry.

Acral-lentiginous melanoma

Acral-lentiginous melanoma occurs mainly on the palms and soles — especially on the tip of a finger or toe or in the nail fold or bed; sometimes, it's seen on mucosal surfaces, such as the vulva or vagina. It appears as an irregular, enlarging black macule and has a prolonged nonvinvasive stage. Although relatively rare, it's the most common melanoma type in nonwhite persons.

Lentigo malignant melanoma

Lentigo malignant melanoma, a relatively rare type, develops over many years from a lentigo maligna (a black or brown, mottled, slowly enlarging lesion with irregular borders) on an exposed skin surface. Usually diagnosed between ages 60 and 70, the lesion looks like a flat, large (2.5 to 6.5 cm) freckle.

A neutral palette

The lesion may be tan, brown, black, white, or slate; and may have scattered black nodules on the surface. Eventually, it may become ulcerated.

What tests tell you

- A skin biopsy with histologic examination distinguishes malignant melanoma from a benign nevus, seborrheic keratosis, or pigmented basal cell epithelioma. It also determines tumor thickness.
- Chest X-ray aids staging.
- Blood studies may show anemia and an elevated erythrocyte sedimentation rate. With metastasis, these tests also may reveal an abnormal platelet count and abnormal liver function studies.

How it's treated

Wide surgical resection is imperative in treating malignant melanoma. The extent of resection depends on the size and location of the primary lesion. Surgery may include regional lymphadenectomy.

Chemotherapy and biotherapy

Deep primary lesions may merit adjuvant chemotherapy with dacarbazine and the nitrosureas carmustine and lomustine. Biotherapy with interferons, interleukin-2, and tumor necrosis factor is being studied.

Radiation therapy

Radiation therapy is usually reserved for metastatic disease. It doesn't prolong survival but may reduce tumor size and relieve pain. Prognosis depends on tumor thickness.

What to do

• After surgery, take steps to prevent infection. Check the wound often for excessive drainage, foul odor, redness, and swelling. If surgery involved lymphadenectomy, minimize lymphedema by applying a compression stocking, and instruct the patient to keep the extremity elevated.
• During chemotherapy, know which adverse reactions to expect, and do what you can to minimize these. For instance, give an antiemetic, as ordered, to reduce nausea and vomiting.
• For advanced metastatic disease, control and prevent pain by giving an analgesic around the clock. Don't wait until pain begins to initiate pain relief.
• Provide psychological support to help the patient cope with anxiety. Encourage him to express his fears. Answer his questions honestly without destroying hope.
• Evaluate the patient. He should recover uneventfully from surgery. He should also understand risk factors and the importance of getting careful treatment follow-up, preventing sun exposure, and performing monthly skin self-examinations. (See *Malignant melanoma teaching tips.*)

Prostate cancer

The most common cancer in men over age 50, prostate cancer is the second leading cause of cancer deaths among males. Incidence is highest among Blacks and men with blood type A and

Education edge

Malignant melanoma teaching tips

• Inform the patient with malignant melanoma that the donor site for a skin graft may be as painful as (or even more painful than) the tumor excision site itself.
• When preparing the patient for discharge, emphasize the need for close follow-up care to detect recurrences early. Explain that recurrences and melanoma spread (if they occur) are commonly delayed, so follow-up must continue for years.
• Teach the patient how to recognize signs of melanoma recurrence.
• To help prevent malignant melanoma, stress the hazards of exposure to sunlight. Recommend that the patient use sunblock or sunscreen whenever he's outdoors. Teach him and his family to conduct monthly skin self-examinations and to have yearly screenings by a dermatologist.

lowest in Asians. Incidence isn't affected by socioeconomic status or fertility.

PSA in the spotlight

To detect prostate cancer early, all males over age 40 should undergo a DRE and serum prostate-specific antigen (PSA) testing as part of their annual physical examination.

Prognoses and predictions

When prostate cancer is treated in its localized form, the 5-year survival rate is 84%. After metastasis occurs, the rate drops below 35%. Death typically results from widespread bone metastasis.

What causes it

The cause of prostate cancer is unknown. Risk factors may include:
- age over 40
- diet high in saturated fats
- hormonal factors (testosterone may initiate or promote prostate cancer).

Pathophysiology

Prostate cancer grows slowly. When primary lesions spread beyond the prostate, they invade the prostatic capsule and spread along the ejaculatory ducts in the space between the seminal vesicles.

Prostate cancer grows slowly. Eventually, it may invade the prostatic capsule and the ejaculatory ducts.

What to look for

Signs and symptoms of prostate cancer appear only in advanced disease stages and may include:
- difficult urination
- urinary dribbling
- urine retention
- unexplained cystitis (urinary bladder inflammation)
- hematuria (blood in the urine), a rare sign.

DRE may reveal a hard nodule, which may be felt before other signs and symptoms develop.

What tests tell you

- PSA testing may be used to detect cancer. (The ACS recommends PSA testing and a DRE annually for men age 50 and older

who have a life expectancy of at least 10 years as well as for younger men at high risk.)
• Transrectal prostatic ultrasonography can detect a mass.
• Biopsy confirms the diagnosis.
• Serum acid phosphatase levels are elevated in two-thirds of patients with metastasized prostate cancer. Successful therapy restores a normal enzyme level; a subsequent rise points to cancer recurrence.
• Increased alkaline phosphatase levels and a positive bone scan suggest bone metastasis. However, routine bone X-rays don't always show evidence of metastasis.

How it's treated

Treatment varies with each disease stage, but generally includes:
• radiation
• prostatectomy (prostate removal)
• orchiectomy (removal of one or both testes) to decrease androgen production
• cryoablation (tumor removal by freezing)
• hormone therapy with synthetic estrogen (diethylstilbestrol [DES]) or leuprolide and flutamide.

Radical measures

For localized lesions with no evidence of metastasis, radical prostatectomy (removal of the prostate with its capsule, seminal vesicles, ductus deferens, some pelvic fasciae, and sometimes, pelvic lymph nodes) is usually effective.

Radiation therapy

Radiation therapy is used in the early stages to relieve bone pain from metastatic skeletal involvement, or prophylactically for patients with regional lymph node tumors.

Planting a seed

Alternatively, implantation of radioactive seeds (brachytherapy) focuses radiation on the prostate while minimizing exposure of surrounding tissue.

Chemotherapy

If hormone or radiation therapy and surgery can't be done or prove ineffective, chemotherapy may be tried. Common combinations include cyclophosphamide, vinblastine, doxorubicin, bleomycin, cisplatin, and vindesine.

A radioactive seed may be implanted to focus radiation on the prostate while minimizing the effects on surrounding tissue.

What to do

• Provide supportive care if the patient is scheduled for prostatectomy, along with good postoperative care and symptomatic treatment of radiation and postsurgical complications.

• If incontinence or impotence follows treatment, the patient and his significant other should be informed about corrective techniques and educational and support groups. Encourage the patient to contact the ACS for information.

• If the patient has received radiation or hormonal therapy, watch for and treat nausea, vomiting, dry skin, and alopecia. Also watch for adverse effects of DES (such as gynecomastia, fluid retention, nausea, and vomiting) and thrombophlebitis (such as pain, tenderness, swelling, warmth, and redness in a calf).

• Evaluate the patient. He should understand the treatment regimen and be aware of adverse effects that require immediate medical attention (such as thrombophlebitis). He should also express his feelings about potential sexual dysfunction. (See *Prostate cancer teaching tips.*)

Education edge

Prostate cancer teaching tips

• If your patient has prostate cancer, explain the expected aftereffects of surgery (such as impotence and incontinence) and radiation therapy. Discuss tube placement and dressing changes.

• Teach the patient to perform perineal exercises 1 to 10 times an hour. Have him squeeze his buttocks together, hold this position for a few seconds, and then relax. Encourage him to begin perineal exercises within 24 to 48 hours after surgery.

Squamous cell carcinoma

Squamous cell carcinoma is an invasive tumor with metastatic potential that arises from squamous cells — thin, flat cells on the outer layer of the skin. The disease commonly develops on sun-damaged areas.

Except for those on the lower lip and the ears, lesions on sun-damaged skin are less likely to metastasize as readily as lesions arising on unexposed skin. With treatment, prognosis is excellent for well-differentiated lesions on sun-damaged areas.

What causes it

Squamous cell carcinoma may result from overexposure to UV rays, radiation, chronic skin irritation and inflammation, ingestion of herbicides containing arsenic, and exposure to local carcinogens (such as tar and oil).

Overexposure to ultraviolet rays, as from sunlight, may lead to squamous cell carcinoma.

Sunbathing sequelae

Risk factors for squamous cell carcinoma include:

• being white, male, and over age 60
• having an outdoor job
• living in a sunny, warm climate
• premalignant lesions

- such hereditary diseases as xeroderma pigmentosum or albinism
- psoriasis or chronic discoid lupus erythematosus
- smallpox vaccination.

Pathophysiology

Transformation from a premalignant lesion to squamous cell carcinoma may start with hardening and inflammation of a preexisting lesion. When the disease arises from normal skin, the nodule grows slowly on a firm, hardened base. If untreated, this nodule eventually ulcerates and invades underlying tissues.

What to look for

Physical findings may include lesions on the face, ears, or backs of the hands and forearms as well as on other sun-damaged skin areas. Lesions may be scaly and keratotic (marked by excessive growth of horny skin tissue), with raised, irregular borders.

Powder and crust

In late disease, lesions grow outward from the epithelium, are friable (easily reduced to powder), and tend toward chronic crusting.

What tests tell you

Excisional biopsy of the lesion confirms the diagnosis.

How it's treated

Depending on the lesion, treatment may consist of wide surgical excision or electrodesiccation (destruction by electrical current) followed by curettage (tissue removal). These procedures offer good cosmetic results for smaller lesions.

Other treatments

Radiation therapy is usually used for older or debilitated patients. Mohs' surgery (serial excision and histologic analysis of cancerous tissues) also may be indicated.

What to do

- Disfiguring lesions may be distressing to the patient. Try to accept him as he is, increase his self-esteem, and strengthen a caring relationship.
- Develop a consistent care plan for changing the patient's dressings. A standard routine helps the patient and family learn how to

Education edge

Squamous cell carcinoma teaching tips

To help prevent recurrence of squamous cell carcinoma, cover these topics when providing patient teaching:
- Avoid excessive sun exposure.
- Apply sunscreen 30 to 60 minutes before sun exposure. Use a strong sunscreen containing para-aminobenzoic acid, oxybenzone, and zinc oxide.
- Wear protective clothing, such as a hat and long sleeves, when outdoors.
- Use a lipscreen to protect the lips from sun damage.
- Periodically examine the skin for precancerous lesions, which should be removed promptly.

care for the surgical wound. Keep the wound dry and clean. Try to control odor with balsam of Peru, yogurt flakes, oil of cloves, or other odor-masking substances (although they're usually ineffective for long-term use). Topical or systemic antibiotics also temporarily control odor and eventually alter the lesion's bacterial flora.

• Be prepared to deal with other problems that accompany metastatic disease, such as pain, fatigue, weakness, and anorexia.

• Evaluate the patient. He should recover from surgery uneventfully. He should also demonstrate an understanding of sun protection methods and the importance of follow-up care. (See *Squamous cell carcinoma teaching tips*.)

Quick quiz

1. Reed-Sternberg cells are associated with:
   A. prostate cancer.
   B. malignant melanoma.
   C. Hodgkin's disease.
   D. multiple myeloma.

Answer: C. The diagnosis of Hodgkin's disease hinges on the presence of Reed-Sternberg cells.

2. According to the ACS, how often should a woman have a mammogram?
   A. Once every 3 years starting at age 21
   B. Once a year starting at age 35
   C. Every 5 years starting at age 30
   D. Once a year starting at age 40

Answer: D. The ACS recommends a yearly mammogram for all women age 40 and older.

3. One risk factor for prostate cancer is:
   A. a history of infertility.
   B. poverty.
   C. age 15 to 34.
   D. over age 40.

Answer: D. Prostate cancer seldom develops before age 40. Socioeconomic status and infertility don't appear to affect the risk of this cancer.

4. The leading cause of death in women is:
   A. breast cancer.
   B. lung cancer.
   C. cervical cancer.
   D. ovarian cancer.

Answer: B. Lung cancer is the most common cancer among females in the United States and is leading cause of death in women.

Scoring

☆☆☆ If you answered all four questions correctly, congratulations! You've conquered the cancer chapter and are ready to move on with your life.

☆☆ If you answered three questions correctly, pat yourself on the back! Your cancer comprehension is nearly complete.

☆ If you answered fewer than three questions correctly, don't withdraw. Just review the chapter again, and your knowledge deficit is bound to go into remission.

Gerontologic care

Just the facts

In this chapter, you'll learn:

♦ normal physiologic changes associated with aging

♦ how to perform a thorough assessment on an older adult

♦ how to prevent adverse drug effects and interactions in older adults

♦ how to help older adults deal with urinary incontinence

♦ how to prevent falls in older adults.

People age 65 and older require health care services more often than any other age-group. Chances are, you'll care for a great many older adults — especially if you practice in California, New York, Florida, Illinois, Texas, Ohio, Pennsylvania, Michigan, or New Jersey, where 52% of people age 65 and older live.

Attitudes about aging are improving among the general public and health care professionals alike. More people have come to view aging as a normal lifelong process that begins at conception and culminates with old age.

The American Nurses Association (ANA) emphasizes holistic care and treatment of elderly patients. Significantly, ANA now uses the term *gerontologic* rather than *geriatric* to describe the process of providing nursing care for older adults. Not just a matter of semantics, this change acknowledges the need to address not only age-related diseases but also associated physiologic, pathologic, psychological, economic, and sociologic issues.

Demographic trends

The older adult population is growing rapidly and becoming more racially and ethnically diverse. In 2000, the number of people age 65 and older grew by 12%.

The old get older

What's more, the older adult population of the United States is getting progressively older. In 1980, nearly 40% of the elderly population was age 75 or older. By 2000, 47% were age 75 or older. By the middle of the next century, the number of people age 84 and over is expected to increase fivefold.

Gender trends

The majority of older adults are women, who now outnumber elderly men three to two. The gender disparity is even greater among persons age 85 and older, with just 40 men for every 100 women in this age group.

Health perceptions among the elderly

Contrary to stereotypes, most older adults view their health positively. Even if they have chronic illnesses, four out of five describe their health as good or excellent.

Still, the likelihood of having a chronic illness rises with age. More than 20% of people age 65 and over have at least one chronic condition, and many have multiple chronic conditions.

Implications for nursing

These demographic trends have important implications for health care. For one thing, they show a need for increased long-term care services and more gerontologic nurses, especially in states with high percentages of elderly people.

Also, as the number of elderly women increases, so does the need for information about women's health across the entire life span.

Four out of five older adults describe their health as good or excellent — even those who have chronic illnesses.

Normal changes of aging

With aging comes the loss of some body cells and reduced metabolism in others. These changes lead to altered body composition and reductions in certain body functions. For instance, adipose (fatty) tissue stores typically increase with age, whereas lean body mass and bone mineral content diminish.

Older but not necessarily ill

Although an older person's body tends to work less efficiently than a younger person's, illness doesn't inevitably accompany old age. Certainly, the heart, lungs, kidneys, and other organs are less

Aging and its effect on the body

Although the effects of aging vary with the specific tissue or organ, all older adults eventually become more susceptible to fatigue and disease. Here are some of the physiologic changes that occur with aging.

• Gradual loss of subcutaneous fat and elastin causes the skin to wrinkle and sag.
• After about age 50, brain cells decrease at a rate of 1% per year.

• Between ages 30 and 75, the heart's efficiency decreases by about 30%, and the lungs' by about 40%
• Between ages 40 and 90, renal function and bladder size and capacity decrease by as much as 50%.
• The liver's efficiency decreases by 10%.

efficient at age 60 than at age 20 but that doesn't mean aging always leads to the breakdown of body systems.

As a nurse, you must recognize these gradual changes in body function so you can adjust your assessment techniques accordingly. (See *Aging and its effect on the body.*) It's also important to understand how aging increases the risk of developing certain diseases and sustaining certain types of injuries.

Nutritional aspects of aging

Protein, vitamin, and mineral requirements usually remain stable as we age, but caloric needs decrease. Diminished activity may lower daily energy requirements by about 200 calories for men and women between ages 51 and 75, by 400 calories for women over age 75, and by 500 calories for men over age 75.

Notes on nutrition

Other physiologic changes that can affect an elderly patient's nutritional status include:

• decreased renal function, which heightens susceptibility to dehydration and renal calculi formation
• loss of calcium and nitrogen (in patients who aren't ambulatory)
• diminished enzyme activity
• reduced pepsin and hydrochloric acid secretion, which may reduce the absorption of calcium and vitamins B_1 and B_2
• decreased salivary flow and a reduced taste sensation, which may diminish the appetite and lead to greater consumption of sweet and spicy foods
• reduced intestinal motility and intestinal peristalsis
• thinning of tooth enamel, causing teeth to become more brittle
• decreased biting force
• diminished gag reflex
• limited mobility (in persons with certain health conditions), which may hamper the ability to prepare food or feed oneself.

Some older adults eat more sweet or spicy foods because taste sensation diminishes with age.

GI problems

Reduced intestinal motility may lead to such GI disorders as constipation and fecal incontinence. Other factors that may contribute to constipation in older adults include:
• nutritionally inadequate diets that are high in soft, refined foods and low in dietary fiber
• physical inactivity
• emotional stress
• use of certain medications.

Laxative overload

Some older adults abuse laxatives, resulting in rapid transport of food through the GI tract. This, in turn, decreases digestion and absorption.

Socioeconomic and psychological factors

Socioeconomic and psychological factors that can affect an older person's nutritional status include:
• loneliness
• perceived decline in his importance to the family
• susceptibility to nutritional quackery
• lack of money to buy nutritionally beneficial foods.

Skin, hair, and nails

Age-related subcutaneous fat loss, dermal thinning, and decreasing collagen lead to the development of facial lines (crow's feet) around the eyes, mouth, and nose. Women's skin, which is thinner and drier than men's, shows signs of aging about 10 years earlier.

Also, the supraclavicular and axillary regions, knuckles, and hand tendons and vessels become more prominent, as do fat pads over bony prominences. Cell replacement decreases by 50%.

High and relatively dry

Mucous membranes become dry, and sweat gland output lessens as the number of active sweat glands decreases. Body temperature grows harder to regulate as sweat glands decrease in size, number, and function and subcutaneous fat is lost.

Pigmentary plotlines

Skin also loses elasticity with age, to the point where it may seem almost transparent. Although the production of melanocytes (skin cells that produce the pigment melanin) decreases, localized melanocyte proliferation is common. Thus, older people tend to have brown spots (senile lentigo), especially in areas regularly exposed to the sun.

Hair pigment decreases with age as the number of melanocytes declines, so the hair may turn gray or white. Hair also thins; by age 70, it may be baby fine.

Hormonal changes cause pubic hair loss. Facial hair generally increases in postmenopausal women and decreases in aging men.

The naked truth about nails

With age, nail growth slows and longitudinal ridges, thickening, brittleness, and malformations may increase. Toenails may become discolored.

Tags, tumors, and keratosis

Other common skin conditions in elderly people include:
• senile keratosis — overgrowth and thickening of the horny epithelium
• acrochordon — benign skin tags
• senile angiomas — benign tumors made up of blood vessels or lymph vessels.

Also, wounds take longer to heal.

With age, body temperature gets harder to regulate, partly because the sweat glands decrease in size, number, and function.

Eyes and vision

Aging brings changes to both the eye structure and visual acuity. With advancing age, the eyes sit deeper in the bony orbits and the eyelids lose their elasticity, becoming baggy and wrinkled. The conjunctiva (the membrane coating the eye's outer surface) becomes thinner and yellow, and pingueculae (yellowish spots) may develop on the bulbar conjunctiva.

No more tears?

As the lacrimal apparatus gradually loses fatty tissue, tears diminish in quantity. Tears also tend to evaporate more quickly, increasing the risk of eye infection.

The cornea loses its luster and flattens. The iris fades or develops irregular pigmentation, turning pale. Increased connective tissue may cause hardening of the eye sphincter muscles.

Let there be (more) light

The pupil shrinks, decreasing the amount of light that reaches the retina. To see objects clearly, older adults need about three times as much light as younger people.

Aging also diminishes night vision and depth perception. The sclera becomes thick and rigid, and fat deposits cause yellowing. Senile hyaline plaques may develop.

Floaters and rings

The vitreous humor (the glassy substance behind the lens) may degenerate over time, revealing opacities and floating vitreous debris on examination. Also, the vitreous may detach from the retina, appearing as an empty space. Through an ophthalmoscope, the detached vitreous looks like a dark ring in front of the optic disk.

Lens lessons

The lens enlarges and loses transparency with age. Accommodation diminishes from decreased lens elasticity. This leads to presbyopia, a vision defect in which objects very close to the eye can't be seen clearly without corrective lenses.

Color curtailment

Many older adults have impaired color vision, especially in the blue and green ranges, as the photoreceptive retinal cones deteriorate. Decreased reabsorption of intraocular fluid may predispose older adults to glaucoma.

Don't be surprised if an older adult has poor color vision. With age, the photoreceptive retinal cones deteriorate.

Ears and hearing

Many elderly persons lose some degree of hearing. Hearing loss sometimes results from gradual cerumen buildup in the ear. More often, though, hearing loss progresses slowly, resulting in presbycusis (sometimes called *senile deafness*). This irreversible, bilateral, sensorineural hearing loss usually starts during middle age and slowly worsens. Presbycusis affects men more than women.

A hush at high pitches

The most common form of presbycusis, called *sensory presbycusis*, results from atrophy of the organ of Corti (which contains special hearing receptors) and the auditory nerve. Hearing loss occurs mostly in the higher pitch ranges.

By age 60, most adults have difficulty hearing above 4,000 Hz. (The normal range for speech recognition is 500 to 2,000 Hz.) Many older adults have trouble distinguishing higher-pitched consonants, such as s, sh, f, ph, ch, z, t, and g.

No dearth of deafness

Aging results in degenerative structural changes in the entire auditory system. In fact, hearing loss in elderly people may be more common than statistics indicate. Some people may not be immediately aware of the onset or progression of a hearing defect. Others may recognize the problem but view it as a natural part of aging — and thus not seek medical help.

Respiratory system

Age-related anatomic changes in the upper airways include nose enlargement from continued cartilage growth, tonsil atrophy, and tracheal deviations caused by changes in the aging spine.

In the thorax, anteroposterior chest diameter may increase from altered calcium metabolism and costal cartilage calcification. This, in turn, reduces chest wall mobility. Kyphosis (curvature of the thoracic spine) advances with age from such factors as osteoporosis and vertebral collapse. Respiratory muscle degeneration or atrophy also may occur, reducing pulmonary function.

Lung changes

Ventilatory capacity diminishes as the lungs' diffusing capacity declines. Also, decreased inspiratory and expiratory muscle strength diminish vital capacity. Lung tissue degeneration reduces the lungs' elastic recoil, causing higher residual volume. (In fact, aging alone can cause emphysema.)

Red ink in the oxygen column

What's more, closing of some airways impairs ventilation of the basal areas, decreasing both the surface area available for gas exchange and the partial pressure of arterial oxygen (Pao_2).

Thus, maximum breathing capacity, forced vital capacity, vital capacity, and inspiratory reserve volume all diminish, reducing the tolerance for oxygen debt. The normal Pao_2 decreases to 70 to 85 mm Hg, and oxygen saturation drops 5%.

Aging and alveoli

With age, the lungs become more rigid and the number and size of alveoli decline. A 30% reduction in respiratory fluids and a decrease in ciliary action increases the risk of respiratory tract infection and mucus plugs.

Cardiovascular system

With age, the heart usually becomes slightly smaller (except in people with hypertension or heart disease). By age 70, many people experience a 35% decrease in cardiac output at rest.

Stiffer valves, thicker walls

As the heart muscle becomes less efficient and loses contractile strength, fibrotic and sclerotic changes thicken the heart valves and reduce their flexibility. The valves may become rigid and unable to close completely, leading to systolic murmurs. Also, the left ventricular wall grows 25% thicker between ages 30 and 80.

The heart's ability to respond to physical and emotional stress may diminish markedly with age; for instance, the heart rate takes longer to return to normal after exercise. Also, elderly adults may develop obstructive coronary disease and fibrosis of the cardiac skeleton.

Vessels in distress

Aging commonly contributes to arterial and venous insufficiency, as blood vessels lose strength and elasticity. These factors contribute to a higher incidence of cardiovascular disease, especially coronary artery disease.

As myocardial irritability increases with age, extra systoles may occur, along with sinus arrhythmias and sinus bradycardias. Increased fibrous tissue infiltrates the sinoatrial node and internodal atrial tracts, possibly causing atrial fibrillation and flutter.

Pressure surge

Veins dilate and stretch with age, and coronary artery blood flow decreases 35% between ages 20 and 60. The aorta grows more rigid, causing systolic blood pressure to rise proportionately more than diastolic blood pressure (resulting in a widened pulse pressure).

Electrocardiographic changes may include increased PR and QT intervals, decreased QRS complexes, and a leftward shift of the QRS axis.

With age, coronary blood flow decreases and the aorta grows more rigid.

GI system

When assessing the elderly patient's GI system, pay special attention to the physiologic changes that accompany aging. Normal changes include diminished mucosal elasticity and reduced GI secretions, which in turn may alter digestion and absorption.

Dawdling digestion

GI tract motility, lower esophageal sphincter tone, bowel wall and anal sphincter tone, and abdominal muscle strength may decrease with age. These changes may cause signs and symptoms ranging from appetite loss to esophageal reflux to constipation.

Losses of the liver

In the liver, normal age-related changes include decreased liver weight, reduced regenerative capacity, and diminished blood flow.

Urologic system

After age 40, renal function may diminish; by age 90, it may decrease by up to 50%. Age-related changes in renal vasculature that disturb glomerular hemodynamics reduce the glomerular filtration rate.

Renal blood flow decreases 53% from reduced cardiac output and age-related atherosclerotic changes. Tubular reabsorption and renal concentrating ability also decline as the size and number of functioning nephrons decrease.

Also, the bladder muscles weaken, possibly causing incomplete bladder emptying and chronic urine retention — conditions that set the stage for bladder infection. Residual urine, urinary frequency, and nocturia also grow more common.

Renal reductions

Other age-related changes affecting renal function include diminished kidney size, impaired renal clearance of drugs, reduced bladder size and capacity, and decreased renal ability to respond to variations in sodium intake. Blood urea nitrogen levels rise about 20% by age 70.

Female reproductive system

Declining estrogen and progesterone levels cause various physical changes in aging women. As estrogen levels decrease and menopause approaches (usually at about age 50), a host of physiologic changes occur.

As menopause approaches, estrogen and progesterone levels decrease and various physical changes occur.

Breasts

The breast's glandular, supporting, and fatty tissues atrophy with age. As Cooper's ligaments lose their elasticity, the breasts become pendulous. The nipples become smaller, flatter, and nonerect. Inframammary ridges grow more pronounced.

Farewell to fibrocystic breasts

Any fibrocystic breast disease present at menopause usually diminishes and disappears.

Ovaries

Ovulation usually stops 1 to 2 years before menopause. As the ovaries reach the end of their productive cycle, they become unresponsive to gonadotropic stimulation.

Pelvic support structures

Pelvic support structures typically relax after menopause. Such relaxation may first occur with labor and delivery—but clinical effects may go unnoticed until menopause, when relaxation is accelerated by estrogen depletion and loss of connective tissue elasticity and tone.

Signs and symptoms include pressure and pulling in the area above the inguinal ligaments, low backache, a feeling of pelvic heaviness, and difficulty rising from a chair. Urinary stress incontinence may become a problem if urethrovesical ligaments weaken.

Uterus

After menopause, the uterus atrophies rapidly to one-half its premenstrual weight. Uterine regression continues until the organ reaches about one-fourth of its premenstrual size. The cervix shrinks and no longer produces mucus for lubrication, and the endometrium and myometrium become thinner.

Vagina

Atrophy causes the vagina to shorten and the mucous lining to become thin, dry, pale, and less elastic. In this state, the vaginal mucosa is highly susceptible to abrasion. Also, the pH of vaginal secretions rises.

Vulva

The vulva atrophies with age. Pubic hair loss occurs, and the labia majora flatten. Vulval tissue shrinks, exposing the sensitive area around the urethra and vagina to abrasions and irritation (for instance, from undergarments). With age, the introitus (vaginal opening) constricts, vaginal tissues lose their elasticity, and the epidermis thins from 20 layers to about 5.

Male reproductive system

In elderly men, reduced testosterone production may cause a decline in libido, atrophy and softening of the testes, and decreased sperm production.

Normally, the prostate gland enlarges with age, while its secretions diminish. Seminal fluid decreases in volume and viscosity.

Sluggish but still sexual

During intercourse, elderly men experience slower and weaker physiologic reactions. However, these changes don't necessarily weaken the sex drive or reduce sexual satisfaction. (See *Characteristics of the male climacteric*.)

Musculoskeletal system

Decreasing height is the most apparent age-related musculoskeletal change. This decrease results from exaggerated spinal curvatures and narrowing intervertebral spaces, which shorten the trunk and make the arms appear relatively long.

Other musculoskeletal changes include:
- decreased bone mass
- reduced muscle mass, which may lead to muscle weakness
- diminished collagen formation, which causes loss of resilience and elasticity in joints and supporting structures
- greater viscosity of synovial fluid
- increased fibrosis of synovial membranes.

Walking woes

An older adult may have difficulty performing tandem walking (walking heel-to-toe in a straight line). Also, he may take shorter

Characteristics of the male climacteric

Here's a list of the physiologic changes that characterize the male climacteric:
- Erections require more time and stimulation to achieve.
- Erections aren't as full or as hard as they were before.
- Testosterone production declines.
- The prostate gland enlarges and its secretions diminish.
- Seminal fluid decreases.
- Ejaculatory force diminishes.
- Contractions in the prostate gland and penile urethra during orgasm vary in length and quality.
- The refractory period following ejaculation may lengthen from minutes to days.
- Pleasure sensations become less genitally localized and more generalized.

steps and use a wider leg stance to achieve better balance and a more stable weight distribution.

Nervous system

Aging affects the nervous system in many ways. Neurons in the central and peripheral nervous systems undergo degenerative changes. Nerve transmission slows, causing the elderly adult to react more sluggishly to external stimuli.

Brain cell drain

After about age 50, the brain loses cells at a rate of about 1% per year. However, clinical effects usually aren't noticeable until aging is more advanced.

> After about age 50, the brain loses cells at a rate of about 1% per year.

Other neurologic changes

Here are other effects of age on the nervous system:
• The hypothalamus becomes less effective at regulating body temperature.
• The corneal reflex becomes slower, so the lids close more slowly in reaction to corneal irritation.
• The pain threshold increases.
• Certain sleep stages (including rapid-eye-movement sleep) shorten.

System overlap

When testing an elderly patient's nervous system, keep in mind that neurologic changes stemming from alterations in other body systems may affect assessment findings. For instance, sensory receptor changes may lead to hearing and vision loss, cerebrovascular dysfunction, and mental status changes induced by medications.

Other factors that can influence an elderly patient's test results include fatigue, lack of sleep, depression, hyperactivity, fear, and anxiety. The patient may seem disinterested or preoccupied or he may be slow to respond.

Endocrine system

A common—and important—endocrine change in elderly adults is a decreased ability to tolerate stress. The most serious sign of a diminished stress response is altered glucose metabolism.

Stress and sugar spikes

Normally, fasting blood glucose levels don't differ significantly in young and older adults. However, in an older adult, stress stimulates a rise in blood glucose that lasts longer than it does in a younger adult. In part, this stems from decreased insulin secretion and reduced responsiveness of insulin receptors. Approximately 25% of older people develop diabetes.

Thyroid slowdown

The thyroid hormones triiodothyronine and thyroxine decrease by 25% in older adults. Ordinarily, the remaining secretion of thyroid hormones is adequate for homeostasis. However, the basal metabolic rate and oxygen consumption slow.

Menstrual finale

During menopause, ovarian senescence causes permanent cessation of menstrual activity. Although changes in endocrine function during menopause vary from one woman to the next, estrogen and progesterone levels normally diminish and follicle-stimulating hormone production increases.

Estrogen deficiency may lead to coronary thrombosis and osteoporosis. Signs and symptoms commonly associated with menopause (such as depression, insomnia, headaches, fatigue, palpitations, and irritability) may also be linked to other endocrine disorders. In men, the climacteric stage lowers testosterone levels and seminal fluid production.

Other normal variations in endocrine function include a 50% decline in serum aldosterone levels and a 25% decrease in cortisol secretion rate.

Hematologic and immune systems

Total and differential white blood cell (WBC) counts don't change significantly with age. However, after age 65, some people have a slight decrease in the range of normal WBC counts. When this happens, B cell and total lymphocyte counts decrease and T cells decrease in number and become less effective.

Me, myself, and non-self

Immune function starts to decline at sexual maturity and continues to diminish with age. The incidence of autoimmune disease rises as the immune system starts to lose the ability to differentiate between self and non-self.

The cancer incidence increases, too, as the immune system grows less proficient at recognizing and destroying mutant cells. Decreased antibody response in elderly adults heightens suscepti-

After age 65, T cells may decrease in number and become less effective.

bility to infection. Tonsillar atrophy and lymphadenopathy are common.

Assessment

Comprehensive health assessment of the older adult focuses on medical history and current health status, including a review of body systems and evaluation of the patient's dietary regimen and ability to function. Besides establishing the patient's health status, the information you obtain during assessment aids your evaluation of improvements or declines in his condition over time and helps determine whether he needs support services.

Health history

The information you elicit during the health history and interview alerts you to key areas to focus on during the physical examination. To begin the history, establish the patient's well-being as your primary concern. Talking with him about health concerns promotes his health awareness, helps identify knowledge deficits, and allows you to launch your patient teaching.

Move along methodically

Because the patient may overlook some important health information, be sure to interview him methodically. When necessary, gather additional or corroborating information from his family or friends.

Current health status

Begin with the patient's current health status. Record his full name, address, age, date of birth, birthplace, and persons to contact in an emergency. Be sure to document this information on an appropriate patient history form.

Next, record the reason he's seeking treatment (chief complaint). Ask him about current medication use and treatments, his diet, and any devices he uses (such as a cane, walker, or hearing aid).

If he seems confused or shows signs or symptoms of dementia, consider asking his permission to include a spouse, child, or significant other in the interview.

Ask the patient what medications he's taking and find out if he uses a cane, hearing aid, or other medical device.

Medical history

During the medical history, obtain an overview of the patient's general health status, a history of his adult illnesses, record of past hospitalizations, frequency of doctor visits, and previous use of drugs and other treatments and their purpose.

Review of body systems

When reviewing an older adult's body systems, consider the physiologic changes normally associated with aging. Also keep in mind that older adults commonly have atypical disease presentations. For example, subtle changes in appetite and mental status may be the only signs and symptoms of certain disorders.

From the top down?

Assess specific body areas and systems using either the head-to-toe approach or the major body system approach. Both methods provide a systematic and organized framework, so choose the one that works best for you.

Physical examination

During the physical examination, use inspection, palpation, percussion, and auscultation to gather objective data that help validate the subjective data obtained from the health history.

General survey

Begin the physical examination with a general head-to-toe observation to gain an overall impression of your patient's status. Be sure to observe:
• overall appearance, including body build, skin, hygiene, and grooming
• general mobility status
• level of consciousness (LOC), affect, and mood
• overt signs of distress.
   Then take the patient's vital signs. Keep in mind that in an older adult, normal body temperature ranges from 96° to 98.6° F (35.6° to 37° C).

Skin

Inspect the skin on the patient's scalp, head, neck, trunk, and limbs. Be sure to note its color, temperature, texture, tone, turgor, thickness, and moisture. Remember that areas such as the knees and elbows may look a bit darker because of sun exposure and that calloused areas may look yellow.

Turgor testing

When assessing skin turgor, keep in mind that turgor may not reliably reflect hydration in older people, who have less subcutaneous tissue. For more accurate results, check turgor by pinching the subcutaneous tissue of the forehead or over the xiphoid process, and then watching for a quick return to baseline.

Inspect the patient's skin for tears, lacerations, scars, lesions, and ulcerations.

Skin scrutiny

Inspect the skin for tears, lacerations, scars, lesions, and ulcerations. Look for early signs of pressure ulcers such as local redness over pressure sites.

Stay alert for common benign skin lesions found in older adults; these must be differentiated from precancerous or malignant lesions. Note lesion size, distribution pattern, shape, color, consistency, and borders. Also ask about the lesion's onset. Any suspicious lesion warrants further evaluation.

Hair and nails

Inspect and palpate the patient's hair, noting its color, quantity, distribution, and texture (fine, silky, or coarse). Know that hair thinning and sparseness are common around the axillae and symphysis pubis.

Nail ailments worth noting

Inspect fingernails and toenails, noting their color, shape, thickness, capillary refill, and presence of any lesions. Some distortion of the normally flat or slightly curved nail surface is normal with aging, but other changes in color, shape, or angle may indicate a pathologic condition.

Head and face

Inspect the patient's head, noting its size, contour, and symmetry. Skull size and shape don't normally change with age. Soft-tissue swelling or cranial bulging may indicate recent head trauma.

Palpate the skull, noting tenderness, masses, or lesions. Localized cranial enlargement requires further evaluation.

Reading faces

Inspect the face and neck for skin color and proportion. Skin color should be evenly distributed. Facial features should be proportionate to head size. Also observe the patient's facial expression and movements.

Nose and mouth

Examine the external portion of the patient's nose, noting any asymmetry or abnormality such as a structural deformity. Inspect the internal mucosa, noting its color and any discharge, swelling, bleeding, or lesions. The area should be pink and moist, with clear mucus and no crusting or lesions. Palpate the frontal and maxillary sinuses for tenderness, which should be absent.

Oral observations

Inspect the mouth, starting with the lips. Note their color, symmetry, and hydration status as well as any lesions or ulcers. Dry, parched lips indicate dehydration.

Note whether the patient wears a dental appliance. Inspect his mouth with the appliance in place, noting its fit and observing for sores or abscesses resulting from friction.

Then inspect the oral mucosa, noting color, texture, hydration status, and any exudate. The mucosa and gums should be pink, smooth, and moist — although in a dark-skinned person, the mucosa normally may be slightly bluish.

Palpate the oral mucosa for lesions and nodules, noting tenderness, pain, or bleeding. Inspect the gums for color, inflammation, lesions, and bleeding. They should be pink and moist. If your patient has his natural teeth, note their number and condition.

Tales of the tongue

Next, observe tongue color, size, texture, and coating. The tongue is normally pink to red, smooth, and free from involuntary movement. Assess tongue position; deviation to one side suggests a neurologic disorder.

Observe the pharynx for signs of inflammation, discoloration, exudate, and lesions. It should be pink to pale pink, without discharge or lesions.

Eyes

When examining an older adult's eyes, keep in mind that ocular signs of aging can affect the appearance of the entire eye. Also know that age-induced fatty tissue loss may cause the eyes to sit deeper in the bony orbits.

Lids and lacrimation

Compare eyelid color to facial skin color; the lid should be free from redness and other color changes. Check for lesions and edema, and note the direction of the eyelashes. Determine whether the upper eyelid partially or completely covers the pupil — which indicates ptosis, an abnormal finding.

Inspect the lacrimal apparatus, noting discharge, redness, edema, excessive tearing, or tenderness. Examine the sclera and conjunctiva; the sclera should appear creamy white.

Pointers on pupils

Next, inspect the pupils, noting their size, shape, and reaction to light. Observe the iris, noting any margin aberrations. You may see bilateral irregular iris pigmentation, with the normal pigment replaced by a pale brown color.

Acuity analysis

Test the patient's visual acuity with and without corrective lenses, and note differences. Perform an ophthalmoscopic examination to inspect internal eye structures.

Ears

Inspect the auricle of the ears, noting color and temperature changes, discharge, or lesions. Palpate the auricle for tenderness.

Inspect internal ear structures with an otoscope. Examine the external canal and tympanic membrane, and observe for the light reflex. Note lesions, bulging of the tympanic membrane, cerumen (earwax) buildup, or (in a male) hair growth.

Can you hear me now?

To detect hearing loss early, perform the Weber and Rinne tuning fork tests. Also evaluate the patient's ability to hear and understand speech, in case you need to recommend rehabilitative therapy. If the patient wears a hearing aid, inspect it closely for proper functioning.

Neck

Inspect the patient's neck, noting scars, masses, or asymmetry. Gently palpate any masses, noting their consistency, size, shape, mobility, and tenderness. Repeat this inspection for the lymph nodes.

Check the trachea for alignment. Normally, the trachea is midline at the suprasternal notch. Note any displacement or masses.

Spying on the thyroid

Inspect the thyroid gland while your patient sips water. Note any masses or bulging. Normally, the thyroid can't be seen or palpated.

Chest and respiratory system

Inspect the shape and symmetry of the patient's chest, both anteriorly and posteriorly. Note the anteroposterior-to-lateral diameter. During respirations, listen for inspiratory or expiratory wheezing, which may be audible from the oral airways.

Palpate the anterior and posterior chest for tenderness, masses, and lumps. Assess diaphragmatic excursion. Palpate the anterior and posterior chest symmetrically for tactile fremitus. Usually, fremitus is most evident near the tracheal bifurcation.

A percussion discussion

Percuss the patient's lung fields anteriorly and posteriorly from the bases to apices. Be sure to percuss in a symmetrical pattern for comparison. Normal lung fields sound resonant. Bony prominences, organs, or consolidated tissue sound dull.

Next, auscultate from the lung bases to the apices, anteriorly and posteriorly. Ask the patient to take some deep breaths, in and out, with his mouth open. You may hear diminished sounds at the lung bases if some of the airways are closed. Inspiration is significantly more audible than expiration.

Auscultate from the lung bases to the apices as the patient breathes deeply through his mouth.

Cardiovascular system

Inspect and palpate the point of maximal impulse (PMI, or apical pulse), normally located in the fourth or fifth intercostal space just medial to the midclavicular line. In an older adult, the PMI may be displaced downward to the left.

Using the ball of your hand, palpate over the aortic, pulmonic, and mitral areas for thrills, heaves, or vibrations. You may detect a palpable thrill in a patient with valvular heart disease.

Heart sound symphony

Auscultate the heart over the aortic, pulmonic, tricuspid, and mitral areas and Erb's point, listening for the first and second heart sounds (S_1 and S_2) over each area. Also listen for extra diastolic heart sounds, or third and fourth heart sounds (S_3 and S_4).

In an older adult, S_3 heard between S_1 and S_2 (usually at the lower sternal border) isn't a reliable indicator of heart failure. Instead, it may be physiologic or occur in response to an increased diastolic flow. You may hear S_4 after S_2 and before S_1 — most audibly over the heart's apex.

Vessel investigation

Next, assess blood vessels of the patient's head, neck, trunk, and extremities. Palpate the carotid arteries one at a time, pressing lightly so you don't obliterate the carotid pulse. Note the rate, rhythm, strength, and equality of both pulses. Auscultate each carotid artery for bruits — high-pitched sounds that represent narrowing of the arterial or venous lumen.

Evaluate for jugular vein distention. Identify the level of venous pulsation and measure its height relative to the sternal angle.

A height exceeding 1⅛" (3 cm) is considered abnormal and indicates right-sided heart failure.

Palpate the peripheral arteries, noting the rate, rhythm, strength, and equality of pulses and checking for bruits. In an older adult, expect the arteries to be tortuous, kinked and, possibly, stiffer. However, pulses should be symmetrical in strength.

Limb look-see

When inspecting the legs, note their color and temperature and check for edema, varicosities, and trophic changes of the toes.

Using the ball of your hand, assess the temperature of the arms and legs, which should be equal bilaterally. Thrombosis is usually associated with a sensation of heat, although this response may be reduced in an older adult.

Edema exploration

Finally, check for edema, best assessed over bony prominences or the sacrum. Typically, edema is more pronounced in the most dependent body areas. Determine if the edema is pitting or nonpitting, and grade the degree of edema.

> Edema may occur over bony prominences in dependent body areas, like the ankles.

GI system

When examining the GI system, be aware that older adults are more likely to have abdominal distention and less likely to have abdominal rigidity than younger adults. Inspect the abdomen, noting its shape and symmetry and any scars, masses, pulsations, distention, or striae. Describe the abdomen as obese, scaphoid, or distended.

Auscultate all four abdominal quadrants for bowel sounds. Listen over the abdominal aorta for bruits.

Next, percuss the abdomen to determine the presence of air or fluid, assess liver size, and check for bladder distention. Air in the large bowel sounds tympanic, whereas fluid sounds dull.

Palpation implications

Palpate the belly, noting masses or tenderness on light or deep palpation. Watch for peritoneal signs, such as rigidity or rebound tenderness. Masses in the lower quadrants may be impacted stool. Try to palpate the liver; normally it isn't palpable.

Genitourinary system

When you assess the patient's genitourinary system, use the same basic technique as you would in a younger patient. Note that pubic hair becomes sparse and gray with age. Normally, the testes of an older male are slightly smaller than adult size. However, they should be equal, smooth, soft, and freely movable, without nodules.

Musculoskeletal system

Assessing the musculoskeletal system helps determine the older adult's overall ability to function. Limitations in range of motion (ROM), difficulty in ambulation, and diffuse or localized joint pain can be detected easily during the physical examination.

Stay alert for signs and symptoms of motor and sensory dysfunction, such as weakness, spasticity, tremors, rigidity, and sensory disturbances.

Rating the gait

Observe the patient's walk, noting his gait and posture. Gait reflects integration of reflexes as well as motor function. Assess static balance and station by gently pushing on his shoulders while he's standing.

Then observe the patient's tandem (heel-to-toe) walking, watching for exaggerated ataxia (coordination difficulties) and observing the position of his head and neck relative to the shoulders and legs.

To evaluate posture and balance, elicit Romberg's sign by noting whether the patient sways or falls when standing with his feet close together and eyes closed. Swaying indicates a positive Romberg's sign.

Watch for exaggerated ataxia as the patient performs tandem (heel-to-toe) walking.

Judging joints

Inspect the joints of the hands, wrists, elbows, shoulders, neck, hips, knees, and ankles. Note any joint enlargement, swelling, tenderness, crepitus, temperature changes, or deformities.

Following the feet

Assess the feet for common deformities, such as:
• hallux valgus—angulation of the great toe away from the midline or toward the other toes
• metatarsal (forefoot) prolapse
• hammer toe—bending of the second, third, or fourth toe at the middle joint.

Taking measure of muscles

Inspect each muscle group for atrophy, fasciculations, involuntary movements, and tremor. Move the joints through passive ROM exercises, and palpate the muscles for tone and strength.

Then assess for rigidity and spasticity. Rigidity is best detected in the wrist or elbow joint.

Appraising zip and grasp

Throughout the physical examination, ask the patient to show you how he buttons or zippers his clothing. This allows you to directly observe his ability to perform selected activities of daily living. Also observe him grasping items, such as a doorknob or water faucet.

Neurologic system

The neurologic examination includes assessment of LOC or awareness, affect, mood, cognition, orientation, speech, general knowledge, memory, reasoning, object recognition and higher cognitive functions, cranial nerves, motor and sensory systems, and reflexes.

Cool screening tools

To assess the older adult's cognitive status, consider using a screening tool, such as the Mini-Mental Status Examination, the Short Portable Mental Status Questionnaire, or the Mental Status Questionnaire.

Monitoring mood

Start by observing your patient's general appearance, including mood, affect, and grooming. An older adult who seems depressed may require further evaluation, as with the Geriatric Depression Scale. Note whether the patient is dressed appropriately, responds to questions appropriately, and is oriented to person, time, and place.

Next, assess the patient's speech. Evaluate his vocabulary and general knowledge level by discussing current news items or family events.

Memory, reason, and recognition

To evaluate memory, assess the patient's immediate, recent, and remote recall.
• Check *immediate* recall by naming a certain number of objects or reciting a group of numbers and having him repeat them immediately.
• To elicit *recent* memory, ask him about events that occurred during the past 24 to 48 hours.
• To assess *remote* memory, ask him to recall significant events that occurred many years ago.

You may want to use a screening tool, like the Mini-Mental Status Exam I'm holding, to evaluate your patient's cognitive status.

Reasoning and reckoning

Next, evaluate the patient's ability to reason by asking questions that require judgment, insight, and abstraction to answer.

To assess his object recognition, point to two objects and ask him to identify each one. Grade his response as normal or agnosia (inability to name objects).

Cranial nerves

Assess each cranial nerve sequentially, beginning with cranial nerve I and progressing to cranial nerve XII.

Motor and sensory systems

Evaluate the patient's muscle and joint function. Assess for rapid, rhythmic, alternating movements, which reflect coordination. Observe whether he can repeat maneuvers, and watch for smoothness in executing them. Expect an older adult to respond more slowly than a younger person.

Probing perception

Next, check the patient's pain perception, using the sharp and dull ends of a safety pin; temperature perception, using hot and cold substances; touch perception, using a light touch of the hand; and vibration perception, using a vibrating tuning fork.

Also evaluate his two-point discrimination and position sense. His perceptions should be accurate and symmetrical.

Reflexes

Assess an older adult's reflexes as you would in any other patient. Be sure to check for the plantar and Babinski's reflexes, which may suggest upper motor neuron disease.

Special considerations

Older adults have special health needs that require skilled, knowledgeable care. For instance, people over age 65 use twice as many medications annually as people under age 65. What's more, age-related physiologic changes may influence drug actions, so you need to understand how drugs affect elderly patients to promote compliance and minimize adverse reactions.

You may also need to help an older adult learn to deal with such age-related concerns as managing incontinence and preventing falls.

Drug therapy

Four out of five older adults have chronic medical conditions. Accordingly, they buy approximately 400 million prescriptions per year—twice the number bought by people under age 65.

For elderly patients with chronic disorders, drug therapy may extend life and enhance its quality. One or more drugs may successfully manage arthritis, diabetes, heart disease, glaucoma, osteoporosis, and hypertension.

The polypharmacy predicament

However, if your patient has multiple diseases and takes several different drugs, be sure to watch for problems stemming from polypharmacy (concomitant use of multiple medications) such as drug interactions.

Age-related changes in pharmacokinetics

Drug therapy in elderly people is complicated by age-related changes in body functions, which may influence a drug's action— how a drug is absorbed into the bloodstream, distributed throughout the body, metabolized, and eliminated. (See *How aging influences drug actions*.)

Age-related changes in pharmacodynamics

Pharmacodynamic changes can significantly alter a drug's action and effect in an older adult. Aging alters tissue sensitivity to drugs, enhancing certain drug effects. This is especially true for barbiturates such as pentobarbital; benzodiazepines such as diazepam; and alcohol.

Dearth of drug receptors

Age-related changes in the number or function of tissue and organ receptors may also alter a drug's effect. For instance, the number of beta-adrenergic receptors decreases with age, reducing beta-adrenergic receptor function and influencing the effects of drugs that stimulate or block these receptors (for example, metaproterenol and propranolol).

Similarly, changes in cholinergic and dopaminergic receptors may influence the effect of such drugs as phenothiazines, chlorpromazine, and other psychoactive agents. These changes may contribute to such adverse neurologic reactions as extrapyramidal effects and tardive dyskinesia. To compensate for these pharmacodynamic changes, prescribers usually reduce drug dosages for elderly patients.

How aging influences drug actions

The physiologic changes that come with aging cause changes in how the body absorbs, distributes, metabolizes and eliminates drugs. Awareness of these changes can help you better predict the outcome of your patient's drug therapy.

Action	Physiologic change
Absorption	• Increased gastric pH • Slower gastric emptying • Decreased gastric blood flow and motility
Distribution	• More fatty tissue • Less lean body mass
Metabolism	• Decreased total body water • Smaller liver • Less liver blood flow and enzymatic activity • Less air exchange • Decreased renal mass
Elimination	• Decreased nephron function • Decreased glomerular filtration rate, tubular secretion, and creatinine clearance and reabsorption

Caregivers may mistakenly attribute drowsiness and other adverse effects of drugs to aging.

Adverse drug effects

Adverse drug effects and unwanted drug interactions are common in elderly patients, and result mainly from physiologic changes and multiple medication use.

One troublesome aspect of drug therapy in elderly adults is the potential for misdiagnosing or failing to detect adverse reactions, such as confusion, depression, drowsiness, and urine retention. Caregivers may mistakenly attribute these problems to aging.

Spotting adverse reactions

Careful nursing assessment can help identify adverse reactions, so that the offending drug's dosage may be lowered or the drug can be replaced with a safer one. To recognize common adverse reactions, make sure you know both the intended and adverse effects of all the drugs your patient takes. (See *Recognizing common adverse drug effects in elderly patients*, page 862.)

Recognizing common adverse drug effects in elderly patients

Signs and symptoms of common adverse drug effects include hives, impotence, incontinence, stomach upset, and rashes. Elderly patients are especially susceptible to adverse effects, and may even experience more serious ones such as orthostatic hypotension, altered mental status, anorexia, dehydration, blood disorders, and tardive dyskinesia.

Also, other adverse effects—such as anxiety, confusion, and forgetfulness—may mistakenly be dismissed as typical effects of aging rather than correctly identified as drug reactions.

To help recognize bad reactions to drugs, be sure you know the potential adverse effects of the drugs your patient is taking.

Pharmacologic class	Potential adverse effects
Angiotensin-converting enzyme inhibitors	Dizziness, headache, fatigue, orthostatic hypotension, nasal congestion, cough
Alpha-adrenergic blockers	Dizziness, palpitation, nausea
Aminoglycosides	Ototoxicity, nephrotoxicity
Antiarrhythmics	Dizziness, tremors, blurred vision, nausea, vomiting, dry mouth
Anticholinergics, antihistamines	Drowsiness, blurred vision, fatigue, constipation, dry mouth
Anticoagulants	Bleeding
Antispasmodics, phenothiazines, tricyclic antidepressants	Sedation, extrapyramidal movements, anticholinergic effects
Beta-adrenergic blockers	Bradycardia, fatigue, hypotension, central nervous system (CNS) disturbances, impotence
Antidiabetics	Hypoglycemia, weight gain, nausea
Diuretics	Electrolyte disturbances, urinary frequency, dehydration
Histamine-2 blockers	Diarrhea, fatigue, dizziness, neutropenia
Narcotics	CNS depression, respiratory depression, dependency
Nonsteroidal anti-inflammatory drugs	Bleeding, GI upset, renal compromise

Drug interactions

Many potent drugs commonly used by elderly adults can interact, resulting in hazardous consequences. For example, cimetidine interacts with aminophylline, phenytoin, antidepressants, propranolol, and other drugs.

Anticholinergics, such as some antidepressants and tranquilizers, may have additive effects when used together. Digoxin may have increased toxic effects when taken with a diuretic or other drug that decreases body potassium levels.

Hindering interactions

To help prevent harmful drug interactions, make sure you know all the drugs your patient is taking. Keep in mind that he may be taking several drugs prescribed independently by several doctors.

Adherence with drug therapy

An elderly adult may have any number of reasons for not adhering to the treatment regimen—for example, poor vision or hearing, physical disability, inability to afford drugs, cultural beliefs, or failure to understand the importance of taking a particular drug.

Augmenting adherence

Nonadherence can lead to treatment failure. If the doctor misinterprets this failure as ineffective drug therapy, he may mistakenly increase the dosage or prescribe a second drug, compounding the problem.

Helping the patient overcome obstacles to adherence is an important nursing responsibility. To meet it, make sure your patient understands the purpose of each prescribed drug and knows how to take each one correctly.

> To promote adherence to drug therapy, make sure your patient understands the purpose and administration method for each drug.

Urinary incontinence

Incontinence, the uncontrollable passage of urine, is common among the elderly—but it shouldn't be considered a normal part of aging. Incontinence can result from bladder abnormalities or neurologic disorders. It may be transient or permanent, and may involve large volumes of urine or scant dribbling.

Incontinence categories

Urinary incontinence occurs in four main forms.
- *Stress* incontinence refers to loss of less than 50 ml of urine triggered by increased abdominal pressure—for example, from coughing or sneezing.
- *Overflow* incontinence is an involuntary urine loss occurring at somewhat predictable intervals when a specific bladder volume is reached.
- *Urge* incontinence involves a strong, sudden need to urinate, followed immediately by a bladder contraction that leads to involuntary urine loss.

• *Total* incontinence is complete lack of urinary control, resulting from the bladder's inability to retain urine.

What causes it

Urinary incontinence may result from a wide range of conditions, including:
• benign prostatic hyperplasia
• bladder calculi (stones)
• bladder cancer
• stroke
• chronic prostatitis
• diabetic neuropathy
• drugs, such as diuretics, sedatives, hypnotics, antipsychotics, anticholinergics, and alpha-adrenergic blockers
• Guillain-Barré syndrome
• multiple sclerosis
• prostate cancer
• spinal cord injury
• urethral stricture.
    In some patients, incontinence follows a prostatectomy (prostate removal) that damaged the urethral sphincter.

What to look for

If your patient has urinary incontinence, be sure to cover these factors in your assessment:
• Ask the patient when he first noticed the problem and whether it began suddenly or gradually.
• Have him describe his typical urinary pattern: Does incontinence usually occur during the day or night? Does he have any urinary control or is he totally incontinent? If he sometimes urinates with control, what are the usual times he voids and the amounts of urine voided?
• Ask about other urinary problems, such as hesitancy, frequency, urgency, nocturia, and decreased force or interruption of the urine stream.
• Evaluate the patient's fluid intake.
• Obtain a medical history, especially noting urinary tract infection, prostate conditions, spinal injury or tumor, stroke, or surgery involving the bladder, prostate, or pelvic floor.
• Determine if the patient is taking any medications, particularly sedative-hypnotics, anticholinergics, or diuretics.
• After completing the history, have the patient empty his bladder. Inspect the urethral meatus for obvious inflammation or anatomic defects. Have a female patient bear down; note any urine leakage.

Memory jogger

The mnemonic OUTS helps you remember the main forms of urinary incontinence.

O Overflow incontinence: urine loss occurring when a specific bladder volume is reached

U Urge incontinence: urine loss from a bladder contraction that follows a strong, sudden need to urinate

T Total incontinence: complete loss of urinary control, as from a nonfunctioning urethral sphincter muscle

S Stress incontinence: loss of small amounts of urine (less than 50 ml) when abdominal pressure increases, such as when a person coughs, sneezes, or lifts a heavy object.

Correcting incontinence with bladder retraining

An incontinent patient typically feels frustrated and embarrassed—sometimes even hopeless. Fortunately, bladder retraining—a program that aims to establish a regular voiding pattern—may help correct the problem. Here are some guidelines for establishing such a program.

Assess elimination patterns

Before you start the program, assess the patient's fluid intake pattern, voiding pattern, and behavior (for example, restlessness or talkativeness) before each voiding episode.

Establish a voiding schedule

Encourage the patient to use the toilet 30 minutes before he's usually incontinent. If this isn't successful, readjust the schedule.

Once he can stay dry for 2 hours, increase the time between voidings by 30 minutes each day until he achieves a 3- to 4-hour voiding schedule.

Provide consistency and privacy

When the patient voids, make sure the sequence of conditioning stimuli is always the same. Also, ensure his privacy while voiding; any inhibiting stimuli should be avoided.

Record results and stay positive

Keep a record of continence and incontinence for 5 days to help reinforce the patient's efforts to remain continent. Remem-

ber, your positive attitude—and the patient's—are crucial to successful bladder retraining.

Here are some additional tips that may help your patient succeed.
• Make sure the patient is near a bathroom or portable toilet.
• Leave a light on at night. If the patient needs help getting out of his bed or chair, promptly answer his call for help.
• Encourage him to wear his accustomed clothing, which conveys that you're confident he can remain continent. Acceptable alternatives to diapers include condoms for a male patient and incontinence pads or panties for a female patient.
• Encourage the patient to drink 2 to 2½ qt (2 to 2.5 L) of fluid each day. A lower fluid intake doesn't prevent incontinence—but does promote infection. To help him stay continent overnight, limit his intake after 6 p.m.
• Reassure the patient that if he has an episode of incontinence, that doesn't mean the program has failed. Encourage him to maintain a persistent, positive attitude.

• Gently palpate the abdomen for bladder distention, which signals urine retention.
• Perform a complete neurologic assessment, noting motor and sensory function and muscle atrophy.

Nursing interventions

• Prepare the patient for diagnostic tests, such as cystoscopy, cystometry, and a complete neurologic workup.
• As appropriate, implement a bladder retraining program. (See *Correcting incontinence with bladder retraining.*)
• Make sure the patient receives an adequate fluid intake.
• Have him void regularly.
• If his incontinence has a neurologic basis, monitor him for urine retention, which may warrant periodic catheterizations.
• If appropriate, teach the patient how to catheterize himself.

Falls

In people age 75 and older, falls cause three times as many accidental deaths as motor vehicle accidents. Several factors can make falls ominous for elderly patients—lengthy convalescence, the risk of incomplete recovery, and inability to cope physiologically. Also, injuries caused by falls can be psychologically devastating, leading to loss of independence and self-confidence.

A fall can be ominous to an elderly patient. She may lose her independence and self-confidence.

Accident or omen?

Falls can be accidental or result from temporary muscle paralysis, vertigo, postural hypotension, or central nervous system (CNS) lesions. Accidental falls commonly result from environmental factors, such as poorly lighted stairs, throw rugs, and highly waxed floors. Sometimes, an accidental fall stems from physiologic factors, such as decreased visual acuity, loss of muscle strength, or poor coordination.

Temporary muscle paralysis may explain falls that occur with no apparent cause. This phenomenon presumably results from compromised blood supply to the reticular formation in the brain's medulla, caused by spondylosis (vertebral joint fixation or stiffness)—resulting from head and neck movement in the presence of cervical arthritis.

Other falling factors

Vertigo, as from a middle-ear disturbance or infection, may cause the patient to lose his balance and fall. Orthostatic hypotension may cause dizziness, which leads to a fall when he rises too quickly from a lying or sitting position. CNS lesions, as from a stroke, may affect nerve impulses and set the stage for falls.

What to look for

If your patient is found on the floor or reports falling, don't move him until he has been evaluated. Relieve his anxiety as you rapidly assess his vital signs, mental status, and functional capacity.

Note such signs and symptoms as confusion, tremors, weakness, pain, dizziness, or shortening of one leg. Take steps to control any bleeding, and assess whether the patient hit his head. Obtain an X-ray if you suspect a fracture. Observe and monitor the patient's status for the next 24 hours.

Chasing down clues

After the patient's condition is stabilized, include these factors in your assessment:
• Review events that preceded the fall to help avoid future episodes. Did the patient make an abrupt position change or other movement? If he normally wears corrective lenses, was he wearing them when he fell?
• Review his use of such medications as tranquilizers and opioids, which can cause drowsiness that leads to a fall.
• Assess for other contributing factors, such as gait disturbances, poor vision, improper use of assistive devices, and environmental hazards.

Obtain an X-ray to find out if your patient suffered a fracture during the fall.

What to do

• Provide measures to relieve pain and discomfort. Give an analgesic, if ordered. Apply cold compresses for the first 24 hours and warm compresses thereafter to reduce the pain and swelling of bruises.
• If the patient is bedridden, encourage him to stay as active as possible to avoid becoming bedbound and immobile.
• Provide appropriate care for the patient who has sustained a fracture.
• If indicated, arrange for visiting nurse services for the recovery period after the patient's release.

Baby needs a new pair of shoes

• Teach the patient how to reduce the risk of accidental falls by wearing well-fitting shoes with nonskid soles, avoiding long robes, and wearing eyeglasses if he needs them.
• Advise him to sit on the edge of the bed for a few minutes before rising and to use a walking stick, cane, or walker if he feels even slightly unsteady on his feet.
• Suggest ways he can adapt his home to guard against accidental falls — for instance, applying nonskid treads to stairs and installing handrails to walls around the bathtub, shower, and toilet.
• Teach the patient how to fall safely by protecting his hands and face. If he uses a walker or wheelchair, make sure he knows how to cope with a fall, should one occur. Teach him to survey the room for a low, sturdy piece of furniture (for example, a coffee table) he can use for support. Then teach him the proper procedure for lifting himself off the floor and either standing up with the walker or getting into the wheelchair.

Quick quiz

1. What isn't a normal age-related change?
   A. Difficulty regulating body temperature
   B. Blurred vision caused by corneal flattening and loss of corneal luster
   C. Enlargement of the heart
   D. Decreased pulmonary function

Answer: C. As a person ages, the heart usually becomes slightly smaller, not larger.

2. Which statement about urinary incontinence is *not* true?
   A. It's a normal result of aging.
   B. It may be associated with certain medications.
   C. It may be transient or permanent.
   D. It may result from conditions such as prostate cancer.

Answer: A. Urinary incontinence is *not* a normal result of aging.

3. Which cardiovascular changes in the older adult isn't normal?
   A. Loss of efficiency and strength of the heart muscle
   B. Hypotension
   C. Decreased cardiac output at rest
   D. Displacement of the PMI and heart sounds

Answer: B. Aging causes the arterial walls to thicken and lose elasticity, leading to higher-than-normal blood pressure, not hypotension.

4. Which instruction may *increase* a patient's risk for falling?
   A. "Use a cane or walker if you feel even slightly unsteady."
   B. "Wear well-fitting shoes with nonskid soles."
   C. "Rise quickly when getting out of bed."
   D. "Install handrails around your bathtub, shower, and toilet."

Answer: C. Rather than rise quickly out of bed, you should advise the patient to sit on the bed's edge for a few minutes before rising to avoid orthostatic hypotension and consequent dizziness.

Scoring

☆☆☆ If you answered all four items correctly, glorious! You're a genius when it comes to gerontologic care.

☆☆ If you answered three items correctly, good job! Your elder-care expertise is maturing quite nicely.

☆ If you answered fewer than three items correctly, don't go gray with worry! If you read this chapter again, your understanding of aging is sure to ripen.

Appendices and index

Glossary

anemia
reduction in the number and volume of red blood cells, the amount of hemoglobin, or the volume of packed red cells

aneurysm
sac formed by the dilation of the wall of an artery, a vein, or the heart

angiography
radiographic visualization of blood vessels after injection of radiopaque contrast material

anorexia
loss of appetite

aphasia
loss or impairment of the ability to communicate through speech, written language, or signs, resulting from brain disease or trauma

apraxia
complete or partial inability to perform purposeful movements in the absence of sensory or motor impairment

ascites
fluid in the peritoneal cavity

ataxia
impairment of the ability to coordinate voluntary muscle movement

aura
sensations that occur before a paroxysmal attack, such as a seizure or migraine headache

auscultation
physical assessment technique by which the examiner listens (usually with a stethoscope) for sounds coming from the heart, lungs, abdomen, or other organs

autoimmune disorder
disorder in which the body launches an immunologic response against itself

bruit
abnormal sound heard over peripheral vessels on auscultation that indicates turbulent blood flow

cardiac output
volume of blood ejected from the heart per minute

constipation
decreased passage of stools; stools are characteristically hard and dry

crepitation
grating sound produced by bone rubbing against bone

decerebrate posturing
associated with a lesion of the upper brain stem or severe bilateral lesions in the cerebrum; the patient typically lies with legs extended, head retracted, arms adducted and extended, wrists pronated, and the fingers, ankles, and toes flexed

decorticate posturing
associated with a lesion of the frontal lobes, cerebral peduncles, or internal capsule; the patient lies with arms adducted and flexed, wrists and fingers flexed on the chest, legs stiffly extended and internally rotated, and feet plantar flexed

diarrhea
rapid movement of fecal material through the intestines that causes poor absorption of water and nutrients; stools are watery and frequent

disease
pathologic condition that occurs when the body can't maintain homeostasis

distal
farthest away

dysmenorrhea
painful menstruation

dyspepsia
gastric discomfort, such as fullness, heartburn, bloating, and nausea, that occurs after eating

dysphagia
difficulty swallowing

dysphasia
impairment of speech involving failure to arrange words in their proper order, usually resulting from injury to the speech area in the cerebral cortex

dyspnea
difficult, labored breathing

ecchymosis
bruise

embolism
sudden obstruction of a blood vessel by foreign substances or a blood clot

exacerbation
increase in the severity of a disease

fasciculation
involuntary twitching or contraction of the muscle

Fowler's position
patient positioning with head of bed raised, knees slightly flexed

hematuria
blood in the urine

hemoglobin
iron-containing pigment in red blood cells that carries oxygen from the lungs to the tissues

hemoptysis
expectoration of bloody sputum

hemorrhage
escape of blood from a ruptured vessel

hirsutism
excessive hair growth or unusual distribution of hair

hormone
chemical substance produced in the body that has a specific regulatory effect on the activity of specific cells or organs

hypertension
high arterial blood pressure

hypotension
abnormally low blood pressure

hypoxia
reduction of oxygen in body tissues to below normal levels

idiopathic
disease with no known cause

inspection
critical observation of the patient during which the examiner may use sight, hearing, or smell to make informed observations

insulin
hormone secreted into the blood by the islets of Langerhans of the pancreas; promotes the storage of glucose, among other functions

ischemia
decreased blood supply to a body organ or tissue

jugular vein distention
distended neck veins that may indicate increased central venous pressure

lateral recumbent position
patient positioning lying on the left side with the right thigh and knee drawn up

lethargy
slowed responses, sluggish speech, and slowed mental and motor processes in a person oriented to time, place, and person

lichenification
thickening and hardening of the epidermis

lithotomy position
lying on the back with the hips and knees flexed and the thighs abducted and externally rotated

lymphadenopathy
enlargement of the lymph nodes

melena
passage of black, tarry stools

murmur
abnormal sound heard on auscultation of the heart; caused by abnormal blood flow through a valve

necrosis
tissue death

nocturia
excessive urination at night

oliguria
urine output of less than 30 ml/hour

orthopnea
respiratory distress that's relieved by sitting upright

palpation
physical assessment technique by which the examiner uses the sense of touch to feel pulsations and vibrations or to locate body structures and assess their texture, size, consistency, mobility, and tenderness

pathogen
disease producing agent or microorganism

percussion
physical assessment technique by which the examiner taps on the skin surface with his fingers to assess the size, border, and consistency of internal organs and to detect and evaluate fluid in a body cavity

peristalsis
intestinal contractions, or waves, that propel food toward the stomach and into and through the intestine

petechiae
multiple, small, hemorrhagic areas on the skin

plasma
liquid part of the blood that carries antibodies and nutrients to tissues and carries wastes away from tissues

platelet
disk-shaped structure in blood that plays a crucial role in blood coagulation

polydipsia
excessive thirst

polyphagia
consuming abnormally large amounts of food

polyuria
excessive production of urine

prone position
lying face down

proximal
nearest to

pruritus
severe itching

ptosis
drooping of the eyelid

renal colic
flank pain that radiates to the groin

reverse Trendelenburg's position
lying flat with the head higher than the body or legs

subluxation
partial dislocation of a joint

supine position
lying flat on the back

thrombosis
the development of a thrombus (blood clot)

tophi
clusters of urate crystals surrounded by inflamed tissue; occur in gout

Trendelenburg's position
lying flat with the head lower than the body or legs

vasopressor
drug that stimulates contraction of the muscular tissue of the capillaries and arteries

virus
microscopic, infectious parasite that contains genetic material and needs a host cell to replicate

Selected references

Bickley, L.S., and Szilagyi, P.G. *Bates' Guide to Physical Examination and History Taking*, 8th ed. Philadelphia: Lippincott Williams & Wilkins, 2003.

Black, J.M., et al. *Medical-Surgical Nursing: Clinical Management for Positive Outcomes*, 6th ed. Philadelphia: W.B. Saunders Co., 2001.

Bullock, B.L., and Henze, R.L. *Focus on Pathophysiology*. Philadelphia: Lippincott Williams & Wilkins, 2000.

Burns, N., and Grove, S.K. *The Practice of Nursing Research: Conduct, Critique, and Utilization*, 4th ed. Philadelphia: W.B. Saunders Co., 2001.

Connolly, M.A. "Chest X-Rays. Completing the Picture," *RN* 64(6):56-62, June 2001.

Craven, R.F., and Hirnle, C.J. *Fundamentals of Nursing Human Health and Function*, 4th ed. Philadelphia: Lippincott Williams & Wilkins, 2003.

Fetter, M.S. "Medical Errors: Medical-Surgical Nurses Speak," *Medsurg Nursing* 9(2):58-68, April 2000.

Greggs-McQuilkin, D. "The Specialty of Medical-Surgical Nursing: The Solid Rock, Not the Stepping Stone," *Medsurg Nursing* 12(1):25-26, February 2003.

Ignatavicius, D.D., and Workman, M.L. *Medical-Surgical Nursing: Critical Thinking for Collaborative Care*, 4th ed. Philadelphia: W.B. Saunders Co., 2001.

Lewis, S.M., et al., eds. *Medical-Surgical Nursing: Assessment and Management of Clinical Problems*, 5th ed. St. Louis: Mosby–Year Book, Inc., 2000.

Morrison, E.F., et al. "Managing the Care of Complex, Difficult Patients in the Medical-Surgical Setting," *Medsurg Nursing* 9(1):21-26, February 2000.

Nurse's 3 Minute Clinical Reference. Springhouse, Pa.: Lippincott Williams & Wilkins, 2003.

Nursing2003 Drug Handbook, 23rd ed. Springhouse, Pa.: Lippincott Williams & Wilkins, 2003.

Portable RN: The All-in-One Nursing Reference. Springhouse, Pa.: Springhouse Corp., 2002.

Professional Guide to Pathophysiology. Springhouse, Pa.: Lippincott Williams & Wilkins, 2003.

Smeltzer, S., and Bare, B.G., eds. *Brunner and Suddarth's Textbook of Medical-Surgical Nursing*, 9th ed. Philadelphia: Lippincott Williams & Wilkins, 2000.

Springhouse Review for Medical-Surgical Nursing Certification: An Indispensable Study Guide for the A.N.A. Exam, 3rd ed. Philadelphia: Lippincott Williams & Wilkins, 2002.

Springhouse Review for NCLEX-RN, 5th ed. Springhouse, Pa.: Springhouse Corp., 2002.

Wang, C.E. "Knowing and Approaching Hope as Human Experience: Implications for the Medical-Surgical Nurse," *Medsurg Nursing* 9(4):189-92, August 2000.

Yoder, L.H., and Wassum, E. "Medical-Surgical Nurses in the Military," *Medsurg Nursing* 11(4):203, August 2002.

Index

i refers to an illustration; t refers to a table; boldface refers to full-color pages.

i refers to an illustration; t refers to a table; boldface refers to full-color pages.

i refers to an illustration; t refers to a table; boldface refers to full-color pages.

i refers to an illustration; t refers to a table; boldface refers to full-color pages.

i refers to an illustration; t refers to a table; boldface refers to full-color pages.

i refers to an illustration; t refers to a table; boldface refers to full-color pages.

i refers to an illustration; t refers to a table; boldface refers to full-color pages.

Notes

Notes

Notes